Practical Orthopaedic Medicine

To Monica and Anne for all the disruption in their lives

Practical Orthopaedic Medicine

Brian Corrigan
MB, BS, MRCP, MRCPE, FRACP, FACRM, DPhysMed
Rheumatologist, Concord Hospital, Sydney, Australia

G.D. Maitland
MBE, AUA, FCSP, FACP, FACP (Specialist in Manipulative Physiotherapy)
Senior Lecturer, Royal Adelaide Hospital, Australia

Butterworths

London Boston Singapore Sydney Toronto Wellington

First published, 1983
Reprinted 1985, 1986, 1987, 1988

© **Butterworth & Co (Publishers) Ltd, 1983**

British Library Cataloguing in Publication Data
Corrigan, Brian
   Practical orthopaedic medicine.
   1. Orthopedia
   I. Title   II. Maitland, G.D.
   617′.3   RD731
   ISBN 0–407–00238–3 (cased)
   ISBN 0–407–00440.8. (limp)

Filmset by Northumberland Press Ltd, Gateshead, Tyne and Wear
Printed in England at the University Press, Cambridge

Preface

This book has developed as a result of post-graduate teaching by the authors on the clinical aspects of medical disorders of the musculoskeletal system. Orthopaedic medicine is still a relatively new specialty that is concerned mainly with soft-tissue lesions. It covers a wide range of conditions that tend to fall between orthopaedic surgery and rheumatology and some aspects of each of these specialties will necessarily overlap. Interest in these conditions and in the role of manipulative procedures in their overall management is increasing. The first part of this book considers disorders of the peripheral joints. In the second part, disorders of the spine are discussed.

Management of musculoskeletal disorders usually requires a total rehabilitation programme based on the patients' requirements and expectations and depends on assessment of the whole patient. Great reliance is placed on clinical examination to assess the patient and evaluate the treatment techniques and their effects. Many of the views expressed about these are derived from the authors' clinical experiences. Emphasis in treatment is placed on physical methods; particularly on the use of passive-movement techniques, such as mobilization and manipulation, which are based completely on the concepts of Geoff Maitland and now enjoy world-wide recognition. One problem has been to determine how much detail of his methods should be included, since much of it is properly the concern of the physiotherapist. However, the referring physician needs to have an appreciation of the types of treatment available, their indications and possible results; the physiotherapist needs to apply the treatment techniques available to a specific diagnosis. In general, only the principles

of these techniques are discussed, and for further details the reader is referred to the books *Peripheral Manipulation* (Maitland, 1977) and *Vertebral Manipulation* (Maitland, 1977).

Other methods of treatment will be discussed, including the indications for surgery. However, strictly surgical conditions and techniques are not the province of this book.

One of the purposes of this book is to provide a practical guide to clinical management and to interest general practitioners, rheumatologists, orthopaedic-medicine specialists and physiotherapists in the role of manipulative methods in the types of clinical problems that are encountered so commonly.

The authors acknowledge their many associates. These include: Dr Carson Dick and the Staff at Royal Victoria Infirmary, whose help has been invaluable; members of the Australian Association of Manipulative Medicine and the Manipulative Therapists Association of Australia, with whom ideas in the text have been discussed; Dr J. Bertouch, Dr G. Byth, Dr G. Carr, Dr D. Champion, Dr M. Cross, Mr Brian Edwards, Dr H. Francis, Dr W. Hargrave-Wilson, Dr M. Ingpen, Dr F. Johnson, Dr S. Kannangara, Mr Paul Kelly, Mr Neil Munro, Dr R. Robinson, Dr W. Walter, Dr J. Webb, Dr C. Winer, Dr Hugh Burry in New Zealand, Professor Derrick Brewerton, and Dr John Williams in England; Mrs J. Homan and our secretaries for repeated retyping of the manuscript; the artists, Anne Maitland and Julie Eichorn; Roger Hanssen, Department of Clinical Photography, Concord Hospital; and the publishers, Butterworth and Company, whose representatives have been of invaluable assistance.

Contents

Part I—Peripheral Joints

1 Classification

Orthopaedic medicine is concerned mainly with soft-tissue lesions. These include lesions in: the joint capsule, lined by a synovial membrane and strengthened by surrounding ligaments; bursae; muscles; and tendons and their tenosynovial sheaths.

Pain and disability arise from the traumatic, degenerative, and inflammatory conditions— often present in varying combinations—to which these tissues are subject. Although common, these conditions are often poorly diagnosed and inadequately managed. However, most of these lesions can be diagnosed accurately with the standard medical practice of taking an adequate history and conducting a careful clinical examination (Cyriax, 1978; Polley and Hunder, 1978). These conditions are interesting because a diagnosis and assessment of their degree can be made clinically, and because when the lesion has been accurately localized appropriate therapy can be instituted—often very successfully.

Peripheral joints

Although the minute structure of the peripheral joints is complex, their basic design is relatively simple. The bone ends forming the joint are lined by avascular articular cartilage, nourished by synovial fluid derived from the vascular synovial membrane. Five joints—the knee, wrist, sternoclavicular, temporomandibular, and acromioclavicular—contain an intra-articular fibrocartilaginous meniscus.

Synovial joints are movable joints and normal movement depends on several factors. Each peripheral joint has a normal or physiological range of movement determined to some extent by the configuration of the opposing joint surfaces. On joint movement, these opposing surfaces can slide, roll, and spin on one another (Gray, 1973). This normal range also depends on the integrated action of the surrounding soft tissues, which is under voluntary neurological control, and on a series of involuntary, or accessory, joint movements that vary for each joint. Pain and disability may be associated with loss of accessory movements, which is often associated with lesions in the surrounding soft tissues. Considerable attention will be given later to a description of normal accessory movements and their clinical assessment.

Joint stability is essential for normal movement and the joint must remain within the constraints that hold it together but allow movement to the limit of these constraints (Wright and Dowson, 1975). Joint stability depends on many factors, including the shape of the joint surfaces, the integrity of the surrounding soft tissue—e.g. the capsule, ligaments and muscles—and atmospheric pressure.

Link system

The joints in a limb may be looked upon as forming links in a chain, moved by muscles whose action is integrated through this system of links. During activity, large internal forces may be generated around a joint, which then acts as a fulcrum both for proximal and for distal lever arms. Musculoskeletal pain may develop as the result of an alteration in other parts of the system of links. Accordingly, when examining a patient with joint pain the whole of the limb must be examined to determine whether any abnormality is present in another part of the link. These abnormalities include joint stiffness; muscular weakness or tightness; and postural abnormalities and misalignments, such as knee or foot deformities.

Joint pain

The causes of joint pain may be considered under two headings:

(1) The arthropathies, or diseases of joints. Since this book is not a rheumatology text, a classification and description of all of these will not be attempted. Some of the more common diseases will be described, mainly because they may need to be differentiated from disorders of joint movement, which will be considered in more detail.
(2) Disorders of joint movement. Joint pain may be associated with an alteration in the range of joint movement. This may be:

  (a) Decreased due to a loss of accessory joint movements (hypomobility).
  (b) Increased (hypermobility).
  (c) Abnormal due to joint instability.
  (d) Blocked due to an internal derangement of a joint (e.g. a torn intra-articular meniscus).

Bone pain

Disorders of the bones—such as fractures, dislocations, tumours and infections—are also important causes of musculoskeletal pain. This book is not concerned with these orthopaedic conditions; however, some conditions—e.g. stress fractures—that often need to be differentiated from causes of soft-tissue pain will be described.

Neurogenic pain

Pain in the limbs caused by neurological lesions may be due to spinal disorders causing either nerve-root compression or referred pain. These are discussed in Chapter 19. Peripheral joint lesions may also refer pain more distally; a common example is pain in the knee referred from disease of the hip. Limb pain may also be caused by an entrapment neuropathy of a peripheral nerve. The nerve is usually compressed as it runs through its normal anatomical confines, such as fibro-osseous canals or ligaments. It also runs through soft tissues and entrapment may complicate soft-tissue lesions—e.g. tenosynovitis due to overuse, trauma, or rheumatoid arthritis.

Psychogenic causes

Psychogenic causes must also be considered in any discussion of limb pain. Symptoms are most commonly due to tension which may be associated with an underlying anxiety neurosis or depression. In addition, a psychogenic overlay to the patient's symptoms may be associated with a secondary gain, either emotional or financial, or may be related to a fear that the patient will eventually become crippled, especially if there is a family history of arthritis.

2 Subjective assessment

History taking in musculoskeletal disorders is, as in the whole of medicine, of paramount importance and well repays the time spent in recording it accurately. This may allow an accurate assessment of the diagnosis, or at least narrow down the different diagnostic possibilities, before undertaking the clinical examination. It is always a worthwhile practice to have a printed form containing a body chart on which the site and distribution of the patient's symptoms can be charted.

History taking requires a capacity to listen sympathetically to the patient and not to ask leading questions. However, some patients—because of either a natural reticence or circumlocution—need to be led to, and kept firmly on, the main points at issue. Nevertheless, even these patients should, as much as possible, tell the history in their own words. The actual events should be recorded and should not be confused with opinions of the patient or other interested parties.

The main consideration in this lengthy process is for the examiner to build up a pattern so that the behaviour of the patient's symptoms and his reactions to them can be identified. This includes an appreciation of the time relationship of the various symptoms, and their onset and variability (considered more fully below). It should also allow some assessment of the patient as a person, his pain threshold, and the presence of any non-organic pattern or psychogenic overlay to his symptoms. This may be possible by observing the relationship between the patient's behaviour while speaking about his pain and the degree of pain complained of.

It is most important to start taking the history by asking the patient to describe his major complaint. Pain is nearly always the main reason for the patient to seek advice.

Pain

A detailed description of the patient's pain includes the following points.

Site

The patient's original statement about his site of pain can be misleading. For example, although he may complain of pain in the shoulder, this may represent to the patient any area from the neck to the upper arm. Similarly, the patient may complain of pain in the hip but really be suffering from buttock pain; whereas hip pain may be referred over a wide area of the upper leg. Accordingly, the patient should be asked to point and map out the area of pain as accurately as possible. As a general rule, pain in the distal joints can be more accurately localized than pain in the proximal joints. It is also necessary to enquire whether pain is felt within the joint; some patients often have difficulty in relating whether pain is felt in the joint or in surrounding parts. Moreover, pain may be felt in several different sites in an area or limb; this again requires careful charting.

Radiation

The area where the pain began, where it is most felt, and where it radiates should also be mapped out. It is also important to remember that pain may be felt in one area of a limb but is referred from a more proximal site, which may also be associated with referred tenderness.

Quality of pain

The patient should be encouraged to describe the quality and character of his pain in his own words. Musculoskeletal pain is usually described as being deep, dull, and aching. Other descriptive titles that may be used include sharp, throbbing, or stabbing. The patient is usually unable to differentiate between different qualities of pain originating from the various structures that make up the musculoskeletal system. However, bone pain is usually described as severe, boring pain, often worse at night.

Severity

The severity may be difficult to assess as it depends mainly on the patient's description of and reaction to the pain. The degree of functional incapacity that results may be a good guide to severity; the patient may recognize that it is of nuisance value only or it may seriously interfere with and limit function.

Time relationships

The patient is first asked the total length of time that pain has been present. He is then asked whether pain is constantly, variably or intermittently present. In addition, pain of musculoskeletal origin typically has a diurnal variation. Hence the duration of pain and the pain-free periods or the variation in pain throughout a 24-hour period is of considerable relevance. For example, pain due to osteoarthritis is usually worse at the end of the day; in inflammatory arthritis it is often worse early in the morning.

Night pain

Pain of musculoskeletal origin may be worse at night and, if sufficiently severe, may disturb the patient's sleep. As a general rule, this reflects the intensity of the underlying inflammation. Thus this symptom may occur in:

(1) Inflammatory arthropathy such as rheumatoid arthritis or ankylosing spondylitis.
(2) Gout.
(3) Septic arthritis.
(4) Polymyalgia rheumatica.
(5) Peripheral nerve entrapments, particularly of the median nerve in the carpal tunnel.
(6) Bone disorder, including avascular necrosis, Sudeck's atrophy, and malignancy.

In individual joints, nocturnal pain is particularly common in:

(1) Capsulitis of the shoulder.
(2) Osteoarthritis of the hip.
(3) Cysts of the meniscus in the knee.

Finally, it should be remembered that this symptom may also occur in patients with a depressive illness.

Onset

The onset of pain may be spontaneous, either sudden or gradual, or follow trauma. In the latter a detailed history is necessary describing the position of the joint at the time of injury and the type of stress applied to the joint. In many patients with chronic degenerative or inflammatory conditions, the onset is gradual. However, symptoms often follow overuse and an assessment should be made of the total load applied by the patient to a joint, both at work and at play. A sudden onset of severe pain and swelling commonly occurs in patients with crystal synovitis or avascular necrosis of bone.

Aggravating and relieving factors

The relationship of several factors to the patient's pain is of major significance. These include rest, movements of the affected part, exercise, and posture.

In general, musculoskeletal pain of mechanical origin is relieved by rest and aggravated by movement. In addition, mechanical factors such as stretching or compressing the joint (for example, by lying on it) may also cause pain. If the joint is painful at rest it usually is because of the severity of the underlying inflammation.

Pain may also be related to posture and develop only after the patient has adopted a particular posture and maintained it over a considerable period. At times pain may also be related to several different positions; or holding a joint comfortable in one position over a length of time and then moving from this position may produce sudden, sharp pain.

It is also necessary to enquire if pain varies either in site or in intensity, and how long it takes for these symptoms to subside. If pain is aggravated or relieved by certain postures or movements it may be helpful to have the patient demonstrate these movements.

Patients with psychogenically determined pain often lack the characteristic pattern of pain relief and aggravation described above.

Pattern of joint involvement

Whether one joint, several or multiple joints are involved is important. Hence one must first enquire about the number of joints involved; the first joint and subsequent joints involved; the pattern of joint involvement, e.g. migratory, additive, or simultaneous; and whether the joint involvement is symmetrical or asymmetrical.

Effects of treatment

The patient should be questioned about the results of any form of previous or current treatment on the pain and whether it has relieved or aggravated the pain. In particular, the patient should be asked about the name, dosage, duration of use, effects, and side effects of any medications or injections; and the results of any physiotherapy, including the type of therapy given, its duration, and its effects; and whether it was beneficial or caused any exacerbation of symptoms.

Joint 'irritability'

This is a most useful concept, especially for therapy. 'Irritability' may be defined as the relationship of the degree of activity to the pain subsequently evoked; this pain is assessed both by its degree and by the length of time taken for this increased pain to subside to its usual level. Hence, a joint is 'irritable' if only a moderate degree of activity provokes an increase in pain lasting for approximately an hour. Examination should not then be prolonged and subsequent treatment by passive movements must be gentle. Alternatively, a patient may suffer only a sharp momentary pain after a sudden jarring. This condition is not 'irritable' and subsequent examination and management by passive movements can be more forceful. 'Irritability' is also an important assessment to make during therapy. If a previously 'irritable' joint becomes non-irritable during treatment it is patently improving.

Progress

The progress of the underlying condition may be:

(1) Intermittently present.
(2) Constantly present.
(3) Present in recurrent attacks, in which case the frequency, regularity, and duration of attacks needs to be known.
(4) Progressively worse.

Worst problem

The patient should be asked about the worst clinical problem that he currently has in terms of pain and loss of function.

Related signs and symptoms

Related signs and symptoms include stiffness, swelling, crepitus, locking, instability, weakness, and neurological symptoms. Stiffness and neurological symptoms will be discussed here, as the other signs and symptoms are described in some detail later in the book. Stiffness is a symptom that implies an increased resistance to movement of a part throughout a given range. This range may not necessarily be restricted and so it is differentiated from limitation of movement, which is an objective sign. Hence it may be possible to demonstrate a restriction of movement in one direction—for example, rotation of the neck to the right—but the patient may be more conscious of stiffness of movement in another direction— rotation of the neck to the left.

Points in the history include the distribution of the stiffness, how long it has been present, and its relationship to pain. The duration of stiffness, especially the length of time that stiffness persists in the morning, is of prime importance. It is, moreover, an objective test of the degree of under-lying inflammation in the joint; the duration of morning stiffness correlates well with this inflammatory change. Stiffness or 'articular gelling' may occur in patients with osteoarthritis or tendinitis; it lasts for only a few minutes and follows a period of prolonged immobilization, such as sitting in a chair.

Neurological symptoms include sensory symptoms such as pins and needles or numbness. In patients who present with pain in the limb, the presence of such sensory symptoms is of major significance since it points to the diagnosis of neural compression, either in the spine or as a peripheral nerve entrapment.

Important points in the history include:

(1) The distribution of the sensory symptoms.
(2) Their relationship to the onset and distribution of pain.
(3) Aggravating and relieving factors, especially spinal movements of posturing.

General history

This includes the history related to:

(1) Other systems; symptoms that may arise from the other bodily systems and any medications they may require should be enquired into.
(2) Previous health; this includes details of previous trauma, operations, medical illnesses, and their investigations and treatments.
(3) Precipitating factors; besides trauma, these may include infections, illnesses, surgery, and stress.
(4) Family history of any joint or systemic disorders.
(5) Social history; the type of work that the patient does and any difficulty encountered in its performance; the type and intensity of any recreational or sporting activities.
(6) Functional assessment; the loss of any function as the result of the current illness and its effect upon the patient must be assessed.

3 Examination

Clinical signs in patients who complain of musculoskeletal pain are nearly always present and readily detectable. Emphasis in this book is mainly on the diagnosis of soft-tissue lesions; this diagnosis can usually be made on clinical grounds, and the methods follow the pioneering work of Cyriax (1978). The main purpose of clinical examination is to localize accurately the anatomical site which is involved. This depends on a knowledge of the anatomy and surface anatomy of the moving parts; it also requires an understanding of the usual traumatic, inflammatory and/or degenerative lesions which commonly involve these structures. The possible underlying pathological basis is determined to some extent from the patient's history and also from ancillary tests, such as X-rays, blood tests and occasionally by a biopsy. X-rays of the affected area are usually of such importance that their use may also be considered as part of the normal joint examination.

Clinical examination to reveal the anatomical site of the lesion must be carried out using an orderly system comprising inspection, movement and palpation.

The limbs must be fully exposed and, in all of the tests to be described, the unaffected limb is always examined before the affected one to gain the patient's confidence and assess the normal pain-free range of movement. It should be remembered that the joints of a limb form part of a link system so that any alteration, weakness or tightness of one part of the link may be reflected in an alteration of another part. Also, pain may be referred from another, usually proximal, site. A common example is pain in the knee referred from a lesion in the hip joint, and pain in a limb may be referred from spinal joints. Hence the whole of the limb and the relevant part of the spine, referred to by Maitland (1979) as the 'other joints in plan', should also be examined. A general physical examination is also necessary and, in the limbs, special attention is given to the neurological and vascular systems. To summarize, the clinical examination comprises:

(1) Adequate exposure of the parts to be examined.
(2) Examination of the normal side before the affected one.
(3) Use of an orderly system comprising:

    (a) Inspection.
    (b) Movement.
    (c) Palpation.

(4) Contraction, stretching or compression of the musculoskeletal parts by movements designed to be:

    (a) Active.
    (b) Passive.
    (c) Isometric.
    (d) Accessory.

(5) Examination of other joints in 'plan'.
(6) General physical examination.
(7) X-rays.

Inspection

General examination

A great deal of information can be obtained from inspection, which should commence as soon as the patient is first met; even the fact that he is in bed or in a wheel-chair is of obvious significance. If the patient is mobile his posture; gait; need to use supports or aids; deformities; ability or willingness to use certain joints; and how he sits down, undresses, or gets on and off a couch may provide valuable information. The patient's personality should also be assessed and an attempt made to gain a knowledge of his pain threshold and reaction to pain.

Inspection of the posture may provide a clue to an underlying disorder. For example, a patient with ankylosing spondylitis may have stiffness of spinal movements, kyphosis and forward flexion of the head. Patients with polymyalgia rheumatica, a condition found usually in an elderly female, may have great difficulty in rising from a chair and may require someone to help them as movements are so painfully stiff. Inspection of the hand, described by Hench as the arthritic's call-card, can reveal considerable information before the formal examination begins. A patient with gout in the metatarsophalangeal joint of the feet may have a classic sign—he may be well dressed except for wearing a shoe with a hole cut in it, or a sandshoe.

The skin

The skin over the joint should be examined for any scars, sinuses, colour changes or rashes. An erythematous rash may occur over the joint in any of the connective-tissue diseases and redness may also indicate an underlying inflammation. The skin over a joint involved with gout is red, hot and dry and may desquamate, indicating the intensity of the inflammation, whereas the skin over the joints involved with rheumatoid arthritis is often moist. Rashes may be due to psoriasis or other skin diseases and areas of pigmentation or depigmentation may be found.

Swelling

The presence of any swelling is often best appreciated by comparing the two limbs. A synovial effusion is usually better recognized by inspection than by palpation as it tends to bulge the synovium in a manner which is characteristic for each joint and is determined by the anatomical confines of the synovial membrane.

Deformities

Deformities of the joint are best seen on inspection and in the lower limb may be more apparent when the patient is weight bearing. Examination usually reveals the site of the deformity which may be caused by alterations in the bones, joints or the soft tissues around them. A fixed deformity is due to a structural abnormality so that the joint cannot be voluntarily restored to its normal anatomical position. Fixed-flexion deformities are commonly present with diseases of the joints. The terms valgus and varus refer to angulation of the distal bone of the joint from the midline; valgus is a lateral inclination and varus a medial inclination.

Muscle wasting

With any severe degree of joint disease, especially in the hip, the surrounding muscles will become wasted and this is usually obvious on inspection. Wasting of the small muscles in the hand is very common in rheumatoid arthritis. Muscle wasting also occurs in lower motor-neurone lesions.

Movements

The musculoskeletal system is made up of movable structures, hence it should be possible to reproduce the patient's symptoms by testing various movements. The fundamental rule in musculoskeletal examination is that the parts should be moved so as to reproduce the patient's pain. This may not necessarily be experienced to the same degree and in exactly the same distribution as the patient's description, but the patient must at least recognize that it is the same type of pain of which he complains. Testing needs to be done in an orderly fashion; tension is applied to each of the structures around a joint so that it is moved by being contracted, stretched, or compressed. The tension can be achieved by clinical testing using a sequence of active, passive, and isometric contractions. Accessory movements, described later, form an essential part of normal joint movements and should also be tested routinely.

The patient needs first to undress so that the whole limb being examined can be observed. The unaffected limb is examined first before the affected one to provide a basis for comparison and allow the normal range of movement to be assessed. The patient is usually examined first while standing, but may also be sitting or lying down. The examiner ensures that the patient is as relaxed as possible and enquires if any pain is felt in the standing position; if so, the patient is asked to point to its site and distribution. The joint is then moved in each of its appropriate directions and the patient is asked to report any alteration in his symptoms.

With this series of tests, a pattern of movement emerges. These consist of positive signs—the movements that are restricted and reproduce pain—and negative signs—movements that are of full range and painless. These movements will now be described.

Active movements

As this name implies, the patient moves the parts himself. Active movements are performed within the patient's own limits of pain and should always be tested before the passive movements, as they indicate the degree of disability present and act as a guide to the examiner of the range of passive movement that can be reached without causing the patient any undue discomfort. Active movements indicate that the musculotendinous structures that produce the movement are intact, and if they are completely ruptured active movement in the desired direction is usually impossible. They also indicate the patient's willingness to perform them. While the active movements are being performed, the following observations are made by the examiner:

(1) The range of movement.
(2) Whether these movements reproduce the patient's pain.
(3) The behaviour of pain.
(4) The rhythm of the movement.
(5) The effect of rapid movements.
(6) The effects of compression.

The range of movement is best measured with a goniometer and may be normal, decreased, increased or abnormal. The normal range depends mainly on anatomical features and varies according to age, sex and individual variation. The type of movement and its range in each joint will be stressed later in this book. Various methods have been used both to chart this measurement and to describe the position of rest from which the joint is moved. The system used here follows that described by the American Academy of Orthopedic Surgeons (1965). The joint range may be decreased by pain, muscle spasm or stiffness in either joint or its surrounding soft tissues. A decrease in the joint range may be either in all directions of the joint movement or else in one or a few directions only. Decreased movement in all directions is usually due to arthritis or capsulitis of the joint. Decreased movement in only one or a few directions indicates an intra-articular lesion, such as a loose body, or an extra-articular soft-tissue lesion. It may also occur with loss of accessory joint movements; when this is the only clinical finding detectable it is known as a hypomobility lesion. Finally, the joint may be ankylosed and no movement at all will be possible. Hypermobility, an increase in the normal range of joint movement, may be a cause of joint pain. Instability results in abnormal joint motion and often follows disruption of the ligamentous support of the joint.

The patient is asked to report whether the movements are painless or whether his pain is reproduced on certain movements. If so it is important to relate the pain to the joint range in which it is felt.

The relationship of pain to any loss of joint movement should always be assessed. The site, type, degree of pain, and any alteration in pain throughout the joint range is recorded and one of three patterns may emerge. Pain may be felt before the limit of the range; pain may be felt at the limit of the range; or the range may be limited but not painful unless over-pressure to the joint is applied. These patterns are mentioned here even though they add little to the clinical diagnosis, but they are of importance when considering the type of treatment to be used.

An arc of pain may sometimes be present. This means that no pain is present with the joint at rest, but commences after the joint is moved, persists through the middle range and then ceases on further movement. The common example is in the shoulder when an arc of pain may be felt on abduction of the shoulder through the range of approximately 60–120 degrees, but no pain is felt on abduction before or after this middle range.

The rhythm of the movement should be assessed. This involves the changes in relationships between the moving parts and the movements usually need to be repeated several times while observing the normal joint rhythm. It may not be possible, however, to perform repeated movements if the movement is very painful.

Rapid movements: if pain in a suspected joint is not provoked by a full range of movement performed at the usual speed the movements should be retested using a series of rapid movements, as these may then reproduce the pain.

Compression: the effect of compression on the joint may be tested. As an example, knee movements may be tested by having the patient squat and it may then be demonstrated that this movement is limited and may reproduce pain.

Passive movements

Passive movements, as their name implies, are performed by the examiner. Since the patient plays no active role in producing these movements, they can also be performed in the presence of a ruptured musculotendinous structure and the effects of any compression of the joint surfaces by the contraction of surrounding muscle is also eliminated. The starting position in which the joint is positioned is similar to that used for active movements and again the patient should be as relaxed as possible, preferably while lying supine. It should be stressed that extreme care and gentleness is always necessary when handling the joints to ensure that undue pain is not provoked and to allow a proper 'feel' of the parts being moved.

On passive movement, the following observations are made:

(1) The range of movement: as described, the range may be normal, increased, or decreased in one or all directions.
(2) Whether any of these movements reproduce the patient's pain.
(3) The position in the range where pain and muscular spasm is first felt and their subsequent behaviour on passively increasing the range. In general, the more rapidly and the earlier in the range that the pain increases, the more severe is the underlying lesion and the greater the need for more care and gentleness in performing the examination.
(4) The end-feel of the movement: the range of

passive movements is usually somewhat greater than the range of active movements and is associated with a normal amount of 'give' in the musculoskeletal structures. This elasticity may be felt as a sense of end-feel and practice is necessary to develop an appreciation for the normal characteristic type of end-feel in each joint. The normal types of end-feel may be caused by approximation of the normal soft tissues around the joint, which gives a soft, springy type of feel; or by a bony block due to approximation of the bones around the joint or to ligamentous tightening.

Abnormal types of end-feel may be produced by:

(a) Muscular spasm.
(b) Joint stiffness, due to capsular thickening, ligamentous adhesions or adaptive muscular shortening.
(c) A cartilaginous loose body.

(5) Over-pressure may be applied at the end of the passive range by using small oscillatory movements. It tests the small extra range normally available in the passive movements. At times, this may be the only movement that reproduces the patient's pain and so no joint can be assessed as being normal unless over-pressure at the end of the range can be applied painlessly. A common example is a sprain of an ankle ligament when active plantar flexion of the ankle may appear to be full and painless, but over-pressure applied at the end of the passive range reproduces pain.
(6) Ligaments: the strength and stability of the ligaments are tested by applying a passive stretching force to the joint.

Isometric tests

The musculotendinous structures and their insertions around a joint are tested by the use of isometric contractions in which the muscle is contracted strongly but the joint itself does not move. The joint being examined first needs to be positioned accurately and so it may be necessary first to explain and demonstrate to the patient what is required.

Starting position

To test a musculotendinous structure three positions of the joint may be used as the starting position:

(1) The joint is placed in the neutral position and the examiner resists the patient's attempt to move it in the desired direction.

(2) The examiner initially passively stretches the musculotendinous structure being tested and he then actively resists the patient's attempt to return the joint to the neutral position.

(3) The examiner places the joint in a position midway through its active range and the patient holds it steady in this position while the examiner attempts to return it to the neutral position.

It is also important for the examiner to palpate with his other hand the patient's muscle and its tendinous attachment while carrying out this test, in order to assess its bulk and continuity.

The observations to be made from this test are:

(1) The strength of the movement.
(2) Whether it reproduces the patient's pain.

In this way, one of three patterns should then emerge:

(1) The resisted movements may be strong and painless; if so the musculotendinous structure involved in that movement can be considered to be normal.

(2) The movement may be weak and painless; this may be due either to a complete rupture of the musculotendinous apparatus being tested or to an interruption in its motor-nerve supply.

(3) The movement may reproduce the patient's pain; this indicates that the musculotendinous structure being tested is at fault. An assessment of the degree of the underlying lesion may be obtained from the strength of the contraction, for if the movement is weak and painful it usually indicates a more severe degree of damage than if the movement is strong and painful.

Patterns of movement

By testing the active, passive, and isometric contractions a pattern of movement emerges that should allow the anatomical site and type of lesion to be identified. The usual or typical findings in the more common types of diagnoses will now be summarized.

In arthritis and capsulitis the usual patterns are:

(1) The active and passive ranges of movement are decreased and usually painful, especially at the limits of the range. However, there are exceptions to this finding, especially in early cases of arthritis when movement may be lost mainly in one or two directions only. Ultimately, however, movements are lost in a proportionate degree that varies depending on the severity of the underlying inflammation.

(2) Resisted movements should be painless.

In tendinitis:

(1) Pain is best reproduced by fully resisted movements.

(2) Pain may also be reproduced by stretching the tendon.

(3) The range of active movement is often normal, but pain may also be produced during or at the end of the range.

With complete rupture of musculotendinous structure:

(1) Active range of movement is lost.
(2) Passive range is normal.
(3) Resisted movements are weak and painless.

With ligament sprains:

(1) Pain is reproduced on passively stretching the ligament, especially if over-pressure is applied.

(2) The range of active and passive movements is usually decreased and painful.

(3) Resisted movements are normal. With complete ligamentous rupture, abnormal joint movement is present on passive movement of the joint.

With muscle lesions:

Pain may be present on resisted movement, and stretching the muscle produces a painful loss of movement.

With hypermobility: the active and passive range is increased but resisted movements are normal.

With an intra-articular loose body: pain is of sudden onset; active and passive movements in one direction, usually extension, are blocked but other movements are full.

Accessory movements

These joint movements, which cannot be performed voluntarily or in isolation by a patient, are a necessary component of normal joint function. Although their range of movement is small, a full range of accessory movements is essential for normal active and passive joint movements. Accordingly, a loss of an accessory movement produces a restriction in the normal range of joint motion. An example of a normal accessory movement may be observed when the hand grasps an object such as a ball, and as the grip is tightened rotation occurs at the metacarpophalangeal joints. The normal physiological movements in this joint are flexion, extension, adduction and abduction, whereas rotation is an accessory movement. In this situation, rotation is produced during the active movement. However, rotation can also be tested for passively and the range of motion produced is then greater. To test this range passively, the left index finger is held relaxed in a position midway between the limits of flexion, extension, abduction and adduction. The proximal phalanx is supported by the thumb and forefinger of the right hand, which are then used to move the proximal phalanx through quite an appreciable range of either medial or lateral rotation.

Another example of accessory movement is that in the glenohumeral joint. With the arm hanging loosely by the side, the head of the humerus occupies the upper portion of the pear-shaped glenoid cavity, from which it is separated by a small gap. To move the arm into flexion, the surrounding muscles contract and the first accessory movement in the joint is a compression of the joint surfaces. When the shoulder is flexed, the humeral head is involved in a second accessory movement as it slides downwards and slightly backwards in the glenoid fossa. There are, in addition, some accessory movements that can never be produced actively. One such movement is a distraction of one joint surface away from another.

The articular surfaces of many joints are normally incongruent in most positions of the joint. They become congruent only at one extreme of the joint ranges as tension in the capsule and ligaments is increased, so that the joint surfaces are brought in maximal contact and are tightly compressed. No movement is then possible; this is known as the close-packed position. In all other positions of the joint the articular surfaces are not congruent, the capsule is more lax, and the joint is in a loose-packed position so that movement at the joint surfaces can more readily take place, usually by sliding, rolling or spinning (Gray, 1973). Similarly, the range of accessory joint movements is greatest when the muscles acting over the joint are relaxed and the joint is positioned midway between the limits of its different directions of active movements.

Clinical testing

The patient is placed in a relaxed position with the joint to be tested adequately supported. It is first placed in a starting position that ensures relaxation of the surrounding muscles and of the joint, usually the position in which the joint capsule has its greatest laxity. Usually the proximal bone forming the joint is fixed and the more distal bone is moved. The different accessory movements present in each joint and their method of clinical testing will be described later.

When testing accessory movements, different areas of adjacent surfaces of hyaline cartilage will be opposed when the joint is positioned in different ranges. For example, if the arm is kept by the side and a posteroanterior accessory movement of the head of the humerus in the glenoid cavity is tested, particular areas of the articular surface of the humerus will be opposed to particular areas of the articular surface of the glenoid cavity. However, if the arm is then abducted by thirty degrees and the same posteroanterior accessory movement is produced a different area on the articular surface of the head of the humerus will now contact the same or different areas of the articular surface of the glenoid cavity. Thus different positions of the arm will yield different relationships of the opposed adjacent articular surfaces between the head of the humerus and the glenoid cavity while any one accessory movement is being tested.

It is also important to realize that when the accessory movements are performed in different positions of the joint, different joint structures or parts of structures are placed on stretch. Accordingly, when testing accessory movements of a joint it is sometimes necessary to perform each accessory movement with the joint placed in different positions. This is necessary if restrictions of movement, pain with movement (perhaps reproducing the patient's pain) and smoothness of movement between the opposing joint surfaces are to be determined accurately.

Clinical importance

The importance of accessory movements:

(1) They play an essential role in the production of normal joint movement.
(2) Loss of accessory movements is associated with loss of normal joint movement.
(3) Normal or restricted accessory movements can be detected by appropriate clinical testing.

(4) At times, a restriction in their range (hypo-mobility) may be the only relevant clinical finding detectable.

(5) They are used to treat painful or stiff joints by a passive movement technique using gentle rhythmical oscillations (mobilization). The range of joint movement is increased by this method, rather than by directly trying to force an increase in the passive joint range.

The clinical importance of accessory movements may be considered in three different types of joint:

(1) In joints such as the shoulder or knee, where a large range of physiological movement is normally possible; a lesion of these joints is usually associated with loss of the normal range of active and passive movements. If so the accessory movements will also be lost and testing them by suitably applied pressures should also reveal a painful restriction in their range.

(2) In small single joints such as the sternoclavicular, acromioclavicular or temporomandibular joints, active and passive joint movements may not be painful but testing of accessory movements may reveal that accessory movements are restricted and reproduce the patient's pain. This may be the only abnormal clinical sign that can be elicited.

(3) In the integrated movements of several small joints, such as in the carpus, active and passive wrist movements may reproduce the patient's pain but do not accurately localize the affected joint. However, this may be localized by testing the accessory movements of all the small intercarpal joints.

An example of the importance and differing relationships between accessory movements may be given by considering movements between the capitate and hamate bones, which can easily be grasped by the examiner. He places one hand over the radial surface of the patient's hand so that his middle finger is over the palmar surface and his thumb is over the dorsal surface of the capitate. The examiner's other hand is placed over the ulnar side of the patient's hand to hold the hamate bone between the examiner's finger and thumb. These two bones can then easily be made to glide backwards and forwards against each other, and the joint movement—which is normally pain free—can be readily felt. However, in some patients with wrist pain the pain may be produced with movement either of the capitate or the hamate. In theory, if movement of the hamate on the capitate produces pain then movement of the capitate on the hamate should also produce pain, but clinically this is not necessarily so.

Assessment

During the testing of accessory movements three factors need to be assessed: stiffness, smoothness, and pain.

Stiffness—The available range of accessory movement is assessed and any restriction in the range noted. This is tested with the joint placed in two positions: firstly, midway between the limits of all active ranges; and secondly, with the joint placed at the limit of any one or all directions of active movement.

Smoothness—Smoothness implies the friction-free feel of the accessory movements through the full amplitude of joint range from the limit of the range in one direction to the limit of the range in its opposite direction. The test for normal smoothness of movement is performed with the joint positioned midway between the limits of all its active ranges and the joint surfaces in a relaxed relationship to each other. The smoothness of their movement should be compared also with that which can be felt when the joint surfaces are compressed and then moved through the same range.

Pain—An assessment should be made of any pain or discomfort that a patient may experience as the accessory movement is taken from one limit of its range to the other. Once again, an assessment of pain through the range should be first made when the joint surfaces are in a relaxed relationship to each other, and this should then be compared with pain or discomfort experienced throughout the same range with the joint surfaces compressed.

Palpation

Palpation forms an essential part of examination and requires a knowledge of the surface anatomy of each of the joint structures. These are palpated in an orderly sequence and the examiner confirms the presence of any alterations, such as deformity or muscle wasting, that have been noted on inspection. On palpation, the examiner also detects the presence of any warmth, swellings, crepitus, and tenderness.

Warmth

The presence of any warmth over the joint surface should always be sought by palpation as it indicates the presence of an underlying inflammation or haemarthrosis. The customary teaching is to elicit this sign with the dorsal surface of the fingers but it is often better appreciated by palpating the area with the palmar surface of the whole hand.

Swellings

Swelling may be either intra- or extra-articular. Intra-articular swellings may be either soft or hard. Soft-tissue swellings may be due either to fluid or to synovial thickening. The presence of synovial effusion is usually better recognized on inspection than on palpation, but palpation is necessary to confirm its presence and that the swelling is due to fluid. Synovial thickening due to a chronically inflamed synovium produces a characteristically firm and 'doughy' feel, best felt by rolling the fingers across the area of attachment of synovium to the underlying bone.

Hard intra-articular swellings are usually due to bone and may be caused by osteophytic outgrowths around the edge of the joint, joint subluxations, intra-articular bony foreign bodies, bone tumours, or bone deformities. An example of the last cause occurs in Freiberg's disease, an osteochondrosis involving the head of the second metatarsal, where the irregular and deformed bone ends may be easily palpable.

Extra-articular swellings may be due to oedema, haematoma formation, fat deposits, synovial swellings in bursae or tendon sheaths, calcific deposits, nodules or tophi. Swellings should be palpated to record their size, shape, consistency, surface, edges, and attachments to superficial or deeper structures.

The tendons and their muscle bellies should also be palpated for the presence of any localized swelling. Tears in muscles or tendons may be felt as a localized gap often with a nearby swelling from the rolled-up portion of the torn muscle or tendon tissue. Localized areas of thickenings in the muscle belly may be found with healing of recent tears. The bones around the joint are palpated for the presence of any swellings, irregularities or thickening.

Crepitus

Crepitus is a noise that may be heard or felt on a movement. A course, grating crepitus palpable with the hand placed over the joint surface indicates articular-cartilage degeneration and is often best felt in the knee. A fine crepitus is felt with synovial thickening and is often best felt in patients with tenosynovitis. Clicks such as the normal vacuum click may be felt in the joint and are usually of no significance. They are particularly common in hypermobile joints. A painful click may indicate the presence of a torn meniscus. Snapping may be heard or felt around joints as tendons or ligaments slip over bony prominences. This is often loud and disturbing to the patient but is usually of no clinical significance. A coarse 'clunking' type of noise may accompany joint subluxation or instability. This may be produced by degenerative changes in the joint or can be found particularly in the knee with rotary instability due to ligamentous damage.

Tenderness

The structure being examined should be carefully palpated for tenderness while simultaneously observing the patient's face to gauge the degree of any painful reaction. Palpation is usually carried out by the examiner using his thumb or forefinger and it is essential that a firm even pressure be used. This can usually be judged to be sufficient if a blanching of the distal aspect of the examiner's thumb becomes apparent during the palpation.

However, considerable difficulties arise in the correct assessment of tenderness. The point at issue is not that locally inflamed or damaged tissues may be tender but that correct interpretation of this sign requires considerable experience and expertise. Tenderness can often be a misleading sign, because it is in part subjective. Also, many normal structures can often be made to feel tender, especially if the patient is not sufficiently relaxed. Moreover, tenderness may at times be referred when it is associated with referred pain, so the site of the causative lesion may be more proximal.

Hence, the mistake most commonly made is to seek for tenderness as the first sign in the clinical examination. As a general rule, tenderness should be used only as a confirmatory test after the site of the underlying lesion has been indentified with the appropriate movement tests described. For example, if clinical examination of a joint with active, passive and isometric test movements has demonstrated the presence of tendinitis then tenderness over the involved tendon is most useful as a confirmatory sign. But to commence the examination of a patient with joint pain by first palpating for tenderness will often lead to an incorrect diagnosis.

4 Management

Treatment may be classified under the following headings:

(1) Rest.
(2) Aids and supports.
(3) Medications.
(4) Injections.
(5) Physical therapy. This includes:

  (a) Heat.
  (b) Ice.
  (c) Exercise therapy.
  (d) Deep-friction massage.
  (e) Transcutaneous nerve stimulation.
  (f) Interferential therapy.

(6) Manipulative therapy. This includes:

  (a) Mobilization.
  (b) Manipulation.

(7) Surgery.
(8) Aftercare and prophylaxis.

Most of these will now be discussed in some detail.

Rest

For over a century, there has been considerable medical controversy regarding the value of rest in the treatment of musculoskeletal disorders. The pendulum of opinion has swung backwards and forwards since John Hilton in 1863 published his famous book *Rest and Pain*, in which he advocated a system of prolonged uninterrupted rest and splinting for inflamed joints. Since infective causes

of arthritis, especially tuberculosis, were then so prevalent this system of treatment was undoubtedly a major advance and subsequently prolonged rest was advocated as the treatment of most musculoskeletal diseases.

Unfortunately this regimen was advocated to an extreme, so that many other types of joint conditions—which could well have been managed with early mobilization of the patient—were treated with splinting for prolonged periods, often with disastrous results. During the Second World War, opinion again shifted so that more active exercises and rehabilitation programmes were undertaken, particularly in patients with injuries. This has been well typified in the management both of direct and of indirect sporting injuries where prolonged rest leads to a longer period of disability, whereas quite vigorous treatment programmes involving active exercises and passive stretching that enable the athlete to return to his sport more rapidly without having lost any general level of fitness can be instituted soon after the original injury.

However, it is probably correct to say that many patients with soft-tissue or joint disorders caused by an underlying degenerative process with an associated inflammatory reaction are encouraged to exercise too early and too vigorously. This applies particularly to those with the overuse type of soft-tissue disorder, or an inflammatory polyarthritis such as rheumatoid arthritis, who believe that 'exercise is good for you' and that it can hence overcome the effects of inflammation. Most patients with overuse type of injuries require rest from the prolonged or repetitive activities that are responsible for their symptoms.

The degree of rest needed will vary according to the degree of inflammatory reaction and also to the expectations of the patient. Thus, in many athletes or if the patient is the breadwinner a prescription for complete rest is most likely to go unheeded. However, it may be possible to arrange rest to the overused musculoskeletal structures while not inhibiting more generalized activities.

Aids and supports

These may be used to support a painful joint or to help to transfer the body weight from one leg to the pain-free one. The large variety of supports will not be considered here, but some general examples only will be given. In the lower limb, these include:

(1) Crutches, walking frames and sticks.
(2) Knee cages with side bars and a locking device may help to support a painful, weakened or unstable knee.
(3) Callipers may be long leg and weight bearing under the ischial tuberosity or used to support the ankle or subtalar joint with a T strap.

In the upper limb slings, triangular bandages or a collar and cuff bandage may be used to rest the shoulder or elbow.

Aids to improve the patient's functional activities can be supplied by an occupational therapy department based on an Aids to Daily Living (ADL) assessment.

Orthotics

Orthotic devices are used to obtain a functional control of any biomechanical deformity that may be present during the different phases of stance by providing normal muscular action about a stable lever system. As an example, orthotics may be considered in the treatment of foot disorders. Here their advantage over conventional types of arch supports is in controlling the function of both the rear-foot and the forefoot simultaneously so that the angular relationship between the bones of the rear-foot to the forefoot is retained. The orthotic forms a system with the foot that moves with it and not against it and also permits the rear-foot to act as a shock absorber. Orthotic devices are available in different forms of increasing rigidity

that vary in effectiveness and patient acceptability (Rinaldi and Sabia, 1978):

(1) Soft devices are usually made of felt or rubber and are used particularly in running-shoes.
(2) Semi-flexible devices are usually made of leather or firmer rubber.
(3) Rigid devices are made of thermally pliable plastic that is constructed from a neutral balanced cast of the patient's foot.

They extend from the heel to behind the metatarsal head and provide stability during the heel-strike and mid-stance phases of gait. They also allow the foot to supinate during mid-stance. They may need to be balanced by posts or wedges at either the rear-foot or forefoot, or both. For example, patients with either rear-foot varus or valgus deformities will require pronatory or supinatory wedging of the heel. Care must be taken during the making of the cast to ensure that the foot is in a neutral position relative to the lower leg—that is, not supinated or pronated, or altered in shape by the body weight.

Medications

Medication may be used to produce either an analgesic or an anti-inflammatory effect. Since pain is such a common problem in musculoskeletal disorders, it is not unreasonable to prescribe simple non-narcotic drugs for pain relief. Paracetamol, salicylates or dextropropoxyphene are commonly used, often in combination tablets.

The non-steroidal antiflammatory (NSAI) drugs have a role in overall management. All of them cause analgesic and antipyretic effects and modify and reduce the effects of experimentally produced inflammation in animal models. Inflammation in musculoskeletal diseases is usually mediated by a complex chemical process and the exact site of action of these drugs in modifying it is largely determined. As they influence to a varying extent the chemical mediators of inflammation, such as the kinin peptides, lysosomal enzymes and prostaglandins, they may help to prevent vasodilatation, capillary permeability, oedema, swelling and pain.

In general these drugs are readily absorbed from the gastrointestinal tract and enter the circulation, where they are extensively (up to 99 per cent) bound to albumin and so can displace other drugs such as warfarin, which are also highly bound to albumin. Most of the NSAI drugs are metabolized in the liver and are excreted mainly through the kidney. Most of them also have short half-lives—except for sulindac and naproxen, which can be given twice daily. All of these drugs produce a maximal effect within 2 weeks of starting treatment. They all have potent side effects, especially on the gastrointestinal tract; these include nausea, vomiting, indigestion, gastric bleeding and occasionally abdominal cramps and diarrhoea or constipation. They may also be associated with varying degrees of bone-marrow suppression, central nervous system disturbance, and fluid retention; hence they may precipitate congestive cardiac failure, rashes, stomatitis, hepatotoxicity and hypersensitivity reactions. They may also induce an attack of asthma in susceptible individuals. An iron-deficiency anaemia may develop due to their effect on the gut, and these drugs must be used with great caution in patients with impaired renal function.

Mainly because of the side effects of the more potent anti-inflammatory drugs—aspirin, phenylbutazone and indomethacin—considerable research has gone into producing newer compounds. The first propionic acid drugs to be manufactured were shown to cause fewer side effects but this may also correlate with their having less of an anti-inflammatory action. Of some significance is the pro-drug sulindac, which is not converted to its active metabolite until after it has been absorbed and metabolized in the liver. A pro-drug could have a minimal effect on the gut both before and after absorption.

Salicylates in one of the many available preparations of aspirin are often the first choice in the treatment of inflammatory polyarthritis, such as rheumatoid arthritis. It is rapidly absorbed from the stomach and small intestine but to produce an anti-inflammatory effect at least 4 g daily are necessary, given four times daily in divided doses. Unfortunately, at this high dosage side effects are common and patient compliance is poor.

Phenylbutazone and indomethacin are of greater efficacy in spondyloarthritis, where they may produce significant improvement in small dosages, and in acute crystal synovitis, where they need to be given in a dosage of at least eight tablets daily for a few days until inflammation is controlled; the dose is then gradually reduced.

In the soft-tissue inflammatory diseases with which this book is mainly concerned, aspirin is not as useful as the other NSAI drugs which are especially indicated in the overuse syndromes but may also help in relieving pain and inflammation in other types of injury (Muckle, 1980). They should be given in a dosage sufficient to produce the required anti-inflammatory effect, usually two or three times a day after meals. However, the choice of drug in these conditions should be influenced largely by the problem of side effects, and so simpler agents—such as the propionic acid group—should be the first choice of treatment. If a response is being obtained after a week their use is continued but in as small a dose as is compatible with relief. If no response is obtained after a week other drugs in the propionic acid group may be substituted; and if still no response is obtained one of the other group of drugs may be tried, such as sulindac. Only if these are also unsuccessful should the more potent drugs such as phenylbutazone or indomethacin be used.

Injection therapy

Shortly after corticosteroids were first introduced in 1949, it was realized that a low dose of this preparation, deposited at an affected site of inflammation, could obviate some of the problems caused by a large oral dose. The original corticosteroid used, cortisone, was ineffective for local use as it needs to be converted in the liver to hydrocortisone. Several synthetic analogues of hydrocortisone have since been manufactured. Taken by mouth, these drugs have different degrees of potency and side effects that are not necessarily reflected in their usefulness as local preparations either topically or as local injections; for example, triamcinolone given by mouth has considerable side effects but is a most useful form of local injection. In general acetate, tertiary butyl acetate, or phosphate salts are used in local injections; their different properties are related to their solubility and chemical preparation. Crystalline forms, which may themselves produce an intense crystal synovitis, and long-acting preparations are available.

Injections must be given using thorough aseptic precautions, including scrubbing of the hands and sterilization of the skin. Similarly, local injections must never be given in the presence of any skin infections. It is good practice to swab the skin at least twice with an antiseptic skin solution, and an alcohol swab may be left on the skin with the finger placed over it to palpate the site of the injection. The use of disposable syringes and needles and small phials of local anaesthetic and corticosteroid preparations have undoubtedly been major advancements. The injections may be given either into joints or into surrounding soft tissues. They are especially useful in traumatic or inflammatory synovitis and are of great value in treating crystal synovitis, particularly if it involves the larger joints. The joint surfaces are palpated and the patient suitably postured so that the synovium bulges at the site of injection. The optimum site for injection varies with each joint but is usually found on the extensor surface and will be described in subsequent chapters. The size of the needle used varies with the size of the joint, but in small joints a 25-gauge needle may be used and in large joints, such as the knee, a 20-gauge needle is usually sufficient for aspiration and injection.

If the bony outlines of the joint have been carefully palpated it is usually possible, with sufficient practice, to insert the needle directly into the synovial cavity without having to guide it along the bony surfaces so that entering a distended synovial space can be as easy as puncturing an inflated balloon. Any synovial fluid present should be aspirated and submitted for routine analysis of its cell count, protein content and the presence of any crystals.

Occasionally, folds of synovium or fibrinous intrasynovial deposits block the tip of the needle and prevent easy withdrawal of fluid. Should this happen, the needle is withdrawn slightly and moved about within the joint gently. Any fluid that has already been aspirated may be reinjected through the needle to clear it; if not, a few ml of 1% local anaesthetic solution may be injected.

The dose of corticosteroid given is best measured as the volume of injected solution. For example, small joints such as the finger joints can usually take approximately 0.5 ml of solution, the wrist and elbow about 1 ml, larger joints such as the elbow or ankle about 2 ml and a large synovial joint such as the knee 2–3 ml. Thus the total dosage of corticosteroid will also vary with the pharmacological composition of the steroid preparation being used.

If the needle has been correctly placed inside the cavity the injection of corticosteroid can be made easily without any sense of resistance. If not, the needle has probably been placed outside the synovial cavity. Inside the synovial cavity the corticosteroid solution spreads evenly, mixes with the synovial fluid and bathes the cells of the synovial membrane. It acts by blocking the inflammatory reaction and this action may be related to its effect in stabilizing lysosomal membranes. Hence, it is important in treating joint diseases that the corticosteroid preparation is deposited within the synovial cavity. Once the injection has been given, the needle is rapidly withdrawn, the skin area again swabbed and a small protective dressing applied.

In the soft tissues, local corticosteroid injections are of most value in the overuse type of inflammatory lesions involving the bursae, ligaments or musculotendinous structures and in the nerve entrapment syndromes. In injuries due to direct or indirect trauma, their use is much more limited. They certainly should never be given in the early stages of these injuries since they may induce further bleeding. However, at a later stage in the healing of these lesions a small area of fibrous tissue thickening may form that limits movement and promotes an inflammatory reaction with use of the part. These areas in muscles, tendons or ligaments can usually be readily felt with careful palpation and often respond well to local corticosteroid injection.

In soft-tissue lesions the injection must be deposited accurately at or around the involved site and this presupposes an accurate clinical diagnosis and knowledge of the anatomy and surface landmarks. For soft-tissue injections the optimum position for injection depends on suitable posturing of the patient so that the area to be injected can be accurately palpated. As a general rule, they should be given with the structure to be injected put on stretch. Soft-tissue landmarks and the site of injection varies for each joint and will be considered in greater detail in succeeding chapters. Local anaesthetic, usually 1% Xylocaine (lignocaine), is also added to the corticosteroid solution as it eases any pain from the local injection. Moreover, if this injection has been accurately sited the patient's pain should be relieved so that retesting the active, passive or resisted movements should no longer reproduce the patient's pain.

The patient should be warned, however, that as the effect of the local anaesthetic wears off, some pain or discomfort may be experienced for 1 or possibly 2 days, but that subsequently there should be considerable improvement in their symptoms. Also, to prevent further damage they should not overuse the part while the analgesic effect of the local anaesthetic is still present.

It is important to stress that the injection therapy forms only a part of the overall management and that the injected area should be rested after the injection is given. For this reason the practice of giving a local corticosteroid injection and allowing the patient to exercise immediately afterwards should be condemned.

There is no absolute rule as to how often an injection should be repeated. It was originally believed that repeated injections at frequent intervals were preferable, but as a general rule injections are best given with as long an interval as possible between the injections. In the weight-bearing joints injections should be limited to two or at the most three times yearly.

Contraindications

Injections should never be given:

(1) In the presence of any infections.
(2) At a late stage of articular diseases when irreparable joint damage is present.
(3) If a haemarthrosis is present.
(4) If a fracture involves the joint surfaces.
(5) Before a definitive diagnosis has been reached.
(6) If a psychogenic cause of the patient's symptoms is suspected.
(7) If previous injections have failed to produce any prolonged benefit.

Advantages

In most of the soft-tissue lesions for which local corticosteroid injections are indicated, a considerable degree of relief of symptoms can usually be expected. In the chronic joint diseases these injections obviously do not represent a cure but, since they help to suppress the inflammatory reaction, they can provide at least a temporary relief of pain and swelling. This may permit the use of other pharmacological and physical methods to improve the functional status of the patient.

In inflammatory arthritis injections are of considerable value in the total management of the patient. They should be used only if:

(1) A few joints are affected.
(2) A few joints are actively inflamed.
(3) A few involved joints prevent active rehabilitation of the patient. For example, a patient may have severe joint disease but only synovitis in the knee prevents him from becoming ambulant.
(4) The use of anti-inflammatories by mouth is contraindicated.

In degenerative joint disease, injections are most unlikely to produce any lasting effect or alter the underlying pathological process. They may occasionally be of value when there is a superadded inflammatory element, such as in Heberden's node.

Complications

The complications of intra-articular injections should always be remembered, particularly since these injections are so easy to perform.

Infection

Infection introduced with the injection is a major tragedy, although fortunately quite rare. Hollander (1970) reported an incidence of only one infection in 14 000 injections. Since *Staphylococcus aureus* is the most common infecting organism, the need for constant attention to maintaining asepsis is of paramount importance.

Acute crystal synovitis

If the corticosteroid solution is microcrystalline an intense crystal synovitis may be produced, which lasts for a few days. This has been estimated to occur in 2 per cent of injections with these types of preparations.

Systemic absorption

The synovial cavity is a highly vascular structure so the local injection is never retained wholly within the joint cavity but is partly absorbed.

Articular cartilage damage

Corticosteroids, whether given by mouth or injection, can inhibit the metabolism of cartilage, probably by their effect on chondrocytes and glycosaminoglycan metabolism. Damage to hyaline cartilage of the joint after the use of local hydrocortisone injections was first reported clinically by Chandler and Wright (1958). Of 25 knees so treated, 13 showed radiological evidence of loss of joint space; Chandler and Wright concluded that the alleviation of the patient's pain may result in overuse of the joint. Most reports of cartilage damage have followed repeated intra-articular injections and Salter, Gross and Hall (1967) were able to produce degenerative articular cartilage changes in rabbits given frequent injections. Hollander (1970), however, studied a series of 8000 patients given repeated intra-articular injections and followed up. In these, less than 1 per cent showed any marked evidence of joint deterioration. Gibson *et al.* (1977) injected a large dose of methylprednisolone into Macaca monkeys over 12 weeks and failed to demonstrate any significant degree of cartilage damage. They suggested that in man infrequent injections would probably not accelerate cartilage damage, and that its benefits in reducing synovial inflammation could far outweigh any problems caused by cartilage damage.

A further complication of this type of damage may result in cartilage and bone destruction, producing an aseptic necrosis of the bone, or a destructive Charcot type of arthropathy. This appears to be more common in the hip but tends to follow repeated injections in any joint; for example, Steinberg, Duthie and Pina (1962) reported a case of a Charcot type of arthropathy in a patient with rheumatoid arthritis whose knee was injected 22 times over 2 years.

Tendon rupture

An injection should never be directly into the tendon substance, as there is at least a theoretical consideration that it may weaken the collagen fibres. Of more significance, it may cause swelling and so compress the relatively tenuous vascular supply which runs beside the tendon. The area of tenderness, usually near the tendon origin or on its surface, should be found by careful palpation and the needle is then directed obliquely alongside this area.

To summarize; the use of local corticosteroid injections is still controversial but it seems reasonable to conclude that:

(1) In soft-tissue injuries after trauma or overuse, they are of immense value if properly administered into the locally affected area.

(2) In degenerative joint disease their use is short lasting and add little to the total management of the patient.

(3) In chronic inflammatory arthritis they are of considerable value as an adjunct to the total management of the patient, especially when combined with joint aspiration.

(4) In acute crystal synovitis involving large joints, such as the knee, their use —combined with aspiration of the joint—is usually the treatment of choice.

(5) The advantages of their use outweigh their complications, which must none the less never be ignored.

(6) They must be used only as one part of a total programme of management.

Physical therapy

Physical methods of therapy have a time-honoured role in the management of musculoskeletal disorders. Those considered here are: heat; ice; exercise therapy; deep-friction massage; and methods of inducing analgesia, such as transcutaneous nerve stimulation and interferential therapy.

Heat

Heat may be used to relieve the symptoms of musculoskeletal disorders, but it seems obvious that it will play little part in their cure. Hence it may be used for its analgesic properties, and is especially useful when given before exercise therapy (Wright, Dowson and Longfield, 1969). The physical intricacies of the various forms of therapeutic heat will not be considered here, but factors in its form of application include its depth of penetration beneath the skin and the convenience and availability of application.

Simple methods of producing heat for home treatment include infrared lamps, hot packs, showers or contrast baths in which heat is alternated with the use of cold. More complex methods used by the physiotherapist include the following:

Paraffin-wax baths

These are used with commercially available paraffin wax which melts at 52–53 °C. All clothing and jewellery are removed from the parts to be treated, nearly always the hands. They are then dipped up to ten times in the melted wax to provide a coating of wax that stays on for about 20 minutes.

Microwaves

These are electromagnetic radiations with a wide frequency range produced by a microwave machine with applicators placed a few centimetres from the skin surface to direct a beam of radiation. It is an easy method to use but the depth of heating is largely superficial.

Ultrasound

This employs an acoustic vibration that is produced when a high-frequency oscillatory voltage is passed through a quartz crystal to produce a piezoelectrical effect. The crystal is contained in a metal head that produces a cylindrical beam and so allows optimal ultrasound transmission.

Ultrasonic therapy is believed to increase the permeability of semi-permeable membranes and so disperse any accumulation of fluid. Dyson *et al.* (1968) found that ultrasound improved the rate of healing of injured rabbit ears, independent of any heating effect. Harvey *et al.* (1975) reported that ultrasound given to tissue culture stimulated an increased protein synthesis in fibroblasts. It also may produce a local micromassaging effect that may help to disperse fibrous tissue and so is useful in the chronic stage of many soft-tissue injuries. However, its main effect is probably as a form of heat produced particularly at the inter-surface between tissues such as muscle layers.

Its concentrated use can produce tissue damage from a localized mechanical destructive force, but this potential danger is overcome by moving the point of application gradually over a field of several square centimetres at any one time. It may, however, produce a rapid rise in the temperature of the deep tissues without producing any skin heating or sensation of warmth, so that a correct knowledge of its use and method of application is essential. It is also helpful to ask the patient whether the therapy causes any discomfort.

Short-wave diathermy

This undoubtedly produces the deepest penetration of heat but requires expensive equipment and supervision by a physiotherapist. It uses high-frequency currents and the patient is placed within the electrical circuit to produce an impedance. Two methods are available, which use either an induction coil or a condenser field. The machine needs to be tuned to adjust the total impedance so that the frequency of oscillation in the machine resonates with the patient's circuit.

All clothing, jewellery and metallic objects must be removed from the patient before treatment and this form of therapy cannot be used if the patient has had a metal implant inserted surgically. The accumulation of any sweat on the skin can also result in local burning.

Ice therapy

Ice has been used as a therapeutic agent for many years but interest in its use has increased since Grant (1964) reported good results in treating musculoskeletal disorders. Its main indication would appear to be in the immediate treatment of sporting injuries, where the rationale for its use is cooling of the deeper tissues with vasoconstriction and reduction of the localized bleeding. Hartviksen (1962) has shown that the depth of cooling depends on the length of time that the ice is applied. For the first 10 minutes after application to the gastrocnemius the intramuscular temperature did not alter, but after that time the temperature dropped rapidly from 35 to 28 °C for the next 40 minutes even though the ice-pack had been removed. Laing, Dalley and Kirk (1973) reported that surface cooling for 20 minutes produced a cooling effect in the deeper muscles which lasted for up to 2 hours. However, ice may also be used in the treatment of chronic musculoskeletal conditions, including the healing phase of musculotendinous injuries, and often replaces the traditional role played by heat. There is also some evidence that surface ice increases the temperature in articular structures (Hollander and Horvath, 1949) and that it may act in the same way as locally applied heat by increasing articular blood flow (Kirk and Kersley, 1968); the clinical use of cold produces the same results as does heat.

Method of application

The ice is finely crushed and placed in a wet towel, which is then placed over the area to be treated and kept in place with a crêpe bandage for approximately 20 minutes. Some patients cannot tolerate this because of an intense burning sensation, but most report only minor, tolerable, discomfort or numbness. The ice is taken off after 20 minutes but may be reapplied every 4 hours.

Ice is easy, safe, simple to apply, cheap, convenient and may be used as a home treatment.

Indications

(1) The immediate treatment of most sports injuries.
(2) Acute bursitis, e.g. acute subacromial bursitis where heat often produces an exacerbation of the pain.
(3) To reduce oedematous swelling, e.g. in the hand.
(4) Preparatory to exercise therapy or stretching.
(5) To relieve muscular spasm.
(6) In most overuse injuries.

Precautions

Prolonged or often repeated ice therapy should not be used. Complications of its use cannot be predicted. It may damage the skin, the so-called 'ice burn', which produces painful, red skin blotches that usually disappear within a few days if ice is not reapplied. More extensive damage may occur in the subcutaneous tissues due to a fat necrosis and persists for some weeks. In one series of 1000 cases (Laing *et al.*, 1973), 15 patients had a skin reaction but only one developed subcutaneous fat damage.

Contraindications

Ice should never be used if there is any impairment of the local blood supply, such as peripheral vascular disease or Raynaud's phenomenon, or if the patient is known to be unduly sensitive to the effects of cold.

Exercise therapy

Exercise therapy has an important role to play in the management of musculoskeletal disorders and may be used:

(1) To restore strength in muscles weakened by disuse, for example around an inflamed joint, or after injury.
(2) To restore mobility or increase the range of movement. This occurs especially after a muscle injury with a loss of extensibility.
(3) To correct postural faults.
(4) To prevent joint deformity.
(5) To improve joint stability. For example, if a patient has cruciate ligament rupture increased knee stability may be obtained by use of quadriceps exercises. This is even more important if the quadriceps have become rapidly wasted, as usually happens.

The major indication for exercise therapy in the management of musculoskeletal disorders then is to restore function and it should be noted that exercises have little role to play while joint pain is the major problem. They may also be used after passive-movement techniques have relieved joint pain in order to restore a full range of physiological movement.

Classification of exercises

Exercises may be active or passive.

Active exercises

These are performed by the patient who moves the part himself. They are classified as:

(1) Active–assisted: the patient moves the part partly by himself but is assisted in this movement by a therapist or by apparatus such as pulleys.
(2) Active–resisted: the part is moved by the patient but some form of resistance to the movement is offered.
(3) Progressive–resisted: as the strength of the muscle increases the amount of resistance offered is also increased.
(4) Isometric: the muscle is exercised by contraction but without moving the joint on which the muscle acts.

Passive exercises

In these the part is carried through a full range of movement by the therapist without any help or resistance by the patient. They have little or no role to play in musculoskeletal diseases, but a variation using passive stretching is considered at more length later.

Relaxation exercises

These are usually based on the technique described by Jacobson (1938) and are of particular value in patients with musculoskeletal pain associated with psychogenic or tension states. A minimal contraction of each muscle is followed by a period of maximum relaxation.

Requirements of an exercise regimen

The practice of handing a patient a sheet of printed exercises and giving the general advice that exercises should be performed is to be deplored. To be effective, an exercise regimen requires:

(1) A medical prescription.
(2) Assessment.
(3) Individualization.
(4) Motivation.
(5) Supervision.
(6) Progression.
(7) Effectiveness.

The first requirement is a proper medical prescription because, as with drug medication, too little exercise therapy can be of no value and too much harmful.

This prescription can only be made after a proper assessment of the patient's disabilities, deformities and muscle strength. This assessment then needs to be related to the patient's future needs, work requirements and capacity to undertake such work.

An exercise regimen needs to be prepared and tailored to these individual deficits and requirements.

The patient must be properly motivated. This can be difficult at times, as a long period of therapy is necessary before any great degree of improvement can be observed. A detailed explanation of the aims of therapy is required and often great enthusiasm on the part of the physiotherapist.

The exercise programme needs to be supervised by a physiotherapist to ensure that they are properly taught and carried out.

The exercise programme needs to be gradually progressed and increased in its intensity.

The regimen should produce its desired result without producing any prolonged period of pain or undue fatigue; should it do so, the treatment programme needs to be revised.

The exercises also should be done, if possible, with the minimum use of equipment, but active assisted exercises may require the use of slings and pulleys, and weights may also be used to provide resistance. Occupational therapy techniques in which functional type of activities are used can also be of great assistance, especially in people with an inflammatory arthritis. A hydrotherapy pool can also be of great assistance in allowing exercises without the effect of gravity and may be assisted by the physiotherapist in a warm and relatively frictionless environment. Proprioceptive neuromuscular facilitation (PNF) was originally introduced for treating neuromuscular disorders by stimulating motor neurones by transmission of voluntary impulses through new detour pathways in the central nervous system (Kabat, 1965). However, the use of similar rotational patterns of movement can also help to improve muscle function in musculoskeletal disorders.

Massage

Massage by rubbing a painful area has the longest history among the physical methods of treatment. It is used in different forms but these are variants of a single theme and have been glorified by the use of French names. These include stroking (effleurage), kneading (pétrissage) and percussion (tapotement). They will not be described here as they are of little practical value, but one form of massage that may be useful, is deep friction.

Deep-friction massage uses intermittent pressures over the soft tissues in which the therapist's finger and the patient's skin and subcutaneous tissues are moved simultaneously over the deeper structures in a transverse direction. The pad of the operator's index finger is usually used and force is supplied by the flexor tendon and not by pressure from the terminal interphalangeal joint. This action may be strengthened by laying the pad of the middle finger over the dorsum of the index finger (Cyriax, 1978).

The action of deep-friction massage appears to be mainly as a form of counter-irritation but it may improve the local blood supply and provide some degree of reaction in chronic ligamentous sprains or in chronic tendinitis. It should never be used in the early stages of healing of an injury or in the presence of acute inflammation.

Transcutaneous nerve stimulation

Transcutaneous nerve stimulation is a simple and safe method used to control pain. An electric current is applied to the skin through electrodes connected to a small battery-operated pulse generator. This apparatus was originally developed as a screening device to test patient's responses to electrical stimulation before surgical implantation of a nerve stimulator, but was found to relieve pain itself in many cases. It has since been used in the control of chronic pain arising from many different disorders. Its method of action seems to be by stimulating peripheral nerves and so modulating pain sensation. This may be because stimulation of the large myelinated nerve fibres inhibits pain impulses carried along the small unmyelinated fibres, or by alteration in the gate control mechanism in the spinal chord.

The electric current is produced by a small pulse generator, which can be carried by the patient and has controls for adjusting the electrical output, frequency and duration. This is connected to two cables attached to flexible electrodes that are strapped to the patient's skin over a painful area or over a peripheral nerve proximal to it. An electrode gel is first applied to the skin and the electrodes are then taped in place. The stimulator is switched on and the output control slowly adjusted until stimulation is felt. This is then adjusted so that the most comfortable sensation with the maximum pain relief is obtained. Pain relief may be obtained on the first application or only after several weeks. It may last only while the current is turned on or it may last for hours or days after the current is turned off.

Interferential therapy

This form of electrotherapy was introduced in 1959. The machine used is electrically operated and is small, light and easily portable. It uses a wide variety of low-frequency currents delivered into the deeper structures but without any sensory stimulation of the skin. The intensity of the combined current increases and decreases rhythmically so that in the area of the body where the currents mix a medium-frequency current is produced that changes in intensity as a low-frequency rhythmical beat. By adjusting these low-frequency rhythms, different structures are stimulated and varying therapeutic effects produced. Thus these rhythms may be used to produce analgesia, whereas at another frequency swelling and oedema may be assessed. Hence this form of therapy may be useful in treating pain and swelling arising as a result of various musculo-

skeletal conditions or as a precursor to more active therapy.

Manipulative therapy

Manipulative therapy is a passive-movement technique that can be classified into either joint manipulation or mobilization.

Manipulation is a sudden movement or thrust of small amplitude; it is performed at the end of the joint range at such a speed that the patient is unable to prevent it. In disorders of the peripheral joints, a joint is usually manipulated while the patient is anaesthetized. However, a similar type of movement can be produced in unanaesthetized patients. Without anaesthesia, the procedure may be modified using a steady, controlled movement to stretch a stiff joint in an attempt to increase the joint range.

Mobilization is defined as a passive-movement technique that is performed so that the movements are at all times within the control of the patient, who can prevent them if he wishes. They are performed mainly as oscillatory movements in either the physiological or accessory range of a joint and the joint surfaces may be held either distracted, compressed or midway between these two positions. Distraction is applied by pulling the bone ends apart at right angles to their joint surfaces. Compression is applied in the opposite direction so as to push the joint surfaces together. The oscillatory movements are usually used in one or two methods, either:

(1) as large- or small-amplitude movements, at a rate of two or three per second, and applied anywhere within the joint range; or
(2) combined with sustained stretching as small-amplitude oscillations applied at the limit of the joint range.

Method

The patient should be as relaxed and comfortable as possible. The therapist holds and stabilizes the joint to be moved in a firm grasp so that the joint movement can be appreciated. This requires the therapist to be comfortably positioned, so as to control the movement with a minimum of effort and ensure that no undue pain is produced. The joint to be mobilized is placed in a starting position that ensures relaxation of the joint and its surrounding muscles, usually in the mid-position of the joint. The proximal bone forming the joint surface is usually fixed and the distal bone is moved. The movements produced must be very gentle and the amount of treatment given in the first few sessions limited.

Grades of movement

Any part of a range of movement may be used in treatment, and widely varying amplitudes may be chosen. It is time consuming to refer to a treatment movement as a 'large-amplitude movement performed in the early part of the range' or as a 'small-amplitude movement performed firmly at the limit of the range'. To overcome this and make the recording of treatment quicker and simpler, a system of grading the movement is used. Grades I and IV are used to describe the treatment movements but, like all similar gradings (for example, rating of muscle power), the values overlap, and so there is also a place for plus and minus values. The grades of movement described below can be depicted by a straight line representing a full range of movement (*see Figure 4.1*).

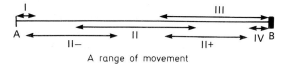

A range of movement

Figure 4.1 Grades of movement. A = Beginning of range of movement; B = end of normal, average range of movement

Grade I is a small-amplitude movement performed at the beginning of the range.

Grade II is a large-amplitude movement performed within the free range but not moving into any resistance or stiffness. If the movement is performed near the beginning of the range it is expressed as II −; if it is taken deeply into the

range but is still free of resistance it is expressed as II +.

Grade III is a large-amplitude movement performed up to the limit of the range. This movement can also be expressed with plus and minus values. If the movement knocks vigorously at the limit of the range it is expressed III + but if it nudges gently at the limit of the range it is expressed as III −.

Grade IV is a small-amplitude movement performed at the limit of the range. This too can be expressed as IV+ or IV− depending on the vigour with which it is used.

If a joint disorder limits the normal range of joint movement grades III and IV are restricted to smaller amplitudes (*see Figure 4.2*).

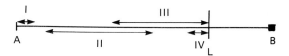

Figure 4.2 Restricted grades of movement. A = Beginning of range of movement; B = average anatomical limit; L = pathological limit of range

Similarly, pain may arise from a hypermobile joint that has become slightly stiff. This alters the positions of grade III and IV movements, as shown in *Figure 4.3*.

The oscillatory treatment movements may be smooth and regular or performed with an irregular rhythm. When the treatment movement is carried into the painful range and the patient finds it difficult to relax, the treatment movement must be regular; it should be performed a little slower than usual with an even rhythm. The patient will then realize exactly how his joint is to be moved and will find it easier to relax. Some patients have difficulty in relaxing completely even when pain is minimal and may periodically tense their muscles without realizing they do so. If large-amplitude treatment movements are hindered by this tension, movements of broken rhythm and changing amplitude should be employed in an attempt to trick the muscles. Some-

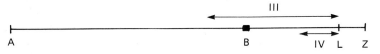

Figure 4.3 Grades of movement in a hypermobile joint. A = Beginning of range of movement; B = average anatomical limit; L = pathological limit of range; Z = limit of normal hypermobile range

times the movements need to be performed almost as a flick. A technique initially used in treatment is to move the joint in an exploratory manner to determine the response of the joint. In this way the treatment movement is continually modified to meet the changing circumstances. The movements used will vary in depth, gradually moving deeper or receding, according to what the therapist feels at different depths.

Many techniques are performed in positions similar to those used for the joint examination. The therapist tests many directions of movement during examination, each movement being performed only once or twice. This usually indicates the best position for treatment. In treatment the movement is repeated many times in only one direction, although the position may be altered after such a sequence.

Assessment of mobilization

A balance needs to be maintained between the firmness of the treatment, the amount of improvement produced in the patient's symptoms and any reaction suffered by the patient. This requires constant reassessment of symptoms and signs, which are checked after each treatment and again before the next treatment session. Symptoms should not be checked by asking the patient direct questions, but indirect questioning should be used to seek the spontaneous statements of the patient. The active and passive ranges of movements are retested to determine any increase in their range and whether pain is reproduced. Provided that joint range is improving, treatment may be continued but constant reassessment is still necessary. If there is no improvement, or if the patient's pain is aggravated, a different treatment technique should be selected.

Indications for manipulative therapy

(1) Replacement of a joint dislocation—for example, a dislocated shoulder—or a joint subluxation—for example, in a child with a pulled elbow.
(2) Reduction of an internal derangement of a joint; for example, in the knee, where a torn meniscus or loose body produces blocking of joint movements, and manipulation can re-

position the torn meniscus to allow normal movements.
(3) Stretching or breaking down adhesions. Joint stiffness may follow a sprained ligament and is then associated with pain and tenderness over the ligament. In capsulitis of the shoulder, mobilization and manipulation may be used to break down periarticular adhesions and increase joint mobility.
(4) Restoring the normal joint range in patients with painful and/or stiff joints in which there is an associated loss of the normal accessory movements that may also be associated with some degree of spasm in the surrounding muscles.

Choice of techniques

The choice of techniques depends on whether the patient suffers from joint stiffness, pain, spasm, or combinations of these.

Treatment of joint stiffness

A patient with joint stiffness alone may be treated by mobilization using either the physiological or accessory joint movements; in practice both of these movements are usually used. The physiological movements are used first and any of the normal movements for the particular joint may be employed. All normal joint movements are used if the degree of stiffness is marked. Alternatively only one of the reduced physiological movements may be used in treatment, and if so it is often found that as the range of this movement increases the range of all the other joint movements also increases.

Treatment is first performed using physiological movements at the limit of the available joint range with small-amplitude oscillatory movements for approximately 2 minutes. Then, while still holding the joint at the limit of the range, the accessory joint movements are also mobilized with small-amplitude movements. This cycle of treatment with physiological and then accessory movements may be repeated three or four times in a treatment session. If this technique causes any subsequent soreness in the joint it can be relieved by repeating the physiological movement and using a large-amplitude movement within the pain-free joint range.

Treatment of joint pain

A patient with joint pain alone, or joint pain and stiffness in which pain is the predominant symptom, is treated mainly by mobilization using accessory movements. When the pain is the dominant factor the joint being treated needs to be supported in a neutral position at first and accessory movements should be performed in the pain-free range. If pain or discomfort is provoked during the first treatment session treatment must continue in the pain-free range and smaller-amplitude movements must be used. As the condition improves, movements may be increased and taken into the painful range and the movements increased in amplitude. Provided that improvement is maintained, physiological movements can be introduced in the treatment technique, performed slowly through a large amplitude.

Treatment of painful and stiff joints

Most patients requiring treatment will have both painful and stiff joints. The painful component is best treated first, using the accessory joint movements with small-amplitude movements and with the joint positioned in a neutral and pain-free position. These movements are initially used in a range that does not provoke pain but their range may be increased as the patient's pain improves and ultimately they may be performed in the painful range also. The direction of the treatment movement is selected according to the type of accessory movement lost, as found on clinical examination.

Stiffness in the painful joint may also be treated with gentle grade IV movements applied at the limit of the range, so stretching the joint. If these are not successful manipulation of the joint under anaesthetic should be considered.

Treatment of muscular spasm

Patients with joint pain may be found to have a marked muscle spasm at the limit of the available range. This is best treated by moving the joint at the limit of the physiological range until spasm commences and using small-amplitude grade IV movements; this may also be combined with active relaxation techniques.

5 The shoulder

The glenohumeral joint is a ball-and-socket joint surrounded by a loose capsule, which inferiorly forms a wide pouch-like axillary recess. This arrangement allows the shoulder greater mobility than any other joint. The shoulder is also unique in that it has an accessory joint, the subacromial joint, formed between the humerus and a superior arch made up of the acromion process and the coracoid process of the scapula which are joined by the stout coracoacromial ligament (*see Figure 5.1*). This arch is lined by the synovial membrane of the subacromial bursa. In this space runs the rotator cuff, which comprises the tendinous insertions of the subscapularis, supraspinatus, infraspinatus and teres minor muscles (*see Figure 5.2*). These tendons blend intimately with the shoulder capsule, help to provide shoulder stability and are involved in most shoulder movements. They function in a relatively confined space where they are subject to trauma and attrition, and their movement is aided by the presence of the subacromial bursa.

Movement of the shoulder depends on a complex series of movements in the glenohumeral, clavicular and scapulothoracic joints (Lucas, 1973). All these joints are involved, for example, in abduction in which the arm is carried outwards in the coronal plane first to a right angle and is then raised to the side of the head through a range of 180 degrees. In this position the palm of the hand faces medially with the thumb facing posteriorly. This position of the hand is also the

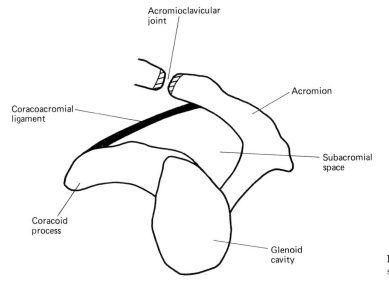

Acromioclavicular joint

Coracoacromial ligament

Acromion

Subacromial space

Coracoid process

Glenoid cavity

Figure 5.1 Components of the subacromial joint

31

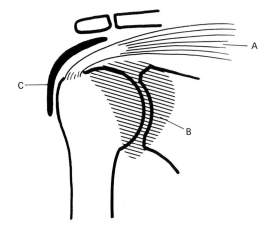

Figure 5.2 The supraspinatus muscle (A) runs through the subacromial space and its tendon, which is inserted into the greater tuberosity. The tendon blends with the capsule of the joint (B) and the subacromial bursa (C)

same as that reached on forward flexion of the arm.

The position of palm of the hand during abduction shows readily that the shoulder rotates laterally after approximately 90 degrees of abduction. This rotation is necessary to prevent impingement between the bony surfaces of the acromion and the greater tuberosity and it allows the tuberosity to slide under the more spacious posterior part of the subacromial arch. The joint capsule is both lax and voluminous to accommodate lateral rotation of the head of the humerus, which amounts to almost 180 degrees.

Concomitant movements in the scapulothoracic, acromioclavicular and sternoclavicular joints are necessary to achieve full elevation of the arm. This movement requires a smooth integration of all of these joints, which function simultaneously once movement is initiated. The scapula glides smoothly over the thoracic wall, which is made up of the ribs and intercostal muscles, and this scapulothoracic area may be looked on as a joint. The plane of the scapula runs obliquely in an anteroposterior and mediolateral direction to form an angle of 30 degrees with the frontal plane. The proportion of glenohumeral to scapulothoracic joint movement in attaining full elevation is of the order of two to one, but in the range of abduction from 0 to 30 degrees this ratio is five to four (Poppen and Walker, 1976). After 30 degrees, rotation of the scapula becomes more marked, and the scapulothoracic movement contributes approximately 60 degrees to full elevation of the arm in abduction. As the arm is abducted the scapula rotates so that its inferior angle moves laterally and the glenoid fossa now faces upwards.

Simultaneous movements take place in the clavicle, which acts as a strut to prevent the scapula moving medially. The clavicle is attached to the scapula through the acromioclavicular joint and also through two strong ligaments, the conoid and trapezoid, that bind the outer third of the clavicle to the coracoid process of the scapula. Thirty degrees of rotation about the long axis of the clavicle can occur in each of these two clavicular joints. So, as the arm is abducted, the clavicle rolls upwards and backwards and the clavicular joints are elevated. This clavicular movement takes place mainly after shoulder abduction has reached 90 degrees.

Codman (1934) first used the term scapulohumeral rhythm to describe the smooth transition between all of these movements. For ease of description, the component parts are usually taken separately, but in the normal shoulder with a full and painless range at each joint and normal musculotendinous co-ordination one observes a smooth integrated movement as the arm is moved. A disturbance of this normal rhythm may readily be observed in patients with lesions of these structures, which results in an altered or 'jerky' type scapulohumeral rhythm.

The rotator cuff

The rotator cuff is made up of four strap-like muscles: the subscapularis, supraspinatus, infraspinatus, and teres minor, which pass from the

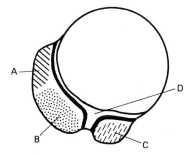

Figure 5.3 Upper end of humerus, showing insertion of: (A) infraspinatus tendon; (B) supraspinatus tendon into greater tuberosity; (C) subscapularis tendon into lesser tuberosity; and (D) bicipital groove

scapula to be inserted into the humerus (*see Figure 5.3*). The tendons converge so that they are connected together to form a cap (or cuff) over the shoulder joint, which is intimately blended with the lateral aspect of the capsule. One of its main functions is to produce rotation of the shoulder, and hence its more common name of rotator cuff.

The supraspinatus muscle plays only a minor role in rotation but has a greater role in shoulder abduction. It holds the head of the humerus in the glenoid cavity, thus allowing the deltoid to exert maximal pull and move the arm into abduction. This is achieved by pulling the greater tuberosity, to which it is attached, upwards and inwards under the acromial arch, so pulling the head of the humerus into the glenoid fossa and preventing any tendency for the humeral head to sublux upwards. Electromyography has shown that the supraspinatus and deltoid muscles act simultaneously as a functional unit and not singly, so that their resultant forces produce abduction.

An additional function of the rotator cuff is to stabilize the upper part of the shoulder joint, and degenerative changes with thinning or rupture of the cuff will allow the head of the humerus to sublux upwards. The cause of these degenerative changes may be related to the wear and tear that accompanies friction and attrition of the cuff tendons as they run in the subacromial space. During abduction of the arm the greater tuberosity and the supraspinatus tendon approximate the obstruction of the overhanging acromion and must slide laterally beneath it. The earliest changes involve a hyaline degeneration of the collagen fibres of the tendon, associated with alterations and disintegration of the cell nuclei.

Peculiarities in the microvascular supply also play a role (Lindblom, 1939) as there is an area of relative avascularity in the tendon just proximal to its insertion. Moseley and Goldie (1963) called this the 'critical zone' (*see Figure 5.4*) as it is the site at which degenerative changes, tendinitis, calcification and spontaneous rupture tend to occur. Rathbun and Macnab (1970) demonstrated that the vascular bed of the supraspinatus was markedly different from that of the other rotator-cuff tendons. At post-mortem they confirmed this area of relative avascularity, which was present even in people under the age of 20. They also showed that vascular compression occurred when the arm was held up by the side, so stretching the tendon over the head of the humerus, but when the arm was held in abduction the circulation was restored. They concluded that the 'critical zone' of reduced vascularity precedes and not follows degenerative changes in the supraspinatus tendon. As degenerative changes progress, the tendon becomes attenuated and the zone of relative avascularity extends. Also, in patients with complete spontaneous rupture of the tendon the tendon proximal to the rupture site was avascular and markedly degenerated.

Shoulder pain

Shoulder pain is a very common symptom. In part this may be because the glenohumeral joint normally enjoys considerable mobility and stability but degenerative changes commonly develop in its surrounding soft-tissue structures. Pain in this region may arise not only from intrinsic disorders of the glenohumeral joint but be referred from extrinsic causes outside the shoulder and arise either from the cervical spine or visceral structures. Patients with lesions of the cervical spine may present clinically either with neck pain alone, or neck and arm pain or else arm pain alone. These may produce shoulder pain either on the basis of a referred pain or else as the result of a compression neuropathy of the cervical nerve root in the intervertebral foramen. In the latter case, pain is usually felt down the arm and is associated with neurological symptoms such as paraesthesias or weakness. In patients who have a disorder of the cervical spine with pain referred to the shoulder, one of the following clinical settings may be found:

(1) The patient may present with pain in the

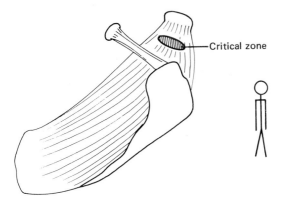

Critical zone

Figure 5.4 The supraspinatus tendon viewed from above, with arm by the side

neck radiating to the shoulder. This usually causes no great clinical confusion since neck movements reproduce the patient's pain whereas shoulder movements are normal and painless.

(2) The patient may have shoulder pain alone in the absence of any neck pain. Clinical examination should provide the necessary diagnostic clues, since neck movements will reproduce pain whereas shoulder movements do not. This finding is often associated with a hypomobility lesion at the C4–5 or C5–6 level and appropriate clinical testing of the movements of these joints reveals that they are restricted and painful. Treatment to the neck, especially mobilization techniques, should alleviate the shoulder symptoms.

(3) An uncommon and unexplained variation of this presentation is shoulder pain alone, when clinical testing of the shoulder reveals that shoulder movements do cause pain at the limits of range. Active neck movements are either normal or produce only a slight degree of pain or restriction of movement. Testing of the passive intervertebral movements of C4–5 or C5–6 produce pain and reveal a local restriction of movement of the intervertebral joint on the same side as the painful shoulder. In this group, treatment to the neck by traction and mobilization techniques for up to 3 consecutive days should relieve the patient's shoulder symptoms. If treatment has not produced any marked improvement within 3 days it should be abandoned and treatment confined to the shoulder.

Shoulder pain may also be the presenting symptom in visceral diseases and so is an important, though uncommon, cause of confusion. These visceral causes arise from intrathoracic or intra-abdominal diseases and it will be remembered that the phrenic nerve arises from the C3, 4, 5 nerve roots which also share in the innervation of the shoulder structures.

To differentiate between these disorders, associated symptoms such as cough, chest pain or abdominal symptoms should be enquired into and a full clinical examination, including X-ray, undertaken.

This chapter is concerned mainly with intrinsic disorders arising around the glenohumeral joint, and strictly orthopaedic disorders such as fractures, dislocation, tumours and infectious arthritis will not be considered. The majority of lesions to be discussed are soft-tissue lesions involving the musculotendinous structures and capsule surrounding the shoulder. It should also be remembered that although arthropathies may involve the shoulder as part of a generalized disease or may even commence in the shoulder, they are relatively uncommon and accounted for only 5 per cent of one large series (Graham, 1960).

The site of pain may also provide a clue to the source of the underlying lesion. For example, the patient with shoulder pain referred from the neck often clasps his opposite hand over the trapezius area. With pain referred from visceral structures the pain may be localized diffusely in the scapular region. In disorders of the acromioclavicular joint the patient usually places one finger over the upper part of this joint. Pain from intrinsic disorders of the glenohumeral joint may be felt deeply inside the joint, in which case the patient clasps his hand over the lateral aspect of the joint, or occasionally over the shoulder tip. However, in many patients with an intrinsic disorder of the glenohumeral joint the patient indicates that the site of pain is felt around the area of the deltoid insertion and it may be difficult to dissuade him that this is not really the source of pain. Pain felt in this region is referred and, typically with referred pain, the further the pain radiates distally the greater the degree of the underlying inflammation in the involved structure is likely to be. Hence pain may at times radiate down the outer side of the arm.

The patient usually describes pain arising from an intrinsic shoulder lesion as having a deep aching quality, made worse by shoulder movements. Night pain that disturbs the patient's sleep is commonly found with glenohumeral joint lesions and reflects the degree of the underlying inflammatory process. Hence it is a common symptom in patients who have capsulitis or arthritis, but it may also arise in patients with supraspinatus tendinitis when the patient rolls onto the affected shoulder.

The painful arc

This refers to pain which is felt in the middle range of abduction (*see Figure 5.5*). The patient experiences no pain with the arm by the side but as the shoulder is moved into abduction in the coronal plane the greater tuberosity approaches the acromion, and painful structures between these two bony prominences are impinged and

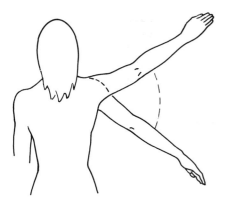

Figure 5.5 The painful arc on abduction

cause pain (*see Figure 5.6*). As the arm is raised further the painful tissues are accommodated beneath the coracoacromial ligament and pain ceases. The essential clinical feature, then, is a painless range of movement up to approximately 70 degrees of abduction, followed by an arc of pain to approximately 120 degrees, after which movement again becomes painless.

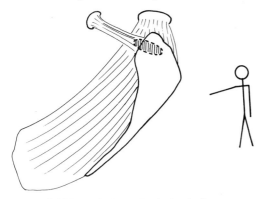

Figure 5.6 The critical zone impinging in the subacromial space on abduction

Pain may be felt on active or passive abduction, or as the arm is raised or lowered. It is also usually accompanied by a disturbance of scapulohumeral rhythm, and a jerky type of movement occurs during the painful arc. This is often best observed while the patient is lowering the arm to the neutral position; a sudden hitch in the movement is produced as the shoulder passes through the painful area. The patient may have learnt a trick movement in which the arm is carried forwards at this point from the coronal plane. Local anaesthetic injected into the tender area usually abolishes the source of the painful arc (Kessel and Watson, 1977).

Soft-tissue lesions include posterior structures such as the infraspinatus tendon; superior structures such as the supraspinatus tendon; and anterior structures such as the subscapularis tendon. Degenerative changes in the inferior aspect of the acromioclavicular joint or, rarely, lesions of the acromion and greater tuberosity may also cause a painful arc.

Examination of the shoulder

At times, considerable information may be obtained from the patient's ability to move the shoulder while undressing to bare the neck, arms, and scapular regions. The neck should first be examined to assess its range and whether movement reproduces shoulder pain. It is also important to examine the whole arm for evidence of any neurological or vascular abnormality. The hands should also be examined for any evidence of arthritis, swelling, vasomotor disturbances, skin diseases or Dupuytren's contracture.

Examination of the shoulder joint

(1) Inspection—observe:
    (a) The shape and contour of the shoulder.
    (b) Muscle wasting.
    (c) Swelling.
(2) Movements:
    (a) Active.
    (b) Passive.
    (c) Accessory.
    (d) Isometric.
    (e) Special tests.
(3) Palpation.

Inspection

The examiner should stand at first behind and then in front of the patient to compare the soft-tissue contours of the shoulder, and to observe any muscular wasting that may be evident over either the deltoid or the supraspinous or infraspinous fossae of the scapula. Synovial effusion, if present in small amounts, is usually difficult to detect, but a moderate degree of synovial fluid is usually seen to bulge anteriorly. A synovial swelling localized over the lateral aspect of the joint due to an effusion into the subacromial bursa is rare; more commonly there is a combined swelling involving the glenohumeral joint itself and the subacromial bursa around the shoulder.

Movements

Active

The patient stands with the arms by the side in neutral rotation so that the thumbs are placed anteriorly. The examiner should stand behind the patient and ask whether any pain or discomfort is experienced in this position and if so its site. Seven active movements are tested routinely: forward flexion, abduction, extension, lateral and medial rotation and combined movements.

FORWARD FLEXION
This is tested first. The patient is asked to move the arm forwards to a position of 180 degrees with the palm facing inwards. The examiner observes:

(1) The range of this movement.
(2) Whether the patient's pain is reproduced.
(3) Scapulohumeral rhythm.
(4) Whether the affected arm can be moved as quickly as the unaffected one or is now moved more slowly because of pain.
(5) Whether the patient needs to carry the arm into some degree of abduction to perform the movement.
(6) If this abnormal movement is produced the patient should repeat this movement but this time with the examiner applying gentle pressure with his hand placed over the lateral aspect of the patient's elbow so that the arm is now flexed forwards directly in the sagittal plane. The range of this movement may now be found to be restricted and reproduce the patient's pain.

ABDUCTION
The examiner stands behind the patient who is asked to raise the arm sideways to above the head. This combined glenohumeral and scapulothoracic movement should approach 180 degrees. During this movement the examiner should make six observations:

(1) The extent of this range.
(2) Whether pain is reproduced.

(3) The presence of an arc of pain.
(4) The scapulohumeral rhythm.
(5) Whether the patient needs to carry the arm into a degree of horizontal flexion so that the arm is abducted forwards of the frontal plane.
(6) If this abnormal movement is produced the patient should repeat the movement but this time the examiner applies gentle pressure with his hand placed anteriorly over the elbow so that the arm is now abducted directly in the coronal plane. By preventing horizontal flexion of the arm, the range of abduction may be found to be reduced and painful.

EXTENSION
The patient stands with the arm by the side and the elbow extended. He then carries the arm backwards into extension and the range is observed.

MEDIAL ROTATION
This is tested with the arm by the side and the elbow flexed to 90 degrees. The hand is then carried inwards towards the abdomen.

LATERAL ROTATION
This is tested with the arm by the side and the elbow flexed to 90 degrees. The hand is then carried outwards.

COMBINED MOVEMENTS
These are useful as a screening test and to measure the progress of several shoulder conditions. The patient is asked to place the hand behind the back and reach upwards as far as possible. This involves mainly medial rotation. The patient is then asked to abduct the shoulder, place the hand behind the neck and reach downwards as far as possible. This involves lateral rotation.

Passive movements

Five passive shoulder movements are tested: flexion, abduction, medial rotation, lateral rotation and horizontal flexion.

The first four movements are again tested by the examiner moving the patient's arm in the same direction as described above for active movements. Horizontal flexion is also tested by a movement in which the examiner places his hand over the posterior aspect of the patient's elbow joint and passively flexes the glenohumeral joint to ninety degrees. The patient's arm is then passively abducted across the chest so that his hand reaches towards the opposite shoulder (*see Figure 5.7*).

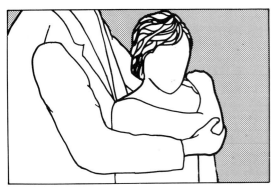

Figure 5.7 Passive horizontal flexion

While performing these passive movements, the following five findings are noted:

(1) The range of each movement.
(2) Whether pain is reproduced.
(3) The presence of an arc of pain.
(4) Over-pressure is applied at the limit of the normal range to assess:
   (a) Whether pain is now reproduced; and
   (b) the end-feel of movement, which is normally felt as a springing type sensation.
(5) Compression—the movements should also be tested while compressing the head and the humerus into the glenoid cavity.

Accessory movements

There are five accessory movements in the shoulder:

(1) Posteroanterior movement, which is produced by pressure on the posterior surface of the humeral head (*see Figure 5.8*).
(2) Anteroposterior movement, produced by the heel of the hand over the anterior surface of the humeral head (*see Figure 5.9*).
(3) Longitudinal caudad movement, produced by pressure over the head of the humerus (*see Figure 5.10*).
(4) Longitudinal cephalad movement, produced by compression upwards of the humerus (*see Figure 5.11*).
(5) Lateral movement, produced by movement

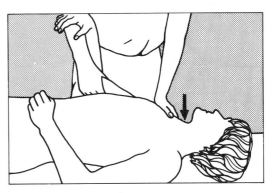

Figure 5.9 Anteroposterior accessory movement

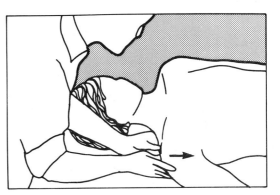

Figure 5.10 Longitudinal caudad accessory movement

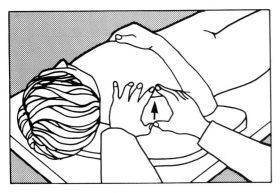

Figure 5.8 Posteroanterior accessory movement

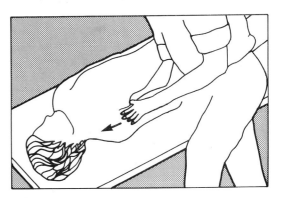

Figure 5.11 Longitudinal cephalad accessory movement

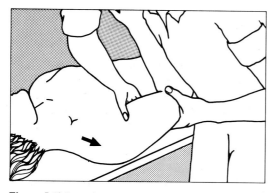

Figure 5.12 Lateral accessory movement

of the humeral head away from the glenoid cavity (*see Figure 5.12*).

It may also be necessary to test all of these accessory movements in other positions of the glenohumeral joint, e.g. 90 degrees of abduction or 90 degrees of flexion.

Isometric tests

Four isometric tests are assessed routinely: abduction, medial rotation, lateral rotation, and flexion. These tests apply an isometric contraction to the shoulder tendons. The examiner notes the strength of these movements and whether they reproduce the patient's pain; at the same time, he should also carefully palpate the tendon being tested with his other hand.

RESISTED ABDUCTION

This tests primarily the supraspinatus tendon.

Starting position—The patient sits with the glenohumeral joint abducted to 30 degrees and the elbow flexed to 90 degrees. The examiner stands behind the patient and places one hand on the lateral side of the elbow.

Method—The patient's attempt to move the arm outwards into abduction is fully resisted by the examiner, who simultaneously palpates the supraspinatus tendon over its insertion into the greater tuberosity.

RESISTED MEDIAL ROTATION

This tests primarily the subscapularis tendon.

Starting position—The patient stands with the upper arm by the side, the elbow flexed to 90 degrees and held firmly by the side with the palm of the hand facing inwards. The examiner stands in front of the patient and places the palm of his hand over the palmar surface of the patient's wrist.

Method—The patient is asked to attempt to move the forearm medially and this movement is fully resisted by the examiner while palpating the subscapularis tendon over its insertion into the lesser tuberosity.

RESISTED LATERAL ROTATION

This tests primarily the infraspinatus tendon. There are two methods of testing this movement:

(1) The patient stands with the arm by the side; the elbow is flexed to 90 degrees and held firmly against the side with the palm of the hand facing inwards. The examiner stands in front of the patient and places the palm of his hand over the dorsal surface of the patient's wrist. The patient is then asked to attempt to move the forearm outwards into the lateral rotation but this movement is fully resisted by the examiner.

(2) Alternatively, the patient stands with the shoulder abducted to 90 degrees and the elbow flexed to 90 degrees. The patient's shoulder is then fully medially rotated so that the palm of the hand faces backwards. The examiner then places the palm of his hand over the dorsal surface of the patient's wrist (*see Figure 5.13*). The patient attempts to bring the hand forwards, so laterally rotating the shoulder, but this movement is fully resisted by the examiner.

FORWARD FLEXION

This tests primarily the biceps tendon and is best performed by first placing the biceps tendon on the stretch (*see Figure 5.23*).

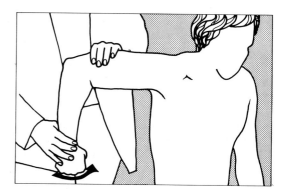

Figure 5.13 Resisted lateral rotation

Starting position—The patient stands with the shoulder fully extended; the elbow is also fully extended with the forearm pronated so that the hand faces backwards. The examiner places his hand over the dorsal aspect of the patient's wrist.

Method—The patient is asked to attempt to move the arm forwards but this movement is fully resisted by the examiner, who simultaneously palpates the biceps tendon in the bicipital groove.

Additional tests of the biceps muscle may be carried out at the elbow by making use of this muscle's action of flexing the elbow and supinating the forearm.

Patterns of movement

Clinical examination of the shoulder usually allows the anatomical site of the underlying lesion to be localized. By the use of active, passive and isometric tests, certain patterns of shoulder movements can be built up. Three distinct patterns can usually be differentiated. These are:

(1) Pain on active and passive movement, usually with restriction of shoulder movement in each plane, which may be of sudden or gradual onset. A sudden onset of severe shoulder pain and restriction of movement in each plane is usually caused by an acute calcific bursitis. A more gradual onset of shoulder pain and restriction of movement in each plane may be due to either a capsulitis or arthritis of the shoulder. Ancillary tests, including X-rays, should help to differentiate between these two conditions.

(2) Pain may be present on movement in only one of the planes tested, usually both on active and on passive movements. It may also be associated with a painful weakness or restriction on isometric testing of the movement. This pattern is produced by a tendon lesion.

(3) A painless weakness of movement in one plane only may be due to either a rupture of the musculotendinous insertion or else a neurological lesion, e.g. a painless weakness of shoulder abduction usually indicates a complete rupture of the supraspinatus tendon. Less commonly, it is due to a C5 nerve-root palsy with paralysis of the deltoid muscle.

Undiagnosed cases

By the systematic use of these clinical methods and ancillary tests, such as X-ray, an accurate diagnosis may be made in a vast majority of patients. There does remain, however, a small percentage of patients in whom definitive diagnosis cannot be readily made. This includes patients in whom signs are equivocal or difficult to detect. Usually a prolonged period of observation and repeated clinical retesting or arthrography is necessary to elucidate the cause of these problems. In addition, some patients may have shoulder pain without obvious clinical signs. In this group of patients, testing of two other positions of the glenohumeral joint, called the locking and the quadrant positions (Maitland, 1977), is often of value.

Locking and quadrant tests

Both these tests refer to the position of the greater tuberosity of the humerus in relation to the acromion and the posterior margin of the glenoid. In the locking position the greater tuberosity is caught within the subacromial space so that any further movement into lateral rotation, abduction or flexion is impossible. The shoulder joint is then locked and hence the title used for this position. The term quadrant position is derived from the fact that the arm can normally be circumducted through an arc of 360 degrees, which requires the greater tuberosity of the humerous to move so that it does not impinge on the acromion. The area being tested forms one quadrant of this total 360 degrees.

These movements are usually the first to be lost during the early stages of many shoulder conditions. A normal painless range of these movements must be present if the glenohumeral joint is to be considered normal. Their clinical significance is in patients with intermittent or minor degrees of shoulder pain in whom routine testing of shoulder movements does not reproduce their pain. Examination of these two positions may then reproduce the pain and demonstrate a small but significant loss of movement. Accordingly, the importance of these two tests lies in the fact that the movements may be found to be painfully restricted in many shoulder conditions, but they may at times be the only clinical abnormality found. Also, they may be used as the starting position for several of the passive-movement techniques used for treating the shoulder, as discussed later.

Locking position

STARTING POSITION
The patient lies supine and the examiner stands by the side with his forearm placed medial to the patient's scapula and the fingers extended over the patient's trapezius to prevent any shoulder shrugging. With his other hand he first flexes the patient's elbow and places the shoulder joint in a slight degree of medial rotation and extension.

METHODS
The arm is moved from alongside the patient's side into abduction and towards a position of full flexion. It is moved until the humerus reaches a position where it becomes locked and further movement is impossible (*see Figure 5.14*).

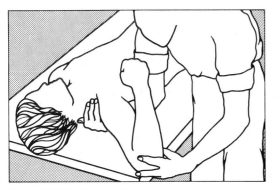

Figure 5.14 Locking position

SIGNIFICANCE
The normal shoulder can easily be placed in this locking position without pain. In some shoulder abnormalities the locking position may not be attainable, usually because of pain.

Quadrant position

This small arc of movement may be felt by the examiner as the arm is released from the locking position and is taken towards full flexion.

STARTING POSITION
The locking position is obtained, as described.

METHOD
The arm is carried towards full flexion by first relaxing the pressure on the abducted arm so that it can be moved anteriorly from the coronal plane.

Lateral rotation of the shoulder can then take place as the movement into abduction continues. The small arc of movement that can be felt during this anterior and rotational movement is known as the quadrant position. Thus the quadrant position is felt at approximately 30 degrees lateral to the fully flexed position when the arm moves anteriorly from the locked position. The humeral head is now unlocked and the arm can continue its normal movement into full flexion (*see Figure 5.15*).

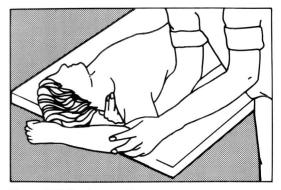

Figure 5.15 Quadrant position

The following observations are made in the quadrant position: the site and degree of pain with this movement, and then on applying over-pressure; the range of this movement in the sagittal plane between the humerus and the plane of the scapula; the degree of prominence of the head of the humerus in the axilla.

Palpation

Many of the bony landmarks and the soft-tissue structures around the shoulder that are involved clinically can be readily palpated. The spine of the scapula is subcutaneous and ends laterally in the broad, rectangular-shaped acromion process. This process articulates with the clavicle (which is subcutaneous) at the acromioclavicular joint, which can be palpated easily just lateral to the enlarged outer end of the clavicle. By palpating two finger-breadths medially and two finger-breadths caudally from this joint the bony outline of the coracoid process may be felt. The anterior part of the glenohumeral capsule lies just lateral to this process and overlies the joint line.

A finger-breadth distal to the lateral border of the acromion lies the greater tuberosity of the humerus to which is attached the tendinous insertions of the rotator cuff. Two finger-breadths medial to the anterior aspect of the greater tuberosity lies the tendon of the long head of the biceps in the bicipital groove and the tendon can be easily felt to move if the shoulder is abducted to 90 degrees and then rotated medially and laterally. Just medial to the biceps tendon lies the lesser tuberosity of the humerus and its attached subscapularis tendon.

Palpation is used to confirm the presence of any crepitus, heat, swelling, or tenderness.

Soft-tissue crepitus may be palpable in patients with degeneration of the rotator cuff and a bony crepitus in patients with osteoarthritis. Both shoulders should be palpated for comparison to determine the presence of any heat in the abnormal shoulder. The presence of synovial swelling may also be confirmed by palpation. Tenderness around the shoulder is sought but it must be remembered that this is used only as a confirmatory test of the presence of a soft-tissue lesion. The supraspinatus tendon insertion is palpated easily as the examiner stands behind the patient and places two fingers of one hand over the greater tuberosity (*see Figure 5.16*); with the other hand he passively rotates the patient's arm medially and laterally, while also applying a distraction force downwards. The normal tendon insertion can be felt to move as a firm cord. This area should be palpated carefully for an area of tenderness and at times a gap may be felt if the tendon has been ruptured.

The infraspinatus tendon is best palpated while the patient's arm is held with the glenohumeral joint at 90 degrees of forward flexion and the elbow also flexed to 90 degrees. Two fingers of the examiner's hand are then placed over the posterior aspect of the joint just below the acromion process and behind the posterior border of the deltoid. The arm is then passively rotated medially and laterally while the examiner palpates deeply over the humeral head for any tenderness (*see Figure 5.21*).

The tendinous insertion of the subscapularis is palpated over the lesser tuberosity just medial to the tendon of the long head of the biceps. The patient's arm should be held in about 20 degrees of extension. The long head of the biceps is easily palpated in its bicipital groove. The patient's glenohumeral joint is firstly abducted to 90 degrees with the elbow held flexed also at 90 degrees. The examiner places two fingers of his other hand over the bicipital groove while the patient's arm is medially and laterally rotated and palpates for the presence of any tenderness (*see Figure 5.24*).

Classification of shoulder lesions

(1) Tendon lesions, involving either:
  (a) rotator-cuff tendons—tendinitis, incomplete rupture, complete rupture, and calcification; or
  (b) the biceps tendon—tendinitis, tenosynovitis, subluxation, and rupture.
(2) Bursitis:
  (a) Subacromial bursitis—chronic or acute calcific bursitis.
  (b) Subcoracoid bursitis.
(3) Capsulitis.
(4) Instability of the shoulder joint.
(5) The shoulder–hand syndrome.
(6) Entrapment neuropathies.

Lesions of the supraspinatus tendon

These are the most common cause of shoulder pain. The basic lesion is degeneration in the supraspinatus tendon, the causes of which have been discussed above, which may remain asymptomatic for a considerable length of time. Clinically, however, symptoms may arise due to:

(1) Supraspinatus tendinitis.
(2) Subacromial bursitis.
(3) Incomplete rupture of the tendon.
(4) Complete rupture of the tendon.
(5) Calcification.

Supraspinatus tendinitis

This condition usually follows overuse or trauma involving a degenerated supraspinatus tendon. The patient complains of pain, usually over the outer aspect of the shoulder but which may radiate down the arm to the region of the deltoid insertion or may be felt in this site only when severe pain radiates down to the elbow and is then very likely to disturb the patient's sleep. The natural history of this condition is often one of exacerbations and remissions over several years.

MAJOR SIGNS
Pain is reproduced on active and/or passive abduc-

tion of the shoulder. It is usually felt as an arc of pain in the mid-range of this movement, between approximately 60 and 120 degrees, as the tendon is compressed between the tuberosity of the humerus and the acromion. When the patient brings the arm down from full abduction to the side, pain is again usually felt in this range of the arc due to the same mechanism. At this point a characteristic sign may be present in which the patient suddenly allows his shoulder to drop past this painful spot.

Pain may also be reproduced on isometric contraction of the supraspinatus, which is tested by having the examiner fully resist the patient's attempt to abduct the shoulder.

CONFIRMATORY SIGNS

There may be a disturbance of scapulohumeral rhythm during abduction. The supraspinatus tendon may be palpated easily as a tender cord between the examiner's finger and the patient's greater tuberosity while the shoulder is depressed by applying traction to the arm and then laterally and medially rotating the humerus (*see Figure 5.16*).

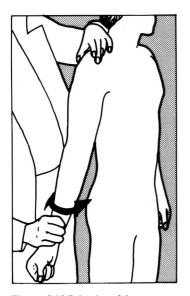

Figure 5.16 Palpation of the supraspinatus tendon

X-ray of the shoulder is usually normal, but degenerative changes in the tendon may lead to an area of sclerosis, roughening and sometimes pitting on the greater tuberosity.

MANAGEMENT

(1) Rest from movements known to aggravate the pain is usually required. Activities with the shoulder in a position of either abduction or abduction and external rotation, such as serving at tennis or swimming, often provoke or prolong the patient's pain.

(2) Non-steroidal anti-inflammatory drugs are used to control the inflammatory component and provide relief of pain.

(3) Local infiltration of corticosteroids around the tendon may be expected to control the inflammatory component (Richardson, 1975), even though they have no effect on the underlying degenerative changes. For the starting position the patient sits with the arm hanging loosely by the side and the shoulder in full lateral rotation and a slight degree of abduction. The tendon can be palpated a finger breadth lateral to the acromion and towards the anterior surface of the tuberosity by passively rotating the arm medially and laterally. A 23-gauge needle is used and is inserted under the lateral surface of the acromion along the line of supraspinatus tendon. If the needle strikes the humerus it should be withdrawn slightly and then angled upwards so that it lies between the tendon and the acromion. 1 ml of corticosteroid solution with 2–3 ml of local anaesthetic are injected. The injection may be repeated several times at intervals of 1–4 weeks, depending upon the degree of improvement.

(4) Physical therapy, ice or ultrasound applied directly over the site of local tenderness can produce an improvement in symptoms. Exercises into the painful range of movements are contraindicated.

(5) For manipulative therapy three passive-movement techniques may be used. The first involves accessory movements of the head of the humerus, especially posteroanterior movement (*see Figure 5.8*). It is essential to position the patient's arm first in a pain-free neutral position, and the movement should also be pain free. Its effectiveness is assessed by comparing the behaviour of the patient's pain during shoulder movement before and after mobilization. The second accessory-movement technique is a movement of the head of the humerus away from and then towards the under-surface of the acromion process (*see Figure 5.12*). This procedure should also be painless. If accessory movements do not produce sufficient improvement the quadrant position should be used; the technique is performed as very small range movements carried into some degree of discomfort

for 1 minute. While it is being performed, any increase of pain should be reported and any changes in shoulder flexion and abduction are assessed at the completion of treatment.

(6) With conservative therapy, symptoms gradually improve. However, tendinitis may subsequently recur when the patient returns to activity. In the small percentage of patients with chronic disability or frequent recurrences, various surgical procedures have been advocated. Their main aim is to increase the subacromial space and prevent impingement of the tendon. Operations include removal of the anterior acromion (Neer, 1972) and division of the coracoacromial ligament. Excision arthroplasty of the acromio-clavicular joint may be necessary if there is coincidental osteoarthritis of that joint.

Chronic subacromial bursitis

The subacromial bursa is a serous sac that is intimately connected with the rotator cuff. The supraspinatus tendon forms the major part of its floor and the tendon and bursa work together as a functional unit in the subacromial space. Hence the chronic form of subacromial bursitis is usually found to occur in association with an underlying supraspinatus tendinitis.

Incomplete rupture of the supraspinatus tendon

The supraspinatus tendon runs through the subacromial space where it may be subjected to degenerative changes and ultimately becomes roughened and frayed. The degenerated tendon is then easily torn, causing a partial rupture either on its superior or inferior aspect. This tends to occur in one or two age groups: it is much more common in the elderly but it may also occur in younger people who consistently overuse their shoulder, such as labourers or sportsmen.

The clinical findings are usually indistinguishable from those previously described in supraspinatus tendinitis, as the same symptoms and signs are common to both. Arthrography of the shoulder is indicated if a precise diagnosis is necessary and may demonstrate the presence of an incomplete rupture involving the inferior surface of the tendon.

MANAGEMENT
This is also similar to that of supraspinatus tendinitis. Local corticosteroid injections are also

helpful in relieving pain, although they may not alter the physical signs (Darlington and Coomes, 1977). Surgery is not indicated in the elderly to repair the tendon; but in younger patients it should be considered as the tear is apt to produce chronic disability. Primary suture is usually possible if necessary after excision of any degenerative areas of tendon (Post, 1978).

Complete rupture

A complete rupture may occur in elderly patients with long-standing degenerative changes in the tendon who often have a previous history of recurrent attacks of supraspinatus tendinitis. The onset may be spontaneous or follow a sudden movement or injury. However, in athletes there may be no such previous history. The site of the rupture is usually through the 'critical zone' of the tendon (*see Figure 5.4*) although occasionally the tendon may be avulsed from its insertion into the greater tuberosity. The patient may be conscious of having heard or felt a sudden painful 'snap' in the shoulder. Pain remains for some time afterwards and usually eases gradually. The patient is usually conscious of a loss of strength and mobility in the shoulder (Samilson and Binder, 1977).

MAJOR SIGNS
This lesion is diagnosed by finding a marked disparity between the active, passive and isometric tests.

There is loss of active range of shoulder abduction, so that the shoulder can be abducted to only

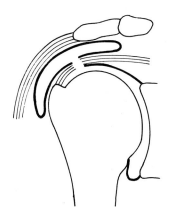

Figure 5.17 Complete rupture of the supraspinatus tendon allows a communication between the synovial cavities of the glenohumeral joint and the subacromial bursa

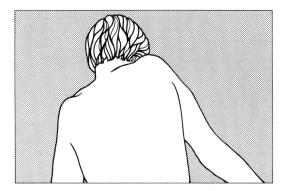

Figure 5.18 Complete rupture of the supraspinatus tendon
—active movement

approximately 20 degrees. This movement is also accompanied by a considerable degree of scapular movement with an upward shrugging of the shoulder (*see Figure 5.18*). This movement was thought to be produced by the action of the deltoid, which, since it was acting without the stabilizing effect of the supraspinatus tendon, resulted in elevation of the shoulder. However, this movement may be due to the action of the serratus anterior muscle, which rotates the scapula and produces an abduction movement of 20 degrees at the glenohumeral joint.

On testing the passive movements the shoulder can be fully passively abducted by the examiner (*see Figure 5.19*).

On testing isometric shoulder movements a marked painless weakness of abduction is found.

CONFIRMATORY SIGNS
A gap in the tendon may be felt by palpation of the shoulder area between the acromion and the greater tuberosity. After some time atrophy of the supraspinatus muscle can be observed as a hollowing in the supraspinous fossa.

VARIATIONS
A complete rupture may present with other clinical features. Pain may be the dominant feature and be prolonged (Samilson and Binder, 1977). Also, the clinical findings described above, with a marked difference between the active and passive shoulder movements, may not be so clear cut. In some patients a greater range of active abduction is possible; in others a block to full passive abduction of the shoulder is present, presumably due to a rolled-up portion of the ruptured tendon interfering with the mechanics of this movement.

X-RAYS
Plain X-rays of the shoulder will usually be normal unless the tendon has been avulsed with a small fragment of bone. Arthrography demonstrates the rupture, which allows a communication between the glenohumeral joint and the subacromial bursa.

MANAGEMENT
In the elderly, pain usually settles with conservative treatment and, although the physical signs do not alter, the resultant functional disability may not be sufficient to warrant surgery. In younger patients, surgery is indicated and primary suture of the rupture attempted. If this is not possible the supraspinatus muscle should be detached from its scapular fossa and relocated more laterally. This allows the tendon to be repaired by suturing its proximal divided end to the greater tuberosity of the humerus (Debyre, Patte and Elmelik, 1965). Partial acromionectomy may also be necessary (Neer, 1972).

LATE COMPLICATIONS OF COMPLETE TENDON RUPTURE
The supraspinatus is responsible for the superior stabilization of the glenohumeral joint and when its integrity is lost the humeral head can sublux upwards. The greater tuberosity of the humerus becomes attenuated as it loses the traction from the supraspinatus tendon. In time, degenerative changes may be found in the glenohumeral joint itself and there is erosion and a thinning out of the lower surface of the acromion with osteophyte formation. Degenerative changes may also develop in the acromioclavicular joint.

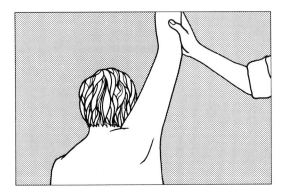

Figure 5.19 Complete rupture of the supraspinatus tendon
—passive movement

Calcification

Calcification in the supraspinatus tendon is present in approximately 8 per cent of routine shoulder X-rays (*see Figure 5.20*). It develops in the area of degenerated tendon just proximal to the tendon insertion. The calcific deposits are usually firm and granular in texture, single or multiple, about 10 mm in size, but may at times have a linear appearance spreading along the tendon. If found in one shoulder there is a 25 per cent chance that it is also present in the other shoulder (Welfling, 1969). Similar calcific deposits may also be found in the trochanteric bursa or gluteal medius tendon on X-ray of the hip.

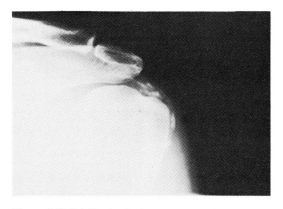

Figure 5.20 Calcification in the supraspinatus tendon and subacromial bursa

Calcification may:

(1) Be asymptomatic and a chance finding only on X-ray.
(2) Be associated with supraspinatus tendinitis. The signs and symptoms of this calcific tendinitis are identical with those of uncomplicated tendinitis, as described above.
(3) Be of a sufficient size to produce a mechanical block to full shoulder abduction, as the calcified mass catches beneath the acromion.
(4) Produce an acute calcific bursitis. This is one of the most painful and dramatic events in clinical practice. It is a relatively common condition and may occur in the younger, more active age group. It appears to follow an acute calcific tendinitis with rupture of microcrystals of calcium hydroxyapatite into the subacromial bursa, producing an acute inflammatory synovitis. There is no adequate explanation for this sudden rupture, as the

calcific deposits may have been present in the tendon for some years.

Patients present with an intense pain in the shoulder, often radiating down the upper arm, which usually starts suddenly and rapidly becomes worse. Pain is made worse by any shoulder movement and disturbs sleep. Patients are unable to use their arm and clinical examination reveals that this is due to a painful limitation of shoulder movements in all directions, and the arm usually needs to be supported in a sling. Indeed, it is usually impossible to attempt to examine these movements properly but some swelling may be obvious over the lateral aspect of the joint, which is exquisitely tender and warm on palpation.

X-rays will confirm the presence of the calcific deposits, which may still be present as a granular deposit but are more commonly seen as a hazy, poorly defined appearance within the bursa. The size of the calcific deposit on X-ray does not usually bear any direct relationship with the acuteness or severity of the attack and at times only small deposits are visible. Enlargement of the soft-tissue shadow of the subacromial bursa and a displacement downwards of the humeral head may also be evident. An X-ray taken after the condition has resolved often shows that the calcific deposit has disappeared. If so it may reaccumulate over several years so that another acute attack may occur.

MANAGEMENT

The patient presents with a sudden onset of intense pain made worse by movement of the shoulder in any direction. Hence rest to the shoulder is essential and may be provided by the use of a sling, which needs to be worn constantly for several days. This does not produce subsequent stiffness of the shoulder.

Anti-inflammatory drugs must be given in a relatively high dosage to control the intense crystal synovitis. Phenylbutazone or indomethacin is used in a dose of eight tablets per day for 2 or 3 days until the intense pain begins to settle and should then be continued in a dosage of three or four tablets a day until pain is controlled. Analgesics are also usually needed to control pain and ensure sleep.

The following injections may be used:

(1) Local anaesthetic and corticosteroid may be injected directly into the subacromial bursa. The technique will be described later. Although this may be painful at the time, the

patient is usually grateful for the relief obtained.

(2) Two wide-bore 19-gauge needles may be inserted into the calcific mass. A lateral approach is used, after first anaesthetizing the skin. An injection of 10 ml of local anaesthetic is given rapidly into one of the needles. The calcific deposit, which resembles gritty tooth-paste, may be extruded through the other needle; even if this does not happen the patient often experiences some degree of relief, possibly due to dispersion of the calcific deposit.

Heat, exercises or massage are contraindicated, but ice applied locally to the shoulder region may provide pain relief.

With conservative treatment most cases resolve over a period of 4 or 5 days. A subsequent X-ray usually shows that the calcific deposit has disappeared. Surgery may be indicated if the acute bursitis does not resolve as rapidly as indicated above or if it fails to resolve completely. The calcific mass is evacuated by curettage. At operation, an inflamed bursa is found with a granular deposit of calcific material bulging into it.

Infraspinatus tendinitis

This is not as common as supraspinatus tendinitis and is associated with underlying degenerative changes involving the infraspinatus tendon and pain, usually after overuse of the shoulder. Infraspinatus tendinitis occurs most commonly in labourers or in patients involved in sports such as swimming or tennis. The site of the lesion may be either over the insertion of the tendon into the posterior aspect of the greater tuberosity or at its musculotendinous junction. The patient usually presents with pain over the posterior aspect of the shoulder, which is made worse by most shoulder movements and when severe may radiate down the posterior aspect of the upper arm.

Major signs

The patient's pain may be reproduced by either contracting or stretching the infraspinatus tendon.

Isometric contractions of the tendon are tested by the examiner fully resisting lateral rotation of the shoulder; a painful weakness of this movement may be demonstrated.

The tendon is stretched by first placing the glenohumeral joint in 90 degrees of abduction with the elbow flexed at 90 degrees and the forearm pronated so that the palm of the hand faces the floor. By moving the forearm downwards towards the floor, the infraspinatus tendon is stretched and pain may be reproduced. In this last position the patient attempts to move the forearm back to its original position, thus laterally rotating the shoulder. If this movement is fully resisted by the examiner by placing one hand over the dorsal aspect of the patient's wrist, pain may then be reproduced (*see Figure 5.13*).

Confirmatory signs

The patient may feel an arc of pain in the middle range of abduction as the tendon catches under the acromion. Also, the infraspinatus tendon may be palpated by placing the shoulder at 90 degrees of forward flexion with the elbow also at 90 degrees of flexion and rotating the arm medially and laterally (*see Figure 5.21*). Tenderness may be felt either at the tendon insertion or at the musculotendinous junction. In patients with a lesion at the musculotendinous junction, a tender area of thickening or swelling may be palable at this site.

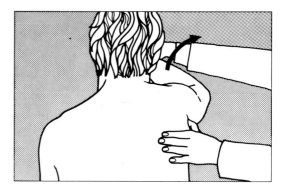

Figure 5.21 Palpating the infraspinatus tendon. The shoulder is in medial rotation

Management

This is similar to that outlined for supraspinatus tendinitis and includes local injections.

Injection of the infraspinatus tendon

The patient sits with the arm held across the lower chest. This brings the posterior portion of the greater tuberosity into prominence and stretches the tendon. The insertion may then be palpated deep to the deltoid about a finger-breadth lateral to the posterolateral border of the acromion. A 23-gauge needle should be used and is directed under the lateral surface of the acromion, and the area around the tendon is injected with 1 ml of corticosteroid solution and 2–3 ml of local anaesthetic.

Complications of infraspinatus tendinitis

The complications are similar to those described above for supraspinatus tendinitis: a partial rupture or a complete rupture of the infraspinatus tendon.

Complete rupture of this tendon usually occurs suddenly and the patient complains of pain over the posterior aspect of the shoulder. The clinical findings reveal a marked disparity between active, passive and resisted movements. The normal range of active lateral rotation of the shoulder is lost but the passive range remains full. Testing the resisted movement by isometric contraction reveals a painless weakness of lateral rotation. After a time, wasting of this muscle in the infraspinous fossa of the scapula becomes evident.

Bicipital tendinitis

The biceps tendon is the second most common cause of shoulder tendinitis and the usual site of involvement is in the bicipital groove (*see Figure 5.22*). Here, the tendon takes part in all shoulder movements, and as the groove slides along the tendon it is subjected to the same type of degenerative processes of wear and tear and attrition which involve the rotator cuff. The tendon may also be impinged against the acromial arch during many of the functional patterns of

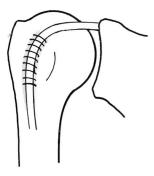

Figure 5.22 The long head of the biceps running in the bicipital groove

shoulder movement. Tendinitis usually occurs in a degenerated tendon after overuse or trauma to the shoulder. It may also be associated with a tenosynovitis of the synovial sheath that invests the biceps tendon, which will produce the same symptoms and signs as tendinitis.

The patient presents with pain in the shoulder, which is usually well localized anteriorly over the joint but may radiate down the anterior aspect of the upper arm. It is usually chronic and recurrent. Pain may be produced on shoulder movement but especially when the arm is abducted with the shoulder laterally rotated as in the action of throwing a ball or in overarm swimming.

Major signs

The patient's pain may be reproduced by stretching or contracting the biceps tendon. Stretching the tendon is usually best achieved by having the patient stand with the elbow extended and the forearm pronated so that the hand faces backwards and the examiner fully passively extends the shoulder. Pain may then be reproduced by this manoeuvre; if it is not the patient should remain standing with the shoulder in this extended position and the examiner should place one hand over the dorsum of the patient's wrist and actively resist the patient's attempt to move the arm into forward flexion. Simultaneously the examiner should palpate over the bicipital groove with his

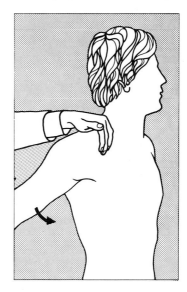

Figure 5.23 Palpation of the biceps tendon. The shoulder is extended and the examiner simultaneously resists forward flexion of the shoulder

other hand (*see Figure 5.23*); pain and tenderness, well localized over the bicipital groove, is then usually reproduced.

Confirmatory signs

Two other tests using isometric contraction of the biceps may be used but do not consistently reproduce pain. They rely on the action of the biceps, which flexes the elbow and supinates the forearm. In the first, the examiner resists active flexion of the elbow while the patient stands with the elbow at 90 degrees and the forearm supinated. In the second, the patient stands with the elbow flexed to 90 degrees and the forearm in the midposition while the examiner resists active supination of the forearm (Yergason's sign).

The tendon may also be stretched by first abducting the arm to 60 degrees with the elbow flexed at a right angle and then passively rotating the shoulder laterally. Pain may be reproduced at the extreme of this movement.

Finally, the biceps tendon can be palpated in most patients unless they are obese or have an hypertrophied deltoid muscle. This is best tested

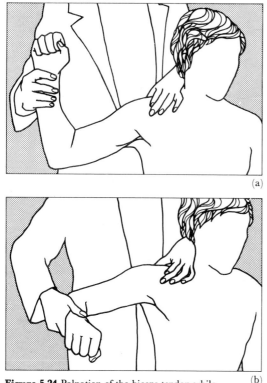

(a)

(b)

Figure 5.24 Palpation of the biceps tendon while rotating the shoulder

with the patient's arm abducted to approximately 90 degrees and the elbow flexed to 90 degrees (*see Figure 5.24(a)*). The shoulder is then medially and laterally rotated by the examiner using one hand while palpating the biceps tendon with the fingers of his other hand (*see Figure 5.24(b)*). The tendon may be felt to roll under the examiner's fingers as a tender cord-like structure in the bicipital groove. X-rays of the shoulder are usually normal, but an oblique radiograph projection taken along the bicipital groove may show evidence of a bony abnormality such as roughening of the groove.

Management

The general management of a patient with bicipital tendinitis is basically similar to that of supraspinatus tendinitis and includes the use of rest, anti-inflammatories and ice.

Injections

The site of maximal tenderness should be found (*see Figure 5.24*) and the patient then sits with the arm hanging loosely by the side and the palm facing forwards. The examiner stands behind the patient and again locates the tender area in the bicipital groove. A 23-gauge needle is inserted at the proximal end of the bicipital groove above the tender area and is then slid down the groove until the tender area is reached. 1 ml of corticosteroid solution and 2 ml of local anaesthetic are injected around this site.

Surgery

If the symptoms persist or are recurrent the tendon may be divided and its distal end transplanted either to the short head of the biceps or to the coracoid process. This procedure gives good results (de Palma, 1957).

Rupture of the biceps tendon

Rupture of the long head of the biceps tendon in its groove is not uncommon. It usually occurs in male patients, middle aged or older, who may have a history of bicipital tendinitis. The rupture may occur spontaneously or the patient may have been lifting or may have fallen on the outstretched hand. The patient is usually conscious of a sudden tearing or snapping sensation in the shoulder. The shoulder may be painful or difficult to move and bruising may appear over the upper arm after some days. Pain usually settles over a short period of time; there is little functional disability since the short head of the biceps remains intact so only rarely does the patient complain of any significant degree of weakness. The distal belly of the biceps muscle rolls up and the patient may notice it as a lump in the anterior part of the upper arm.

Major signs

The rolled-up belly of the muscle may be seen to bulge when the muscle is made to contract, as by bringing the hand up to the mouth or by resisting flexion of the elbow (*see Figure 5.25*). The gap in the tendon is easily seen and felt by palpation over the bicipital groove.

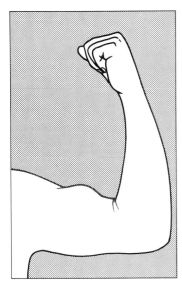

Figure 5.25 Ruptured long head of biceps

Management

This injury usually occurs in patients aged over 40, and since little functional incapacity is caused active treatment is not indicated.

Subluxation of the biceps tendon

The long head of the biceps tendon lies in the bicipital groove, roofed over by the strong transverse humeral ligament, which maintains the tendon in position and prevents it bowstringing on contraction. The transverse ligament may be ruptured after an injury in which the shoulder is suddenly forcibly extended while it is abducted (O'Donoghue, 1973a) and commonly occurs in a rugby football tackle. The ligament fibres may also rupture after a sudden, forceful, active contraction of the biceps while the arm is simultaneously abducted and laterally rotated, such as in bending over and lifting a heavy weight from the ground. Anatomical factors, such as a shallow bicipital groove, may also contribute.

When the transverse ligament is ruptured the biceps is free to sublux out of its groove. The movement that most commonly produces this sudden subluxation is when the shoulder is abducted and laterally rotated and the elbow flexed, as in serving at tennis (*see Figure 5.26*). The patient feels a sudden severe painful click over the front of the shoulder and is virtually unable to use his arm for a short period of time afterwards.

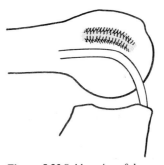

Figure 5.26 Subluxation of the biceps tendon

Major signs

The patient's symptoms should be reproduced by the examiner holding the arm in about 90 degrees of abduction with the elbow flexed. The tendon can usually be felt to slip in and out of its groove while the arm is rotated laterally and medially and the bicipital groove is palpated.

X-rays of the shoulder are normal but a view taken along the bicipital groove may demonstrate abnormal shallowness.

Management

In most patients with this condition, pain and disability are such that surgery is indicated. The operative procedure used depends on the extent of any degenerative changes in the biceps tendon. Since most patients are relatively young, degenerative changes may be absent or minimal. If so the tendon is positioned in its groove and the transverse ligament reconstituted with deep fascia. If the tendon is degenerated it may be divided and repositioned by suturing it to the short head of the biceps.

Subscapularis tendinitis

This condition is not uncommon. The patient presents with pain in the front of the shoulder, usually after an overuse type injury that involves excessive internal rotation of the shoulder.

Major signs

Pain should be reproduced on isometric contraction of the subscapularis muscle if the examiner fully resists medial rotation of the patient's arm. A painful arc may be present, especially on abduction and lateral rotation.

Confirmatory signs

On palpation, tenderness is found in a localized area medial to the lesser tuberosity of the humerus. Routine X-rays are usually normal and calcification if present may only be evident on an axial view. Management is as outlined for patients with supraspinatus tendinitis. These patients usually respond readily to local corticosteroid injections.

Bursitis

Subacromial bursitis

A diagnosis of subacromial bursitis is commonly made but it is rarely found as a primary disorder and is secondary to lesions in the rotator cuff. It was previously considered that chronic bursitis with adhesion formation caused capsulitis of the shoulder but this has not been supported by subsequent studies.

Major signs

The patient experiences a painful arc in the midrange of active and passive shoulder abduction. However, resisted abduction of the shoulder should not reproduce the patient's pain, which should distinguish it from supraspinatus tendinitis.

Management

Chronic subacromial bursitis is usually associated with supraspinatus tendinitis and its management is similar. Injection into the subacromial bursa is easy to perform. The patient sits on a chair with the arm hanging loosely by his side. A posterior approach is used and the posterolateral angle of the acromion is identified by palpation.

A 23-gauge needle is slid under the posterolateral angle of the acromion in an anterior direction so that it lies free in the subacromial space. 1 ml of local corticosteroid and 3 ml of 1% local anaesthetic can be injected easily without encountering any resistance.

Subcoracoid bursitis

This rare condition may follow overuse associated with repeated shoulder rotation and may occur in table-tennis players or people driving heavy trucks. Pain is usually well localized over the anterior aspect of the shoulder, just distal to the coracoid process of the scapula.

The patient's pain may be reproduced by two passive shoulder movements. One involves lateral rotation of the shoulder, when pain is felt at the extreme of the movement. The other occurs on passive horizontal flexion of the arm across the patient's chest. Resisted movements are usually painless. Palpation usually reveals an area of tenderness well localized to just below the tip of the coracoid process; injection of corticosteroid into this area usually produces marked relief of symptoms.

Capsulitis

Capsulitis is an inflammatory lesion of the glenohumeral joint capsule that leads to thickening and contraction with consequent loss of joint volume. Clinically it results in a painful stiffness of the active and passive range of all the shoulder movements. X-rays are essentially normal but may show at times a disuse osteoporosis or small cystic inclusions along the line of the capsule insertion into the humeral head. X-rays are, however, necessary to differentiate this condition from arthritis of the shoulder joint, which may have similar clinical findings.

The pathology of capsulitis was demonstrated by Welfling (1969). The shoulder capsule was thickened and retracted so that glenohumeral

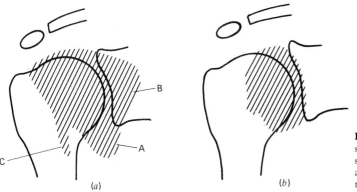

Figure 5.27 Outlines of arthrograms: (*a*) showing (A) the axillary recess, (B) the subscapularis recess, and (C) extension around the biceps tendon; (*b*) in capsulitis of the shoulder

movement was markedly restricted. The joint surfaces and surrounding tissue such as the subacromial bursa and tendons were all normal. These findings can be confirmed by arthrography, which demonstrates contracture of the joint capsule with loss of joint volume. In these cases only 5–10 ml of contrast medium can be injected instead of the usual 20–30 ml and more pressure is needed to effect the injection. The arthrogram demonstrates a marked reduction in joint volume together with a loss of the normal capsular recesses such as the axillary recess (*see Figure 5.27*).

It occurs most commonly in middle-aged females and its aetiology is unknown. No theory has been evinced for its relative frequency in the shoulder joint, whereas it is quite rare in other joints. Degenerative changes in the joint capsule or surrounding structures have been suggested (Bateman, 1972) but since it is not associated with an increased incidence after middle age such an explanation seems most unlikely. Also, contrary to most standard teaching, capsulitis almost never arises as a complication of existing intrinsic shoulder lesions such as supraspinatus or bicipital tendinitis and is quite a different condition to either of them. Previous theories have also ascribed capsulitis to the presence of adhesion between the layers of the subacromial bursa, across the biceps tendon or between the joint surfaces but these were never found by Welfling (1969). It is considered to be a primary condition affecting the capsule but it may follow conditions that result in prolonged immobilization such as trauma to the arm, neurological lesions such as hemiplegia, herpes zoster or Parkinson's disease and myocardial infarction or other intrathoracic disease.

Psychogenic factors were considered to be of major importance by Coventry (1953), who thought that these patients had what he described as a 'periarthritic personality'. This was a peculiar emotional and constitutional state, characterized by apathy, passivity, an exaggerated response to pain and hyperactive vasomotor responses, which predisposed to 'periarthritis'. Fleming *et al.* (1976) examined the premorbid personality of 56 patients, whose mean age was 58 years, by use of the Middlesex Hospital Questionnaire. They found in the 40 females in this series a statistically significant increase in somatic anxiety. However, Wright and Haq (1976) studied 186 patients with a peak age of onset in their late fifties using a Maudsley Personality Inventory and showed no statistical difference between any of the scores used in these patients and a normal control. As Codman (1934) states, any personality changes in patients with chronic shoulder pain may be the result of the pain rather than the cause of the condition.

Clinical findings

The onset of capsulitis is usually gradual, although it may at times be sudden or even rarely come on overnight. It may occur in one shoulder and then after a variable time involve the other shoulder or much more rarely it may commence in both shoulders simultaneously. However, once an attack has resolved, second attacks of this condition in the same shoulder are quite rare. Capsulitis usually goes through four stages and the typical findings of pain and restriction of movement in all planes will be present in varying proportions according to the particular stage that has been reached (*see Figure 5.28*).

Stage one

Pain is experienced usually in or around the glenohumeral joint and is made worse by shoulder

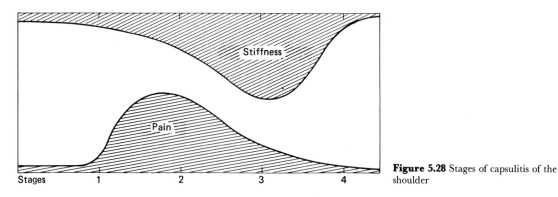

Figure 5.28 Stages of capsulitis of the shoulder

movements, but stiffness is not usually noticed by the patient.

MAJOR SIGNS

Active and passive movements are of almost full range but pain is reproduced at the extremes of all movements and over-pressure applied at the limits of the passive range produces increased pain. Isometric resisted movement tests at this stage are strong and do not produce pain. Testing of the accessory shoulder movements at the limit of the physiological range is important because in this position they are nearly always found to be restricted and painful.

Stage two

Pain becomes more intense, is present at night and disturbs the patient's sleep, especially if he rolls onto the affected shoulder. Most shoulder movements produce pain and sudden movements or jarring are intensely painful. Pain is commonly felt deep in the shoulder or in the region of the deltoid insertion and may radiate further down the arm to the elbow. In addition, the shoulder becomes increasingly stiffer. This painful restriction of shoulder movement results in a severe functional disability; the patient experiences great difficulty in dressing; working, driving a car, or hanging clothes on the line.

MAJOR SIGNS

Active movements become more limited and painful in every plane of movement. Passive movements are similarly restricted and over-pressure produces considerably more pain. The accessory shoulder movements become more restricted. Fully resisted movements should remain painless. In this stage, active flexion is performed with a degree of lateral drift, and abduction with forward drift. Both movements also include some hitching of the shoulder.

Stage three

There is now little spontaneous pain at rest, although pain still may be experienced on suddenly stretching the joint. However, the degree of shoulder stiffness has now become much more pronounced due to adhesion formation and contracture of the thickened shoulder joint capsule. Muscles surrounding the shoulder such as the supraspinatus and infraspinatus become wasted and atrophic. The term 'frozen shoulder' is an unfortunate one as it has led to considerable confusion about the nature and management of this condition. However, if it is to be used it should be reserved to describe this stage in which pain is not a feature but there is marked restriction of shoulder movements.

MAJOR SIGNS

The range of the active and passive glenohumeral movements is greatly restricted in all planes and, as in Stage 2, has drift and hitch, but even in its most severe degree, some degree of scapular movement remains so that some movement at the shoulder is possible.

Stage four

In this stage there is a gradual resolution of the shoulder stiffness with a gradual return of shoulder mobility in most patients.

Course

Capsulitis runs a protracted course, which varies in length from about 9 to about 18 months; accordingly the length of any one of the above four stages is also variable. As an approximation, each of the first three stages lasts from a few weeks up to about 2 months and the fourth stage starts about the fourth or fifth month of the disease and lasts approximately 6–12 months. However, there are variations to this general scheme so that capsulitis may occasionally commence at the second or even third of these stages without having gone through the previous one and it may also rarely resolve spontaneously at any stage. It would appear that such alterations represent only different clinical presentations of the same disease, though it does remain a possibility that a different underlying pathology is involved. Finally, although the natural tendency of capsulitis is towards complete resolution, nevertheless up to 20 per cent of patients may be left with some degree of residual shoulder stiffness.

Management

The management of capsulitis remains controversial. Many different therapeutic regimens have been advocated and no single method of treatment will cure this condition. More importantly, management of capsulitis should be considered in relation to its natural history which involves four distinct stages as described above. It appears that much of the controversy results from the failure to relate the treatments available to each of these stages. In the first two stages pain is the dominant problem and in the next two stages stiffness is the major problem. The therapeutic approach to these two different clinical problems should be varied accordingly.

Stages one and two

REST
Rest to the shoulder is essential as forced movements will increase the patient's pain, especially at night. In stage one, when pain and restriction of movement are not yet marked, this may consist of rest from excessive use of the shoulder, especially from activities that use the shoulder at the limit of the range. In stage two, pain is usually severe. Rest is obtained with a sling, which needs to be worn continuously, with the arm held next to the skin so that it is not disturbed while dressing and undressing. The arm may be supported in any position that provides maximal relief and the hand may be used by placing it through a blouse or shirt. The sling needs to be worn for approximately three weeks until the nocturnal pain has abated. This treatment will undoubtedly also increase the

shoulder stiffness but if active exercises are given with the aim of relieving stiffness at this stage they will inevitably increase the degree of the patient's pain.

MEDICATIONS
Analgesics are needed to control pain. Non-steroidal anti-inflammatory drugs are also usually prescribed but are not often very successful in controlling pain. Oral corticosteroids may then be used and prednisolone, 20 mg daily, is given for approximately 2 weeks, when the dose is then gradually reduced until pain settles. If oral or injected corticosteroids are used they should only be given in the first two stages of this disorder to control inflammation as they will not assist in the last two stages with fibrosis and stiffness.

INJECTIONS
Intra-articular injections of corticosteroids may be given once a week for several weeks to help control symptoms. Various techniques have been advocated, including injections into the bicipital tendon or into painfully tender areas around the shoulder. Multiple injections into three sites—the subacromial bursa, the long head of the biceps tendon and the shoulder joint via the posterior route—were assessed by Steinbrocker and Argyros (1974). Forty-two shoulders were injected at intervals varying from 3 to 7 days. They reported that pain was abolished in 1–3 sessions and function was restored to at least 85 per cent of normal in 40 shoulders. The best method is an intra-articular injection with a posterior approach.

Starting position—The patient sits on a chair with the arm hanging by his side. The examiner palpates the acromial process and places the left thumb under its inferior angle. The index finger of the left hand is then placed anteriorly over the patient's coracoid process.

Method—A 22-gauge needle is inserted from a point just medial to the inferior angle of the acromion and directed in a line towards the coracoid process. The needle passes through soft tissue and may then be felt to enter the joint space, where it lies free. The injection must be given without encountering any sense of resistance.

PHYSICAL METHODS
Ice may also be used to control pain but heat to the shoulder is usually of no benefit; exercises, massage and forcible movements are contraindicated.

MOBILIZATION TECHNIQUES

Treatment with mobilization techniques in the first two stages of capsulitis must be extremely gentle. These techniques are designed to ease the degree of pain. They should be discontinued if they produce any exacerbation of pain. No treatment is given on the day the patient is first seen and examined lest the initial clinical examination causes any exacerbation of pain. Subsequently, treatment is given on a daily basis but the amount of treatment given is limited by the degree of any reaction provoked in the joint.

Two techniques may be used and selection is determined by the range of pain-free forward flexion of the arm. If this range is limited to less than 90 degrees the physiological glenohumeral movements are used as a large-amplitude oscillatory movement performed without causing any discomfort.

Stages three and four

In the third and fourth stages of capsulitis pain is not the major problem, but the shoulder is now stiff. Routine physical methods used to increase the joint range include mobilization techniques, stretching and exercises. Heat or ice may be applied to the shoulder before their use. Rarely, a manipulation under anaesthetic may be indicated.

MOBILIZATION TECHNIQUE

These are the main method of treatment in stages three and four. Forward flexion is usually chosen first as the treatment position.

Starting position—The patient lies supine without a pillow under the head and the therapist supports the patient's fully flexed arm. Longitudinal, posteroanterior and anteroposterior accessory movements are used as small-amplitude movements at the limit of the available range. Treatments should not provoke any excessive pain and are carried out for approximately 3 minutes. The patient is then asked to stand and the range of shoulder movement reassessed. Provided that there has been some improvement in the range, this technique may be repeated once or twice. This whole cycle is repeated daily if no painful reaction is provoked.

STRETCHING

The patient lies supine and the therapist first stabilizes the scapula with one hand and then fully flexes the shoulder by the elbow with the other hand.

Technique—Small-amplitude oscillatory move-

ments are used at the end of the range and then by gradually increasing the pressure the shoulder is stretched to a limit tolerated by the patient. The stretching is maintained for approximately 1 minute. This technique is then changed to the use of accessory movements applied at the end of the range, as described above. These two treatments, used alternately, may be repeated two or three times in a treatment session.

EXERCISES

These increase or maintain any increase in range obtained by the passive techniques and also increase the strength of the shoulder muscles. Exercise programmes should be carried out in a set routine, supervised by a physiotherapist. Several different methods are available:

(1) Isometric exercises: The therapist fully resists the patient's attempt to move the arm into flexion, abduction, lateral rotation and medial rotation.
(2) PNF techniques, using rotary movements in the normal patterns of motion for the upper limb. These consist first of flexion–abduction, lateral-rotation patterns, followed later by extension–abduction, medial-rotation patterns, in which the patient contracts and then relaxes the agonist and then the antagonist muscles.
(3) Pendular exercises are antigravity exercises with the patient flexed forward at the hips so that the arm hangs freely down. A weight is carried in the hand to produce traction on the glenohumeral joint, so stretching the capsule. By moving the trunk the shoulder can be moved so that there is no muscular activity around the glenohumeral joint. The arm can then be moved like a pendulum in a forwards and backwards, lateral or circumduction plane.
(4) Active assisted exercises may be given, using either an apparatus such as a pulley or a rotation disc.
(5) The patient may also force the movements of flexion and abduction by supporting the affected arm against a wall and 'climbing up' the wall with the fingers. These movements should not be accomplished by any 'trick' movements, such as shoulder shrugging. However, the patient should elevate the arm as high as possible up the wall even if the trick movements are used. This point is marked and the patient should lift or swing

the arm to this level without any support from the wall and hold it there to maintain the range.

MANIPULATION

In most patients, a slow steady increase in the range of shoulder movements may be expected. Occasionally, treatment produces an early improvement but after some weeks it fails to effect any further improvement in the range. Should this occur, a manipulation under anaesthetic may be used in an attempt to stretch the shoulder capsule. The advantage of this technique is that the shoulder muscles are relaxed and no great force is needed. It is indicated if there is no continuing improvement in the range of shoulder movement with mobilization and active-exercise techniques; or if there is a loss of range that prevents functional shoulder activities.

TECHNIQUE

Movements are controlled by the therapist, who holds the patient's shoulder in one hand with his palm under the posterior aspect of the patient's shoulder and his thumb over the anterior aspect of the joint. The manipulation consists of a gentle forced–passive stretching of the capsule in which adhesions can be felt to tear. The following movements are used in an orderly routine using great care and gentleness:

(1) Traction on the arm while held at approximately 10 degrees of abduction.
(2) Forward flexion of the shoulder.
(3) Full adduction of the shoulder across the patient's chest.
(4) Abduction of the shoulder.
(5) Lateral rotation of the shoulder with the patient's arm at 90 degrees of abduction and the elbow held at a right angle.
(6) Medial rotation of the shoulder with the arm in the same position as in (5).

An intra-articular injection of corticosteroid is given after the manipulation to dampen any subsequent inflammatory reaction in the joint.

Bloch and Fischer (1961) reported 2000 cases of capsulitis so treated and emphasized that great force must never be used, since it may rupture the joint capsule or subscapularis tendon (Reeves, 1966) or fracture or dislocate the humerus. A single manipulation will only rarely result in a full range of shoulder movements being restored. More commonly, the manipulation will allow the range of movements to start to improve once again

and this improvement can then be maintained with the continued use of mobilization techniques. Accordingly, mobilization techniques are reinstituted daily to maintain and improve the newly acquired range of movement. They are combined with an active routine of exercises.

Prophylaxis

Prevention of capsulitis should always be considered, especially since any condition that produces prolonged immobilization of the shoulder may result in capsular contraction with shoulder stiffness. This is especially apt to occur in patients with cardiac or thoracic diseases or with neurological disorders. It is important to recognize that stiffness may occur as a complication of these disorders so that prophylactic measures, such as encouraging the patient to move the shoulder and passive shoulder movements, can be undertaken.

Instability of the shoulder joint

Instability or recurrent subluxation of the shoulder is not uncommon and results from a similar type of capsular tear found in recurrent dislocation of the shoulder. The shoulder usually subluxes anteriorly, and recurrent posterior subluxation is extremely rare. The original injury suffered by the patient may have been a dislocation of the shoulder, but recurrent subluxation can occur in the absence of a previous dislocation if the capsule has been torn.

The patient presents with a history of recurrent, sudden attacks of shoulder pain that occur with shoulder movements and are usually so severe that he is unable to use his arm. The attack may last for only a short time and the patient is often conscious of a clicking sensation or that the shoulder slips out. However, in some cases the history is not nearly so definite, so that the patient is unaware of the abnormal shoulder movement and complains rather of a sudden onset of shoulder pain, followed by a more generalized feeling of 'soreness' in the upper arm.

Major signs

The abnormal shoulder movement may be demonstrated by the examiner positioning the patient's arm in abduction and lateral rotation and then applying pressure in an anterior direction to the back of the head of the humerus (*see Figure 5.29*). This manoeuvre may reproduce the patient's pain and the shoulder joint may be felt to begin to sublux. This may produce an inhibition of the movement similar to the pain inhibition test for recurrent patellar subluxation. This test should also be performed by placing the shoulder in the quadrant position and the examiner pushing the humeral head anteriorly. Rarely, the patient may be seen at the time of subluxation and it may be possible to feel the humeral head rock back on the glenoid rim and slip back into place.

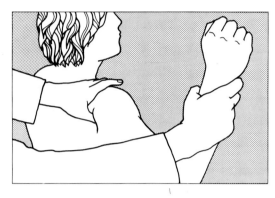

Figure 5.29 Testing recurrent subluxation of the shoulder

Routine X-rays of the shoulder are usually normal but an axial view should be taken as this may show a stripping up of the inferior glenoid rim. Arthrography has been used to demonstrate a ballooning of the capsule anteriorly and inferiorly (Bateman, 1972) but it usually adds little to the clinical assessment. Treatment is surgical.

The shoulder–hand syndrome

The essential clinical features of the shoulder–hand syndrome are shoulder pain, usually associated with stiffness of the shoulder, and pain and vasomotor disturbances in the corresponding hand. This combination of clinical features allows this condition to be differentiated from other conditions causing pain that radiates down the arm from the shoulder. The underlying cause appears to be related to disturbance of the sympathetic nerve control of the vascular supply to the hand.

The shoulder–hand syndrome has three distinct phases (Steinbrocker, 1968). In the first stage there is pain and stiffness in the shoulder that may precede, accompany or follow pain in the hand. The hand is painful, stiff, extremely tender, sweaty, oedematous and warm. The palm is usually pink, red or cyanotic. This stage, which is due to a state of increased vasodilatation, lasts for approximately 3–6 months. Although it may resolve spontaneously it usually proceeds to the second stage. In the second stage the hand becomes less swollen and painful but stiffness becomes more marked. The palm appears pale and dry with atrophy of skin, its appendages and muscles. The shoulder becomes increasingly more painful and stiff and clinically behaves like a capsulitis. This stage lasts approximately 3–6 months. In the third stage the hand becomes stiff and atrophic without any vasomotor changes and a flexion deformity of the fingers develops. The shoulder remains stiff and there is wasting of the muscles around the joint. This stage varies in duration but it may last for some years.

X-ray changes in the shoulder and hand are due to osteoporosis. Blood studies are usually normal but the erythrocyte sedimentation rate may be elevated. A bone scan shows an increased uptake in the involved hand.

The aetiology of this condition is unknown but is believed to be due to a reflex sympathetic disturbance with consequent vasomotor disturbances. This may follow bombardment of the internuncial neurones in the spinal cord, which initiates a reflex cycle of impulses throughout the cord and leads to stimulation of the autonomic fibres originating in the lateral horn. These in turn produce the vasomotor reactions with pain and swelling in the hand, so that pain fibres are stimulated, thereby producing a feed-back circuit into the cord. This condition may have a variety of causes, most of which are either painful in themselves or involve neurological structures. Thus, it has been reported as a complication of myocardial infarct, cervical disorders, trauma to the arm (including surgery), hemiplegia, herpes zoster and lung tumours. In 23 per cent of 146 cases, no initiating cause was found (Steinbrocker, 1972).

Entrapment neuropathy

An entrapment neuropathy causing shoulder pain may arise from the thoracic-outlet syndrome or entrapment of suprascapular nerve.

Thoracic-outlet syndrome

The neurovascular bundle, comprising the subclavian artery and the brachial plexus, may be compressed in its course through the thoracic outlet in the neck. This will produce varying combinations of pain in shoulder and arm, with neurological and vascular symptoms. Pain and paraesthesias are most commonly found on the ulnar side of the arm. The onset of symptoms is usually spontaneous but they may sometimes follow trauma to the neck or arm (Rosati and Lord, 1961). The thoracic-outlet syndromes may be classified as:

(1) The costoclavicular syndrome.
(2) The cervical rib syndrome.
(3) The scalenus anterior syndrome.

Costoclavicular compression results from a decrease in the size of the space between the clavicle and the first rib. This area may be congenitally narrowed, but symptoms are produced usually as the result of a postural sagging of the shoulder girdle. Rarely a space-occupying lesion, such as a tumour or a malunited fracture, may be present.

Cervical ribs may be demonstrated radiologically in about 1 per cent of the population but are less commonly the source of symptoms. They represent either a supernumerary rib or an enlarged transverse process of the 7th cervical vertebra. Compression of the subclavian artery and the brachial plexus may be due to the presence of such an abnormally placed rib or to a fibrous band passing from the 7th cervical vertebra down to the first rib.

The anterior scalene syndrome is quite rare and is produced if the neurovascular bundle is compressed between the scalenus anterior and scalenus medius muscles.

Major signs

Arm pain and paraesthesias should be reproducible by suitable posturing of the patient. Sustained traction on the shoulder by pulling on the patient's wrist may reproduce the patient's symptoms and passive elevation of the shoulder girdle may then relieve them. Conversely, some patients experience their pain only on shoulder elevation.

Adson's test must be carefully performed to give reproducible results. The radial pulse is first palpated by the examiner while the patient's arm hangs loosely by the side. The patient then turns the head towards the ipsilateral side, at the same time taking in and holding a deep breath. The shoulder is passively abducted to just beyond 90 degrees, care being taken to avoid any degree of glenohumeral joint extension. The test is considered to be positive if there is loss of the radial pulse. However, there are many false positives associated with this test since the radial pulse may become obliterated in normal people or in the patient's pain-free arm.

A bruit may be heard on auscultation of the subclavian artery just above the clavicle, either at rest or on performing these postural tests.

Investigations

Routine X-rays of the neck and chest are essential and may demonstrate the presence of a cervical rib. Other investigations including cervical myelograms, subclavian arteriograms and electromyography may be necessary to exclude other causes before a definite diagnosis is made.

Management

Physical therapy is designed firstly to restore pain-free movements at the site of the compression and then to correct any postural abnormalities that may be present. Exercises to strengthen the shoulder-girdle muscles or to stretch any soft-tissue tightness should be given but need to be carried out for a prolonged period of time. Attention to the type of brassiere worn and avoidance of bra-straps may help if the patient has large, pendulous breasts. If these measures fail an operation may be indicated to relieve the site of compression. Surgery may consist of removal of the first rib or a cervical rib and only rarely is an anterior scalenotomy indicated.

Suprascapular nerve entrapment

The suprascapular nerve, derived from C5 and C6, supplies motor innervation to the supraspinatus and infraspinatus muscles and sensory innervation to the posterior shoulder capsule and the acromioclavicular joints. At the upper border of the scapula it runs through the suprascapular notch before entering the supraspinous fossa. The site of compression of this nerve is in the suprascapular notch, which is enclosed by a transverse ligament. Entrapment may follow trauma, especially traction (Clein, 1975) or overuse of the shoulder—as, for example, from painting a house. Pain is felt mainly in the posterolateral aspect of the shoulder but may also radiate down the arm. It is often severe but may be only vaguely localized. When entrapment has been prolonged it is usual to find wasting of the supraspinatus and infraspinatus muscles.

Major signs

Pain should be reproduced by compressing the nerve. This is achieved by passively adducting the arm fully across the chest and applying overpressure at the end of the range. Alternatively, it may be produced by elevating the arm above the head and then depressing the shoulder girdle.

Confirmatory signs

Pressure over the site of the nerve reproduces the patient's pain. The site of the nerve in its suprascapular notch is found at the junction of the outer quarter of the spine of the scapula with the inner three-quarters. Prolonged downwards pressure by the examiner's thumb over this site should reproduce the patient's pain. The diagnosis may be confirmed by electromyography (Khalili, 1974). The suprascapular nerve is stimulated at the suprascapular space and potentials picked up in the supraspinatus muscle may show an increased latency or a decreased amplitude.

Management

Rest to the shoulder is essential. An injection of 5 ml of local anaesthetic and 1 ml of corticosteroid solution may be given around the nerve as it runs through the suprascapular fossa. The patient sits with the arm hanging by the side, the spine of the scapula is palpated and a point marked on its inner and outer ends. The site of injection is located just above the spine of the scapula at the junction of the outer quarter with the inner three-quarters of the spine.

A 23-gauge needle is used and inserted distally in the supraspinous fossa until it hits the scapular spine. The needle is then withdrawn slightly and the injection given over a wide area. Pain should be relieved within a few minutes (Rose and Kelly, 1969). The injection usually needs to be repeated several times at fortnightly intervals.

If conservative measures fail division of the transverse ligament may be necessary.

6 The clavicular joints

The acromioclavicular joint

The acromioclavicular joint moves during all movements of the glenohumeral joint and the scapula. During glenohumeral joint movement, a rotary movement takes place in the acromio-clavicular joint. During movement of the scapula on the thorax, as for example shrugging or depressing the shoulders or protraction or retrac-tion of the scapula, a gliding movement takes place in the acromioclavicular joint.

Acromioclavicular pain

Pain arising from the acromioclavicular joint lesions is usually well localized over the joint and is only rarely referred distally into the upper arm or proximally into the neck. The patient, if asked to put one finger over the site of pain, usually places it accurately over the upper surface of the joint. Pain is usually made worse by movements of the shoulder, especially horizontal flexion.

Clinical examination

(1) Inspection.
(2) Movements:
  (a) Active.
  (b) Passive.
  (c) Accessory.
(3) Palpation.

Inspection

The subcutaneous acromioclavicular joint is easy to inspect. The examiner stands in front of the seated patient to observe the presence of any joint swelling or subluxation upwards of the outer end of the clavicle.

Movements

Active movement is best tested by horizontal flex-ion of the patient's arm across the chest. The examiner stands behind the patient and passively flexes the patient's shoulder to 90 degrees by hold-ing under the flexed elbow (*see Figure 6.1*). He then passively flexes the patient's arm horizontally across the chest so that the hand reaches past the opposite shoulder. The range of this movement is assessed by comparing the patient's two arms and noting the position reached by the point of the elbow in relation to the opposite shoulder.

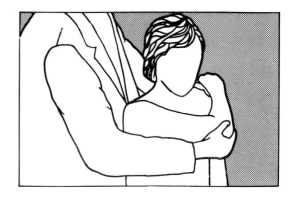

Figure 6.1 Horizontal flexion

Passive movements are tested by the same type of movements and over-pressure is produced by oscillatory movements at the end of the range to reproduce pain. Pain may also be reproduced at times by movement of the glenohumeral joint, especially abduction, or on scapulothoracic movements. These latter movements include elevation, depression, protraction, retraction and rotation of the scapula on the chest wall. Accordingly, in patients who complain of acromioclavicular pain, glenohumeral and scapular movements must always be tested routinely.

There are six accessory movements in the acromioclavicular joint:

(1) Anteroposterior movement, which is produced by pressure over the anterior surface of the outer third of the clavicle and counter-pressure along the spine of the scapula (*see Figure 6.2*).

(2) Posteroanterior movement is produced by pressure over the posterior surface of the clavicle (*see Figure 6.3*).

(3) Rotation is produced when the arm is flexed above the head.

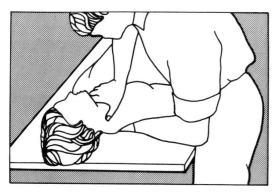

Figure 6.2 Anteroposterior accessory movement

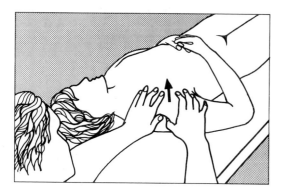

Figure 6.3 Posteroanterior accessory movement

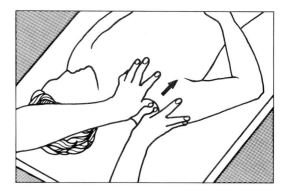

Figure 6.4 Longitudinal caudad accessory movement

(4) Transverse lateral movement is produced by distraction of the joint.

(5) Transverse medial movement is produced by compressing the joint.

(6) Longitudinal movement is produced by pressure over the superior surface of the joint, over the adjacent clavicle and then the adjacent acromiom process (*see Figure 6.4*).

Lesions of the joint

(1) Injuries:
   (a) Ligamentous.
   (b) Intra-articular meniscus.

(2) Arthritis:
   (a) Inflammatory.
   (b) Osteoarthritis.

Injuries

LIGAMENTOUS
The acromioclavicular joint is commonly injured either directly or indirectly. These occur commonly in body-contact sports or after a fall from a speeding object such as a horse or motor cycle. An indirect injury to the joint may follow a fall onto the outstretched hand or a fall onto the outer side of the shoulder, which may follow the patient twisting sideways to avoid a head-on collision. The force is usually transmitted through the glenoid cavity, then to the acromioclavicular ligaments and finally to the coracoclavicular ligaments. Injuries are divided into three grades, or degrees.

Minor or first degree This is produced by a tear of some fibres of the acromioclavicular ligaments but without any joint displacement. Pain, swelling and tenderness are localized over the joint and no obvious deformity is present. Passive shoulder movements, especially horizontal flexion of the arm across the body, usually reproduce the patient's pain.

Management—Treatment consists at first of rest from active shoulder movements or exercises, the use of analgesics and ice. Pain usually settles within a few days after which active exercises can be commenced.

Moderate or second degree A more severe degree of damage is associated with disruption of the capsule and acromioclavicular ligament fibres. This allows the joint to sublux, so that the clavicle moves upwards. A slight step deformity in the joint is present on inspection. Abduction of the arm beyond 80 degrees is usually painful. Pain is also reproduced on horizontal flexion of the shoulder.

Management—Treatment consists of rest from shoulder movements and supporting the arm by a sling or strapping until pain settles. Analgesics are usually required.

Injections are most helpful for relieving pain. The patient sits with the arm hanging loosely by the side and externally rotated. A 25-gauge needle is inserted into the joint space, which is palpable distal to the bony enlargement of the clavicle. The needle needs to be angulated according to the different shapes of the joint surfaces. 1 ml of local anaesthetic and 1 ml of corticosteroid are injected.

Mobilization techniques—Gentle, slow, pain-free accessory movements should also be introduced as early as possible. As pain settles over the next few weeks, active arm exercises should be commenced and the injection may be repeated.

Severe or third degree In this injury, the ligaments that stabilize the acromioclavicular joint are disrupted so that the clavicle becomes dislocated upwards on the acromion. The acromioclavicular ligaments are always involved and usually the coracoclavicular ligaments also. However, Rosenhorn and Pedersen (1974) demonstrated that the coracoclavicular ligament does not have to be completely torn for the joint to be dislocated. The insertions of the deltoid and trapezius muscles are also usually torn, allowing further elevation of the clavicle. The patient complains of a severe degree of pain at first, and shoulder movements are restricted until the pain eventually settles. Ultimately this injury usually causes little pain or functional disability, even in people involved in contact sports, but the dislocation remains unsightly.

Examination—The dislocation is readily obvious on inspection of the shoulder as the patient stands with the arms by the sides and may be made more obvious by holding a weight in the hand on the affected side. The diagnosis is confirmed on X-ray, which shows an increased distance between the acromion process and the clavicle on the affected side. The outer end of the clavicle is elevated so that its inferior border lies level with or above the acromion. An X-ray of both shoulders may be needed for comparison and if so a weight should be carried in the affected arm. At a late stage the ligaments may calcify.

Management—The dislocation may be treated either by conservative methods or by operative reduction; considerable controversy still exists as to which is preferable. Surgical repair designed to restore the rather complex anatomy and function of this joint is neither always successful nor necessary. With conservative treatment reduction of the dislocation is difficult but is preferable to surgery (Glick *et al.*, 1977). Even if this does not produce an effective reduction functional results are usually satisfactory (Jacobs and Wade, 1966). Hence, conservative treatment is indicated in most injuries, including those inflicted in body-contact sports. Surgery needs to be considered mainly in heavy manual workers. However, Nicoll (1954) made the interesting observation that a cosmetic result without an unsightly lump is more important to a model than to a manual worker. Conservative management is aimed at reducing and immobilizing the dislocation but is most difficult to attain. The outer end of the clavicle must be forced downwards and the scapula with its acromion upwards by elevating the elbow. Numerous methods have been described including strapping, slings, braces, harnesses, and a plaster cast (Urist, 1959). A webbing harness applied over the clavicle and under the elbow for 6 weeks provides the most useful compromise in most cases. However, Glick *et al.* (1977) advocated only a short period of complete immobilization until pain settles, followed by active mobilization and early return to sport and reported excellent results in 35 cases. They also stressed that a complete reduction is not necessary for a satisfactory functional result. Surgical procedures are designed to produce fixation of the acromioclavicular joint or coracoclavicular stabilization. Fixation of the joint, achieved with screws, pins, wires and fascial transplants, usually produces unsatisfactory end-results. Coracoclavicular stabilization has been achieved with screws, wire loops, fascial repair, or Mersilene tape. In patients with recurrent acromioclavicular dislocation, removal of the outer end of the clavicle and fixation of the remaining distal end of the clavicle to the coracoid with Mersilene tape has been advocated by Browne, Stanley and Tullos (1977). This is combined with a repair of the origins of the deltoid and trapezius muscles.

INTRA-ARTICULAR MENISCUS

The intra-articular meniscus may be injured, causing recurring joint problems. The patient is usually a young athlete who complains of recurrent attacks of pain and a painful catching sensation on shoulder movements. These can be reproduced on testing passive or accessory acromioclavicular joint movements.

Management—Treatment consists of rest to the shoulder, heat, and injection of local anaesthetic and corticosteroid. Mobilization techniques described below are also helpful. Most patients settle with this regimen but symptoms may recur after vigorous use of the shoulder. Surgery may then be indicated to remove the meniscus; this may be combined with removal of the outer end of the clavicle distal to the attachment of the coraco-acromial ligament.

Arthritis

Degenerative arthritis in this joint is not uncommon. Osteoarthritis is more common here than in the sternoclavicular joint, occurs at an earlier age, develops more rapidly and is more severe (de Palma, 1957). It may be due to previous trauma, form part of a primary generalized osteoarthritis or may follow abnormalities in the glenohumeral joint, such as degeneration and rupture of the rotator cuff, which allows the head of the humerus to sublux upwards. Degenerative changes also occur in calcium pyrophosphate deposition disease and the patient may then present with a large cystic soft-tissue swelling over the joint.

Osteoarthritis may be asymptomatic and pain then usually develops after excessive use of the joint in the middle-aged patient. Pain is often brought on after playing golf or from movements that involve use of the shoulder with the arm above the head. Pain may be reproduced by passive movement of the acromioclavicular joint and crepitus is often palpable over the joint. The diagnosis may be confirmed on X-ray.

MANAGEMENT OF OSTEOARTHRITIS

(1) Rest from those shoulder movements that aggravate pain.
(2) Anti-inflammatory agents.
(3) Local corticosteroid injections, as described above.
(4) Mobilization techniques. Treatment by mobilization techniques uses the accessory acromioclavicular joint movements and should be used within the limits of pain. However, pain and stiffness in the acromioclavicular joint is often associated with disorder of the glenohumeral joint and pain is then also reproduced on shoulder movements. Both of these joints may then require treatment by passive movements and, when so treating the glenohumeral joint, the acromioclavicular joint is also moved. The usual treatment technique is with carefully controlled posteroanterior and anteroposterior movements of the humeral head.
(5) Surgery, with arthroplasty of the joint, is necessary only rarely.

The sternoclavicular joint

The sternoclavicular joint functions as a ball-and-socket joint and the inner end of the clavicle rotates on its long axis during most movements of the shoulder (*see Figure 6.5*). For example, during abduction of the shoulder scapular rotation and movement in the clavicle and the sternoclavicular joint also occur (Lucas, 1973). On abduction or flexion of the shoulder the clavicle rolls upwards and backwards and rotates about

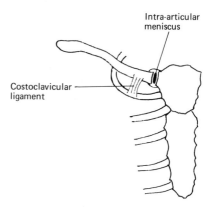

Figure 6.5 The sternoclavicular joint

its longitudinal axis. When the shoulder is returned to the neutral position, opposite movements take place in the clavicle. The total range of this axial rotation is approximately 30 degrees.

Sternoclavicular pain

Pain is usually well localized to the area of the joint or first rib and is usually made worse by shoulder movements such as abduction or flexion that entail rotation of the inner end of the clavicle. Pain from this joint may, however, radiate into the chest wall and so cause confusion with heart or lung diseases. It may also need to be differentiated from disorders affecting the costochondral cartilage. Pain may also be referred to the sternoclavicular area from the cervical spine or shoulder region.

Clinical examination

(1) Inspection; observe:
 (a) Swelling.
 (b) Subluxation.
(2) Movements:
 (a) Active.
 (b) Passive.
 (c) Accessory.
(3) Palpation.

Inspection

The sternoclavicular joint lies subcutaneously and is easy to inspect and palpate. Synovitis is usually evident as a rounded soft-tissue swelling localized over the joint, or just lateral to the joint line filling in the angle between the clavicle and the first rib.

Subluxation of the joint usually occurs in an anterosuperior direction and is best appreciated if the examiner stands behind the seated patient and looks down onto both joints.

Movements

The sternoclavicular joint moves with movements of the shoulder girdle but it is not practical to measure its exact range. In general, movement of the glenohumeral joint beyond 60 degrees will produce pain in the sternoclavicular joint.

ACCESSORY MOVEMENTS

There are six accessory movements in the sternoclavicular joint:

(1) Anteroposterior movement, which is produced by pressure over the sternal end of the clavicle (*see Figure 6.6*).

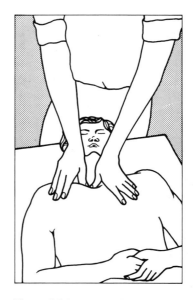

Figure 6.6 Anteroposterior accessory movement of the sternoclavicular joint

(2) Posteroanterior movement is produced by hooking the fingers and thumb around the posterior surface of the clavicle to pull it forwards.
(3) Longitudinal caudad movement is produced by pressure against the superior border of the clavicle adjacent to the joint.
(4) Longitudinal cephalad movement is produced by pressure against the inferior border of the clavicle.
(5) Transverse medial movement is produced by compression along the clavicle from the acromion.
(6) Transverse lateral movement is produced by distracting the joint by pulling the humerus laterally.

Lesions of the sternoclavicular joint

(1) Arthritis:
 (a) Degenerative.
 (b) Inflammatory.

(c) Infective.

(2) Injuries.

Arthritis

Degenerative changes are not found as commonly in the sternoclavicular joint as in the acromio-clavicular joint but may occur as the result of trauma or overuse of the shoulder (Koff *et al.*, 1976). Osteoarthritis is usually unilateral and produces an anterior subluxation of the joint that is easily recognizable on inspection. This may be of concern to the patient as it may be noticed to be gradually increasing in size. Pain may be present on shoulder movement and tenderness is localized over the sternoclavicular joint.

Injuries

The sternoclavicular ligament may be sprained as a result of an injury that usually results from a fall or blow during which the shoulder joint is thrust medially.

A third-degree sprain with disruption of the costoclavicular and sternoclavicular ligaments results in a dislocation of the joint. In the usual type of injury, the inner end of the clavicle dislocates upwards and outwards. Posterior dislocation of the clavicle behind the sternum is rare but potentially much more serious because of damage to the superior mediastinal contents.

Rupture of the intra-articular disc may occur in young athletes. It causes pain and a sensation of catching in the sternoclavicular joint that is brought on by movement of the shoulder.

MANAGEMENT

Management will not be described in detail. The principles of management—including rest, local steroid injection, and mobilization techniques—are similar to those described for the acromio-clavicular joint.

7 The elbow

The elbow comprises three joints functioning as a unit within a single synovial membrane and capsule (*see Figures 7.1 and 7.2*). Its major function is to allow the hand to be positioned; for example, by lifting it to the face while eating. The elbow forms a link between the shoulder and the hand so that the range of motion in the hand also depends upon the position of the elbow. With the elbow flexed to 90 degrees and the arm placed by the side, the total range of supination and pronation in the hand is approximately 180 degrees. But if the arm hangs by the side, the total range of supination and pronation of the hand is 360 degrees, since the shoulder, by rotating laterally and medially, can also participate in this movement. If the range

of elbow movement is restricted, compensatory movements at the shoulder can then help to maintain function. Alternatively, if the range of movement in both the shoulder and elbow is lost the patient may experience marked disturbance of function.

Functionally, the elbow is made up of two primary joints: the elbow joint itself, concerned with flexion and extension; and the superior radioulnar joint concerned with rotation of the forearm. During flexion of the elbow the trochlear notch of the ulna glides around the trochlea of the humerus until blocked by approximation of the muscles and the bony prominence of the coronoid process engaging in the coronoid fossa of the humerus. During extension of the

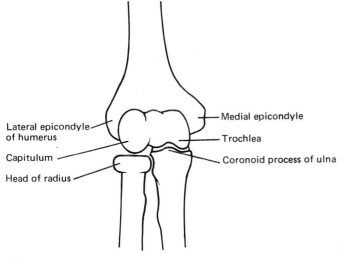

Lateral epicondyle of humerus

Capitulum

Head of radius

Medial epicondyle

Trochlea

Coronoid process of ulna

Figure 7.1 The elbow joint

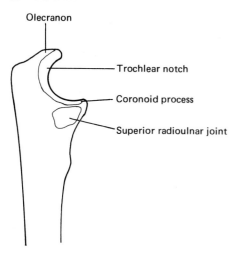

Olecranon

Trochlear notch

Coronoid process

Superior radioulnar joint

Figure 7.2 Upper end of right ulna, viewed from lateral side

elbow the trochlear notch of the ulna glides around the trochlea until the bony prominence of the olecranon process engages the olecranon fossa of the humerus. Simultaneously with these flexion–extension elbow movements, the head of the radius glides backwards and forwards on the capitulum of the humerus. Rotation of the forearm producing either supination or pronation occurs as the concave radial head moves around the lateral side of the stable ulna. As the forearm is moved from supination to pronation the head of the radius is tilted distally and medially and also glides on the capitulum of the humerus.

Elbow pain

Pain in the elbow is usually due to local musculo-skeletal disorders. It may also be produced by lesions of the cervical spine or less commonly as a referred pain from lesions in other areas in the arm. Pain due to shoulder lesions may radiate down the arm, but rarely as far as the elbow, and it is made worse by shoulder and not elbow movements. Occasionally pain may be felt in the elbow from an entrapment neuropathy of the median nerve in the carpal tunnel.

Soft-tissue lesions are the most common cause of elbow pain and the patient is often aware that pain is related to certain movements of the elbow or wrist. Loss of the normal accessory

movements in the elbow joint is also a common but often overlooked cause of painful disability. Of the soft-tissue lesions, epicondylitis is the most common cause of elbow pain but considerable controversy still exists about its basic nature and correct nomenclature. However, epicondylitis is probably the best term to describe a condition that is multifactorial in origin and may involve the lateral or medial epicondyle.

Examination

Examination of a patient with elbow pain should commence by first examining the cervical spine for the presence of any pain or restriction of movement to determine whether the pain can be reproduced by neck movements. It should then include an examination of the whole of the upper limb.

Examination of the elbow

(1) Inspection:
   (a) Deformities.
   (b) Swellings.
   (c) Colour changes.

(2) Movements:
   (a) Active.
   (b) Passive.
   (c) Accessory.
   (d) Isometric.

(3) Palpation.

Inspection

With the arm held in the anatomical position, so that the elbow is fully extended and the forearm supinated with the palm facing forwards, the forearm normally forms a slight degree of valgus at the elbow. This is called the carrying angle and is usually about 5 degrees in males but may be greater in females. It disappears when the arm is placed in full pronation. The carrying angle is of advantage when a heavy object is being carried by allowing the elbow to be tucked in above the iliac crest.

Deformities

Three types of deformity may be present. Firstly, there may be an alteration in the normal carrying angle of the elbow which may be increased, producing cubitus valgus, or decreased, producing cubitus varus. Cubitus valgus may be a sign in Turner's syndrome but more commonly occurs as the result of the previous elbow fracture and may then produce an entrapment neuropathy of the ulnar nerve behind the medial epicondyle. Cubitus varus, a decrease in the carrying angle of the elbow, has been called the 'gunstock deformity' because of its shape and may also occur as the late result of a fracture.

Secondly, flexion deformity of the elbow with loss of full extension may occur. This is the common deformity in patients with arthritis. Thirdly, hyperextension of the elbow or cubitus recurvatus may occur as part of a hypermobility syndrome.

Swellings around the elbow joint

A synovial effusion bulges into the lateral paraolecranon groove (*see Figure 7.10*) and is best seen on inspection with the elbow flexed to less than a right angle. Rheumatoid synovitis may also track down into the forearm or up around the triceps insertion, producing cystic synovial swelling.

Rheumatoid nodules are found in the subcutaneous tissue over the olecranon and extensor surface of the elbow; they feel firm, often rubbery, may be multiple, vary up to 3 cm in size and a small necrotic area may be found in the overlying skin. Nodules, which develop in up to 25 per cent of rheumatoid patients, are caused by a combination of underlying vasculitis and local pressure or friction.

The elbow is also a common site for tophaceous deposits to develop in patients with gout. These can clinically resemble rheumatoid nodules and so, for a correct diagnosis, they should be aspirated to obtain crystals of sodium urate.

Olecranon bursitis presents as a swelling localized to the bursa over the olecranon process. This common condition may be due to trauma, infection or arthritis. Traumatic bursitis may be due to a direct injury to the elbow or follow chronic friction and pressure. A synovial effusion, which tends to be recurrent, develops in the bursa and may at times be haemorrhagic. Olecranon bursitis is common in miners and is known as 'beat elbow'. It is caused by the repetitive nature of their work and may lead to an infected elbow. Two common arthritic conditions—rheumatoid arthritis and gout—may be associated with olecranon bursitis. Swelling may occur as part of the acute inflammatory synovitis in both of these conditions; or the bursa may be chronically involved, showing rheumatoid nodules or gouty tophaceous deposits.

Movements

Active movements

Active movements that are tested at the elbow are flexion, extension, pronation, and supination.

The patient is first asked to extend the elbow by straightening out the arm and then to flex it fully. The active range of extension is normally designated as 0 degrees and is blocked by bony apposition. The active range of flexion is approximately 140 degrees and is blocked by the bulk of the arm muscles.

The active range of supination and pronation is tested in two different positions; firstly, with the elbow in full extension, and next with the elbow held at 90 degrees of flexion.

When performing active movements the patient is requested to move the arm to the limit of each range and then to bounce the arm three or four times into the positions of full flexion, extension, pronation and supination. The range of these movements and whether they reproduce the patient's pain should be noted.

Passive range

The passive range of each of the four elbow movements—flexion, extension, supination and pronation—is tested next. It is usually a few degrees more than the active range. The range of movement is noted, and over-pressure is then applied at the limit of the range to assess the end-feel of each movement.

Accessory movements

The accessory movements in the three separate joints of the elbow are tested separately.

HUMEROULNAR JOINT
The two important accessory movements tested in this joint are:

(1) The range of adduction and abduction of the elbow throughout its last 5 degrees of extension.

(2) The longitudinal caudad movement in the line of the humerus.

(1) With the elbow fully extended, the range of lateral accessory movement can be felt by passive movement of the elbow into adduction and abduction. This may be represented diagrammatically by a straight line X1, Y1—where X1 represents the limit of adduction and Y1 the limit of abduction. If the elbow is now passively flexed by 5 degrees the range between adduction and abduction is increased and may be represented diagrammatically by a line X2, Y2 (*see Figure 7.3*).

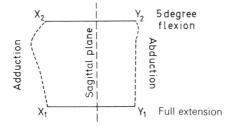

Figure 7.3 Diagrammatic representation of accessory movements in elbow extension

In practice this test is carried out by holding the fully extended elbow firmly in adduction (*see Figure 7.4*) and then moving it from full extension to a position of 5 degrees of flexion (that is, from X1 to X2). During this movement the elbow is felt to move not in a straight line but in a slight curve.

A similar movement is made with the extended elbow held in passive abduction and moving it

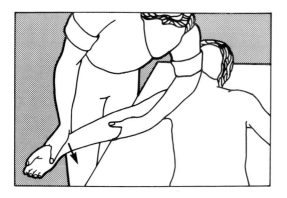

Figure 7.4 The elbow: Extension–adduction

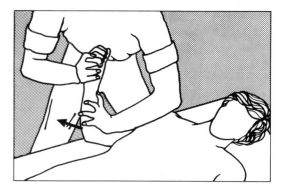

Figure 7.5 Humeroulnar joint; longitudinal caudad accessory movement

from full extension to a position of 5 degrees of flexion (that is, from Y1 to Y2). This movement also follows a slight curve, which is less marked than that felt when the arm is moved while being held in adduction (*see Figure 7.3*).

(2) Longitudinal caudad movement is produced by pressure along the forearm to distract the humeroulnar joint (*see Figure 7.5*).

SUPERIOR RADIOULNAR JOINT

There are four accessory movements in this joint:

(1) Anteroposterior movement, which is produced by pressure over the anterior surface of the head of the radius, which may be placed in supination (*see Figure 7.6*), pronation or midway between them.

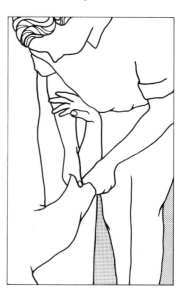

Figure 7.6 Superior radioulnar joint; anteroposterior accessory movement

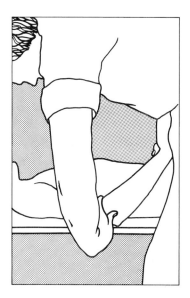

Figure 7.7 Superior radioulnar joint; posteroanterior accessory movement

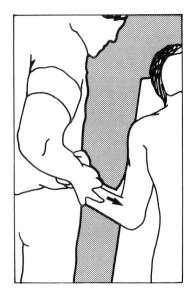

Figure 7.9 Superior radioulnar joint; longitudinal cephalad accessory movement

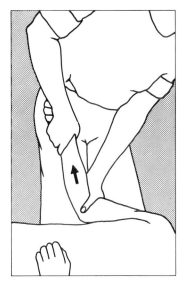

Figure 7.8 Superior radioulnar joint; longitudinal caudad accessory movement

(2) Posteroanterior movement is produced by pressure over the posterior surface of the radial head (*see Figure 7.7*).

(3) Longitudinal caudad movement is produced by pulling along the radius to distract it in relation to the ulna (*see Figure 7.8*).

(4) Longitudinal cephalad movement is produced by compressing along the line of the radius (*see Figure 7.9*).

RADIOHUMERAL JOINT

Four accessory movements are tested in this joint:

(1) Anteroposterior movement, which is a gliding movement applied to the head of the radius.

(2) Posteroanterior movement is also a gliding movement applied to the head of the radius but in an opposite direction.

(3) Longitudinal cephalad movement is produced by compression along the radial shaft.

(4) Longitudinal caudad movement is produced by pulling on the patient's hand to apply a longitudinal movement to the radius.

Isometric tests

Isometric tests should be assessed first at the wrist and then at the elbow. To test resisted movements at the wrist the patient is asked to grip the examiner's hand and squeeze strongly.

If elbow pain is reproduced additional isometric contractions of the wrist are examined. In patients with pain felt over the lateral compartment of the elbow, the isometric movements to be tested are wrist extension, radial deviation of the wrist and finger extension. In patients with pain over the medial compartment of the elbow, the isometric movements to be tested are wrist flexion, ulnar deviation of the wrist and finger flexion.

The four elbow movements of flexion, extension, supination and pronation are next tested using isometric contraction. Flexion is tested while the patient lies supine with the elbow flexed to a right angle and the forearm supinated. The examiner steadies the patient's elbow with one hand. With his other hand, he holds above the flexor aspect of the patient's wrist and fully resists the patient's attempt to lift the hand towards the mouth. A painful weakness of elbow flexion may be present in bicipital tendinitis. A painless weakness may occur in C5 and C6 nerve-root lesions.

Extension is also tested with the patient lying with the elbow flexed to a right angle and the forearm supinated. The examiner places one hand over the extensor aspect of the wrist of the patient, who then attempts to extend the hand towards the floor. A painful weakness of this movement may occur in triceps tendinitis. A painless weakness usually indicates the presence of a C7 nerve-root lesion and may then be associated with a loss or diminution of the triceps reflex.

Supination is tested with the patient lying supine and the elbow flexed to a right angle with the forearm in the mid position. The examiner holds the hand of the patient, who then attempts to turn the palm to face upwards. Pain on resisted supination of the forearm may occur with a bicipital tendinitis.

Pronation is also tested with the patient lying supine and the elbow flexed to right angles with the forearm in the mid position. The examiner grips the hand of the patient, who then attempts to turn the palm face downwards. Pain on pronation may occur in medial epicondylitis.

Palpation

The elbow is best palpated with the patient lying supine and the elbow held in a position of approximately 70 degrees of flexion. If the right elbow is being palpated, the examiner supports the patient's forearm with his left hand and uses the right thumb and fingers to palpate. The olecranon process of the ulna lies subcutaneously and may be easily palpated, as can the triceps tendon which is inserted into it. In front of the olecranon, on the lower end of the humerus, the two small bony protuberances of the medial and lateral epicondyles of humerus are also easily palpable (*see Figure 7.1*). When the elbow is fully extended these three bony landmarks can be felt

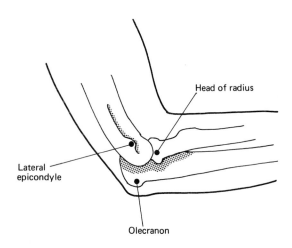

Figure 7.10 Bony landmarks around the elbow. Shading indicates position of the lateral paraolecranon groove

to lie in a straight line. However, when the elbow is flexed to 90 degrees these three bony prominences form an isosceles triangle with its apex over the olecranon and its base between the two epicondyles. The area around both epicondyles should be tested for tenderness.

Above the epicondyles run the medial and lateral supracondylar ridges of the humerus. This ridge is easily felt on the medial side but detection needs deep palpation on the lateral side. The median nerve runs anteriorly to the medial supracondylar ridge. From the anterior aspect of the lateral epicondyle arise the musculotendinous origins of the wrist extensors and from the medial epicondyle arise the wrist flexors and pronators. They can be felt to contract by palpating distally to the epicondyles while the patient clenches his fist.

A finger-breadth below the lateral epicondyle, the head of the radius can easily be felt as it moves while the forearm is rotated. The line of the radiohumeral joint can be palpated just above the radial head. The biceps tendon is easily palpated as it inserts into the radius in the middle of the cubital fossa on the anterior aspect of the elbow joint. The synovial joint between the head of the radius and the cartilagenous lining of the internal surface of the annular ligament, lateral to the head of the radius can also be palpated for swelling, thickening and tenderness.

The space between the olecranon and the epicondyle is known as the paraolecranon groove (*see Figure 7.10*). The synovial membrane lies close to the surface in the lateral paraolecranon groove, and synovitis can be easily palpated here as a slightly tender, soft swelling that bulges against the examining thumb as the elbow is slowly flexed and extended. The medial paraolecranon groove contains the ulnar nerve, which can be rolled in its groove on the back of the medial humeral epicondyle; the nerve is palpated for the presence of any tenderness, swelling or thickening. The supratrochlear lymph nodes should also be palpated just above the medial epicondyle.

Classification of elbow lesions

(1) Soft-tissue lesions:

    (a) Musculotendinous lesions: lateral epicondylitis, medial epicondylitis, bicipital tendinitis and triceps tendinitis.
    (b) Ligamentous sprains.

(2) Joint lesions:
    (a) Pulled elbow.
    (b) Pushed elbow.
    (c) Arthritis.
    (d) Loose bodies.

(3) Nerve entrapments:
    (a) Ulnar nerve.
    (b) Median nerve.
    (c) Radial nerve.

Soft-tissue lesions

Lateral epicondylitis

This condition occurs most often in the dominant arm of middle-aged patients, in females more commonly than males, and is occasionally bilateral. It occurs in patients whose occupation or sport includes excessive use of the wrist or else supination or pronation of the forearm. Its onset may be gradual with an intermittent mild ache, felt first in the elbow or forearm. The onset can also be sudden, and in tennis players may follow either a mis-hit or a change in action. It may also follow a direct blow to the epicondylar region. Pain is felt originally over the lateral aspect of the elbow but then severe pain may radiate down the forearm into the dorsum of the hand and the middle and ring fingers. Only rarely does it radiate up the arm. The pain is made worse especially by movements of the wrist; gripping, e.g. shaking hands, may be particularly difficult. When severe, pain may disturb sleep.

Pain in the lateral aspect of the elbow and forearm may also be caused by C7 nerve-irritation but is usually associated with paraesthesias or other neurological signs, thus helping to differentiate it clinically.

MAJOR SIGNS
Isometric contractions at the wrist are used to reproduce elbow pain and several tests are available:

(1) The patient lies with the elbow extended and grips the examiner's index finger and attempts to lift his hand upwards. Elbow pain is reproduced and the movement cannot be sustained by the patient because of painful weakness in the arm.
(2) The patient lies supine with elbow fully extended and the forearm pronated; the movement of wrist extension is then actively resisted by the examiner.

OTHER SIGNS
Pain may also be reproduced by two additional isometric tests—resisted radial deviation of the patient's wrist and finger extension—and by stretching the extensor muscles of the forearm. The patient lies with the elbow extended and pronated and the examiner passively flexes the patient's wrist and fingers.

Resisted movements of the elbow joint itself do not reproduce the pain.

It has been stated that passive movements of the elbow joint are of full range but this is certainly incorrect in more chronic states; a loss of the last few degrees of passive extension is almost always present in the affected elbow compared with the normal side. The pain response and the end-feel of extension also indicate the loss of normal movement.

Accessory movements, especially adduction in the fully extended position, usually show some restriction of movement and these tests may also reproduce the patient's pain.

Palpation localizes the site of tenderness. This is usually found directly over the anterior aspect of the lateral epicondyle but it may occur more distally over the tendon or at the musculotendinous junction. Rarely, the site of tenderness may be in the muscle belly itself, over the annular ligament of the superior radioulnar joint or over the articular cartilage of the head of the radius.

Elbow X-rays usually are normal for the patient's age, but small areas of calcification may at times be seen in the extensor origin.

AETIOLOGY

A large number of causes have been suggested for this condition, and a single lesion evidently cannot adequately explain the aetiology in all cases. The fibrous origin of the common extensor tendons from the lateral epicondyle is the usual site involved, and so this condition may be looked upon as a form of enthesitis. The most likely explanation appears to be that an area of soft-tissue degeneration develops at this site in the origin of the extensor carpi radialis brevis and that this area develops a tear, an inflammatory change, or both. Degenerative changes commonly occur in this area, probably as a result of ageing, repeated use, or micro-trauma, and are also the basis for the calcification that may ultimately develop. Since the blood supply to this area is relatively poor in middle age, healing is slow and the lesion tends to become chronic.

Muscles that span two joints, such as the hamstrings, are commonly torn as a result of uncoordinated movements. The extensor of the wrist also spans two joints, the elbow and wrist, and uncoordinated movement is even more likely since the extensor arises partly from the surrounding mobile ligaments and aponeuroses. Should a tear occur, the lack of blood supply would again make healing extremely difficult. Coonrad and Hooper (1973) found such tears at the common extensor origin in 28 out of 39 operations.

Inflammatory changes may arise due to overuse after repetitive wrist movements, either occupational or during sporting activity, and involve especially the tenoperiosteal origin from the lateral epicondyle.

Newman and Goodfellow (1975) described 25 patients who underwent arthrotomy; of these, 20 had a chondromalacia of the radial head, similar to that found in the patellofemoral joint. They postulated that repeated pronation and supination of the forearm causes compression of the posteromedial aspect of the radial head and the orbicular ligament under the extensor aponeurosis, producing the degenerative cartilage lesion. Many other causes have been described, and include an entrapment neuropathy, also known as the radial tunnel syndrome (Roles and Maudesley, 1972) and stenosis of the annular ligament (Bosworth, 1965). Finally, the role of cervical-spine degenerative changes in the causation of epicondylitis has always been controversial. One reason is that many reports rely on X-ray changes in the cervical spine alone for confirmatory evidence and in the age group in which this lesion tends to occur, such X-ray changes are a common and often asymptomatic finding. Treatment to the neck only rarely produces any alteration to the symptoms in our experience, but Gunn and Milbrandt (1976) reported on 50 patients with epicondylitis who failed to respond to local elbow therapy, and in whom 43 (86 per cent) responded to suitable therapy to the neck over several weeks.

COURSE

This condition tends to run a protracted course, with exacerbations and remissions often lasting up to 2 years, before most cases undergo natural remission.

MANAGEMENT

Rest The patient needs to rest from those activities that are associated with this condition. These usually involve prolonged gripping with the wrist, such as in tennis. Resting is often difficult for the patient, who should be reassured that the condition tends to be self-limiting over a long period of time and that other treatments will not often be helpful unless activity is curtailed. Immobilization of the forearm and wrist in a cock-up plaster has previously been advocated but is not now recommended. Although the patient's symptoms may settle while the arm is in the plaster, it is a most inconvenient means of treatment and the symptoms usually return after the wrist has been taken out of the plaster and used once again.

Medication Anti-inflammatory drugs are given as there is an inflammatory component to this disorder and they do help to relieve pain.

Injections An injection of corticosteroid is usually the quickest and most effective method of treatment but it must be accurately placed. The patient sits with the elbow flexed to a right angle and the site of maximal tenderness is found by careful palpation with the examiner's thumb. He then places the left thumb over the patient's lateral epicondyle and the fingers are spread out around the elbow to steady it. A 25-gauge needle is used for the injection and so local anaesthetic need not be infiltrated into the overlying skin. An injection of 1 ml of corticosteroid solution and 1 ml of local anaesthetic is injected into and around the tender area. In the tenoperiosteal variety of epicondylitis it is necessary to direct the needle against the epicondyle and inject a small volume of solution into this area.

The patient is advised to rest the wrist and elbow for a week and is warned that there may be a severe exacerbation of pain for a day or two after the injection, which may require analgesics. If after a week the pain is not fully relieved the injection may be repeated at intervals varying from 7 to 14 days. The injection may be repeated several times, but if only transient relief is being obtained this treatment should not continue. If after a week one injection has sufficed and the elbow is pain free the management of the patient is similar to that discussed below for aftercare.

Physical methods Ice, heat and deep-friction massage have been advocated but are rarely successful in the long-term management of this condition.

Mobilization techniques These are helpful especially when, as is usual, examination has demonstrated:

(1) A loss of full passive elbow extension.
(2) A loss of the normal accessory movements, with a painful limitation in the range of extension–adduction.

If the passive range of extension is found to be limited, mobilization techniques using large-amplitude extension movements at the limit of the range should be used first for 20–40 seconds. The passive range is then reassessed to determine whether the pain-free range has increased. On the first day of treatment this technique should be repeated only once, but on subsequent days the amount of treatment given may be increased. It is, however, important to progress this treatment gradually lest it cause an exacerbation of symptoms, and treatment in the painful range should not be performed too early. Treatment is performed daily for about 10 days and then on alternate days until full extension is possible.

If the accessory movement of extension–adduction is painfully limited treatment consists of small-amplitude stretching movements at the limit of the range. This may be achieved by:

(1) Rocking the elbow medially from the abducted to the adducted position while holding the elbow just short of full extension.
(2) Holding the elbow adducted and moving it in an arc through the last 5 degrees of extension, and then back into 5 degrees of flexion.
(3) Moving the elbow in an arc from extension–abduction into extension–adduction, followed by a movement into 5 degrees of

flexion while holding the elbow in adduction and then releasing the adduction strain.

Manipulation This is performed using the technique described by Mills (1928) but it does not often produce lasting benefits. The usual reason given for any success is that it stretches the extensor origin at the lateral epicondyle and separates the edges of any tear or scar tissue that is present. This theory may not be correct and the manipulation may work by restoring normal accessory and physiological movements to the elbow joint. This manipulation must never be performed if the elbow lacks extension due to muscle spasm.

Starting position—The patient is seated with the shoulder abducted and the arm medially rotated so that the lateral epicondyle is facing forwards. The therapist stands behind the patient's shoulder and passively moves the patient's forearm into full pronation and the wrist into flexion with his right hand. He places his thumb over the patient's palm with the fingers spread over the dorsum of the hand. The heel of the left hand is placed over the lower end of the patient's humerus (*see Figure 7.11(a)*).

Method—The patient's elbow is suddenly forced into full extension with the examiner's left hand while maintaining full flexion at the patient's wrist. It is important that the lower end of the patient's humerus is pushed forward and that this movement is not produced by pulling the forearm forwards (*see Figure 7.11(b)*).

Aftercare

(1) The extensor muscles in the forearm should be passively stretched and exercises given to strengthen them before allowing the patient to return to full activity. It is also important to ensure that the return to active sport is gradual.
(2) Any provoking cause, such as a poor sporting technique, should be corrected if possible. This may require consultation with a coach.
(3) The balance of any racquet used may need adjusting; at times this lesion follows an alteration in the type of racquet used.
(4) The grip on the handle of the racquet may also need to be altered. Experiments should be carried out to discover whether the grip has been too large or, more commonly, too small.
(5) A support for the forearm is useful to alter the leverage on the forearm muscles and relieve strain on the elbow. The support is

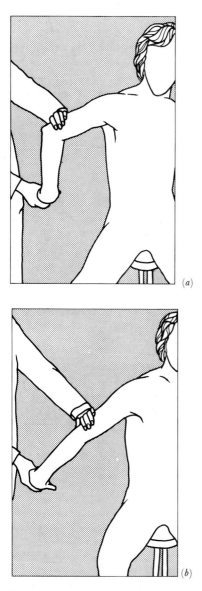

Figure 7.11 (*a*) and (*b*). Mill's manipulation

made of calico and is kept tightly in place with velcro straps. It should only be worn during activities that involve use of the forearm (Froimson, 1971).

Surgery   Surgery, in those patients who are resistant to conservative therapy or have recurrent problems (*British Medical Journal*, 1978), is only rarely indicated. Several operations have been described. The most common is a tenotomy and stripping of the common extensor origin (Spencer and Hernod, 1953) and is usually combined with

debridement of any chronic granulation tissue that is present. Active rehabilitation and an early return to sport postoperatively are essential. A tenotomy may also be performed as a closed procedure under local anaesthesia, using either a beaver-eye blade, a tenotome or even a wide-bore needle. The tenoperiosteal origin is detached by a series of sweeping incisions. Murtagh (1978) reported on this office procedure in 20 patients; of these, 14 showed a total relief of symptoms. Division of the orbicular ligament (Bosworth, 1965) and removal of an area of chondromalacia in the radial head (Newman and Goodfellow, 1975) have also been advised. An acute tear may be successfully repaired (Gardner, 1970).

Medial epicondylitis

A similar but less common condition than lateral epicondylitis occurs over the medial epicondyle, which is the site of origin of the wrist flexors and the pronator of the forearm. It is also known as golfer's elbow but may occur in people who have never played golf. It occurs in middle-aged patients, often those involved in sporting or occupational activities that require a strong hand grip and an adduction movement of the elbow. Pain is experienced over the medial compartment of the elbow and may radiate distally. Pain is made worse by wrist movements, especially gripping or repeated wrist flexion.

Major signs

Pain is reproduced by an isometric contraction of the wrist flexors, which is tested by having the patient lie with the elbow extended and supinated and gripping the examiner's finger. Alternatively, fully resisting flexion of the wrist may reproduce the elbow pain.

Other signs

Pain may also be reproduced by fully resisting pronation of the forearm, or stretching the flexor muscle group by fully extending the supine forearm and then passively hyperextending the wrist. Tenderness on palpation is usually felt under the medial epicondyle.

Management

This is similar to that outlined for lateral epicondylitis; namely rest, medication, local corticosteroid injections and mobilization techniques. A forced manipulation, as with the Mill's technique, is not indicated.

Bicipital tendinitis

This is uncommon. The patient presents with pain that is usually well localized to the middle of the cubital fossa.

Major signs

The patient's pain is reproduced by the examiner fully resisting either elbow flexion or supination of the forearm. Pain may also be reproduced by stretching the tendon, which is best achieved by the examiner extending the elbow and then applying full passive pronation to the forearm. Testing of the accessory movements in the superior radioulnar joint commonly reveals a painful restriction of movement.

Other signs

An area of tenderness may be palpated, with the elbow flexed to 90 degrees, over the insertion of the biceps tendon into the bicipital tuberosity of the radius.

Management

Injection—The patient sits with the forearm supported on the desk and held in slight flexion and supination. The tender area in the tendon insertion into the radial tuberosity is found by palpation. A 25-gauge needle is used and is carefully inserted alongside the tendon insertion, so as not to inject into the tendon substance. 1 ml of corticosteroid solution is injected around the tender area and the patient is advised to avoid excessive use of the elbow for a week.

Deep-friction massage—This may be used across the tendon insertion as an alternative method of treatment.

Accessory movements in the superior radioulnar joint—If these are limited and painful, treatment with passive-movement techniques using pronation are most useful. These consist at first of large-amplitude movements in the pain-free range. The patient lies supine with the elbow flexed to a right angle and the forearm pronated. The therapist places the left hand over the dorsum of the patient's wrist and supports under the elbow with the right hand to stabilize it. The therapist produces the pronation movement by movement of his left arm and shoulder. As movement improves and pain subsides small-amplitude stretching movements are used at the limit of the range of pronation, and compression may be added to this movement.

Triceps tendinitis

This is rare. It follows the sudden severe strain to the triceps tendon, e.g. in javelin throwers, as the arm is fully extended.

Pain is reproduced on fully resisting extension of the elbow while the patient stands with the elbow flexed and forearm fully supinated. An area of tenderness may be palpated over the insertion of the triceps tendon into the olecranon.

Joint lesions

Pulled elbow

This common, dramatic condition occurs in young children who present with a painful inability to use the arm. It is due to a lesion of the radioulnar joint, which is subluxed after a traction injury, and is completely and rapidly cured by manipulation.

CLINICAL FEATURES

The condition of pulled elbow occurs in young children before the age of 8 years, with a peak incidence at between 2 and 3 years. The youngest child we have seen was aged 10 months. It is at least twice as common in the left elbow as the right, and girls are affected twice as commonly as boys (Corrigan, 1965).

The history is of a sudden traction injury that has been applied to the child's arm while held in an extended and pronated position above the head by an adult, who then lifts the child's hand suddenly upwards (*see Figure 7.12*). This may occur in many different situations, such as lifting the child out of the bath or up from the floor, lifting the child's arm as the adult goes up a step or if the child is being swung by the arms in play. Occasionally the child will trip or fall and is grabbed by the arm, which is jerked upwards.

The onset of pain may be accompanied by an audible or palpable click in the elbow. The child cries and refuses to use the arm. Since the

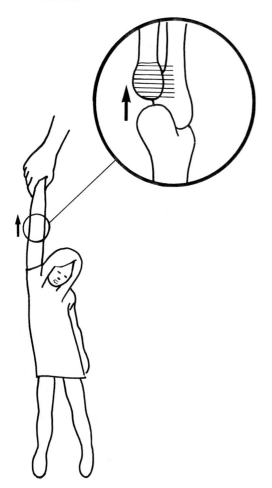

Figure 7.12 Pulled elbow: mechanism of production

beyond the mid position produces tearful and often violent resistance from the child. X-rays are usually normal, but a slight downwards displacement of the proximal end of the radius in relation to the capitulum may be evident.

RECURRENT ATTACKS
Illingworth (1975) reported on a series of 100 children with pulled elbow, of whom 30 had had previous episodes, mainly involving the same arm. This history of recurrent attacks of painful inability to use the arm may cause diagnostic confusion. It may also occur as part of a child-bashing syndrome.

MECHANISM
In this injury, the head of the radius is pulled distally through the normally restraining fibres of the annular radioulnar ligament. Previously, since this lesion occurs only in young children, anatomical factors were considered to be responsible. According to this theory, the head of the radius is smaller than the neck of the radius until the age of 8 and so the annular ligament can easily slip upwards over the radial head. However, Salter and Zahn (1971) have discounted this theory. In a series of post-mortem anatomical dissections they applied traction to the elbow while it was held extended in supination and showed that this type of subluxation could not

pain may be poorly localized, the diagnosis can be difficult; either the neck, shoulder, elbow or wrist may be considered as the site of the problem, and the differential diagnosis may include poliomyelitis or a brachial plexus injury.

Examination usually shows a crying child who carries the affected arm limply by the side or supported on the lap. There is no obvious swelling of the elbow, which is held slightly flexed with the forearm held either pronated or in the mid position. A useful manoeuvre is to stand on the child's painful side and offer him a sweet. The child does not use the nearby, painful arm to take it but reaches across with the other, painless arm. With suitable encouragement normal shoulder and wrist movements may be demonstrated, but there may be a small loss in the range of passive elbow flexion and extension. However, any attempt at producing passive supination

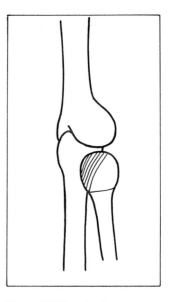

Figure 7.13 Annular ligament displaced over the head of the radius in pulled elbow

be produced. However, when traction was applied to the extended elbow held in pronation (as occurs in the clinical setting) a transverse tear could easily be produced in the distal attachments of the annular ligament to the neck of the radius. The head of the radius can then readily slip through the tear, and the annular ligament becomes detached so that the ligament is interposed between the head of the radius and the capitulum of the humerus (*see Figure 7.13*).

Button-holing of the ligament would then produce pain and a block to active supination. The ligament is released after manipulation and so can heal when it is repositioned in its normal anatomical relationship. The age incidence of pulled elbow is related to the fact that, until about the age of 5 years, the attachments of the ligament are thin and easily disrupted, while above this age the attachments become increasingly thicker.

MANAGEMENT
Manipulation is a simple and effective treatment, which usually produces a dramatic cure. The therapist first needs to gain the child's confidence by gently supporting the injured arm, and a simple manipulation is then performed. The therapist's left hand is placed around the child's elbow to support it with the thumb placed over the head of the radius. The child's hand is held in the therapist's right hand and the forearm is suddenly and firmly forced into full supination. A palpable and often audible click can usually be detected in the region of the radial head as the subluxation is reduced. The child usually stops crying and starts to use the arm again, although this may be delayed for several hours if the lesion has been present for some time. This manipulative reduction is sometimes achieved by a radiology technician when the forearm is forcibly supinated to obtain a true anteroposterior X-ray projection. Only in a very small percentage of patients does the manipulation fail at the first attempt and it is then necessary to repeat the manipulation on the next day. We have never seen a case that needed manipulation under an anaesthetic, but Salter and Zahn (1971) reported one case that required operative reduction. .

The child needs no active treatment after the pulled elbow is reduced but the parents are carefully instructed on the mechanism of the injury to prevent the possibility of a recurrence.

Pushed elbow

This condition follows a fall onto the patient's outstretched hand and the presumed mechanism is that the articular cartilage of the radiohumeral joint is damaged. A common example is in patients who have suffered a Colles' fracture after such a fall and subsequently complain of elbow pain.

Elbow stiffness

This occurs in patients with arthritis or may follow trauma. In the latter it is necessary to exclude myositis ossificans, which follows a haemorrhage into the capsule or the brachial muscle; elbow movements become severely limited and the ossified mass is usually easily palpable. X-rays confirm the diagnosis.

TREATMENT OF ELBOW STIFFNESS
Mobilization techniques with physiological and accessory movements are used. If the range of flexion is limited the following routine is used:

(1) The elbow is flexed to the limit of its range, and small-amplitude oscillatory movements are performed slowly for about 1 minute to stretch the joint. This is followed by accessory movements.
(2) The accessory movements performed at the limit of the flexion range are distraction, flexion–adduction and flexion–abduction as small-amplitude oscillatory movements. On the first day of treatment, the physiological and accessory movements are repeated three times and the range of passive flexion again measured. Next, the patient is reassessed to find whether there has been any painful reaction. If so the strength and amount of treatment must be reduced; if not the same pattern of treatment is repeated more strongly. Over the next few days this routine is repeated, and if the patient is improving active movements are added to increase the range and increase muscle strength. If, however, there is no improvement in the range it is most unlikely that passive-movement techniques will be successful.

If the range of extension is limited the principles of treatment are similar but the physiological movement of extension and the three accessory movements of distraction, extension–adduction and extension–abduction are used.

TREATMENT OF PAINFUL, STIFF ELBOW

If the elbow movements are limited more by pain than by stiffness, large-amplitude flexion movements within the pain-free range are used as the mobilization technique. These are continued for 1 minute and the physiological movements reassessed. If the patient's pain has not been exacerbated this treatment and movement is repeated four times. On the following days, the range of movement and the behaviour of pain throughout this range are reassessed. If they have improved, treatment is continued; if not, the movement should be carried out in the painful range. If this causes an exacerbation of pain this treatment should be discontinued and the treatment outlined above for the stiff elbow substituted.

Loose bodies

AETIOLOGY

(1) Loose, bony foreign bodies may arise as the result of previous trauma to the joint. This happens especially in rugby players and wrestlers, who often fall on to the elbow.
(2) Osteoarthritis may produce either a loose cartilaginous or a bony foreign body.
(3) Osteochondritis dissecans occurs especially in young males, and usually involves the capitulum of the right humerus. At times there may be no history of direct trauma and the patient presents with a gradual onset of pain and stiffness in the elbow.
(4) Synovial osteochondromatosis occasionally occurs in the elbow and produces multiple loose bodies.

Patients present with varying degrees of pain, locking, stiffness and swelling of the elbow. Pain usually comes in sudden attacks associated with locking of the joint. In the usual pattern, there is a block to full extension but flexion remains full and painless. Rarely is this pattern reversed so that extension remains full but there is a block to flexion. Synovial swelling is usually present and X-rays are necessary to confirm the diagnosis.

MANAGEMENT

The elbow is usually locked in extension and manipulation may be used to attempt to free the joint.

The therapist supports the patient's upper arm with his left hand to stabilize it. He grasps the wrist and extends the patient's elbow to the limit of its range. The elbow is then rocked backwards and forwards through the full range of abduction to adduction, and at the same time an attempt is made to ease the elbow into extension. If the loose body is freed the elbow suddenly moves into full extension. If a loose body is producing recurrent or chronic symptoms the joint should be explored surgically and any areas of loose bone or cartilage removed.

Entrapment neuropathies

The ulnar nerve

The ulnar nerve at the elbow passes behind the medial epicondyle in a groove that is converted into a fibro-osseous canal, the cubital tunnel, by the arcuate ligament that runs from the medial epicondyle to the olecranon (Wadsworth and Williams, 1973).

The arcuate ligament is taut at 90 degrees of flexion and lax in extension. The bony floor of this tunnel, formed by the humerus, is lined by the medial ligament of the elbow, which also bulges in flexion. An entrapment neuropathy of the ulnar nerve in the cubital tunnel is common, especially after prolonged flexion of the elbow. The ulnar nerve enters the forearm by passing between the two heads of the flexor carpi ulnaris where it is covered by an aponeurosis and may rarely be the site of an entrapment neuropathy (Kopell and Thompson, 1963).

Aetiology

(1) Acute trauma. The nerve may be damaged by a single traumatic episode as it lies superficially in its groove.
(2) Repeated trauma usually occurs from occupations that involve leaning on the elbow.
(3) Previous trauma to the elbow may result in a cubitus valgus deformity that gradually stretches the nerve. Since the deformity and symptoms take some time to develop this has been called a tardy ulnar palsy.
(4) Cubitus valgus may also be due to arthritis.
(5) Overuse of the elbow can also produce an entrapment neuropathy, since the nerve is tethered in its groove.
(6) The nerve may sometimes sublux in and out of the groove on elbow movements.

Symptoms and signs

Symptoms are mainly sensory with pain and/or paraesthesias in the sensory distribution of the nerve to the medial one and a half fingers. Other sensory symptoms include hyperaesthesia or numbness. Pain may radiate up the forearm to the elbow and may occasionally radiate up as far as the shoulder. Other symptoms include clumsiness of the hand due to weakness of the muscles innervated by the ulnar nerve.

On examination there may be weakness and wasting of the hypothenar eminence and the intrinsic muscles of the hand, often best seen in the first dorsal interosseous space. The typical hand deformity associated with an ulnar nerve lesion is hyperextension at the metacarpophalangeal joints due to intrinsic muscle weakness, and the ulnar two fingers are cocked up because of weakness of their flexor digitorum profundus tendons. Sensation may be disturbed on the palmar or dorsal aspects of the medial one and a half fingers and/or on the ulnar side of the palm of the hand.

Diagnosis

The sensory symptoms may be reproduced by pressure over the ulnar nerve behind the medial epicondyle, where tenderness or thickening of the nerve may be palpable compared with the nerve in the other elbow. Tinel's sign may also be positive and symptoms may be reproduced on sustained full passive flexion of the elbow. Palpation over the ulnar nerve while the elbow is flexed and extended may demonstrate in some patients that the nerve subluxes in and out of its groove.

The diagnosis needs to be confirmed by nerve conduction tests since similar symptoms may arise from lesions in the neck, such as a thoracic-outlet syndrome, or rarely from an entrapment neuropathy of the C8 nerve root in the spinal column.

Management

(1) Avoidance of local extensive trauma and use of foam-rubber elbow pads worn continuously.
(2) Extra rest to the elbow, especially by avoiding repeated or excessive flexion.
(3) Injections: an injection of corticosteroid may be given along the groove behind the medial epicondyle. The therapist inserts the needle so that it travels distally along the canal, being careful not to injure the nerve. If the site of entrapment is between the two heads of the flexor carpi ulnaris, palpation may reveal a localized area of tenderness which can be injected.
(4) Surgery by anterior transposition of the nerve, which may be combined with excision of the medial epicondyle or division of the tendinous origin of the flexor carpi ulnaris from the humerus.

Median nerve

The median nerve crosses the medial side of the lower end of the humerus above the elbow. In this area a vestigial remnant, the ligament of Struthers, may persist and runs from the medial epicondyle upwards to a bony spur on the antero-medial aspect of the humerus. The median nerve runs under this ligament in a fibro-osseous canal when the ligament is present. Below the elbow, the nerve passes through the two heads of origin of the pronator teres muscle, one of which arises from the medial epicondyle and the other from the coronoid process of the ulna. An entrapment neuropathy is rare but may occur in one of these two sites, either above or below the elbow.

Sensory symptoms are similar to those produced by a carpal-tunnel syndrome, as the nerve innervates the lateral three and a half digits. However, motor symptoms are different if compression occurs at the elbow and may include weakness of pronation of the forearm, flexion of the wrist, opposition of the thumb or flexion of the index and middle fingers. If the site of entrapment is in the pronator teres, symptoms may be aggravated by pronation of the forearm.

Radial nerve

The radial nerve at the elbow divides into two branches: one superficial and mainly sensory, the other deep and mainly motor. The latter is also known as the posterior interosseous nerve and it passes under the fibrous origin of the extensor carpi radialis brevis and then pierces the supinator muscles to pass along the interosseous membrane, where it supplies the extensor muscles of the forearm, to reach the wrist.

Entrapment of the superficial branch may

cause pain and altered sensation over the radial aspect of the wrist or thumb. Entrapment of the deep branch may follow direct or indirect trauma to the forearm, or synovitis of the elbow joint. The patient presents with diffuse pain over the forearm and wrist, made worse by supination of the forearm or by wrist movements. There may be wasting of the extensor muscles of the forearm and weakness of wrist and finger extension.

8 The wrist and hand

The wrist is a functional unit made up of the joints between the distal ends of the radius and ulna with the carpal bones. The three joints so formed are:

(1) The radiocarpal joint, between the distal end of the radius and three bones in the proximal row of the carpus (the scaphoid, lunate and triquetrum; *see Figure 8.1*).
(2) The inferior radioulnar joint, formed between the head of the ulna and the radius.
(3) The mid-carpal joint, formed between the proximal and the distal rows of the carpal bones (*see Figure 8.2*).

Movements in the inferior radioulnar joint produce supination and pronation as the radius rotates around the head of the ulna. Movements in the radiocarpal joint produce flexion, extension, radial deviation, ulnar deviation and a combined movement of circumduction. A small but significant degree of these movements also takes place both in the mid-carpal joint and between the carpal bones, mainly in the proximal row

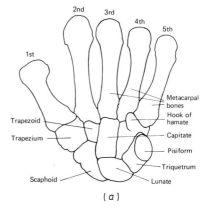

(a)

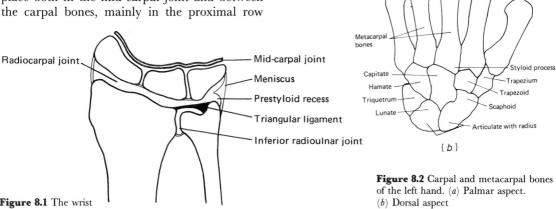

(b)

Figure 8.2 Carpal and metacarpal bones of the left hand. (*a*) Palmar aspect. (*b*) Dorsal aspect

Figure 8.1 The wrist

as the distal row is more firmly attached to the bases of metacarpals. Radiocarpal movements are accompanied by alterations in the shape and direction mainly of the proximal carpal row and the distal carpal row is modified accordingly.

Flexion of the wrist is a combined movement that takes place partly at the radiocarpal joint but mostly at the mid-carpal joints (*see Figure 8.3(a)*). Extension of the wrist (*Figure 8.3(b)*) is also a combined movement but the range is greater at the radiocarpal than at the mid-carpal joint (Gray, 1973). During flexion and extension of the wrist the lunate and capitate bones rotate so that on flexion the space between the dorsal surfaces of the two bones widens and on extension the space between their palmar surfaces widens.

Radial deviation of the radiocarpal joint causes the proximal row of carpal bones and mid-carpal joint to slide reciprocally in an ulnar direction so that the lunate moves to a position under the inferior radioulnar joint. The distal end of the scaphoid partially rotates into the palm and the trapezium slides over its surface. The space

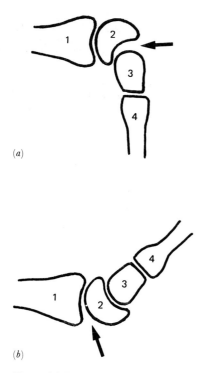

(a)

(b)

Figure 8.3 The wrist, showing: 1, radius; 2, lunate; 3, capitate; 4, metacarpal. Flexion (a) takes place mainly in the mid-carpal joint. Extension (b) takes place mainly in the radiocarpal joint

between the lunate and the triquetrum becomes slightly wider and the capitate slides in an ulnar and proximal direction to produce a tight-packed arrangement. Ulnar deviation of the radiocarpal joint causes the proximal row of carpal bones and the mid-carpal joint to slide reciprocally in a radial direction. In this position the scaphoid becomes elongated and the space between it and the lunate is slightly widened. The capitate moves in a radial and distal direction away from the proximal row of carpal bones, while the hamate moves over the lunate and causes it to rotate into the palm.

Movements of the metacarpophalangeal (MCP) joint

Movements of the MCP joint are flexion, extension, adduction and abduction. The MCP joint is involved in nearly all functional adaptations of the hand and is subjected to a great degree of stress from the surrounding muscles. The movements are not of a simple hinge type and in terms of hand function a pure flexion–extension movement only occurs in the hook grip used in carrying a bag. Flexion of the MCP joint is usually combined with a degree of ulnar deviation and rotation in most functional movements, e.g. when the finger is opposed to the thumb in precision grips or to the thenar eminence in palmar grips. Abduction and adduction are accompanied by a gliding movement of the proximal phalanx on the metacarpal head; the range of this movement is limited by tightening of the collateral ligaments.

Joint stability is supplied by the joint capsule and the collateral ligaments, since the bony surfaces of the joint are incongruous. This provides more effective use of the available power but at the expense of stability (Backhouse, 1969). The MCP joint readily becomes unstable when ligamentous stretching and muscle imbalance occur in an inflammatory arthritis.

Proximal interphalangeal (PIP) joints

The PIP joint is formed between the concave articular head of the proximal phalanx and the convex base of the middle phalanx. It is a hinge joint and the movements of flexion and extension take place by gliding.

Terminal interphalangeal (TIP) joints

These have a similar anatomical arrangement to the PIP joints and the only movements in these hinge joints are flexion and extension.

Hand function

The hand has many functions; for example, it may be used as a tactile organ, a means of expression, and a weapon. Its major musculo-skeletal function lies in its ability to grip objects. Since this requires the hand to function as a unit, grip can never be fully measured in terms of movement of the individual joints. The word grip implies the final static phase of the necessary movements involved; hence prehension, which implies a taking hold or grasping, is a more useful concept. Many classifications of these movements were used until Napier (1956) divided them into two categories, precision grip and power grip. This classification has the advantage of simplicity and a large variety of hand movements can be classified into one or both of these movements.

Precision grip

With precision grip the object has to be picked up and manipulated by the fingers and thumb. This is a dynamic movement and precision handling may be a better descriptive term (Landsmeer, 1962).

It is also mainly a radial-sided movement as the pad of the thumb is manipulated mainly against the next two fingers. This allows three types of grip according to the area of contact:

(1) Tip pinch, in which the pad of the thumb is opposed to the tip of the index finger.
(2) Lateral pinch, in which the pad of the thumb is opposed to the side of the index finger; this is also called a key grip.

(3) Palmar pinch, in which the pad of the thumb is opposed to the pad of one or, more commonly, two pads of the fingers; this is used for picking up and holding an object.

Power grip

With power grip the object is picked up and held tightly as in a clamp. The ulnar two fingers flex across towards the thenar eminence. In the final posture the thenar and hypothenar eminences are used as buttresses and the fingers flex around the object to be grasped. The thumb is used either with its pulp pressed against an object or else wrapped over a heavy object. The crude form of this grip is used while gripping a heavy object such as a hammer and the thumb is used to provide stability and power. A more refined power grip, also called an ulnar grip, is used when a lighter object lying across the palm is gripped mainly by the two ulnar fingers and the thumb is used only for control. With all power grips the hand is kept stable and the power movements are produced by either ulnar and radial deviation of the wrist, as in the action of hammering; supination and pronation of the wrist; or flexion and extension of the elbow.

Examination of the hand and wrist

(1) Inspection:
    (a) Posture.
    (b) Swelling.
    (c) Deformities.
    (d) Muscle wasting.
    (e) Skin changes.

(2) Movements:
    (a) Active.
    (b) Passive.
    (c) Accessory.
    (d) Isometric.

(3) Palpation:
    (a) Warmth.
    (b) Swelling.
    (c) Crepitus.
    (d) Tenderness.

Inspection

Posture

The hand and wrist are first inspected for any abnormalities in posture, which should begin as the patient is first met. The normal hand posture is derived from its three arches, one longitudinal and two transverse, and the hand is normally held slightly flexed. A painful or stiff hand may restrict the normal swinging movement of the arm, as the hand is held stiffly by the side. A patient may be unwilling to use the hand or it may be held splinted across the chest. The hand may also provide a clue to the clinical diagnosis of numerous generalized disease processes.

Swelling

Swelling may be either intra- or extra-articular. Intra-articular swelling may either affect bone, and is then usually due to osteoarthritis, or affect the soft tissues, when it is usually due to inflamed and thickened synovium with a synovial effusion.

Synovitis of the wrist usually presents as a diffuse swelling, commonly on the dorsum of the wrist. It is easily confused with tenosynovitis of the surrounding extensor tendon sheaths, which may also be clinically involved. Synovitis of the MCP and PIP joints bulges onto the looser tissues on the extensor surface of the hand; its shape is determined by the synovial attachments around the joints so that it is limited distally and tends to spread more proximally on either side of the extensor tendon. This gives it a characteristic appearance termed fusiform, spindle or diamond shaped. The effusion is usually evident on inspection; in the early stages of synovitis in the MCP joints the hand should be inspected with the fingers clenched into a fist, when the effusion may become apparent by a filling in of the normal valley between the metacarpal heads. Synovitis produces a diffuse swelling within the synovial joint and so can be easily differentiated from traumatic swellings of the articular structures, which usually form a localized swelling on one side of the joint.

Extra-articular swelling may be either diffuse or localized. Diffuse swelling of the hand is usually due to oedema which may be due to venous or lymphatic obstruction but also occurs in the early stages of rheumatoid arthritis, scleroderma, the shoulder–hand syndrome or Sudeck's atrophy.

Diffuse swelling of a digit produces a sausage-shaped deformity and may be due to psoriatic arthritis or Reiter's disease with synovitis in the PIP joints and the tendon sheaths.

Localized swellings may involve the soft tissues around a joint and tendon sheaths. Tenosynovitis of the wrist may occur in the extensor, flexor or ulnar tendon sheaths. In the palm and fingers it usually involves the flexor tendon sheath and may then be associated with nodule formation and triggering of the finger or thumb. Swelling over the radial styloid occurs in de Quervain's disease. Localized swellings may be due to rheumatoid nodules, tophi, ganglia, granuloma annulare, calcinosis, Garrod's pads, Dupuytren's contracture or cystic swellings associated with Heberden's nodes. A localized bony swelling over the carpus may be due to a dislocated lunate bone.

Deformities

The wrist is normally held in a position midway between flexion–extension and adduction–abduction. Three of the most common deformities that result from inflammatory arthritis in this joint are flexion deformity, palmar subluxation and radial deviation of the wrist. A fixed flexion deformity occurs when the wrist cannot be actively and passively extended to the neutral postion. Palmar subluxation of the carpal bones on the radius results in a bayonet-shaped deformity. Radial deviation of the wrist carries the hand in a radial direction so that the radial styloid approximates to the base of the thumb and there is an undue prominence of the ulnar-sided carpal bones.

Deformity of the inferior radioulnar joint results in a dorsal subluxation or dislocation of the head of the ulna. The head of the ulna becomes prominent and swelling may be accentuated by synovitis in the overlying soft tissue.

THUMB

The three linked joints of the thumb—the carpometacarpal, MCP and IP joints—may be deformed by rheumatoid arthritis, which may produce either a flexion deformity of the MCP joint which is usually associated with a hyperextension deformity of the IP joint; or an adduction deformity of the carpometacarpal joint which may be associated with either a hyperextension deformity of the MCP joint or a hyperextension deformity of the IP joint.

Deformity due to osteoarthritis of the carpometacarpal joint is usually evidenced by a prominence of the base of the metacarpal and adduction deformity of the thumb.

METACARPOPHALANGEAL JOINTS

A flexion deformity of the MCP joints is evidenced by an inability to extend the fingers to the neutral position. In rheumatoid arthritis the most common deformity is a palmar subluxation of the proximal phalanx on the metacarpal bone. It may be associated with an ulnar deviation of the fingers, which may also occur as the sole deformity.

PROXIMAL INTERPHALANGEAL JOINTS

In rheumatoid arthritis either a hyperextension swan-neck deformity or a flexion deformity may occur.

TERMINAL INTERPHALANGEAL JOINT

The common deformity in this joint is a flexion deformity of the terminal phalanx due to a rupture of the extensor tendon.

Muscle wasting

Wasting may be evident in the intrinsic muscles in the hand either between the metacarpals or over the thenar or hypothenar eminences. Small muscle wasting may follow inflammatory arthritis or neurological diseases; for example, peripheral neuropathy, motor-neurone disease or T1 nerve-root lesions. Weakness and wasting of the thenar eminence may occur in median-nerve lesions, e.g. compression in the carpal tunnel.

Skin

Most skin diseases may involve the hand and will be evident on inspection. The hand should also be inspected for any rashes, colour changes, vascular disturbances or nail changes.

Movements

The active and passive movements are tested in all joints of the wrist and hand.

The radiocarpal joint

Four movements—flexion, extension, radial deviation and ulnar deviation—are tested clini-cally. The active range of wrist extension is approximately 70 degrees, flexion 80 or 90 degrees, and the passive range of both these movements is normally a few degrees greater. While the passive range of these movements is tested, the patient's lower arm should be stabilized by the examiner gripping over the dorsal aspect of the lower forearm. However, a quick practical demonstration of the passive range may be made by having the patient adopt two attitudes with the hands. First (*see Figure 8.4*), the wrists are extended by having the patient stand with the elbow flexed and the forearms pronated. The palms of both hands are then approximated into a praying position so that both wrists are passively extended. Second (*see Figure 8.5*), the wrists are passively flexed by having the hands placed back to back.

The range of ulnar deviation is approximately 60 degrees and of radial deviation approximately 20 degrees.

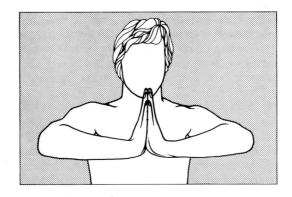

Figure 8.4 Passive dorsiflexion

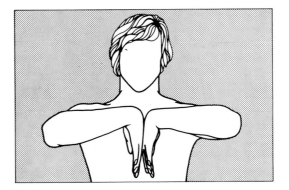

Figure 8.5 Passive palmar flexion

The inferior radioulnar joint

Two movements are tested, supination and pronation, and their range is usually 90 degrees in either direction. The patient is first asked to turn the palm face upwards and then downwards and the examiner then repeats these movements passively.

The thumb

Five movements—flexion, extension, adduction, abduction and opposition—are tested. The thumb movements are tested with the patient's hand supinated, the wrist and fingers held in extension and the thumb in its neutral position.

Active flexion is tested by a combined flexion of the IP joint by asking the patient to carry the thumb across the palm to touch the pad of the thumb against the fat pad at the base of the little finger.

Active extension is tested by having the patient carry the dorsum of the thumb away from the palm. It is more practical to compare the angle formed at the web of the thumb, normally about 90 degrees, in the two hands than to measure the actual range of this movement.

Adduction of the thumb is tested actively by moving the thumb into line with the fingers so that it rests against the second metacarpal.

Abduction of the thumb is tested actively by moving the thumb away from the palmer surface of the hand. It normally forms an angle of about 90 degrees with the web of the thumb.

Opposition of the thumb is tested by rotating the pad of the thumb to touch the pad of the little finger.

Finger joints

Two movements, flexion and extension, are tested while the patient's lower forearm is stabilized by the examiner gripping over it.

(1) The active range of MCP movements is 90 degrees of flexion and 40 degrees of extension. The fingers should be tested together and then individually.
(2) The active range of flexion at the PIP joint is 100 degrees and the range of extension is nought.
(3) The range of flexion at the TIP joint is to approximately 80 degrees and a few degrees of extension are possible.

Joint lesions

The changes produced by joint lesions in the hand and wrist may be summarized as follows.

Terminal interphalangeal joint

(1) Swelling. Soft-tissue swelling may occur in psoriatic arthritis and occasionally in rheumatoid arthritis or tophaceous gout. Bony swelling may be due to Heberden's nodes or an erosive osteoarthritis.
(2) Deformity. The common deformity is a flexion deformity producing a mallet finger.
(3) Instability. Instability may occur in psoriatic arthritis or rheumatoid arthritis and may then form part of the opera-glass hand; it may also occur in osteoarthritis.
(4) Ankylosis. Ankylosis is usually due to psoriatic arthritis but may rarely occur in rheumatoid arthritis or gout.

Proximal interphalangeal joint

(1) Swelling. Soft-tissue swelling is most commonly due to rheumatoid arthritis producing a spindle-shaped swelling. Bony swelling may be due to Bouchard's node or an erosive osteoarthritis.
(2) Deformity. Rheumatoid arthritis may produce a flexion deformity, swan-neck deformity or boutonnière deformity. Flexion deformity of the little finger may be congenital.
(3) Instability. Lateral instability may occur in rheumatoid arthritis or psoriatic arthritis.
(4) Ankylosis is uncommon but may occur in an erosive osteoarthritis and psoriasis.

Metacarpophalangeal joint

(1) Swelling. Soft-tissue swelling is common in rheumatoid arthritis and other forms of arthritis. Bony swelling due to osteoarthritis is rare but may occur with chondrocalcinosis or after trauma.
(2) Deformity. The common deformity due to rheumatoid arthritis is a palmar and/or ulnar subluxation. Flexion deformity may be due to rupture of the extensor tendon.
(3) Instability. Marked instability may occur in the opera-glass hand.

Carpometacarpal joint of the thumb

(1) Swelling. Soft-tissue swelling may be due to rheumatoid arthritis; bony swelling is more common and is due to osteoarthritis.
(2) Deformity. Deformity is common in osteoarthritis. In rheumatoid arthritis the common deformity is an adduction deformity of the thumb.
(3) Instability. Lateral instability occurs as the result of osteoarthritis or inflammatory arthritis.

Wrist and carpus

(1) Swelling. Soft-tissue swelling may be due to an inflammatory or infective arthritis, tenosynovitis, de Quervain's syndrome or a ganglion. Bony swelling of the radiocarpal joint is rare and usually post-traumatic. In the inferior radioulnar joint it may be due to dorsal subluxation of the ulnar head.
(2) Deformity. Deformity may be traumatic as in a Colles' fracture or a Smith's fracture. A flexion deformity occurs in any form of inflammatory arthritis and rheumatoid arthritis may also result in a volar subluxation or radial deviation of the wrist.
(3) Instability of the inferior radioulnar joint may follow rupture of the triangular ligament.
(4) Ankylosis. Ankylosis may follow an inflammatory arthritis.

Accessory movements

INFERIOR RADIOULNAR JOINT
There are five accessory movements routinely tested in this joint:

(1) Posteroanterior movement, which is produced by pressure on the posterior surface of the ulna (*see Figure 8.6*).
(2) Anteroposterior movement, produced by pressure over the anterior surface of the ulna.
(3) Compression, produced by approximating the joint surface (*see Figure 8.7*).

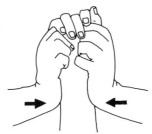

Figure 8.7 Inferior radioulnar joint; compression

(4) Longitudinal cephalad movement, produced in the radius on radial deviation of the wrist.
(5) Longitudinal caudad movement, produced in the radius on ulnar deviation of the wrist.

RADIOCARPAL JOINT
There are eight accessory movements in the radiocarpal joint but only the first six are routinely tested. These are:

(1) Posteroanterior movement, which is produced by pressure over the posterior surface of the carpus (*see Figure 8.8*).

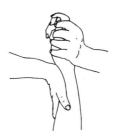

Figure 8.8 Radiocarpal joint; posteroanterior movement

(2) Anteroposterior movement, produced by pressure over the anterior surface of the carpus (*see Figure 8.9*).
(3) Lateral transverse movement, produced by moving the carpus in a lateral direction (*see Figure 8.10*).
(4) Medial transverse movement, produced by moving the carpus medially (*see Figure 8.11*).
(5) Supination, produced by pressure over the

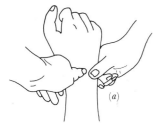

(a)

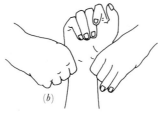

(b)

Figure 8.6 Inferior radioulnar joint; posteroanterior accessory movement; (*a*) posterior view; (*b*) anterior view

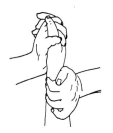

Figure 8.9 Radiocarpal joint; anteroposterior movement

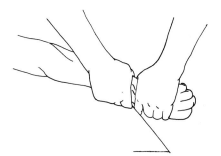

Figure 8.10 Radiocarpal joint; lateral transverse movement

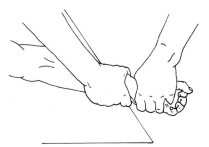

Figure 8.11 Radiocarpal joint; medial transverse movement

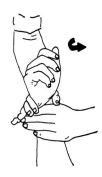

Figure 8.12 Radiocarpal joint; supination

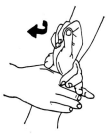

Figure 8.13 Radiocarpal joint; pronation

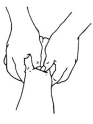

Figure 8.14 Intercarpal joints; posteroanterior movement

anterior surface of the proximal carpus (*see Figure 8.12*).

(6) Pronation, produced by pressure over the posterior surface of the proximal carpus (*see Figure 8.13*).

The two other accessory movements are longitudinal caudad and longitudinal cephalad.

INTERCARPAL JOINTS

There are six accessory intercarpal movements. Their range of movement is small and considerable practice is needed for their assessment;

nevertheless, their importance cannot be too highly stressed. They are:

(1) Posteroanterior movement of one carpal bone on another by pressure over the dorsal surface (*see Figure 8.14*).

(2) Anteroposterior movement, which is produced by pressure over the palmar surface (*see Figure 8.15*).

(3) Horizontal extension, produced by pressure over the dorsal surface of one carpal bone as a fulcrum and extending the other carpal bones around it (*see Figure 8.16*).

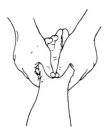

Figure 8.15 Intercarpal joints; anteroposterior movement

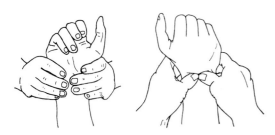

Figure 8.16 Intercarpal joints; horizontal extension

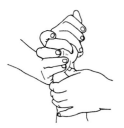

Figure 8.17 Intercarpal movements; horizontal flexion

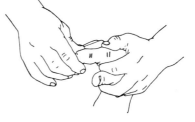

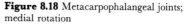

Figure 8.18 Metacarpophalangeal joints; medial rotation

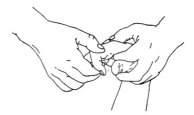

Figure 8.19 Metacarpophalangeal joints; lateral rotation

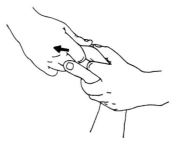

Figure 8.20 Metacarpophalangeal joints; longitudinal caudad movement

(4) Horizontal flexion, produced by pressure over the palmar surface of one carpal bone and cupping the other carpal bones around it (*see Figure 8.17*).
(5) Longitudinal caudad movement, produced by distraction along the metacarpal.
(6) Longitudinal cephalad movement, produced by compression along the metacarpals.

CARPOMETACARPAL JOINTS
There are six accessory movements in the medial four carpometacarpal joints: medial rotation, lateral rotation, anteroposterior, posteroanterior, longitudinal caudad and longitudinal cephalad.

METACARPOPHALANGEAL JOINTS
There are eight accessory movements in the MCP joints:

(1) Medial rotation, which is produced by rotating the proximal phalanx (*see Figure 8.18*).
(2) Lateral rotation, produced by rotating the proximal phalanx (*see Figure 8.19*).
(3) Longitudinal caudad movement, produced by distracting the joint surfaces (*see Figure 8.20*).
(4) Longitudinal cephalad movement, produced by compressing the joint surfaces (*see Figure 8.21*).
(5) Posteroanterior movement, produced by pressure over the posterior surface of the proximal phalanx (*see Figure 8.22*).
(6) Anteroposterior movement, produced by pressure over the anterior surface of the proximal phalanx.

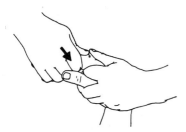

Figure 8.21 Metacarpophalangeal joints; longitudinal cephalad movement

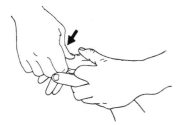

Figure 8.22
Metacarpophalangeal joint; posteroanterior movement

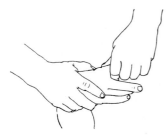

Figure 8.23 Metacarpophalangeal joint; abduction

(7) Abduction, produced by movement of the proximal phalanx away from the middle finger (*see Figure 8.23*).
(8) Adduction, produced by movement of the proximal phalanx towards the middle finger.

Isometric tests

Four isometric contractions are tested at the wrist, three at the thumb, four at the MCP joints and two at the IP joints.

THE WRIST
The four isometric contractions tested are flexion, extension, radial deviation and ulnar deviation.

Pain on resisted flexion may occur in tendinitis of the flexor carpi radialis or of the flexor carpi ulnaris. Pain on resisted extension may occur in tendinitis of the extensor carpi radialis or of the extensor carpi ulnaris. Pain on resisted radial deviation may occur in tendinitis of the flexor carpi radialis or of the extensor carpi radialis. Pain on resisted ulnar deviation may occur in tendinitis of the flexor carpi ulnaris or of the extensor carpi ulnaris.

Thus pain may be reproduced either on wrist flexion or on extension; and with either of these, pain may also be reproduced either on radial or on ulnar deviation of the wrist. From the pattern of movements then built up, the site of tendinitis can be accurately located, as indicated in *Table 8.1*. A painless weakness of any of these four movements usually indicates the presence of a neurological lesion, since rupture of the musculotendinous structures controlling these movements at the wrist is extremely rare.

Table 8.1 Isometric tests in the wrist and hand

Tendon	Flexion	Extension	Radial deviation	Ulnar deviation
Flexor carpi ulnaris	+	−	−	+
Flexor carpi radialis	+	−	+	−
Extensor carpi ulnaris	−	+	−	+
Extensor carpi radialis	−	+	+	−

+ = Painful; − = no pain.

THE THUMB
Pain on resisted flexion of the thumb may occur in flexor tenosynovitis, which may be associated with nodule formation in the tendon. A painless weakness may occur in rupture of the flexor tendon or in C6 nerve-root lesions.

Pain on resisted extension of the thumb may occur with a tenosynovitis of the extensor tendon in the forearm or with a de Quervain's syndrome over the radial styloid. A painless weakness of thumb extension may occur in rupture of the thumb extensor or a C7 nerve-root lesion.

Weakness on resisted abduction of the thumb is usually associated with wasting of the thenar eminence due to a severe degree of compression of the median nerve in the carpal tunnel.

FINGER MOVEMENTS

The four finger movements tested are flexion, extension, adduction and abduction. Finger flexion is tested by having the patient flex all of his fingers at the PIP and TIP joints. The examiner then places his finger-tips against the terminal phalanx of the patient's fingers and attempts to pull them into extension. Normal strength should render this impossible. To differentiate between weakness of the flexor digitorum profundus and the flexor digitorum superficialis the patient's hand is laid flat on the desk, facing palm upwards. To test the profundus tendon the examiner supports the middle phalanx and the patient is asked to bend the TIP joint without bending the other joints of that finger. To test the superficialis tendon, the hand is kept in the same position. The examiner supports the proximal phalanx and asks the patient to bend the PIP joint without bending the MCP or TIP joints of the same finger.

To test finger extension the examiner holds and supports the patient's wrist and asks him to maintain the MCP joints extended with the PIP joint held flexed to prevent the use of intrinsic muscles. The examiner then pushes with his hand over the dorsum of the patient's proximal phalanx and this movement is fully resisted by the patient.

Abduction and adduction of the fingers, controlled by the intrinsic muscles, are best tested with the patient's hand facing palm down, the MCP joint flexed to 90 degrees and the IP joints fully extended. The examiner then fully resists the patient's attempt to push each finger either towards or away from the middle finger. The strength of these movements in the two hands is compared.

Palpation

The wrist and hand should be palpated for the presence of any warmth, crepitus, swelling, deformity or tenderness. The presence of any warmth is detected most easily in the wrist and may be due to inflammatory or infective arthritis. Coarse crepitus due to osteoarthritis may be felt, e.g. in the carpometacarpal joint of the thumb. A fine crepitus occurs in tenosynovitis and a peculiar leathery crepitus is felt over the wrist tendons in scleroderma. Palpation may be also used to confirm the presence of synovitis

which is, as in other areas, often better appreciated by inspection than palpation.

Three bony prominences on the dorsum of the wrist are easily identifiable: the radial styloid; the ulnar styloid; and Lister's tubercle on the radius, about mid-way between the two styloids. The line of the radiocarpal joint lies just distal to this tubercle. The radiocarpal joint is best palpated with two hands so that the thumbs palpate the dorsum of the wrist while the index and middle finger support and palpate its flexor surface. The patient should be relaxed and the wrist held palm downwards in the neutral position. The inferior radioulnar joint is palpated by the thumb and index finger of one of the examiner's hands with the patient's wrist in the same position.

The carpometacarpal compartments of the thumb and fingers should be next palpated with the hand and wrist in the same position. The MCP joints are easily palpable over the dorsal surface of the patient's extended finger by the thumb and index finger of the examiner's hand. The patient's finger is kept stable by the ulnar three fingers of the examiner's hand. Synovitis of the MCP joint is felt as a soft-tissue swelling that bulges on either side of the extensor tendon and may be balloted from side to side. The IP joints are also examined with the finger extended and supported by the examiner, who uses his finger and thumb to palpate any synovial soft-tissue or bony swelling. Tenderness is sought also over the insertions of the tendons into the carpus and in their course in the hand while flexing and extending the fingers.

Classification of musculoskeletal disorders

(1) Soft-tissue lesions:

  (a) Tendon lesions.
  (b) Ligament sprains.
  (c) Dupuytren's contracture.
  (d) Ganglion.
  (e) Volkmann's ischaemic contracture.

(2) Joint diseases.
(3) Bone:

  (a) Osteochondritis of the lunate.

(b) Neurovascular lesions—shoulder–hand syndrome and Sudeck's atropy.

(4) Nerve entrapments:

(a) Median nerve.
(b) Ulnar nerve.
(c) Bowler's thumb.

Tendon lesions

Tendinitis usually involves one of four tendons at the wrist, two of which run on the extensor surface and two on the flexor surface. The two common causes of tendinitis are trauma and overuse. Trauma may follow a fall on the outstretched hand or a strain of the wrist. Overuse occurs most commonly in work that involves repetitive actions and in the racquet sports, squash or tennis. Tendinitis usually occurs just proximal to their insertion or as a tenoperiosteal lesion at their insertion. Tendinitis is also commonly associated with a loss of the normal accessory movements of the intercarpal joints.

Extensor carpi radialis

Two tendons are involved in radial extension of the wrist: the extensor carpi radialis longus, which is inserted into the base of the second metacarpal bone, and the extensor carpi radialis brevis, inserted into the base of the third metacarpal.

Pain is reproduced by an isometric contraction that fully resists:

(1) Radial deviation of the wrist, which is made more pronounced if the wrist is first passively stretched into ulnar deviation and the movement back into radial deviation of the wrist fully resisted.
(2) Wrist extension (*see Table 8.1*). Tenderness is localized over the tendon insertion and is usually best appreciated if the hand is held clenched with the wrist extended.

Extensor carpi ulnaris

This tendon runs over the ulnar styloid and is inserted into the extensor surface of the base of the fifth metacarpal.

Pain is reproduced by isometric contraction that fully resists:

(1) Ulnar deviation of the wrist. This is made

more pronounced if the wrist is first of all passively stretched into full radial deviation and the movement back into ulnar deviation of the wrist is fully resisted.
(2) Wrist extension. Tenderness is usually well localized over the tendon insertion and is best appreciated if the hand is clenched into a fist with the wrist held in extension.

Flexor carpi ulnaris

Tendinitis usually occurs as a tenoperiosteal lesion at the insertion of the tendon into the palmar surface of the base of the pisiform bone. Pain is reproduced by an isometric contraction that fully resists:

(1) Ulnar deviation of the wrist, which is made more pronounced if the wrist is first held in full passive radial deviation and then the movement back into ulnar deviation of the wrist is fully resisted.
(2) Wrist flexion. Localized tenderness over the insertion of this tendon is usually best felt with the wrist held in full extension.

Flexor carpi radialis

Tendinitis of the flexor carpi radialis is the least common of these four tendon lesions and usually occurs as a tenoperiosteal injury at its insertion into the palmar surface of the base of the second metacarpal bone.

Management of tendinitis

(1) Rest from those activities that produce pain is usually necessary.
(2) Non-steroidal anti-inflammatories are given.
(3) Physical methods, such as ultrasound or deep-friction massage, are often helpful.
(4) Injections. The tender area in the tendon is identified by palpation and the wrist is positioned to stretch the tendon. A 25-gauge needle is used and 1 ml of local anaesthetic and corticosteroid injected around the tender area.
(5) Exercise and stretching regimens are taught to the patient to perform himself.
(6) Mobilization techniques; these will be discussed in more detail.

MOBILIZATION TECHNIQUES
In many patients with tendinitis, examination

reveals a restriction in the normal range of accessory movements in the carpal joints. Treatment by mobilization techniques should then be given to ease pain and restore normal joint movement. Careful clinical examination is essential to determine which joint is restricted and treatment techniques are then localized as accurately as possible to that joint. Successful treatment usually depends on using the movement that provokes pain most readily.

When pain is the dominant factor, treatment techniques are used with a large amplitude of movement, performed painlessly at first and then into the most painful direction. For example, if extension of the wrist is painful treatment is started first with the wrist in the fully flexed position. The wrist is then rocked back and forth into extension using large-amplitude grade II movements without provoking pain (*see Figure 8.24*). If this technique is successful and pain-free range of active movement increases treatment is taken further into the range until a degree of discomfort is produced.

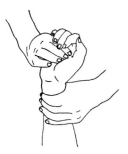

Figure 8.24 Treatment of tendinitis using radiocarpal extension

When stiffness is the dominant factor, treatment is first undertaken using the restricted physiological movement. Strong stretching movements, using small-amplitude oscillatory movements at the end of that range, are necessary. Accessory movements of the carpal bones with anteroposterior or posteroanterior pressures on adjacent carpal bone are then added.

When pain and stiffness are present, treatment usually consists of three stages:

(1) Pain is first treated by the method described above.
(2) Movements are next taken into a degree of stiffness and discomfort, taking care not to provoke any severe exacerbation. If not, treatment is taken further into the most restricted range, using smaller amplitude movements more strongly.
(3) If there is no response treatment needs to be modified, using movements that reproduce pain that are carried slowly further into the range, until pain suddenly becomes sharply exacerbated. Small-amplitude oscillatory movements are used at this point and then eased off into the less painful range, where accessory and physiological movements are used.

Tenosynovitis

Extensor tenosynovitis at the wrist presents as a swelling localized to the anatomical confines of the synovium over the extensor tendons to the fingers that terminates about the middle of the dorsum of the hand. The patient may present with pain over the dorsal aspect of the hand and the swelling is made more obvious by resisted extension of the fingers. It may be difficult to differentiate this swelling clinically from synovitis of the wrist but tenosynovial swelling is usually made more obvious on resisted extension of the fingers and wrist throughout their full range. Crepitus may be present.

Tenosynovitis of the ulnar tendons is common in rheumatoid arthritis, when it may be the first manifestation of this disease and is usually bilateral. Pain may be produced by resisting ulnar deviation of the wrist.

Tenosynovitis of the flexor tendons in the wrist usually occurs as the result of overuse or in inflammatory diseases such as rheumatoid arthritis. It may cause swelling in or proximal to the carpal tunnel or else present as a compound palmar ganglion. Pain and crepitus may be reproduced when the tendon and sheath are held compressed while the tendon is made to move through its full range.

Compound palmar ganglion

This is a chronic inflammatory synovitis of the flexor tendon sheath at the wrist with a swelling that is visible and palpable proximal to the flexor retinaculum in the forearm and distal to it in the palm. Cross-fluctuation between these two sites may be obtained by compressing one or other part of the swelling. It used to be most commonly tuberculous in origin, but nowadays the most common cause is rheumatoid arthritis. The inflamed synovial membrane is thickened and may contain deposits of fibrin formed into rice bodies.

de Quervain's disease

This form of stenosing tendovaginitis involves the thumb tendons at the wrist. The two tendons involved are the abductor pollicis longus and the extensor pollicis brevis, which run in a bony groove across the styloid process of the radius where they are invested in a common synovial sheath which is exposed to repeated friction. Inflammation of the tendon sheath results in thickening that ultimately causes a constriction of the two tendons. In most cases it follows overuse of the wrist.

The patient is usually a middle-aged female who presents with pain over the radial surface of the wrist, often severe and made worse by movements of either the thumb or wrist. Pain brought on by thumb movements usually occurs in a pinch grip during which the tendon of the abductor pollicis stabilizes the base of the thumb. Pain on wrist movements occurs particularly on supination of the wrist while the hand is clenched, as in wringing out clothes. The patient may also be conscious of a tender swelling over the radial styloid at the wrist.

MAJOR SIGN

Pain is reproduced on ulnar deviation of the wrist with the patient's thumb held flexed and adducted and then grasped by the other fingers into the palm of the hand (*see Figure 8.25(a)*). The examiner then holds the patient's forearm with his other hand (*Figure 8.25(b)*). Pain on this movement is also reproduced in patients with osteoarthritis of the carpometacarpal joint of the thumb.

OTHER SIGNS

Swelling localized over the radial styloid process is usually obvious on inspection of the wrist. It is associated with tenderness, at times extreme, over the swelling itself or over the nearby radial styloid process. X-rays of the wrist joint are normal but may show a soft-tissue swelling.

MANAGEMENT

(1) Rest from those movements that aggravate the pain is usually difficult to achieve and splints are usually impractical.
(2) Anti-inflammatory drugs and physical methods usually provide little or temporary benefit.
(3) A local injection of corticosteroid is the treatment of choice as one or two injections

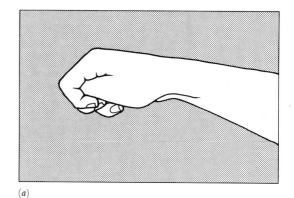

(a)

(b)

Figure 8.25 de Quervain's disease: major sign. (a) The patient's thumb is grasped in his fingers; passive ulnar deviation (b) then reproduces the patient's pain

usually produce complete relief of symptoms. The patient sits with the wrist in ulnar deviation and the thumb flexed to stretch the tendon. A 25-gauge needle is inserted distal to the tender swelling and directed proximally under the tendon sheath. 1 ml corticosteroid solution is injected, which may be repeated in a few weeks if symptoms have not completely resolved. Care must be taken not to inject the solution directly into the tendon itself.

(4) Surgery is indicated in those patients whose symptoms fail to resolve or are recurrent. A small transverse skin incision is used and the thickened tendon sheath is split longitudinally to decompress the tendon. It is important to determine whether the extensor pollicis brevis lies within the same sheath and not in a separate sheath or that anatomical variations in the insertion of abductor pollicis longus are not present. If either of these are present and not corrected the operation will fail.

Tendon rupture

Rupture of the finger tendons is common and usually involves the extensor tendons of the ring and little fingers.

The patient presents with the affected digit held in a position of flexion. Active extension of the affected finger is impossible, passive movement of the digit is normal and resisted extension is weak and painless.

Mallet finger

This common condition is due to rupture of the long extensor of the finger at its insertion into the base of the distal phalanx of the finger. It may occur either as the result of rheumatoid synovitis of the terminal interphalangeal joint of the finger or more commonly follows trauma. A fragment of bone may be avulsed with the tendon from the distal phalanx. The usual mechanism of this injury is a direct blow to the end of the finger while the terminal joint is held extended. Two implements that may produce it are a mallet or a baseball, which has given rise to its more common names of mallet or baseball finger.

The patient presents with a flexion deformity of the terminal joint of the involved finger. Active extension of the flexed terminal interphalangeal joint is impossible and is associated with a painless weakness of resisted terminal joint extension, but passive movement of the joint can straighten the terminal phalanx. The area of the tendon insertion is tender and swollen and an X-ray may reveal an avulsed fragment of bone.

MANAGEMENT
The terminal interphalangeal joint may be splinted in slight hyperextension by a dorsal splint that does not immobilize the proximal joint. The splint needs to be maintained in position undisturbed for approximately 6 weeks and is then applied intermittently over the next few weeks to protect the joint.

Operation is rarely indicated; fixation may be achieved by a Kirschner wire inserted through the terminal phalanx and across the terminal joint. If a large fragment of bone has been avulsed open reduction should be carried out.

Trigger finger

Triggering of the fingers or thumb occurs as a result of nodule formation within a flexor tendon.

This may occur as a complication of either a simple tenosynovitis, usually due to overuse, or of rheumatoid arthritis. The nodule formed within the synovial sheath is usually small, so that on flexion it moves with its tendon under the metacarpophalangeal ligament which binds the flexor tendon.

Most commonly, the nodule is trapped under the metacarpophalangeal ligament as the tendon flexes. The finger is then locked in flexion and active extension is impossible. To unlock the finger and return it to its normal mobility the patient may have to extend it passively, producing a sudden snapping (i.e. triggering) of the digit. This manoeuvre occurs repeatedly, producing a traumatic tenosynovitis in the flexor tendon sheath so that movement becomes even more easily impeded. At times, there may be a painful restriction of finger flexion or the nodule may be so large that it will not pass under the flexor ligament and active flexion of the finger is impossible.

A similar type of triggering may occur in the thumb as the result of nodule formation preventing free movement of the flexor pollicis tendon. This occurs also in children, who usually present with a flexion deformity of the thumb.

MANAGEMENT
Injection of corticosteroid usually relieves symptoms for a prolonged period of time, presumably by decreasing the swelling around the sheath and so relieving the obstruction.

Method—A 25-gauge needle is inserted distal to the nodular swelling and directed proximally under the tendon sheath. 1 ml of corticosteroid solution is injected at this site and may be repeated after a few weeks if symptoms are not completely relieved. If the patient has other evidence of flexor tenosynovitis, with swelling over the proximal phalanx, this area should also be injected.

If injections fail surgery is usually indicated. A transverse skin incision is made proximal to the tendon nodule and the thickened tendon sheath is incised. This operation usually gives permanent relief and it is not necessary to remove the nodule.

Ligament sprains

Inferior radioulnar joint

A tear of the triangular ligament in the inferior radioulnar joint is uncommon. It usually follows an indirect injury in which the forearm is suddenly and forcefully turned into pronation or supination. As a sporting injury, it occurs most commonly in tennis players. The patient complains of pain, usually over the distal end of the ulna, associated with a painful clicking and a sensation of weakness or instability in the wrist. Pain and clicking may be reproduced on circumduction, ulnar or radial deviation of the wrist, or by passive movement of the ulnar head. Diagnosis is confirmed by arthrography of the wrist.

MANAGEMENT

Treatment consists of rest to the wrist in an attempt to promote healing. Physical measures have no role but the inferior radioulnar joint may be injected two or three times with corticosteroid.

If symptoms persist the damaged ligament may be excised, but the wrist is then often left weak and painful on use and it may be difficult for the patient to resume first-class tennis.

Radiocarpal joint

A sprain of either the ulnar or the radial collateral ligaments of the wrist is uncommon. Nevertheless a diagnosis of wrist sprain is commonly made and extreme caution is necessary to differentiate other more serious conditions, such as a fractured scaphoid. Clinically, pain is reproduced on passive stretching of the involved ligament and tenderness is usually localized over the proximal attachment.

Intercarpal joints

Ligamentous sprains of the intercarpal joints may also follow trauma and the scaphoid–lunate ligament is most commonly involved. Pain is reproduced on movement of the wrist or by testing the accessory movements.

MANAGEMENT

The management of sprains of the radiocarpal or intercarpal joints is similar, and consists of:

(1) Rest from those activities that aggravate pain.
(2) Physical methods, such as ultrasound or deep-friction massage.
(3) Mobilization techniques using accessory joint movements are useful both in easing pain and in restoring normal joint movement.
(4) Injections of corticosteroid into locally tender areas.

Rupture of the scaphoid–lunate ligament

Rupture of this ligament is associated with a rotary subluxation of the lunate. Tenderness is felt diffusely over the wrist and the diagnosis is often missed. If it is suspected, an X-ray should be taken with the hand in a position of full supination (Howard and Fahey, 1974). A separation of the scaphoid–lunate joint by more than 2 mm is diagnostic. This has been given the felicitous title of the Terry Thomas sign by Frankel (1977), who likened it to the gap present in the comedian's front teeth. The lunate may sublux intermittently with wrist movements and produce a painful click in the wrist; cineradiography may be used to diagnose this complication.

MANAGEMENT

This injury may be treated by immobilization in a plaster cast with the wrist in a position of radial deviation to approximate the lunate and scaphoid. This needs to be maintained for at least 8 weeks, but results are often unsatisfactory. Surgery is indicated if conservative measures fail to reduce the subluxation or may be used as the treatment of choice. Primary repair of the torn ligament is not usually possible and so fixation of the bone ends with a pin is necessary.

Metacarpophalangeal joints

A sprain of the ulnar collateral ligament of the MCP joint of the thumb is not uncommon after indirect trauma. A complete rupture of this ligament is also known as gamekeeper's thumb because of the action used with the inside of a gamekeeper's thumb to break a rabbit's neck. It is also a common skiing injury which follows a fall onto the hand with the stock held firmly clenched by the thumb. The distal attachment of the ligament is usually avulsed and displaced proximally.

The rupture is diagnosed by keeping the patient's thumb fully extended and applying an abduction strain to the MCP joint to demonstrate any lateral instability.

An X-ray may show that a flake of bone has been avulsed with the ligament.

Dupuytren's contracture

Dupuytren's contracture is a fibrous proliferation in the palmar fascia of the hand that gradually produces a flexion deformity of the MCP and PIP joints. The palmar fascia is continuous with the distal edge of the flexor retinaculum of the wrist into which the palmaris longus tendon is inserted. It forms an expansion of connective tissue covering the palm of the hand with elongations passing distally into the fingers and thumb.

Dupuytren's contracture occurs mainly in white males between the ages of 60 and 70 and usually involves the ring and little fingers in either hand, and less commonly the middle fingers. It is present bilaterally in approximately half of the patients. Its aetiology is unknown but it occurs mainly in male patients of European descent and appears to be inherited by autosomal dominance. It also occurs as a complication of some diseases such as chronic alcoholism and epilepsy and a similar type of contracture may occur in the shoulder–hand syndrome.

The disease begins as a small, fibrous nodular thickening in the palmar fascia usually about the level of the distal palmar skin crease. This increases in size to form a thickened longitudinal fibrous cord-like band. The skin is firmly attached to the fascia by tiny fasciculi and becomes dimpled and puckered as the contracture develops. The nodular thickening also involves the elongation of the palmar fascia into the fingers, and the fingers develop a flexion contracture. The thickening does not directly involve the joints but they may develop a secondary fibrous capsular contracture or degenerative changes in the articular cartilage.

The patient complains at first of a nodular swelling in the palm, which may be painful on use of the hand. Subsequently the condition is painless but the patient complains of loss of function due to the flexor contracture of the involved finger or fingers.

Ganglion

A ganglion is a small, pea-shaped soft-tissue swelling found most commonly over the dorsum of the carpal bones, especially the capitate, or less commonly on the flexor surface of the wrist. It contains mucinous material and is usually soft and cystic to palpate. At times, however, the swelling may be tense and confused with a bony swelling. A ganglion arises from a joint capsule or a tendon sheath and may follow trauma. The patient is usually a young adult who presents with a lump, which may be associated with some degree of pain usually related to movement. The swelling is well defined and may be slightly tender. It may at times spontaneously disappear.

Management

If symptomatic, the swelling may be repeatedly punctured with a 22-gauge needle and injected with 1 ml of corticosteroid.

If this fails, or if the swelling readily recurs and is troublesome, an operation to remove the sac may be required. This often requires quite an extensive dissection, and a pedicle that connects to a tendon or carpal joint should be sought and closed off.

Volkmann's ischaemic contracture

Volkmann's contracture is due to ischaemia of the flexor muscles of the forearm, which become fibrosed after a lesion of the brachial artery which may be damaged in elbow injuries. It usually starts with pain in the forearm and is associated with neurological symptoms and an absent radial pulse. The forearm becomes wasted and the fingers are held flexed, which produces a claw hand. Extension of the fingers is possible only if the wrist is held flexed.

Arthritis

The hand and wrist are involved during the course of most types of arthritis and the differential diagnosis of the more common forms has been considered above. Osteoarthritis commonly involves the interphalangeal joints of the fingers and the carpometacarpal joint of the thumb. Degenerative changes produce bony swellings around the margins of the joint known as Heberden's nodes in the terminal joint, and Bouchard's nodes in the proximal joints. They occur commonly in middle-aged females as part of a primary generalized osteoarthritis. The joint becomes enlarged and tender, and pain may be related to overuse of the joint.

Heberden's nodes:

(1) May begin insidiously with little pain or discomfort and then gradually increase in size.
(2) May develop rapidly with pain, redness and tenderness around the joint.
(3) May present as cystic swelling containing gelatinous mucoid material over the joint margin or over the extensor surface of the distal phalanx.

Similar changes may occur in the PIP joint, known as Bouchard's nodes, and are also found in primary generalized osteoarthritis usually after the terminal joint has been involved. Primary osteoarthritis in the MCP joint is uncommon but may occur secondary to repeated trauma, chondrocalcinosis or haemochromatosis.

Osteoarthritis of the carpometacarpal joint of the thumb

The first carpometacarpal joint plays a major role in positioning the thumb and so is important for normal hand function (Swanson, 1968). The joint has two biconcave saddle-shaped surfaces which allow flexion, extension, abduction, adduction and rotation; combined movements produce opposition and circumduction of the thumb. As the thumb rotates around the long axis of its metacarpal bone the joint surfaces become incongruous, and stability is maintained by tightening of the anterior carpometacarpal ligament. In this position increased pressure is applied to the dorsal aspect of the joint and so the joint has a tendency to sublux dorsally and radially.

Osteoarthritis of this joint occurs most commonly in middle-aged females in whom it may be bilateral and occur as part of a primary generalized osteoarthritis. It may, however, also occur in a young male patient after previous trauma, such as a Bennett's fracture. The patient presents with pain around the base of the thumb, which is made worse by use, especially those activities associated with pinch grip, axial compression of the thumb—for example, in opening the latch of a car door—or rotational movements such as wringing out clothes.

In the early stages, active and passive movements are usually restricted at the limits of their ranges. Pain may be reproduced if the examiner grips the patient's thumb and compresses along the metacarpal shaft in a proximal direction while simultaneously moving the metacarpal into adduction. Crepitus and instability of the carpometacarpal joint may also be felt with the thumb of the other hand placed over the joint. Subsequently, deformities develop with the thumb in a position of adduction. A hyperextension deformity of the MCP or IP joint of the thumb may develop, possibly caused by attempts to increase the range of the hand's grasp. The carpometacarpal joint develops a bony, square enlargement due to the degenerative changes and dorsal subluxation.

Osteoarthritis may need to be differentiated from a de Quervain's syndrome or a carpal-tunnel syndrome, either of which may produce pain in the thumb. It may also occur with either of these conditions and may also be associated with degenerative changes in the joint between the trapezium and scaphoid, especially in patients with hypermobility syndrome who may have practised repetitive trick movements with their thumb.

The diagnosis needs to be confirmed on X-ray, which should include oblique views. In the early stages an X-ray taken while the patient performs a pinch grip may demonstrate dorsal subluxation of the joint.

MANAGEMENT

(1) Rest from those movements that aggravate the pain is important but difficult since this joint is involved in many functional movements of the hand. Various forms of splints have been described but are difficult for the patient to manage and are not often helpful.
(2) Anti-inflammatory drugs and analgesics are given as necessary.
(3) Physical methods are only of limited value.
(4) Manual therapy: treatment consists firstly of large-amplitude movements that are given without provoking any discomfort. As symptoms settle, these movements can be increased further into the range and so may provoke some discomfort. Finally, treatment with small-amplitude movements that provoke pain are used. These may also be used while compressing the joint with pressure along the metacarpal shaft. When indicated by a related pain response, mobilizing may be required to be localized to the joints between the base of the metacarpal, the trapezium and the trapezoid.
(5) Injections of local anaesthetic and corticosteroid into the joint may be given using a 25-gauge needle but do not often provide any lasting relief.
(6) Surgery is indicated if pain and disability are severe. The choice of operation lies between arthrodesis of the joint, removal of the trapezium, or a Silastic implant.

Bone disorders

Osteochondritis of the lunate

This form of avascular necrosis usually occurs in young adults over the age of 15 years. Males are affected more often than females and the right hand more often than the left. It usually follows either acute trauma that produces a compression fracture of the bone or repeated minor trauma, such as in an overuse syndrome. X-ray changes may take some time to develop but eventually the bone appears sclerotic and later becomes fragmented, irregular and altered in shape.

The patient presents with pain and stiffness in the wrist, made worse by use, and usually a gradually progressive swelling may be present. Tenderness is usually localized over the lunate bone. The disease usually runs a course over 2 years, and osteoarthritis of the wrist commonly develops in later life.

MANAGEMENT
Management of this condition is difficult, especially in young players of racquet sports. In the early stages the wrist should be immobilized in a plaster cast for several months to allow pain to settle and attempt repair. Protection may then be given by a reinforced wrist splint, which can be worn when the patient attempts to return to sport. In later life degenerative changes are common. Attempts have been made to replace the bone with a Silastic implant but have not generally been successful. If pain persists an arthrodesis of the wrist may be necessary.

Neurovascular disturbances

Neurovascular disorders associated with a severe degree of osteoporosis of bone include the shoulder–hand syndrome and Sudeck's atrophy.

SUDECK'S ATROPHY
This is a form of reflex sympathetic dystrophy in which the patient presents with severe pain, swelling and disability of the hand. It may occur as an idiopathic condition or follow prolonged immobilization but commonly follows trauma, which may at times be only minor. It may also occur rarely as a complication of neurological disorders. At first, the hand is red and swollen and the skin warm and dry. Subsequently the hand becomes cold, blue, and moist and later appears shiny and stiff with wasting of the small muscles and contractures of the fingers.
Management Management in the early stages is designed to prevent pain, relieve swelling, maintain hand function and prevent future joint stiffness. The patient needs considerable reassurance and support.

(1) Relief from pain must be obtained; dosages of analgesics must be adequate.
(2) The patient must be encouraged to keep using the hand, even though it is painful, as immobilization will make this condition worse. Active exercises should also be given.
(3) Physical methods used to control pain include ice and transcutaneous nerve stimulation.
(4) Passive movements are used to prevent subsequent stiffness in the small joints of the hand and wrist.
(5) In patients with severe pain and swelling, a stellate ganglion block or sympathectomy should be performed.
(6) Corticosteroids have been advocated to prevent inflammatory oedema. If they are to be used they must be given in the early stages, but their use has not been fully evaluated.

Nerve entrapments

Carpal-tunnel syndrome

An entrapment neuropathy of the median nerve in the carpal tunnel of the wrist is common. The convex anterior surface of the carpal bones is converted into a fibro-osseous tunnel by the transverse carpal ligament which runs from the pisiform bone and the hook of the hamate on

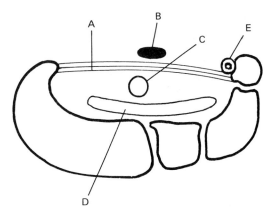

Figure 8.26 The carpal tunnel. (A) Transverse carpal ligament running from the scaphoid to the pisiform. (B) Palmaris longus tendon. (C) The median nerve. (D) Flexor tendons of the fingers. (E) Ulnar nerve and artery

the ulnar side to tubercles on the scaphoid and trapezium on the radial side. The flexor tendons of the fingers and the median nerve run through this tunnel as they pass from the forearm into the hand (*see Figure 8.26*).

Alterations in any of the anatomical structures in the tunnel can result in a loss of volume in the available space in the carpal tunnel and so produce compression of the median nerve. The common cause is swelling due to a tenosynovitis in the flexor tendons. This may follow overuse of the wrist, e.g. in occupational stresses that involve either repeated flexion of the wrist or alternatively gripping movements with the wrist held extended. It may also follow prolonged use of the wrist by arthritic patients who need to use a walking stick. Rheumatoid arthritis produces an inflammatory tenosynovitis of the flexor tendons or synovitis of the wrist joint. This may occur in the early stages of the disease, and so the diagnosis may then be overlooked as the patient's hand pain is presumed to be due to rheumatoid disease alone (Chamberlain and Corbett, 1970).

A carpal-tunnel syndrome may also be associated with previous trauma, such as Colles' fracture or subluxation of the lunate, osteoarthritis of the wrist or ganglion formation (Robbins, 1963). It may also occur during the last trimester of pregnancy or as part of the premenstrual syndrome, presumably due to fluid retention. Various metabolic diseases, including tophaceous gout (Champion, 1969), hypothyroidism, acromegaly or amyloidosis, have also been described as a cause.

CLINICAL FINDINGS

The patient is usually a middle-aged female and one or both hands, but more commonly the dominant hand, may be involved. The symptoms of pain and/or paraesthesias are usually characteristic. Pain is felt in the distribution of the median nerve in the hand and is most severe at night, when it commonly disturbs the patient's sleep. However, pain may also radiate up the arm and may be felt in the elbow or shoulder. Paraesthesias may also occur in the hands, especially at night, and are often relieved by the patient moving the hands about or by posturing them over the edge of the bed or above the shoulder. They are usually felt in the distribution of the median nerve in the hand but the patient often complains that they are present in all fingers. Careful questioning may then determine whether the little finger is spared. The patient may also complain of an unpleasant sensation of fullness or stiffness in the fingers, especially in the morning, or that the fingers feel clumsy or weak.

MAJOR SIGNS

The patient's symptoms may be reproduced by various manoeuvres that are designed to produce increased compression of the median nerve in the carpal tunnel. This may be achieved by the examiner placing his thumb over the patient's wrist and then fully flexing the patient's hand for approximately 1 minute. Alternatively, both wrists may be held fully flexed by compressing the dorsal surfaces of the hands together (Phalen's sign).

OTHER SIGNS

Tapping over the median nerve at the wrist (Tinel's sign) may also reproduce the patient's symptoms. A neurological examination of the hand must be undertaken to determine any loss of sensation in the fingers, by using a pin prick or the two-point discrimination test; wasting of the thenar prominence; and any weakness in opposition or abduction of the thumb.

Examination of the whole of the upper limb and neck is also necessary to exclude a more proximal cause of an entrapment neuropathy. Symptoms of the carpal-tunnel syndrome may be confused with a cervical spondylosis, or the two conditions may occur together. Carpal-tunnel compression may be accompanied by a lateral epicondylitis of the elbow (Murray-Leslie and Wright, 1976).

INVESTIGATIONS

Nerve conduction tests using sensory and motor latencies may be carried out and a comparison made with either the normal limb or with conduction in the ulnar nerve. The most common finding in patients with carpal-tunnel syndrome is a prolongation of the terminal sensory latency. X-rays of the wrist should also include a view to show the bony outlines of the carpal tunnel. It may be necessary to exclude any underlying metabolic disorder or space-occupying lesions of the carpal tunnel by using appropriate investigations. In most patients, however, the entrapment follows overuse of the wrist with a flexor tenosynovitis.

MANAGEMENT

(1) Rest to the wrist. This may require a volar splint that is worn with the wrist held in the neutral position and includes the flexed fingers. It may be worn at night only, or continuously if symptoms are severe.

(2) Anti-inflammatory drugs rarely provide any relief of symptoms.

(3) Injections. An injection of corticosteroid into the carpal tunnel is a simple procedure that usually produces significant symptomatic relief within a day. 1 ml of corticosteroid solution is injected without any local anaesthetic, as this may anaesthetize the nerve. This injection usually produces such good symptomatic relief that it may also be used as a diagnostic test.

Method of injection The patient sits with the wrist extended and fully supinated. The palmaris longus tendon, under which the median nerve is situated, can be easily recognized in most patients by palpation. A site is chosen on the volar aspect of the wrist approximately 3 cm proximal to the transverse crease of the wrist and midway between the palmaris longus tendon and the ulnar artery. A 25-gauge needle is inserted through the skin, being careful to avoid the superficial veins. The needle is then directed distally in almost a horizontal direction so that it runs parallel with the tendons and nerves until it comes to lie in the carpal tunnel. This injection is atraumatic and relatively painless. 1 ml of corticosteroid solution is then injected; this usually produces some exacerbation of pain for a short time only. A single injection will usually produce either complete or considerable relief; however, if the symptoms are not completely relieved this injection should be repeated once or twice at fortnightly intervals.

(4) Physical methods—such as heat, exercise or massage—have no role in the treatment of this condition.

(5) Mobilization. Passive movements aimed at stretching the flexor retinaculum and improving the posteroanterior range of the intercarpal joints may be useful.

(6) Surgery is indicated if:

(a) Conservative methods fail.

(b) Repeated injections are necessary at frequent intervals.

(c) Severe motor impairment of the muscles of the thenar eminence is present.

At operation the transverse carpal ligament must be adequately exposed so that it can be completely divided. This operation may need to be combined with a synovectomy of the flexor tendons.

Ulnar-nerve compression

The ulnar nerve crosses the wrist together with the ulnar artery. In the hand it passes through the tunnel of Guyon, which is bounded on its ulnar side by the pisiform bone and on its radial side by the hook of the hamate; it lies anterior and medial to the transverse carpal ligament. Near the pisiform bone, the nerve divides into a superficial and deep branch. The superficial, mainly sensory, nerve supplies the skin over the hypothenar eminence, the little finger and half of the ring finger. The deep branch supplies the muscles of the hypothenar eminence and most of the intrinsic muscles of the hand.

The ulnar nerve may be compressed in the wrist after trauma, such as a Colles' fracture, or from tendinitis of the flexor carpi ulnaris at its insertion into the pisiform. It may also occur as an acute injury after a blow to the open hand, as in attempting to push upwards a jammed window, or by compression after repeated occupational trauma to the palmar surface of the wrist. The nerve may also be entrapped in the tunnel of Guyon by a ganglion or after repeated overuse of the wrist, such as with a walking stick.

If the superficial division of the nerve is involved it is associated with pain and/or paraesthesias in the sensory distribution of the ulnar nerve to the ring and little fingers. Pressure and percussion over the nerve near the pisiform bone should reproduce the patient's symptoms.

If the deep branch is entrapped patients often complain of a deep aching pain in the palm of the hand but there are no sensory disturbances. Weakness and wasting develop in the hypothenar muscles, the interossei and the adductor pollicis brevis.

MANAGEMENT

The same principles of managing carpal-tunnel compression apply to this condition.

Bowler's thumb

Bowlers use their thumb and index finger inserted into the holes in the bowl for control. This may cause a traumatic neuroma of the digital nerve on the ulnar side of the thumb. Pain is felt in the distribution of the nerve and may be associated with hyperaesthesia and atrophy of the overlying skin. Dobyns *et al.* (1972) reported on 17 patients with this condition. Conservative management, including a protective shell for the thumb, was first used to treat this group but failed to improve symptoms. Surgery to relieve the nerve compression was reported as producing good results.

9   The hip

The hip is a synovial ball-and-socket joint formed between the head of the femur, which normally constitutes two-thirds of a sphere, and the cup-shaped acetabular cavity, which constitutes only one-third of a sphere. Accordingly, there is some incongruence in these surfaces, but this arrangement combines great stability with considerable mobility. Hip mobility, although less than that in the shoulder, is enhanced by co-ordinated movements in the pelvis and lumbar spine.

The pelvis and hips are well adapted to their function of transferring body weight from the trunk to the legs, while at the same time allowing the leg to adopt the numerous positions necessary for standing, walking and running. The spinal column is wedged into the sacrum and the sacroiliac joints are tightly bound by strong ligaments. Weight is transferred through the bony ring of the pelvis to the two lower extremities.

The forces normally applied to the hip have been well described by Pauwels (1973). At rest, the hip is subjected to a constant pressure from the surrounding abductor, adductor, flexor and extensor muscles. When a person stands on two legs, the hips may be compared with a balance, with the pelvis acting as a cross-bar. Body weight is then transmitted equally to each femur, which acts as a supporting pillar (*see Figure 9.1*).

However, when a person stands on one leg, weight distribution is altered and a different type of lever system applies (*see Figure 9.2*). The fulcrum is now at the hip joint of the supporting limb and body weight is carried on the inner arm of the lever. This must be counteracted by a muscular pull on the outer arm of the lever if the pelvis is not to

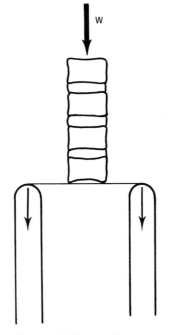

Figure 9.1 When standing on two legs, body weight (W) is distributed equally through the hips

overbalance and tip laterally to the unsupported side. This muscular pull is supplied mainly by the gluteus medius which originates from the ilium and is inserted into the greater trochanter. The lengths of the lever arms are altered so that the ratio between the inner arm of the lever to the outer arm is increased by a factor of three to one. Consequently, the total compressive force on the hip is the sum of the body weight plus three times

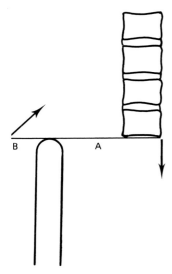

Figure 9.2 When standing on one leg, body weight is redistributed. The ratio of the inner arm A to the outer arm B is now 3:1

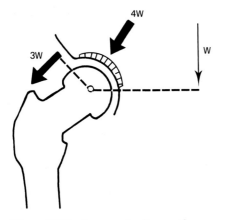

Figure 9.3 Total compressive force on the hip when standing on one leg is 1W + 3W = 4W (W = body weight.)

the body weight; a total force of four times the body weight (*see Figure 9.3*).

The resultant of these forces normally passes in a line running obliquely downwards across the upper and inner part of the roof of the acetabulum and the load is transmitted by the articular cartilage of the acetabular roof to the femoral head. The load on this area of contact is normally about 16 kg. cm^{-2}.

Walking subjects the hip to intermittent loads as body weight is taken alternately on each leg. Theoretically, as body weight is transferred the

pelvis should tilt away from the supporting leg. Tilting is prevented, however, by the action of the gluteus medius muscle which counterbalances this load and maintains the horizontally balanced pelvis steady by approximating the hip and the ilium. Again it can be estimated that the joint must support several times the body weight at each step. If a patient is obese, each extra kilogram of weight imposes a load on the hip, which is again increased by a factor of four with each step.

Hip pain

Pain in the hip region may either be referred from more proximal structures in the spine and pelvis or may be due to local causes in the hip. The site and nature of pain resulting from these various causes are often similar, and care must be taken during the clinical examination to differentiate the intrinsic and extrinsic causes.

Extrinsic causes of hip pain

(1)   Intra-abdominal causes, e.g. appendicitis or intrapelvic diseases.
(2)   Disease in local structures, such as lymphadenopathy or femoral hernia.
(3)   Spinal diseases. Hip pain may be referred from the upper lumbar spine (L2), e.g. secondary deposits or a psoas abscess. L3 nerve-root pressure may present as pain in the hip but usually pain radiates down the front of the thigh and may be exacerbated by coughing, straining or bending; quadriceps weakness or wasting and/or diminished knee jerk is usually present.
(4)   Sacroiliac arthritis may occasionally present as hip pain.

Intrinsic hip disorders

Pain arising from the hip joint may be felt at several different sites, most commonly in the groin or in the lateral aspects of the thigh. Less commonly, pain may be felt deep in the buttock, the back of the thigh, or in the innermost aspects of the thigh. Pain may also radiate down the leg and the greater the degree of underlying inflammation, the further the pain radiates, for example to the knee or even the shin. Pain felt in the knee alone may arise from the hip and is then usually felt just above the knee in the front of the thigh, although when severe this pain may also be felt more proximally in the thigh. This is not a common pattern for pain arising from lesions of the knee joint but a similar pain pattern may occur with pain referred from the lumbar spine.

Pain that is brought on by walking or standing and is relieved by rest suggests the presence of a mechanical derangement of the lumbar spine or hip. Pain that is constantly present and disturbs sleep usually indicates an inflammatory or a neoplastic lesion. Pain in the hip at night is common in patients with osteoarthritis of the hip but again indicates an inflammatory component often related to overuse of the hip during the day.

In adults, the most common cause of pain is osteoarthritis of the hip, but other causes of arthritis and soft-tissue lesions involving the tendons and bursae are not uncommon. In older age groups, polymyalgia rheumatica may commence with bilateral hip pain and stiffness. Hip fractures, sometimes incomplete, are common in the elderly. These require X-rays, including a lateral view of the femoral neck, for diagnosis. The hip region is commonly involved in metastatic deposits or primary tumours, such as multiple myeloma, and pain due to these conditions may be present at night. X-rays or a bone scan of patients presenting with hip pain should always be performed if malignancy is suspected.

Movements of the lumbar spine are tested to determine the presence of any restriction in movement and whether movements reproduce pain in the hip or thigh. However, when the patient stands, extension of the spine will also extend the hip joint. Accordingly, if pain is reproduced on spinal extension it is necessary to test the hip extension, and it should again be tested with the patient lying prone. Routine examination should include examination of the abdomen, the nervous system and the peripheral pulses. The lower leg should also be examined for any musculo-skeletal deformities and the leg length measured.

Examination of the hip joint

(1) Inspection:

  (a) Deformities.

  (b) Gait.

  (c) Swelling.

  (d) Muscle spasm.

  (e) Muscle wasting.

  (f) Trendelenburg test.

(2) Movements:

  (a) Active.

  (b) Passive.

  (c) Accessory.

  (d) Isometric

(3) Palpation:

  (a) Swelling.

  (b) Crepitus.

  (c) Tenderness.

(4) Radiology.

Inspection

The hip and surrounding structures are examined first with the patient standing, then walking and finally lying down.

Deformities

While the patient is standing the examiner looks for deformities in the hip, the lower leg and lumbar spine by inspection from in front, the side and behind. Fixed deformities may occur with the hip held in either flexion, external rotation and adduction or abduction. An extension deformity of the hip does not occur clinically. The most common deformity is a flexion and external rotation of the lower leg, as the hip is usually more comfortable in this position.

FIXED FLEXION DEFORMITY
This may be apparent on inspection, but it may be masked by a compensatory movement in the lumbar spine and pelvis producing an exaggerated lumbar lordosis and anterior rotation of the pelvis. This deformity is best observed with the patient standing, at which time the lumbar lordosis and anterior pelvic tilt become readily evident. When the patient lies supine on the couch the hip may appear to be straight but the underlying flexion deformity may then be revealed by two passive-movement tests: either loss of extension in the affected hip; or Thomas's test, described later.

EXTERNAL ROTATION DEFORMITY

This is usually obvious on examination of the lower leg as the foot and the patella are also rotated laterally. When a fixed lateral rotation deformity is present the leg cannot be rotated to the neutral position. Hence the angle reached by the leg, which is short of the neutral position, is also a measure of the fixed lateral rotational deformity.

ADDUCTION OR ABDUCTION HIP DEFORMITY

These are best observed while standing in front of the patient but they may be masked by a compensatory pelvic tilt. Adduction deformity may follow arthritis, shortening of the leg, or protrusio acetabuli. When severe, the heel of the affected leg may even cross over the opposite leg. This deformity is usually compensated by an elevation of the ipsilateral side of the pelvis, producing a pelvic tilt and an apparent leg shortening. This may be recognized by noting one side of the pelvis or the gluteal fold to be higher than the other. An abduction deformity is less common. It is usually associated with a lateral rotation deformity and occurs in fracture of the femoral neck or anterior dislocation of the head of the femur. It may also be compensated by a pelvic tilt to the opposite side, resulting in an apparent leg lengthening.

Gait

There is a wide variation in gait patterns which is due mainly to differences in anatomical structures. Gait should be observed from the front, the side and from behind with the patient walking both backwards and forwards. This is to assess the stride length, the time spent on each foot and whether the abnormal gait in hip disease is produced by pain, deformity, stiffness or alterations in posture.

Some abnormalities of gait include:

(1) Antalgic gait, produced by a painful hip as the patient stands for as short a time as possible on the affected limb and a correspondingly longer time on the normal limb. This produces a jerky rhythm to movement as the normal hip is moved forward rapidly.
(2) The Trendelenburg gait is produced by an intrinsic disorder of the abductors due either to weakness or to their inability to function properly on an unstable hip. As a result the abductors are unable to stabilize the hip as body weight is transferred to the affected side and so the pelvis tilts or drops towards the opposite side.

(3) A waddling gait or duck gait, occurs when the abductor muscles on both sides are weak and may also be present with bilateral hip disease. As the patient walks the body weight can be seen to shift laterally from side to side.
(4) A swinging gait occurs in ankylosis of the hip when, in order to walk, the patient needs to swing the whole of the lower limb forwards and backwards from the lumbar spine.
(5) An adductor gait occurs with bilateral hip disease, such as advanced osteoarthritis in which marked spasm is present in the adductor muscles so that the legs cannot be adequately separated. It also occurs as a scissors gait due to spasticity.
(6) An uneven gait may be produced by disparity in the leg lengths or because the lumbar spine needs to be extended during locomotion.

Synovial swelling

Synovial swelling involving the hip is only rarely obvious on inspection because the synovium lies deep to the surrounding muscles. It may occasionally become evident on inspection with the patient standing; the effusion bulges anteriorly and the normal concave surface of the front of the thigh becomes convex. Rarely, a synovial cyst may present as a soft-tissue swelling in the front of the thigh.

Muscle spasm

This may be obvious on inspection, especially if it involves the adductor muscles.

Muscle wasting

This occurs early in most hip diseases and involves especially the glutei and quadriceps muscle groups. Wasting is best appreciated by the patient lying on a couch and the examiner standing at the foot of the couch and comparing the development of these muscles on either side.

Trendelenburg test

This tests the ability of the abductor mechanism to stabilize the hip while the patient is standing on one leg. Normally if a person stands on one leg the abductor muscles on that side will contract to maintain pelvic stability. This can be observed by watching the posterior superior iliac spines and the iliac crests which remain level or else are

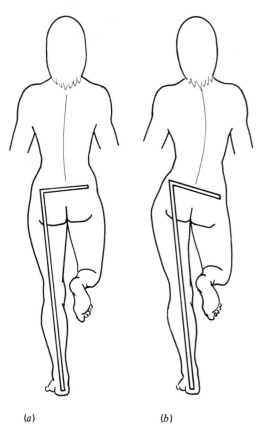

(a)　　　　　　　(b)

Figure 9.4 Trendelenburg test: (a) normal; (b) positive test

slightly raised on the opposite side (*see Figure 9.4(a)*).

The Trendelenburg test is positive when the patient stands on one leg and the opposite side of the pelvis then drops. The test is performed by having the patient stand on the leg to be tested and then raise the opposite leg until the knee is flexed to 90 degrees. At this point, the pelvic level and hence the buttock fold on the side of the elevated leg will drop downwards under the influence of gravity (*see Figure 9.4(b)*).

This indicates that the hip abductors are unable to function properly, which may result from muscular weakness or from an inadequate leverage due to abnormalities of the upper femur such as congenital dislocation of the hip, coxa vara, or non-union of a fractured femoral neck.

Hip movements

The hip movements of flexion, extension, abduc-

tion, adduction, medial rotation and lateral rotation are tested by a series of active, passive, accessory and isometric movements. In the hip the active movements commonly tested are flexion and extension, as more information can usually be obtained from testing passive movements or combined hip movements. While carrying out active and passive movements, it is essential to place one hand over the patient's iliac crest to detect any movement taking place there rather than in the hip joint itself.

The examiner notes:

(1) The range of motion.
(2) Whether movements are painful and reproduce the patient's pain.
(3) The presence of any muscular spasm.
(4) The behaviour of pain and spasm throughout the range of hip movement.
(5) The end-feel of the movement.

In patients whose pain is due to an underlying bone disease, however, testing of hip movements may give confusing results. For example, hip movements may be restricted in patients with bone diseases such as osteomalacia or secondary deposits, whereas in avascular necrosis of the hip the range of movement may remain full but painful.

Active movements

Active hip flexion and extension are best tested with the patient standing and the range of movement is compared between the two sides. The active range of hip flexion should then be tested while the patient is lying supine with the knee flexed to 90 degrees. The normal range of active hip flexion in this position is to 120 degrees, but there is a wide individual variation.

Passive movements

Flexion: passive hip flexion is best tested with the patient lying supine and the knee flexed. The range of passive hip flexion is normally greater than the active range and usually reaches 140 degrees before it is limited by contact between the thigh and the anterior abdominal wall.

THOMAS'S TEST
Thomas's test detects a fixed hip flexion deformity in patients who have developed a compensatory lumbar lordosis that then masks the hip flexion (*see Figure 9.5(a)*). With the patient lying supine

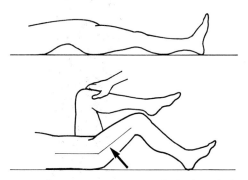

Figure 9.5 Thomas's test. (*a*) Hip flexion is masked by the lumbar lordosis. (*b*) Flexion of normal hip obliterates the lumbar lordosis

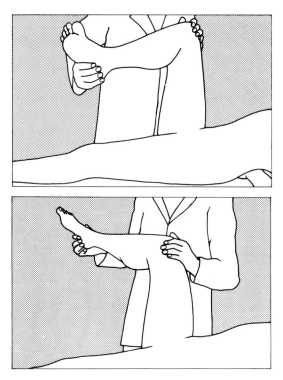

Figure 9.6 (*a*) Passive lateral rotation of the hip: supine. (*b*) Passive medial rotation of the hip: supine

the contralateral hip is fully flexed passively by the examiner. This straightens out the lumbar lordosis and the pelvis will then flex. The affected hip is then observed to develop a degree of flexion deformity (*see Figure 9.5(b)*). This test may also be positive in bilateral hip disease.

Extension: passive hip extension is tested with the patient lying prone with the lower limb fully extended. The examiner first steadies the patient's pelvis with one hand to prevent simultaneous movement in the hip and lumbar spine, and then passively extends the patient's hip by holding under the anterior thigh and lifting the leg upwards. The normal range of hyperextension is 15 degrees.

Abduction: abduction of one hip is normally accompanied by a simultaneous rotation of the pelvis and side flexion of the lumbar spine. Accordingly, to test the true range of hip abduction accurately, the pelvis must first be fixed by the examiner with one hand while the extended leg is then passively abducted with the other hand. The normal range is 45 degrees.

Adduction: adduction of the hip is normally limited by one leg coming into contact with the other. Accordingly, this movement may be tested if one leg is held in slight flexion so as to cross over the other leg. The normal range is 25 degrees.

Rotation: rotation of the hip comprises a rotation of the shaft of the femur and not of the head of the femur which rolls and slides in the acetabulum (Gray, 1973). Passive hip rotation may be tested by three methods:

(1) The patient lies supine with the hip and knee flexed to 90 degrees. The examiner grasps the patient's foot with his right hand and uses the left hand to steady the patient's thigh.

The patient's foot is then moved inwards so that the hip is laterally rotated (*see Figure 9.6(a)*) and then outwards as the hip is medially rotated (*see Figure 9.6(b)*). The normal range is 60 degrees of lateral rotation and 45 degrees of medial rotation.

(2) Rotation is also tested while the patient lies supine with hip and knee extended and the examiner rapidly rotates the leg inwards and outwards. In the early stages of hip disease, before any hip deformity develops, a characteristic end-feel, due to a loss of the normal fluid type of movement, is produced.

(3) Rotation may also be tested with the patient lying prone with the hip extended and the knee flexed to 90 degrees. The examiner rotates the lower leg inwards to measure lateral rotation of the hip (*see Figure 9.7*) then outwards to measure medial rotation.

COMBINED MOVEMENTS

Faber test   The name of this test is derived from the initials for flexion, abduction and external rotation. It is performed as a quick screening test for most forms of hip disease but does not provide detailed knowledge about the loss of a specific hip movement. The lower lumbar spinal

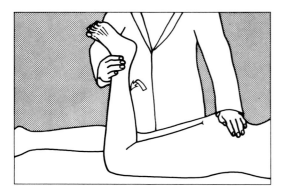

Figure 9.7 Lateral rotation of the hip: prone

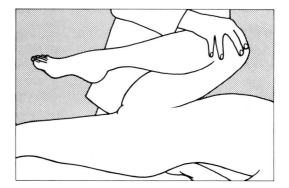

Figure 9.9 Combined flexion, adduction and medial rotation of the hip

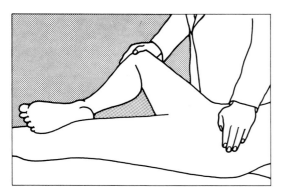

Figure 9.8 The faber test

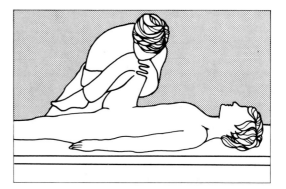

Figure 9.10 Flexion–adduction of the hip joint

joints are also moved during this test and so may produce pain.

Starting position—The patient lies supine with the feet together. The examiner passively flexes the patient's hip and knee and places the heel on the patient's knee.

Method—The knee is then gently moved towards the floor, thus abducting and laterally rotating the hip (*see Figure 9.8*). The range of this movement and whether it reproduces pain is noted. The range may be limited by pain, restriction of hip movements or muscle spasm.

Combined flexion, adduction and rotation The patient lies supine. The examiner fully passively flexes the hip, then adducts and medially rotates it so as to approximate the knee to the opposite side of the patient's chest (*see Figure 9.9*). The distance of the knee from the chest is then measured. It is a useful test for assessing the progress of hip disease. The range and pain response to the

adduction component of this test should also be assessed with the hip in different positions of flexion and rotation.

Bilateral hip abduction The patient lies supine and the examiner abducts both hips. The distance between the ankle malleoli is then measured. Since the bilateral hip abduction cancels the effect of any unilateral pelvic rotation, this test provides a useful measure of any progression or improvement in the range of hip movement.

Flexion–adduction This test is useful when other hip movements are normal or as a mobilization treatment.

Starting position—The patient lies supine near the edge of the couch with the hip flexed to 90 degrees. The examiner stands with the fingers over the top of the patient's knee. The patient's hip is then adducted until the right ilium starts to lift from the couch (*see Figure 9.10*).

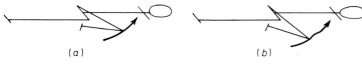

(a)   (b)

Figure 9.11 Diagrammatic representation of hip flexion–adduction

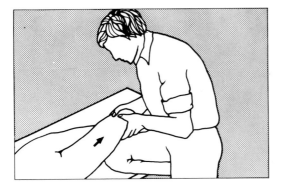

Figure 9.12 Longitudinal caudad accessory movement

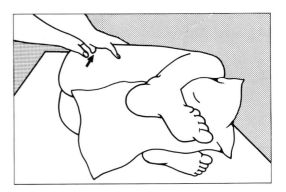

Figure 9.14 Posteroanterior accessory movement

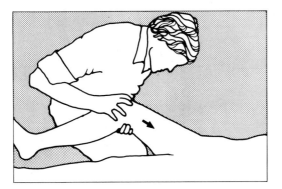

Figure 9.13 Longitudinal cephalad accessory movement

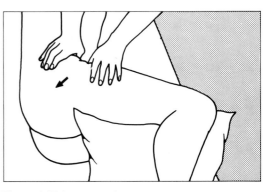

Figure 9.15 Anteroposterior accessory movement

Method—The patient's hip, while maintained in adduction, is moved in an arc from 90 to 140 degrees of flexion. At the same time constant pressure is maintained through the knee along the shaft of the femur. As the knee is moved, it normally follows a smooth arc of a circle (*see Figure 9.11(a)*). An abnormality in this movement is felt as a small hump on the arc which may reproduce pain (*see Figure 9.11(b)*).

ACCESSORY MOVEMENTS
There are five accessory movements in the hip; these are:

(1) Longitudinal caudad. The patient lies supine and the examiner grasps the lower end of the femur. An oscillatory pull is applied along the femur (*see Figure 9.12*).
(2) Longitudinal cephalad. The patient lies supine and an oscillatory compression movement is applied to the femoral head into the acetabulum (*see Figure 9.13*).
(3) Posteroanterior. The patient lies on his side and a posteroanterior movement is applied from behind the greater trochanter (*see Figure 9.14*).

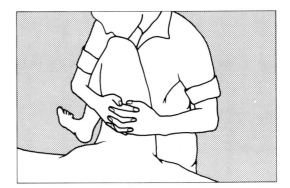

Figure 9.16 Lateral accessory movement

(4) Anteroposterior. The patient lies on the side and the movement is felt by pressure over the greater trochanter (*see Figure 9.15*).
(5) Lateral. The patient lies supine with the hip flexed to 90 degrees. The femoral head is displaced laterally in the acetabulum (*see Figure 9.16*).

Isometric tests

The six isometric tests of the hip are flexion,

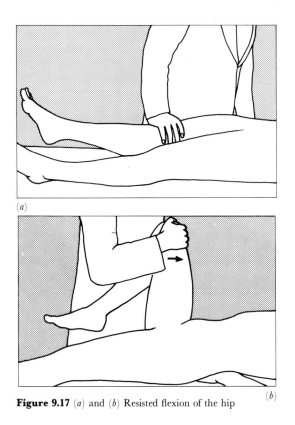

(a)

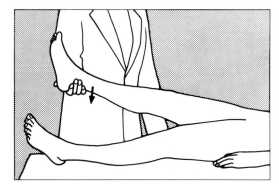

Figure 9.18 Resisted hip extension

Figure 9.17 (*a*) and (*b*) Resisted flexion of the hip   (b)

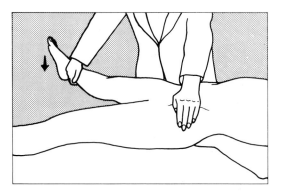

Figure 9.19 Resisted adduction of the hip

extension, abduction, adduction, medial and lateral rotation. Flexion may be tested in one of two positions with the patient lying supine. In the first position (*see Figure 9.17(a)*) both the hip and knee are extended; in the second (*see Figure 9.17(b)*) the hip and knee are flexed with the hip at 90 degrees. In either position the examiner places one hand just above the knee and fully resists the patient's attempt to flex the thigh. A painful weakness of this movement usually indicates a psoas tendinitis; a painless weakness may be due to a rupture of the psoas tendon or to an L2 nerve-root lesion.

Extension of the hip is best tested with the patient supine and the extended leg is moved into approximately 20 degrees of flexion at the hip. The examiner places one hand under the patient's heel and resists the patients's attempt to push the leg downwards towards the couch (*see Figure 9.18*). Pain in the upper part of the posterior thigh on this movement may be caused by a lesion of the hamstring origin.

Adduction is tested with the patient lying supine and the leg extended and fully abducted (*see Figure 9.19*). The examiner places one hand above the medial malleolus of patient's ankle and

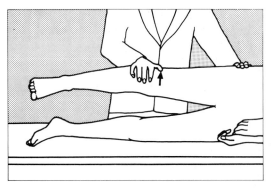

Figure 9.20 Resisted abduction of the hip

resists the patient's attempt to adduct the thigh.

Abduction is best tested with the patient lying on the side with the hip to be tested uppermost and in slight medial rotation and extension.

The examiner places one hand around the patient's knee and resists the patient's attempt to abduct the thigh (*see Figure 9.20*). A painful weakness of this movement is due to a gluteus medius tendinitis. A painless weakness is unusual, but may follow an S1 nerve-root lesion or a rupture of the gluteus medius tendon.

Rotation is best tested with the patient lying prone with the hip extended and the knee flexed to 90 degrees. The examiner places one hand above the ankle and first fully resists the patient's attempt to rotate the thigh medially and then laterally.

Palpation

Many of the bony landmarks and soft tissues around the hip are easily palpable. The iliac crest is subcutaneous and terminates anteriorly at the anterior superior iliac spine from which the tendon of the sartorius muscle arises. The greater trochanter of the femur is easily palpated about a palm's breadth below the iliac crest. The iliac crest terminates posteriorly at the posterior superior iliac spine which lies under the dimple of Venus. The ischial tuberosity is easily palpable under the gluteal fold in the middle of the buttock, especially with the hip flexed. The sciatic nerve runs midway between the ischial tuberosity and the greater trochanter.

The hip joint itself is placed deeply under thick muscles and so synovial swelling is usually appreciated as a vague sensation of fullness or tenderness but may occasionally be detected by placing the thumb over the mid-point of the inguinal ligament with the forefingers placed posteriorly over the buttock opposite to the thumb. In the presence of synovial swelling the fingers may not be able to reach as far posteriorly as do the fingers on the normal side. A synovial cyst may track anteriorly to present as a swelling in the groin and needs to be differentiated from a femoral hernia, a varix of the saphenous vein, arteriovenous aneurysm, psoas abscess, lymphadenopathy, iliopsoas bursitis, haematoma formation and synovial tumours.

Tenderness should be sought by deep palpation over the head of the femur just below the inguinal ligament lateral to the femoral artery. Tenderness over the greater trochanter is commonly found in trochanteric bursitis, over the adductor origin in adductor tendinitis or, in patients with psoas tendinitis, over the psoas insertion into the lesser trochanter.

Radiology

Standard X-ray views of the hip are usually taken in the anteroposterior (*see Figure 9.21*) and lateral positions, but an oblique view with the patient at

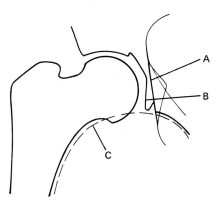

Figure 9.21 Tracing of an X-ray of the hip. (A) Ilioischial line. (B) The acetabular U. (C) Shenton's Line (dotted) is continuous from the neck of the femur to the pubic ramus

a 25 degree angle gives more information than the true lateral (Lesquesne, 1967).

The normal relationship between the acetabulum and the head of the femur is determined by anteroposterior (AP) and oblique X-rays to measure several angles:

(1) In the AP view, the vertical angle is measured using two points, the centre of the femoral head (C) and the lateral edge of the acetabular roof (E). Two lines are then drawn, one a vertical line (V) upwards from the centre of the head and the second joining the centre

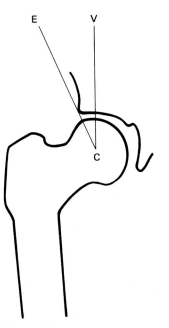

Figure 9.22 (*a*) The vertical angle VCE

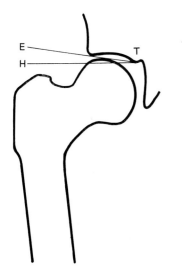

Figure 9.22 (*b*) The horizontal angle HTE

to the acetabular edge. The angle (VCE) measures the degree of envelopment of the femoral head by the acetabular roof and is approximately 25 degrees (*see Figure 9.22(a)*).
(2) In the AP view, the horizontal angle is measured from two points, one the lateral edge of the acetabular roof (E) and the second where the acetabular roof meets the acetabular fossa (T). Two lines are then drawn, one a horizontal line (H) across the femoral head from the point T, and the other a line joining the two points E and T on the acetabulum (*see Figure 9.22(b)*). The angle HTE so formed is normally less than 10 degrees and measures the obliquity of the acetabular roof. An increased obliquity of the acetabular roof is indicated by an increase in the angle HTE above 13 degrees.

Classification of diseases of the hip

(1) Soft-tissue lesions:

  (a) Tendinitis—gluteal, psoas, adductor, hamstring and rectus femoris tendons.
  (b) Bursitis—trochanteric, psoas and ischial.
  (c) Snapping hip.

  (d) Capsulitis of the hip.

(2) Joint lesions:

  (a) Osteoarthritis.
  (b) Monoarthritis of the hip.
  (c) Septic arthritis.
  (d) Instability of the symphysis pubis.

(3) Bone disorders:

  (a) Avascular necrosis.
  (b) Paget's disease.
  (c) Acute osteoporosis.
  (d) Stress fracture.

(4) Entrapment neuropathy—lateral cutaneous nerve of the thigh.

Soft-tissue lesions

Three bursae and five tendons around the hip are commonly involved clinically: the trochanteric, psoas and ischial bursae; the tendinous insertions of the gluteus medius and psoas; and tendon origins of the adductor longus, hamstrings and rectus femoris muscles.

Gluteal tendinitis and trochanteric bursitis

These are the most common soft-tissue lesions around the hip and may occur separately or together. The gluteus medius is a powerful hip abductor which is inserted via its tendon into the lateral aspect of the greater trochanter of the femur. The tendon is separated on its medial aspect from the greater trochanter and the gluteus minimus by a small bursa, and on its lateral aspect the large multilocular trochanteric bursa lies between the gluteus medius and the tensor fascia latae (*see Figure 9.23*).

The patient presents with pain that is usually well localized over the outer aspect of the greater trochanter but when severe it may radiate down the lateral or posterolateral aspect of the thigh. Pain is usually brought on by hip movements, especially while walking or climbing stairs. When severe it may disturb sleep, especially if the patient rolls on to the affected side. It tends to run a protracted course that is punctuated by exacerbations and remissions, often related to activity. This overuse lesion tends to occur in two groups of patients: it occurs in sporting activities that involve extensive running; or in middle-aged, usually female and often overweight patients with

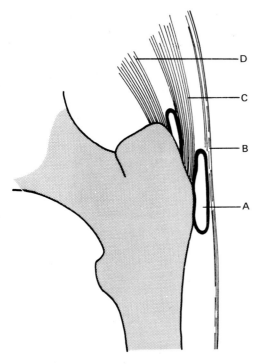

Figure 9.23 The trochanteric bursa (A) lies between the tensor fascia lata (B) and the gluteus medius tendon (C). Another small bursa lies between this tendon and the gluteus minimus (D)

associated degenerative changes in the lower lumbar spine.

MAJOR SIGNS
Pain is reproduced by stretching or contracting the gluteus medius tendon. The tendon is stretched when the hip and knee are flexed to a right angle and the hip is then fully laterally rotated (*see Figure 9.6(a)*). Pain may be reproduced at its extreme range.

Pain may also be reproduced on resisted contraction of the muscle. This is tested by the examiner resisting hip abduction as the patient lies on the unaffected side and attempts to lift the affected leg upwards in abduction (*see Figure 9.20*).

CONFIRMATORY SIGNS
Tenderness is usually well localized over the upper lateral aspect of the trochanter which is palpated with the patient lying on the unaffected side. X-rays of the hip are usually normal but are necessary to exclude any hip joint disease. Calcification in the tendon or bursa may be found on X-ray in up to 20 per cent of cases.

MANAGEMENT
(1) Rest from those activities that produce this condition is necessary.
(2) Anti-inflammatory agents should be prescribed.
(3) Physical methods of treatment including heat, ice, stretching of the tendon and deep-friction massage are useful in relieving pain. Exercises are contraindicated.
(4) Mobilization techniques may be effective and are continued if the pain-free range improves.
(5) Injections of local anaesthetic and corticosteroid are usually necessary to relieve symptoms. The patient lies on the unaffected side and the tender area around the insertion of the gluteus medius tendon and the bursa is found by careful palpation. A 23-gauge needle is used and an injection of 5 ml of local anaesthetic and 1 ml of corticosteroid solution given around this tender area. The injection may need to be repeated several times at fortnightly intervals.

Adductor tendinitis

This common condition occurs most often nowadays in athletes but was previously described in horse riders and was known as 'rider's strain'. Pain is usually well localized either over the tendinous origin of the adductor longus from the pubis or a few centimetres distally at its musculotendinous junction. When it is associated with a tendinitis of the rectus abdominis, pelvic instability should be suspected. Occasionally, adductor tendinitis may be an early sign in spondyloarthritis.

MAJOR SIGN
Pain is reproduced by either stretching or contracting the adductor longus tendon. The tendon is stretched with the patient lying supine and the hip moved into full passive abduction. In this position the examiner fully resists the patient's attempt to adduct the leg back towards the midline.

CONFIRMATORY SIGNS
Tenderness is usually well localized either over the tendon origin or its musculotendinous junction. X-rays are usually normal but may occasionally reveal calcification, or even ossification, in the tendon origin. They should also be taken to exlude other, rare causes of pain in this area—e.g. osteochondritis, stress fracture of the pubis, or secondary metastases.

MANAGEMENT

This includes rest, anti-inflammatories and physical methods. Stretching of the tendon by the physiotherapist is essential and this may also be undertaken in a warm pool. Deep-friction massage applied transversely across the ligament fibres is often useful in this condition. Mobilization techniques can be used to increase the pain-free range of abduction. Response is usually rapid.

Injections of local anaesthetic and corticosteroid must never be given into the tendon but can be given around the tendon or into the musculotendinous junction using a 25-gauge needle.

Psoas tendinitis and bursitis

The iliopsoas muscle is a powerful hip flexor that is inserted via its tendon into the lesser trochanter of the femur. It is separated from the anterior aspect of the hip capsule proximal to its insertion by the psoas bursa which may communicate with the hip joint.

Patients present with pain in the anterior aspect of the thigh that tends to be made worse with activity. Young patients in whom the apophysis has not yet united may suffer a traction injury with separation of part of the lesser trochanter.

MAJOR SIGNS

Pain may be reproduced on contracting or stretching the tendon. The patient lies supine with hip flexed to 90 degrees and the examiner then resists further flexion of the hip (*see Figure 9.17*). Alternatively, the patient lies prone with knee flexed to 90 degrees and the examiner passively hyperextends the hip, so stretching the psoas tendon.

CONFIRMATORY SIGNS

An effusion into the psoas bursa is very rarely of sufficient size to produce a localized swelling. Tenderness may be felt deeply over the tendon insertion which may be palpated with the patient lying supine and hip flexed to 90 degrees. The examiner places one finger just distal to the inguinal ligament over the lesser trochanter and passively abducts the hip with his other hand while palpating for any localized tenderness. X-rays are normal but are necessary to exclude any underlying hip joint or bony pathology.

MANAGEMENT

This condition is treated by rest, anti-inflammatory

drugs and mobilization by oscillatory movements through an arc of the last 40 degrees of hip extension.

Injection—The tendinous insertion of the psoas muscle into the lesser trochanter may be injected with local anaesthetic and corticosteroid, taking great care to avoid the femoral nerve. The patient lies supine with the knee flexed and the hip fully abducted and externally rotated. The tender area is palpated lateral to the femoral artery and nerve and injected with 1 ml of local anaesthetic and 1 ml of corticosteroid solution. This may need to be repeated two or three times at fortnightly intervals.

Hamstring tendinitis

The tendinous origin of the hamstring muscle from the ischial tuberosity may be involved in an overuse sydrome in distance runners, especially if it also involves running up hills, and may occur in occupations such as delivering milk. Pain is reproduced on resisting hip extension or by stretching the tendon origin by fully flexing the hip. Tenderness is well localized over the ischial tuberosity. Separation of part of the bony cortex may occur in young athletes due to an avulsion of the hamstring origin from the ischial tuberosity. It is evident on X-ray and is called 'sprinter's fracture'. The young sprinter usually experiences a sudden severe pain in the back of the thigh while starting from the blocks or while trying to increase speed and often falls over.

Rectus femoris

Tendinitis may involve the origin of the rectus femoris from the anterior inferior iliac spine. In adolescents a traction injury may avulse the spine. This may follow sudden exertion in a patient who has had either a previous tendinitis or a direct contusion injury to the thigh muscles with subsequent loss of muscle extensibility. A similar type of avulsion may occur at the origin of the sartorius muscle from the anterior superior iliac spine.

Ischiogluteal bursitis

The ischiogluteal bursa can become chronically inflamed as the result of prolonged sitting, a condition that has been long recognized as 'weaver's bottom'. An acute bursitis may occur but is also rare (Swarhout and Compere, 1974). The presenting symptom is of pain over the ischial tuberosity, made worse by sitting and relieved by standing. There are no specific signs but tenderness is found localized over the ischial tuberosity and straight leg raising may reproduce pain.

Snapping hip

This refers to a loud snapping noise over the lateral aspect of the hip which may be occasionally associated with pain. It is produced by the fascia lata sliding over the greater trochanter and is usually brought on by active hip flexion or rotation.

MANAGEMENT
No active therapy is required in most cases. The patient needs to be reassured about the benign nature of this condition and advised to limit activities that produce the snapping. If pain is associated with the snapping, mobilization with through-range techniques will usually make the snapping painless.

Capsulitis of the hip

Capsulitis occurs much less commonly in the hip than the shoulder and is found in the middle-aged and younger age groups. The patient presents with a relatively rapid onset of pain and stiffness that comes on for no apparent reason and is made worse by activity.

MAJOR SIGNS
Flexion–adduction, rotation and hyperextension of the hip are usually lost early. In mild cases this may be the only clinical finding but as the disease progresses the range of abduction is also reduced and flexion may be limited to approximately 90 degrees. Accessory joint movements are lost. Pain gradually settles over several months but the stiffness of the hip movements improve more gradually.

CONFIRMATORY SIGNS
Routine hip X-rays and other ancillary tests including blood studies are normal. Arthrography demonstrates a reduction in joint capacity with loss of normal joint recesses (Caroit *et al.*, 1963).

MANAGEMENT
(1) Analgesics and anti-inflammatory drugs are given.
(2) Heat or ice is applied to the hip.

(3) Passive stretching, especially extension, of the hip is necessary.
(4) Passive-mobilization techniques, using flexion–adduction, extension, rotation and accessory movements at the limit of one or more of these movements are essential.
(5) As pain settles, active exercises are commenced and passive mobilization is continued.

Joint lesions

Osteoarthritis of the hip

This is the most common form of hip disease and may be bilateral. It commences in patients of either sex, usually after the age of 50, and any type of body build may be involved. Osteoarthritis of the hip is divided into primary and secondary causes, the former related to an intrinsic disorder of articular cartilage, and a secondary cause after disease or misalignment of the hip joint. However, the hip is subjected to large mechanical forces and the presence of even a slight anomaly or incongruity on the joint surface can predispose to subsequent degenerative changes. Recent studies have suggested that in many cases diagnosed as primary osteoarthritis an underlying abnormality of the joint surfaces can be found that will cause a secondary osteoarthritis. For example, Murray (1965) reviewed 200 X-rays of presumed primary osteoarthritis and demonstrated anatomical abnormalities in 65 per cent. Solomon (1976), in a clinical and radiological survey of 327 patients, found an underlying cause in 300 patients; in the remaining 27 patients the changes were too advanced to allow adequate assessment.

The disorders identified were due either to congenital anomalies such as acetabular dysplasia, subluxation or dislocation of the hip; or to acquired defects after trauma, joint disease, infections or inflammatory arthritis. The three most common causes were acetabular dysplasia, slipped epiphysis and previous inflammatory arthritis.

In acetabular dysplasia the inadequate covering of the femoral head by the acetabular roof leads to an excessive load being placed on the superolateral aspect of the hip and X-ray degenerative changes are found first in this area. The incidence of this deformity in cases of osteoarthritis of the hip varies in the reported series from 13 per cent (Gofton, 1971) to 48 per cent (Lesquesne, 1967). A previous slipped upper femoral epiphysis may present a characteristic deformity with narrowing of the lateral joint compartment, buttressing on both lateral and medial aspects of the neck of the femur and evidence of previous medial migration of the femoral head. A diagnosis of past Perthes' disease cannot always be made from the history, but X-ray changes may show a concentric narrowing of the joint space with a short, wide femoral back and coxa plana.

Disparity in leg length may also play an aetiological role. Gofton and Trueman (1971) described 67 patients with osteoarthritis of the hip in whom 41 had unilateral disease with superolateral subluxation; of these, 29 had an increased leg length on the affected side.

CLINICAL FEATURES
The onset of this disease tends to be insidious and pain is the usual presenting symptom. However, there is no strong correlation between the degree of pain and the radiological changes that are present. This has been demonstrated in several radiological surveys (for example, Lawrence, 1968).

Pain is usually related to weight bearing or movement and may appear first as attacks of hip pain after prolonged or unaccustomed activities. Subsequently, pain tends to become worse as the day goes on and is relieved by rest, but later pain may be present at night and disturb sleep and may be related to the severity of the inflammatory or bony changes. The restricted hip movements in the early stages may be considered by the patient to be part of the normal ageing process until the loss of functional ability becomes more marked. This may be manifested by difficulty in putting on socks or stockings or in tying up shoe-laces—especially in the morning, when hip stiffness is more pronounced. Walking may become more difficult because of the loss of hip extension.

Subsequently, as hip pain and stiffness become more marked, the walking distance is reduced and the patient may need to use a stick and usually develops a limp. Pain in the back may be a feature due to the development of a compensatory lordosis and excessive use of the lumbar spine on walking. Deformity also increases as the patient tends to stand on the unaffected leg and the affected hip is often held in a position of flexion and lateral rotation, producing a characteristic deformity. Less commonly, the hip is held in adduction or medial rotation. There is difficulty both in sitting down and in standing up, going up or down stairs and in sitting forwards in a chair. Disability produced by stiffness and deformity can ultimately become so marked that the patient can only get about with difficulty by using sticks or crutches.

SITE OF INVOLVEMENT
The site of maximal radiological joint-space narrowing may be superolateral, superior or medial. The most common site is superolateral and the head of the femur then tends to sublux upwards. The next most common is the superior aspect of the joint; least commonly, the medial aspect of the joint cavity is narrowed and the head of the femur then tends to migrate inwards, producing a protrusio acetabuli. This classification has some prognostic significance as the superolateral narrowing tends to be more severe and progressive whereas the medial type is more benign; clinical signs may also differ in these types.

CLINICAL EXAMINATION
Gait is usually disturbed, which produces either an antalgic gait; a swinging type of gait if the hip is stiff; a lurching of the trunk towards the affected side if there is any shortening of the limb; or a Trendelenburg gait if any weakness of the abductor muscles is present.

Deformity is looked for first with the patient standing and viewed from in front and the side and then while lying supine. Muscle wasting is almost invariably present in the gluteal and the quadriceps group. Swelling due to synovitis of the hip is usually too deeply placed to become visible on inspection.

HIP MOVEMENTS
The first hip movements lost are medial rotation and extension, and so the hip is held in flexion and lateral rotation. The patient usually compensates for a flexion deformity in the hip by an increased lumbar lordosis. When the patient lies down lordosis can mask the hip flexion unless it is revealed by a positive Thomas's test. An adduction deformity may also be present and results in apparent leg shortening on the affected side. The hip movements ultimately become restricted in all directions. However, the pattern of loss of movement tends to vary according to the site of hip involvement. In the superolateral type there is a progressive loss of medial rotation, extension and abduction so that the common deformity in

flexion, lateral rotation and adduction is produced. In the medial type the head of the femur is displaced into the deepened acetabular cavity, so that rotation in both directions and abduction tend to be most affected.

OTHER TESTS
The leg length on both sides should be measured to determine the presence of any true or apparent shortening, and the thigh girth measured to chart any quadriceps wasting. The lumbar spine should also be examined to determine the presence of any pain and/or restricted movement.

MANAGEMENT
The management of patients with osteoarthritis of the hip has been revolutionized since the introduction of new surgical techniques, such as total hip replacement (Charnley, 1974). However, in its earlier stages much can be achieved by conservative measures to relieve the patient's pain and stiffness, prevent deformity, and maintain functional capacity.

GENERAL MEASURES
(1) It is essential to spend some time with patients explaining the nature of their disability, reassuring them that they need not fear becoming eventually crippled and that the severity of their symptoms is often due to overuse of the joint.
(2) Weight loss, if the patient is obese, is a rational form of therapy designed to take some load off the patient's hip.
(3) Consultation with an occupational therapist is advisable to outline any special problems at work or around the house.
(4) Correction of any other postural problems in the legs or back should be undertaken.

REST
The patient needs to avoid excessive weight bearing and should be advised to stand and walk less on the affected hip if pain, particularly at night, is a problem. The patient should lie down in the prone position for approximately half an hour a day to prevent the tendency for a flexion deformity of the hip to develop. Acute episodes of pain are usually best managed with a few days of complete rest in bed.

AIDS AND SUPPORTS
A walking stick carried in the opposite hand will allow weight to be redistributed on to the normal hip and ease pain in the affected hip. Crutches or a walking frame are only rarely necessary. A heel raise on a shoe may be necessary if there is any disparity in leg length.

ANTI-INFLAMMATORIES
These are given, usually on a long-term basis, and analgesics may be required for pain.

PHYSICAL METHODS
Physical methods of therapy such as heat usually bring only a short-term relief of pain and have little place to play in the long-term management (Clarke *et al.*, 1974). Exercise therapy should be given only with well-defined objectives, is of no value when pain is the dominant feature and should not be persevered with if it causes any exacerbation of pain. Exercises to increase the range of hip movement, particularly rotation, often produce exacerbation of pain. Patients with osteoarthritis of the hip invariably develop weakness and wasting in the thigh and gluteal muscles. They should then be taught isometric exercises, especially if they have difficulty in walking or a feeling of instability in the leg. To overcome stiffness, they may be combined with assisted exercises, e.g. with the use of a sling to stretch the hip in extension.

MANUAL THERAPY
When the pain is dominant, treatment should at first use small-amplitude movements without provoking any further pain. The patient lies on one side with the painful hip uppermost. The therapist places the thumbs over the patient's greater trochanter and uses posteroanterior, anteroposterior and longitudinal movements, together with a lateral movement of the femoral head away from the acetabulum (*see Figure 9.24*). As pain

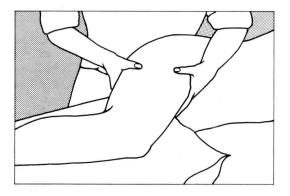

Figure 9.24 Treatment of osteoarthritis of the hip with gentle lateral movement

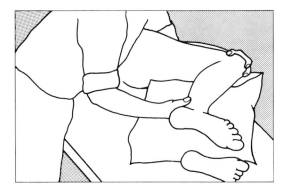

Figure 9.25 Treatment of osteoarthritis of the hip with gentle medial rotation

settles, treatment is progressed by using rotational movements (*see Figure 9.25*) and the amplitude of these movements is gradually progressed until a full rocking from medial to lateral rotation can be attained.

When pain and stiffness are major problems, the hip is first treated in flexion and adduction (*see Figure 9.10*) and accessory movements are used at the end of the range. As the condition improves, medial rotation is usually taken as the treatment method, using large-amplitude movements at the end of the range, and other movements can then be added at the limit of their range.

SURGERY

This should be considered in patients with severe degrees of pain or disability or who fail to respond to conservative measures. Total hip replacement is the treatment of choice in older patients, but in younger patients a femoral osteotomy may still have a role in surgical management.

Monoarthritis of the hip

This rare and apparently unique form of arthritis involves only one hip (Lesquesne and Forestier, 1961). The patient, usually middle aged, presents with a rapid onset of hip pain and stiffness that gradually settle over the next 2–3 years. An X-ray reveals gross narrowing of the joint space with destructive changes in the acetabulum and femoral head but no osteophyte formation. The erythrocyte sedimentation rate (ESR) is always elevated and aspirated samples of synovial fluid show inflammatory changes. Synovial biopsy samples show numerous inflammatory foci in hypertrophic villi and vascular dilatation. This disease is distinct from other important causes of

monoarthritis of the hip—e.g. infections, chondrocalcinosis, rheumatoid arthritis and spondyloarthritis.

Septic arthritis

This is relatively uncommon in the hip and is usually caused by *Staphylococcus aureus*, but other causative organisms include streptococcal, gonococcal and pneumococcal infections. Tuberculosis of the hip has now fortunately become rare.

The patient usually presents with a sudden onset of severe hip pain that is continuous and often worse at night, with marked restriction of hip movement. Associated features include a raised temperature, a leucocytosis and an elevated ESR. Investigations include hip aspiration for cell count and culture, blood cultures and X-rays which may be normal at first but usually go on to severe destructive changes—especially in those patients in whom the diagnosis is delayed, as may easily happen in this joint. Treatment consists of surgical drainage, immobilization in traction and full antibiotic cover for at least three months.

Instability of the symphysis pubis

The pelvis forms a bony ring, with the two sacroiliac joints behind and the symphysis pubis in front. The symphysis pubis is a secondary cartilaginous joint formed between the bony surfaces of the pubis and is lined by a hyaline cartilage and joined by fibrocartilage. Instability of the symphysis may follow operations on the sacroiliac joint (Coventry and Tapper, 1972), confinement or trauma. It is also a common sporting injury (Harris and Murray, 1974) which occurs most commonly in football players but may also occur in runners and has been described in an Olympic road walker (Howse, 1964). Laban and Meerschaert (1975) reported on 50 patients with this condition and noted that 20 had a restriction of ipsilateral hip movements; this has been confirmed by Williams and Sperryn (1976).

The patient complains of pain in one or both groins which may radiate widely to the lower abdomen, adductor region of the thigh, hip, testis or perineum and may also cause low-back pain when it is associated with a lesion of the sacroiliac joint. Pain is usually made worse by exercise, straining, or adopting certain postures (such as standing on one leg) and may be felt while walking upstairs, or thrusting the hip forward. Pain is usually severe, so that running or kicking is virtually impossible, and it may cause the patient to limp. A clicking sensation may also be present on certain movements.

Pain and tenderness can be reproduced by pressure over or springing of the symphysis pubis. Pain and tenderness also occur over the tendons of the adductor longus and the rectus abdominis near their attachments in the pubis and may follow an attempt by these muscles to stabilize the pelvis. Pain may also be reproduced by passively abducting the hip, by resisting the patient's attempt to sit up or by resisting adduction of the hip.

The diagnosis is confirmed by X-ray of the pelvis with the patient first standing on one leg and then on the other and comparing the heights of the two sides of the pubis. Instability is present if their height varies by more than 2 mm. Other X-ray changes include erosions and sclerosis of the bone ends, often with widening of the joint space (*see Figure 9.26*). These changes are similar to those of osteitis pubis.

MANAGEMENT

(1) Rest is essential, since pain is exacerbated by most weight-bearing activities. All sporting activities that involve running or walking must be avoided for several months, although swimming is usually possible.
(2) Anti-inflammatories and analgesics are given for pain relief.
(3) Injections of local anaesthetic and cortico-

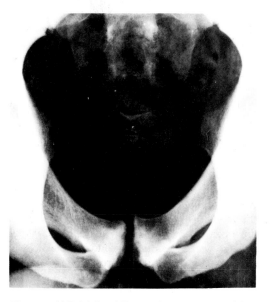

Figure 9.26 Pelvic instability

steroid may be given into painful, tender areas around the pelvis and may be repeated several times if necessary.
(4) When restriction of hip movement, usually internal rotation, is present stretching exercises to the hips are given.
(5) In most patients the condition gradually settles over several months. The patient can then start to resume walking and jogging. Stretching is still continued and abdominal and back exercises commenced. The return to sport needs to be gradual.
(6) Surgery: in those cases that do not respond to conservative therapy, or in which symptoms are recurrent, consideration should be given to fusing the symphysis pubis.

Disorders of the hip bones

Avascular necrosis of the femoral head

Avascular necrosis of the femoral head is believed to follow interruption of its vascular supply. It may follow trauma or occur as a rare complication of many different diseases, but in a proportion of cases no underlying cause can be found and it is then classified as primary or idiopathic.

The initial pathological change is an area of subchondral osteolysis in the femoral head; in the early stages, the articular cartilage remains normal. The underlying subchondral bone rapidly becomes necrotic and liable to collapse and a bony sequestrum may form. Beneath the subchondral bone an area of vascular granulation tissue forms in an attempt at repair as it resorbs the necrotic bone and lays down new bone. As the lesion progresses, the articular cartilage may separate from the femoral head and become re-attached to the collapsed subchondral bone. The femoral head becomes irregular in shape and degenerative changes may ultimately develop.

These changes are consistent with an ischaemic necrosis of bone due to a vascular occlusion but it has not been possible to demonstrate such an occlusion in all cases, including the primary form of this disease. In these cases, it has been proposed that the capillary perfusion pressure becomes insufficient in the rather tenuous microcirculation in this area. Interruption of the arterial blood supply may follow trauma, e.g. a fracture of the femoral neck, slipped femoral epiphysis and dislocation of the hip, but it may follow simple trauma such as a fall on the hip. It may also occur in deep-sea divers, when bubbles of nitrogen gas are formed and cause emboli or direct compression of the vascular channels. Vasculitis, coagulation defects and haemoglobinopathy also produce vascular occlusion. Vasculitis may be the underlying cause in several of the inflammatory arthropathies that may be complicated by an avascular necrosis of bone, especially systemic lupus erythematosus, even if it has not been treated by corticosteroids (Leventhal and Dorfman, 1974).

Fat emboli have been suggested as a cause and may occur in many diseases associated with a disorder of lipid metabolism, such as hyperlipoproteinaemia, Gaucher's disease, gout and chronic alcoholism (Bussere *et al.*, 1975). They may also be the cause in prolonged corticosteroid therapy or Cushing's disease.

CLINICAL FEATURES
Symptoms are identical regardless of the cause. The onset may be gradual, but often there is a sudden, dramatic, onset of hip pain that usually becomes severe and incapacitating and disturbs sleep. Pain may be felt in the hip or thigh but is often felt only at the knee. At first the range of hip movement may remain normal, although pain may be exacerbated by hip movements. After a time, a marked limitation of hip movement and wasting of thigh muscles are usually found.

DIAGNOSIS
Diagnosis is dependent on demonstrating the appropriate X-ray changes. As these usually take some time to develop, a bone scan performed during this period may be useful to demonstrate the presence of a hip abnormality. X-ray changes are found usually in the centre of the femoral head or in its superolateral segment. In the early stages there may be a crescent-shaped area of rarefaction under the subchondral dense bone, which may be more evident if the X-ray is taken while applying traction to the leg. Areas of patchy bony sclerosis develop and the femoral head becomes flattened, irregular or depressed, which produces a step-like appearance. The femoral bone may collapse and appear as an irregular area of sclerosis in the form of an arc with its concavity directed upwards. Subsequent X-ray changes include more extensive sclerosis with destruction and irregularity of the femoral head and the late development of osteoarthritis.

MANAGEMENT
Investigations are necessary to try to establish an underlying cause before appropriate treatment may be given. In its early stages the patient usually needs to be admitted to hospital for bed rest and relief from weight bearing. Analgesics and anti-inflammatory drugs are given for pain relief. If the pain settles the patient can then be mobilized with the aid of crutches and later a walking stick. If pain does not settle surgery is necessary either to replace the femoral head or to give a total hip replacement.

Paget's disease

Paget's disease commonly involves the bones around the hip. Pain is the usual presenting symptom and is often worse at night. Pain may be of bony origin due to the Paget's disease or its complications such as fracture or osteosarcoma. It may also be due to osteoarthritis of the hip. If the juxta-articular bone is involved osteoarthritis of the hip usually develops and produces mechanical hip pain.

Acute osteoporosis

This condition is related to regional migratory osteoporosis (Duncan, Frame and Frost, 1969) and Sudeck's atrophy. It occurs mainly in middle-aged men, usually in the absence of any recognizable cause or rarely after trauma. The patient presents with severe pain and stiffness in the hip or thigh. It is often of sudden onset but becomes gradually progressive over the next few months so that walking becomes increasingly difficult. The course is one of slow resolution over the next 6 months. X-ray changes are necessary for diagnosis and show rarefaction in the hip, especially the femoral head. The joint space remains well preserved, thus helping to differentiate it from arthritis or joint infection. X-ray changes are present for some time after clinical remission.

Stress fractures

Stress fractures of the femoral neck are not uncommon (Devas, 1965) and tend to occur in two types of patient. The first is in young active males, such as army recruits. The second is in the elderly, who may also have osteoporosis. Two types of fracture have also been described. One is a compression fracture that tends to occur at the lower border of the neck in the young and responds well to rest. The second is a transverse fracture across the upper border of the neck in the elderly that tends to become displaced and requires surgical treatment.

Diagnosis is made by X-ray, including tomography of the femoral neck and bone scanning.

Entrapment neuropathy

Lateral cutaneous nerve of the thigh

The lateral cutaneous nerve of the thigh is derived mainly from the L2 and L3 nerve roots and supplies the skin over the anterolateral aspect of the thigh. In the pelvis, the nerve emerges from the lateral border of the psoas, crosses the iliacus muscle and usually enters the thigh by passing through a tunnel in the inguinal ligament near its attachment to the anterior superior iliac spine but may, at times, pass deep to this ligament. The most common site for entrapment of the nerve is found in this tunnel, as the nerve angulates to enter the thigh (Edelson and Nathan, 1977), and it may be compressed or kinked by the inguinal ligament. The degree of angulation is increased by extension of the hip. Many other causes of compression here have been described including direct trauma, pregnancy, alteration in weight or activity after prolonged bed rest. Less commonly, the nerve may be entrapped at other sites along its course from the spinal canal.

Symptoms occur mainly in middle-aged males. The patient describes a typical burning pain with numbness or paraesthesias in the distribution of the nerve over the anterolateral aspect of the thigh to just above the knee. An unusual sensation of itching or formication may be present which leads the patient to rub the area of skin involvement so producing a rash. Symptoms may be intermittent and tend to be brought on by periods of prolonged standing or by alterations of posture which usually involve hip extension.

MANAGEMENT

(1) The patient needs to rest from those movements or positions of the hip that are known to cause exacerbation of symptoms.
(2) Injections of local anaesthetic and corticosteroid may be infiltrated around the nerve as it passes through the inguinal ligament. A tender area may be found approximately one finger-breadth medial to the anterior inferior iliac spine. This site is injected with 5 ml of local anaesthetic and 1 ml of corticosteroid.
(3) Mobilization of the tissues in the entrapment area may relieve the patient's symptoms.
(4) Heat, ice and other physical modalities are of no value.
(5) Surgery to decompress the nerve may be necessary in those patients whose symptoms continue.

Hip diseases in childhood

These include:

(1) Congenital dislocation of the hip and acetabular dysplasia. Failure of normal hip development may result in deformity due to congenital dislocation, subluxation of the hip or acetabular dysplasia, all of which may be associated in later life with osteoarthritis.
(2) Juvenile chronic polyarthritis.
(3) Perthes' disease.
(4) Transient synovitis.
(5) Adolescent coxa vara.

Congenital dislocation of the hip

In this condition the underdeveloped femoral head becomes dislocated upwards into the iliac fossa. A genetic disorder is believed to be at least partly responsible because it is approximately six times more common in females than males and is predominantly a disorder of the caucasian population, especially Scandinavians. It is bilateral in about one-third of cases and the left hip is more commonly and more severely involved. Ideally it should be diagnosed at birth by detecting an abnormal thud on abduction of the affected hip and the diagnosis confirmed on X-ray. If congenital dislocation is detected and reduced early the chances of subsequent osteoarthritis are considerably reduced.

Congenital subluxation

Subluxation is present when the femoral head moves upwards and outwards, losing contact with the underdeveloped acetabulum. X-rays will demonstrate these changes and there is an interruption in Shenton's line (*see Figure 9.21*).

Acetabular dysplasia

In acetabular dysplasia the acetabulum is shallow with an inadequate sloping roof, and it may be associated with coxa valga and anteversion of the femoral neck. Acetabular dysplasia can be measured radiologically as there is a reduction in the vertical angle VCE to less than 20 degrees and an increase in the horizontal angle HTE to more than 10 degrees (*see Figure 9.27*). Inadequate covering of the femoral head may predispose the patient to osteoarthritis of the hip in later life.

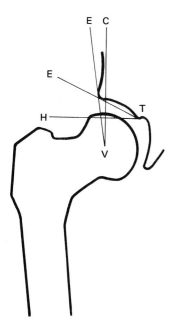

Figure 9.27 In acetabular dysplasia the vertical angle (VCE) is reduced and the horizontal angle (HTE) increased

Juvenile chronic polyarthritis

Hip involvement is an important cause of loss of functional capacity in children with this condition (Isdale, 1970). Hip involvement usually occurs comparatively early in the course of the polyarticular form of this disease, and monarticular hip disease is rare. The radiological features include growth defects in the femoral

head and acetabulum, protrusio acetabuli and coxa valga.

Perthes' disease

Perthes' disease is one of the group of juvenile osteochondroses. It occurs usually in male children aged from 3 to 10 years and may be bilateral. The child presents with a limp, associated usually with a minor degree of pain and a variable degree of limitation of hip movement. The disease runs its natural course over 2–4 years.

The diagnosis is confirmed on X-ray but it may take some time before the typical changes develop. The first change may be a widening of the medial joint space due to an effusion in the hip, and Kemp (1973) has shown that this may even be a causative factor in ischaemia. Later, a line of separation in the subchondral bone develops, the line of the epiphyseal cartilage appears irregular and ragged and the epiphysis becomes necrotic and dense. Healing occurs by revascularization as vascular buds grow out into the epiphysis and produce an appearance of fragmentation of the head. This continues for several years and leaves a residual oval-shaped mushroom deformity of the femoral head—known as coxa plana—and a wide, thick femoral neck. The acetabular fossa becomes oblique and is too small for the femoral head. Osteoarthritis commonly develops in later life.

The aetiology of Perthes' disease is uncertain, but vascular causes due to alteration of the arterial supply producing infarction and necrosis have been implicated. However, a single incident does not usually require such a prolonged period for healing, and McKibbin and Ralis (1974) suggested that repeated episodes of infarction may occur. Robichorv *et al.* (1974), in animal experiments, supported the theory that diminished blood supply to the femoral head caused necrosis of the epiphysis which also resulted in loss of longitudinal but not appositional growth of the femoral neck and that this resulted in the wide, short neck characteristic of this disease. However, Suramo *et al.* (1974), who used intraosseous venography, suggested that the cause of the delayed healing was a disturbance of the venous circulation in the neck. Salter (1973) found in humans and animals that one of the most common factors in pathogenesis was a skeletal immaturity with a progressive subluxation of the femoral head. He also found that deformity of the head could be lessened if it could be contained within the acetabulum.

Management

The orthopaedic management of this condition includes:

(1) Relief from weight bearing, which may be obtained with bed rest combined with continuous traction. This needs to be maintained for a considerable length of time and so is not generally acceptable.
(2) The patient may be kept ambulant by wearing a Snyder's sling.
(3) Management designed to keep the femoral head within the acetabulum, which includes splinting of the lower leg to immobilize it in a hip-to-toe plaster with the hip in abduction and internal rotation. This Whitman splint is, however, not often successful.
(4) Operations designed for the same purpose as (3). These include either a pelvic or a femoral osteotomy to ensure a more complete containment of the femoral head by the acetabulum.

Transient synovitis

This condition is also known as irritable hip or observation hip and results from a benign self-limiting synovial inflammation. The patient is usually a child who presents with a sudden onset of hip pain and a limp with painful limitation of hip movements. There may be a history of minor trauma.

Laboratory tests are always normal but the X-ray may show soft-tissue swelling, especially bulging over the intrapelvic aspect of the acetabulum. Diagnosis may need to be made by exclusion from other conditions such as infective arthritis, Still's disease or Perthes' disease. These conditions usually become evident after repeated investigations whereas transient synovitis settles within a few days' treatment with bed rest and analgesics and without any sequelae.

Adolescent coxa vara

This condition is due to displacement of the upper epiphysis of the femoral head in a medial, posterior and inferior direction. The slip must occur before this epiphysis unites, usually at about the age of 16. It occurs more commonly in males, aged usually 11–15, who are usually either obese with poorly developed secondary sex characteristics or tend to be lean and tall. As this condition is bilateral in approximately 25 per cent of cases, some genetic or hormonal predisposition is considered likely. The onset may be insidious or trauma may produce a shearing strain on the femoral head and then result in an acute slip. The child usually presents with pain, often felt in the knee rather than in the hip, and a limp as the hip is maintained in a position of adduction and lateral rotation. There may be a Trendelenburg gait and clinical examination will reveal restricted hip movements, particularly internal rotation.

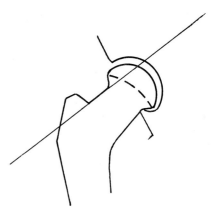

Figure 9.28 Tracing of an X-ray of the right hip. Normally, a line drawn along the superior surface of the femoral neck transects the femoral head

Anteroposterior and lateral X-rays are necessary to confirm the diagnosis (*see Figures 9.28 and 9.29*). In the anteroposterior view the head may appear to be tilted medially so that the medial third of the metaphysis is displaced out of the acetabulum. In this view a line drawn along the superior surface of the femoral neck should transect a portion of the femoral head. If, however, the head has slipped medially a line drawn along the superior aspect of the femoral neck will fall outside the head of the femur. Subsequent bone remodelling occurs as bone is laid down on the medial side of the neck and resorbed on its lateral aspect, producing a characteristic radiological appearance of the femoral head which appears to be tilted.

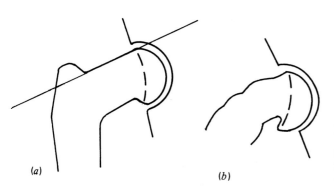

(a)

(b)

Figure 9.29 Tracings of X-rays of the hip.
(*a*) In slipped epiphysis, this line passes above the
femoral head. (*b*) In the lateral view, the slipped
femoral head is extruded from the confines of the
acetabulum

Management

In the acute stages the patient should be admitted
to hospital for bed rest and longitudinal traction
which is applied with the leg in medial rotation.
Manipulative reduction of the displacement
under anaesthesia may be successful, especially in
patients with an acute slip. Once reduced, the
femoral capital epiphysis is held in place by pins
inserted up the femoral neck and across the
epiphyseal plate to stop the epiphysis from again
slipping.

If manipulative reduction is not possible, and
the deformity is marked, it may be necessary to
realign the head and neck of the femur by performing an osteotomy.

Complications

Complications of a slipped femoral epiphysis include cartilage necrosis, avascular necrosis of the
bone and osteoarthritis. The incidence of acute
necrosis involving the cartilage of the femoral
head varies in different series but may be as high
as 28 per cent (Maurer and Larsen, 1970). The
cause is unknown. Osteoarthritis usually develops
in later life if slip has been unrecognized and
becomes chronic. In the chronic condition hip
movements are restricted and an adduction and
external rotation develops, with shortening of the
leg.

10　The knee

The knee joint, the largest synovial joint in the body, combines considerable mobility and strength with the stability necessary to lock the knee in the upright position. The joint is made up of three functional units, the medial and lateral tibiofemoral compartments and the patellofemoral joint, each lined by articular cartilage and all enclosed in a common capsule which is lined by synovial membrane.

The medial and lateral compartments of the knee joint have a similar basic structure (Cross, 1974) and contain an intra-articular meniscus. Each compartment is enclosed by a capsular ligament that runs anteriorly from the patellar ligament to the posterior cruciate ligament. The inner aspects of each capsular ligament are attached to the intra-articular meniscus, and their outer aspect is strengthened and supported by a strong collateral ligament and the surrounding musculotendinous insertions.

Capsular ligaments

The capsular ligaments supporting the two tibiofemoral compartments have a similar anatomical arrangement.

The medial compartment

This is bounded on its medial aspect by the medial capsular ligament and on its lateral aspect by the posterior cruciate ligament. The medial capsular ligament is divided into anterior, middle and posterior thirds (*see Figure 10.1*). The anterior third is thin and loose. The thick middle is attached to the femur above and runs to the medial meniscus as the meniscofemoral ligament and then from the meniscus to the tibia below as the meniscotibial ligament (*see Figure 10.2*). The posterior third is also known as the posterior oblique ligament and is supported by the semimembranosis muscle and its aponeurosis which are also known as the oblique popliteal ligament.

The medial capsular ligament is strengthened

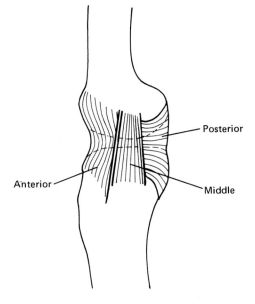

Figure 10.1 Medial aspect of the knee. The medial capsular ligament is made up of three ligaments

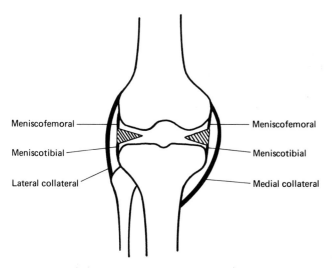

Meniscofemoral ——
Meniscotibial ——
Lateral collateral ——

—— Meniscofemoral
—— Meniscotibial
—— Medial collateral

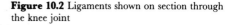

Figure 10.2 Ligaments shown on section through the knee joint

on its medial side by the more superficially placed tibial collateral ligament, which arises from the medial femoral epicondyle and is inserted into the tibia a hand's breadth below the joint line. The collateral ligament is separated from the middle third of the medial capsular ligament by a bursa and at its tibial attachment it is separated from the combined tendons of the semitendinosus, gracilis and sartorius muscles by the pes anserinus bursa.

The lateral joint compartment

This has a somewhat similar arrangement of its capsular ligaments. It is bounded on its lateral aspect by the lateral capsular ligament, and on its medial aspect by the anterior cruciate ligament.

The lateral capsular ligament can also be divided into anterior, middle and posterior thirds. The anterior third is supported on its outside by

the iliotibial band. The middle third is divided into a meniscofemoral and a meniscotibial ligament, and is supported by the fibular collateral ligament which runs from the lateral epicondyle of the femur to the head of the fibula. The posterior third has also been called the arcuate ligament, because of its shape as it arches up across the popliteus muscle. It is supported by the biceps and popliteus muscles.

Cruciate ligaments

The two cruciate ligaments, so named because they cross each other, occupy the central intercondylar area of the knee. They are named according to their tibial attachments, so that the anterior cruciate is inserted more anteriorly on the tibia than the posterior cruciate (*see Figure 10.3*).

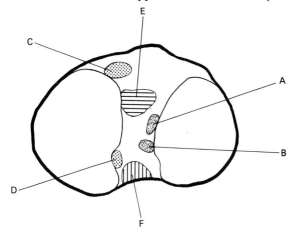

Figure 10.3 Upper surface of right tibia, showing tibial condyles and the intercondylar area with its attachments: (A) anterior horn of lateral meniscus; (B) posterior horn of lateral meniscus; (C) anterior horn of medial meniscus; (D) posterior horn of medial meniscus; (E) anterior cruciate ligament; and (F) posterior cruciate ligament

The anterior cruciate ligament arises from the inner aspect of the lateral condyle of the femur and passes downwards to be inserted on the anterior aspect of the intercondylar area of the tibia between the anterior horns of the two semilunar cartilages. The ligament is composed of three bundles, which are of different lengths and functions: a long anteromedial band, a short posterolateral band, and an intermediate band (Norwood and Cross, 1979).

The normal functions of the anterior cruciate ligament and its degree of tightening during knee movements are still debatable. It is generally agreed that this ligament acts as a guide to the screw-home mechanism by which the femur rotates internally on the tibia during knee extension and plays an important role in maintaining lateral and rotary stability of the knee. Thus it is a stabilizer of the knee against anterior and internal rotational displacements of the knee (Fetto and Marshall, 1979). However, the main function of this ligament is considered by Hughston *et al.* (1976) to be to prevent hyperextension of the knee.

The posterior cruciate ligament arises by a fanlike attachment from the medial condyle of the femur and is inserted into the posterior part of the intercondylar fossa of the tibia, posterior to the posterior horns of the two semilunar cartilages. It receives more ligamentous support than the anterior cruciate by virtue of its attachments to the posterior capsular ligaments and the accessory ligaments of Humphrey and Wrisberg. It is situated in the centre of the knee and is taut in all degrees of flexion and extension. This ligament stabilizes the knee by preventing posterior displacement of the tibia and it appears to be the axis around which the knee moves in flexion, extension and rotation (Hughston *et al.*, 1976).

Knee movements

Two active movements take place in the knee: flexion–extension and axial rotation.

Flexion and extension

These take place around a transverse axis running through the femoral condyles, but as they also involve a spiral action they are not simple hinge movements. Movement involves a complex set of actions in all of the surrounding structures.

Tibiofemoral joints

The articular surfaces of the femur are convex both from front to rear and from side to side. The medial tibial surface is correspondingly concave from side to side and from front to rear but the lateral tibial surface is concave only from side to side and is convex from front to rear. With the knee fully flexed, the extreme posterior portions of the two femoral condyles lie on the posterior portion of the corresponding articular surface of the tibial condyles. Knee extension from this flexed position involves a rolling and sliding action of the femoral condyles on the tibia. However, the two femoral condyles are of unequal sizes, with the medial condyle of the femur being longer, narrower and more curved than the lateral condyle. Accordingly, during extension, the movement on the lateral condyle is completed first while there still remains approximately 1.5 cm of movement available in the medial femoral condyle. Thus, during the last 20 degrees of knee extension the femur can internally rotate on the tibia, so producing the 'screw-home' mechanism. Similarly, on flexion of the knee from the fully extended position the femur must first externally rotate on the tibia. The centre for this condylar motion, the so-called 'instant centre', varies during movements and between individuals.

Patellofemoral joint

During flexion and extension of the knee, the patella moves in its femoral groove. During flexion it moves downwards and backwards on the femoral trochlear surface, which extends down on to the articular surface of the medial and lateral femoral condyles. The patella moves in the deep groove formed by the femoral condyles and comes to lie within the intercondylar notch. The range of patellar excursion is about twice its length, so that on full knee flexion the patella comes to lie under the femoral condyles and faces upwards. Its excursion is controlled by the quadriceps muscle.

Muscles

The muscular control of flexion–extension is supplied by three muscles: the vastus medialis and medial hamstring muscles, which rotate the tibia medially while flexing the knee; and the popliteus, which stabilizes the femur while flexing the knee.

Ligaments

The cruciate ligaments form a functional unit which helps to control flexion and extension and acts as a guide rope to maintain the femur and tibia on their spiral movement. During flexion and extension of the knee they guide the femoral condyles as they slide forwards and backwards.

Menisci

The cruciate ligaments also have firm attachments to the menisci, which are in turn firmly attached to and move with the tibia and are attached to the joint capsule and capsular ligaments. The lateral meniscus is not as firmly attached to its collateral ligament as is its medial counterpart and has greater mobility. In addition the tendon of the popliteus muscle, which is interposed between the lateral meniscus and the capsule, produces an increased excursion of the meniscus. During knee extension the menisci move forwards and on knee flexion they move backwards so that on maximum flexion they are compressed between the posterior aspects of the femur and tibia. The menisci are attached to and controlled in these movements by their attachments to the capsular ligaments.

The infrapatellar fat pad

This lies deep to the patellar ligament and fills in the space between the condyles of the tibia and femur. It lies within the joint capsule but outside the synovial membrane, which is reflected over the lateral margins of the fat pad as the alar ligaments. This mobile cushion plays an important role in aiding knee movements, particularly in flexion and extension, by changes in its shape as it is moved by its alar ligaments.

Axial rotation

Axial rotation of the knee about the long axis of the leg occurs only when the knee is flexed and is normally impossible with the knee extended. This movement can best be observed while the subject is seated with the knee flexed over the edge of a

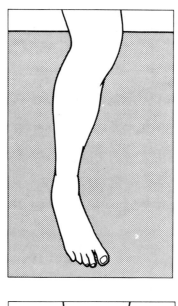

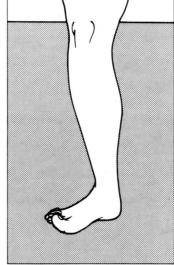

Figure 10.4 Axial rotation in the flexed knee

couch. The active range of internal rotation is normally about 30 degrees and external rotation about 40 degrees (*see Figure 10.4*).

On rotation, the menisci move with the femur; on external rotation, the lateral meniscus moves anteriorly in its tibiofemoral compartment and the medial meniscus moves posteriorly in its compartment. These movements of the menisci are reversed during internal rotation. They can be easily felt to move by palpating the joint line while the flexed knee is externally and internally rotated. A tear in a meniscus is usually produced by a similar type of movement—that is, with the body weight on a slightly flexed knee which is then rotated.

Patellofemoral movements

The retropatellar surface is divided into the smaller, medial and the larger lateral facets by a vertical ridge. The medial patellar facet is also divided by a ridge into two facets, the smaller and more medial facet being given the name of 'the odd facet' because of the peculiarities of its articulation with the femur (*See Figure 10.5*). The lateral facet of the patella articulates with the femur throughout the range of flexion movement, but the odd facet articulates only at 135 degrees of flexion.

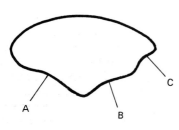

Figure 10.5 The retropatellar surface: (A) the lateral patellar facet; (B) the medial patellar facet with its 'odd facet' (C)

While the patient is standing with the knee extended the patella normally lies above its reciprocal articular margins on the femoral condyle. As the patella descends during flexion of the knee, different areas of its articular surface come into contact with the femur (Goodfellow, Hungerford and Zindel, 1976). At 20 degrees of flexion the medial and lateral facets on its lower pole become apposed and at 90 degrees of flexion the medial and lateral facets of the upper pole of the patella do so. As the knee is flexed past 90 degrees and the patella comes to lie under the femoral condyles the patella rotates and moves laterally. At 135 degrees of flexion the areas of contact are its lateral facet and medially the odd facet now also articulates with the medial femoral condyle.

Symptoms

Perhaps in no other joint is a detailed history as important as in the knee, and it should provide an appreciation of the underlying type and degree of abnormality. Important points in the history include:

(1) Whether the onset of pain is sudden or gradual.
(2) The relationship of pain to any trauma and the mechanism of such trauma.
(3) The presence of any swelling and how rapidly it develops.
(4) A feeling of instability or 'giving way' of the knee on use.
(5) Any locking of the knee.
(6) Clicking of the knee, especially if associated with the patient's pain.
(7) Whether the knee problem is stable, progressive, recurrent or intermittent, or brought on only by certain activities.
(8) The presence of any stiffness.
(9) Whether any other joints are involved.
(10) Any other illnesses that may have been present.
(11) The effects of any previous treatments.

Some of these will be described in more detail.

Knee pain

Since the knee is the largest synovial joint in the body it is a common site for traumatic, degenerative and inflammatory disorders. Pain may also be felt in the knee as the result of disease in more proximal structures. Pain from hip disease may be referred to the knee where it is then experienced as a dull aching pain in the knee or suprapatellar region. Pain from the hip may also radiate down the anterior aspect of the thigh to the knee. Patients with an intervertebral-disc prolapse may also first complain of pain in the knee, which is caused by an L3 or an L4 nerve-root pressure.

Disorders of the knee joint usually produce pain within the knee itself. Pain arising from the tibio-femoral joint is often worse when the patient first stands up and starts to walk or after walking for some distance, is often worse with weight-bearing on the affected leg and is worse on going up or down stairs. Pain may also be associated with stiffness, especially after sitting for a time. Disorders of the patellofemoral joint usually produce pain in the retropatellar area, made worse either by activities that involve this joint such as walking, running, riding a bike or going up stairs; or after a prolonged period of sitting, for example in a car or theatre.

Locking

A history of locking of the knee, if present, is of considerable diagnostic significance but a careful evaluation of this symptom is essential. Locking is usually taken to mean a sudden complete block to full extension of the knee, which is nevertheless able to flex fully. The knee usually lacks about 30 degrees of extension, but this can range from 10 to 45 degrees, and the screw-home mechanism of rotation is lost. The end-feel of extension in a locked knee provides a characteristic rubbery sensation due to the protective muscle spasm. Locking is not an appropriate term since it implies that no movement at all should be possible and also because the patient may use the word to describe an inability to move the knee owing to stiffness or pain.

A history of unlocking of the joint is of considerable value in establishing whether locking has occurred. Unlocking may occur either spontaneously or after manipulation of the knee and the patient reports a sensation of something slipping or snapping back into place. Locking may be due to a torn meniscus, a loose bony fragment from an osteochondritis dissecans, a torn cruciate ligament or avulsed anterior tibial spine, chondromalacia patellae or a dislocated patella.

Instability

A feeling of instability, often described as a 'giving way' or 'buckling' of the knee on use, is a common symptom. It may be produced by several different disorders, including chondromalacia patellae, a torn meniscus, usually a tear of the posterior horn of the medial meniscus (Smillie, 1974), a loose bony foreign body, or arthritis. A feeling of instability may also arise as the result of ligamentous damage resulting in rotatory instability. The knee usually gives way suddenly without any warning or pain but often with a feeling that one bone has moved or slipped on the other. This tends to occur on walking down stairs or over uneven ground when the leg supports the body weight. It is particularly common when a runner suddenly changes direction or steps off the involved leg. Instability may also occur with weakness or inhibition of the action of the quadriceps mechanism, particularly of the vastus medialis; and after injuries to the capsular ligaments of the knee, with subsequent loss of functional stability. This has been called stable instability (Williams and Sperryn, 1976) and is presumably due to pain inhibition or a loss of the normal proprioceptive feedback from the ligamentous structures.

Examination

Before the knee joint itself is tested the lower limb and the lumbar spine should be examined. The knee forms a part of a link system in which the trunk acts as supporting pedestal that transmits forces into the lower leg and foot. As the knee is the mid joint in this link alterations in other lower-limb structures can produce alterations in the biomechanical load on the knee and result in pathological changes (Nicholas, 1970).

Movement in the spine and hip is tested for any limitation in their range and for whether they reproduce pain in the knee. The strength and extensibility of the thigh muscles should be tested routinely. This includes the flexors and abductors of the hip, and the hamstring group for the presence of any 'tightness'. Any deficiency in these structures may be associated with knee pain, especially in the retropatellar area. The patient's gait and the presence of any structural deformities in both lower limbs should also be observed.

Examination of the knee joint

(1) Inspection:

    (a) Deformities.
    (b) Swellings.
    (c) Muscle wasting.

(2) Movements, routine tests:

    (a) Active.
    (b) Passive.
    (c) Accessory.
    (d) Isometric.

(3) Movements, special tests for:

    (a) Ligamentous instability.

(b) Meniscus tears.

(c) The patellofemoral joint.

(4) Palpation.

Inspection

The whole length of both lower limbs is inspected first with the patient standing, then walking, then sitting with knees flexed over the edge of the couch and finally with the patient supine for any deformities, swelling or muscle wasting.

KNEE DEFORMITIES

The knee is inspected for the presence of any deformities, such as genu valgum, genu varum (*see Figure 10.6*), genu recurvatum or flexion deformity. The patella is best inspected with the patient seated and the knees flexed to a right angle over the edge of the couch. The size and shape of the patella, its relationship to the tibiofemoral joint and the direction in which it points is noted.

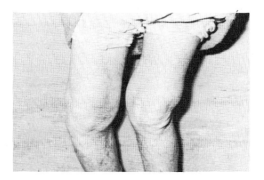

Figure 10.6 Genu varum of right leg and genu valgum of left leg

SWELLINGS

Swellings around the knee are usually evident in certain characteristic sites. A synovial effusion in the knee bulges into the suprapatellar area where the synovium is reflected along the femoral shaft. It obliterates the normal suprapatellar depression and appears as a moon-shaped swelling extending up to 6 cm above the upper border of the patella (*see Figure 10.7*). This swelling is easily seen on inspection especially in the pressure of quadriceps wasting and by comparing the swollen knee with the opposite one.

Swellings in other areas of the knee include: a Pellegrini–Stieda lesion associated with a swelling at the upper attachment of the medial collateral ligament; a prepatellar bursitis, which

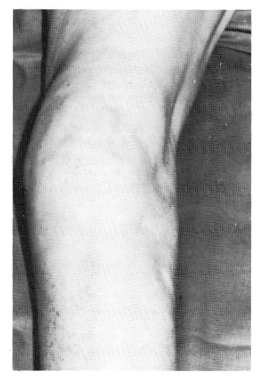

Figure 10.7 Synovial effusion in the knee seen bulging in the suprapatellar area

points forward over the anterior aspect of the patella; cysts of the menisci, which are often best appreciated with the patient sitting with the knees flexed over the edge of the couch and the swelling becomes most apparent over the joint line, with the knees flexed to 45 degrees; Osgood–Schlatter's disease, which is associated with a swelling of the tibial tubercle below the knee; a popliteal cyst, which with the patient standing may be seen bulging into the popliteal space; a calf cyst, which can be easily appreciated, usually as a swelling in the medial aspect of the calf.

MUSCLE WASTING

The size of the quadriceps muscle in each leg is compared and the presence of any muscle wasting is usually detected on inspection.

Movements

These should be first assessed by functional movements such as gait and squatting. The examiner should ask the patient to walk towards him and then away from him and at the same time assess any abnormality or asymmetry in his gait. This test may also be repeated by having the patient walk backwards, at first away from and then towards the examiner. By this method any abnormality or asymmetry of gait and any lack of full knee extension may become evident.

Active movements

The ranges of flexion, extension and axial rotation are tested. The knee should normally extend to a straight line, referred to as nought degrees of extension, and some degree of active hyperextension may at times be possible. The active range of flexion, approximately 140 degrees, may be assessed with the patient lying either supine or prone and then actively flexing the knee. The distance of the heel from the buttock may also be used as a measure of knee flexion.

The degree of axial rotation of the knee is measured with the patient seated with the knee flexed over the edge of the couch. The normal active range is approximately 40 degrees of external rotation of the tibia and 30 degrees of internal rotation.

QUADRICEPS LAG
This is tested by having the patient lie supine with his heel supported on a small block and allowing the knee to sag into full extension but without touching the couch. The patient is then asked to lift his heel off the block. It should be possible to do this before the knee starts to lift. If a quadriceps lag is present the knee will be observed to lift first. Inability to extend the knee fully in this manner is often due to pain inhibition and is usually associated with loss of accessory movements in the knee. Similarly, patients with a quadriceps lag often respond well to manual therapy techniques, which allow a return of pain-free knee movements; the lag then disappears.

Movements

PASSIVE MOVEMENTS
More information may be derived by testing the passive ranges of extension, flexion, and axial rotation. Firstly, the range of hyperextension is tested with the patient lying supine and the examiner holds above the patient's knee with one hand and lifts the lower leg upwards with his other hand around the patient's forefoot. This should also be repeated with the resisting hand being placed over the tibial condyle. The range of this movement is compared in both lower limbs, and normally up to 15 degrees of passive

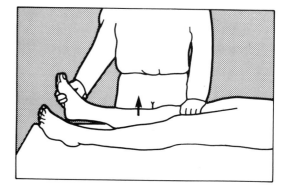

Figure 10.8 Passive hyperextension of the knee

hyperextension is possible (*see Figure 10.8*). The test can be usefully expanded to determine the range and pain response of performing the hyperextension in combination with abduction and adduction.

Secondly, the passive range of flexion is tested. The patient lies prone and the examiner grasps the lower limb above the ankle and moves the heel towards the buttock. Normally the heel should approximate the buttock, as the passive range of this movement is approximately 20 degrees greater than the active range. A decrease in this passive range may be associated either with intrinsic knee disorders or it may indicate a lesion in the quadriceps muscle that is causing a loss of extensibility or a contracture of the muscle.

Thirdly, the degree of hamstring tightness should also be tested with the patient lying supine and the hip flexed to 90 degrees. The examiner then passively extends the knee (*see Figure 10.9*). The normal range of this movement varies with age, physical activity and the normal extensibility of the hamstrings but may also be reduced in disorders of the knee joint.

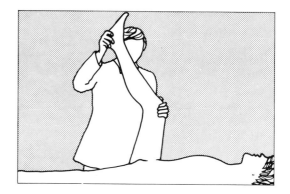

Figure 10.9 Test for the degree of hamstring tightness

Fourthly, the passive range of axial rotation is tested, firstly with the knee in extension and then flexed to 90 degrees. Loss of this range occurs in many intrinsic knee disorders and an increased range with the knee flexed may be associated with a rotary instability of the knee.

ACCESSORY MOVEMENT

There are ten accessory movements in the tibio-femoral joint:

(1) Abduction. The patient lies supine and the examiner produces a valgus movement of the tibia on the femur (*see Figure 10.10*).

(2) Adduction. A varus movement of the tibia is produced.

(3) Anteroposterior. The tibia is moved backwards on the femur (*see Figure 10.11*).

(4) Posteroanterior. The tibia is moved forwards on the femur.

(5) Lateral movement of the tibia on the femur, which is produced by counter-pressure between the examiner's two hands (*see Figure 10.12*).

(6) Medial movement of the tibia on the femur is produced by counter-pressure in the opposite directions (*see Figure 10.13*).

(7) Longitudinal caudad is produced by distraction of the tibia from the femur (*see Figure 10.14*).

(8) Longitudinal cephalad is produced by compression of the tibia.

(9) Medial rotation of the tibia on the femur is

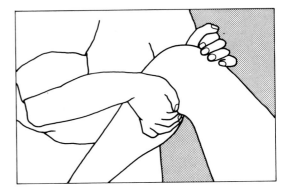

Figure 10.12 Lateral accessory movement

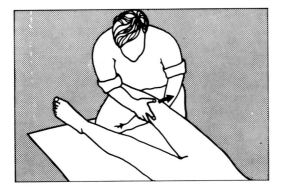

Figure 10.10 Abduction accessory movement

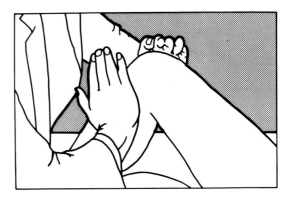

Figure 10.13 Medial accessory movement

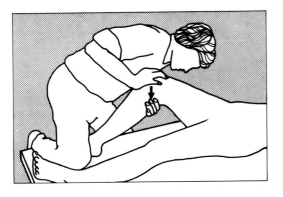

Figure 10.11 Anteroposterior accessory movement

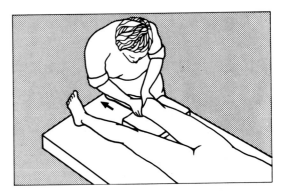

Figure 10.14 Longitudinal caudad accessory movement

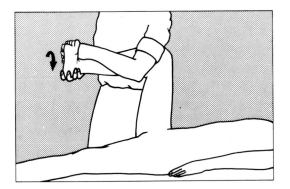

Figure 10.15 Medial rotation accessory movement

produced by the examiner with the patient supine and the knee flexed to 90 degrees (*see Figure 10.15*).

(10) Lateral rotation is produced by the examiner reversing his hands.

ISOMETRIC TESTS

Isometric tests are used to assess the strength of the quadriceps and hamstring muscles. Normal quadriceps development is essential for knee function and is best detected by having the patient sit with the knees flexed over the edge of the couch. The examiner then places one hand above the ankle and resists the patient's attempts to extend the knee. The bulk of the quadriceps muscle can be appreciated on inspection and its tone may be evaluated by palpation. Special attention is given to the size and tone of the vastus medialis muscle, which plays an important role in knee stability.

Hamstring strength is tested with the patient lying prone and the examiner resists the patient's attempt to flex the knee. Finally, as part of the normal knee examination, the strength of the hip flexors and hip abductors should also be tested.

Palpation

The knee joint is palpated for the presence of any fluid; synovial thickening; warmth; swellings; end-feel; crepitus; clicking; and tenderness.

The knee is palpated to confirm the presence of any synovial fluid that bulges into the suprapatellar pouch and has a characteristic fluctuant sensation. In a large effusion this is best appreciated by placing the index finger and thumb of the right hand on either side of the patella and the left hand is placed over the suprapatellar pouch to squeeze the fluid distally. The finger and

thumb of the right hand are separated, which produces a feeling of fluctuation. A small effusion is not so readily appreciated on inspection and is best demonstrated by the bulge sign (*see Figure 10.16*).

THE BULGE SIGN

The examiner first empties the normal gutter over the medial compartment of the knee joint just under the medial border of the patella by stroking out any fluid upwards into the suprapatellar pouch. The left hand is then used to compress

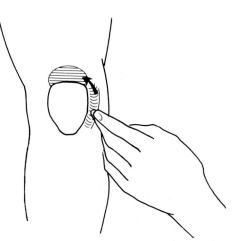

Figure 10.16 (*a*) The bulge sign. Fluid is stroked out of the medial gutter

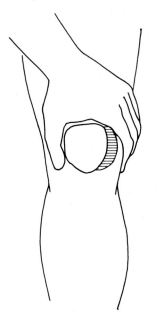

Figure 10.16 (*b*) The bulge sign. The suprapatellar pouch is compressed

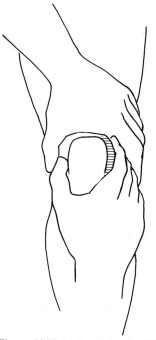

Figure 10.16 (*c*) The bulge sign. Fluid bulges out into the medial gutter

the suprapatellar pouch, which forces any fluid present distally where it can be seen to bulge this gutter outwards in a wave-like motion. This test should then be repeated but this time with the thumb and index finger of the right hand placed on either side of the patella so that the index finger can confirm the presence of fluid.

PATELLAR TAP
To perform this test the examiner first compresses the synovial fluid from the suprapatellar pouch into the knee joint with his left hand and then sharply taps the lower pole of the patella against the underlying femur with the index

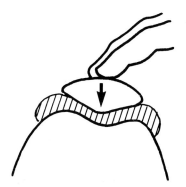

Figure 10.17 Patellar tap

finger of the right hand. When sufficient fluid is present within the joint the patella can be felt to tap against the femur and then float free (*see Figure 10.17*). However, this sign is not of great clinical value since it requires only a certain amount of fluid within the joint and if insufficient or excessive fluid is present the patella cannot be suitably tapped.

Chronic synovial thickening may be palpated about the synovial reflection along the superior margins of the suprapatellar pouch where it presents a characteristic doughy sensation as it is rolled under the fingers. The synovial membrane may also be palpated over the medial joint compartment in the gutter that lies on the medial side of the patella just above the medial tibiofemoral joint line. To palpate the synovium in this area the examiner uses both thumbs, placing one hand below the patella and the other hand above the patella over the suprapatellar pouch.

The synovial membrane in these sites is also palpated for any increased warmth, which is easy to detect by comparison with the opposite knee. An effusion usually produces an increase in temperature, which may also be found in haemarthrosis, infections or malignancy and a routine palpation of the inguinal lymph nodes should also be made at this stage.

Many swellings around the knee can be best appreciated on inspection, but palpation is necessary to confirm their presence and to differentiate them from synovitis or other swellings of the knee. The types of swelling are:

(1) A tender swelling of the tibial tubercle, which is present in Osgood–Schlatter's disease.
(2) Cysts of the menisci, which usually involve the lateral meniscus and produces a tender, tense swelling over the joint line.
(3) A Pellegrini–Stieda lesion, which produces a tender swelling over the upper attachment of the medial collateral ligament to the femoral condyle.
(4) Bursitis, which may be present as a soft-tissue swelling anterior to the patella, known as prepatellar bursitis or housemaid's knee; or bulging on either side of the patellar ligament (infrapatellar bursitis); or as a semimembranosus bursitis with a soft-tissue swelling bulging posteriorly into the popliteal fossa where it may need to be differentiated from an aneurysm of the popliteal artery.
(5) Osteochondromatosis, which can usually be palpated as bony swellings within the syn-

ovial cavity and need to be differentiated from loose bony bodies.

(6) Soft-tissue swellings in the synovial cavity, which may be due to pigmented villonodular synovitis and pedunculated swellings due to a rheumatoid nodule, a ganglion or a benign tumour, such as a fibroma or a giant-cell tumour, are often palpable as they protrude through the joint line.

End-feel is first tested by having the patient lie supine with the knee fully extended and relaxed. The knee is then passively flexed approximately 20 degrees and is then allowed to drop back into full extension. The normal knee can fall into full extension with a typical painless bony end-feel. In patients with osteoarthritis a similar bony end-feel may be found but the joint lacks full extension. In a mechanical block from any cause the tibiofemoral joint has a 'springy' end-feel short of full extension. The end-feel of the movement produced on adduction and abduction of the knee is also characteristic, as the collateral ligaments allow a small range of normal joint movement. If a collateral ligament is ruptured this is replaced by a 'mushy' type of end-feel.

Crepitus is best appreciated by palpating over the patellofemoral joint while flexing and extending the knee. It is present in the young in chondromalacia patellae; in the elderly a fine crepitus is common whereas a coarse crepitus may indicate osteoarthritis. In patients with degenerative changes in the articular cartilage of the tibiofemoral joint, a coarse crepitus may be palpable over the joint line. If osteoarthritis results in instability of the knee a coarse creaking or crunching sensation may be felt.

An audible and palpable click, which may also be painful, may be produced by many of the soft-tissue structures around the knee. The extensor retinaculum may be seen to click over the front of one of the femoral condyles, usually the lateral. Other clicks include that of: the biceps tendon over the head of the fibula; the popliteus tendon in and out of its groove on the lateral femoral condyle; the iliotibial band over the lateral epicondyle of the femur; the normal vacuum joint click associated with the patellofemoral joint; and a torn or discoid meniscus.

Palpation of the knee for tenderness is best achieved by having the patient lie supine with the hip flexed and externally rotated. The examiner then stands beside the couch with one knee flexed and lying on the couch. The patient's flexed knee is then supported over the examiner's knee. In this position the joint line and the upper and lower attachments of the ligaments are easily accessible to the palpating fingers. Injuries of the meniscus may produce tenderness over the anterior, middle or posterior thirds of the joint line. Ligamentous sprains are usually tender over the upper or lower body attachments of the meniscus but tenderness is sometimes found over the middle third of the joint line and so tenderness in this area does not help in differentiating between a ligamentous or meniscus injury. The articular margins of the tibiofemoral joint can also be palpated for tenderness and the presence of osteoarthritic bony lippings.

The retropatellar area is next palpated with the quadriceps relaxed, which is best achieved by having the patient lie supine while the examiner sits on the couch and supports the patient's slightly flexed knee over his thigh. In this position the patella can be readily moved laterally and medially while tenderness is sought in the retropatellar articular surfaces (*see Figure 10.18*).

The popliteal space is examined for the presence of any cystic swellings by having the patient stand with the knee extended and palpating for the presence of any swelling.

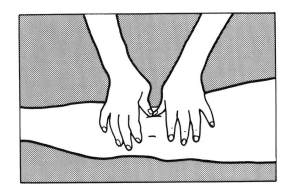

Figure 10.18 Palpation of the retropatellar surface

Classification of knee lesions

(1) Soft tissues:
   (a) Ligament injuries—sprain; ligamentous instability; Pellegrini–Stieda lesion; breast-stroke swimmer's knee.
   (b) Musculotendinous lesions—late effect of quadriceps injury; quadriceps tendon; gastro-

cnemius tendinitis; biceps tendinitis; popliteal tendinitis; iliotibial tract.

(c) Chondromalacia fabellae.

(d) Bursitis.

(2) Joints:

(a) Tibiofemoral joint—meniscus lesions; traumatic synovitis; arthritis; bony lesions (chondral injuries, osteochondritis dissecans, osteonecrosis and haematological diseases); loose body formation, osteochondromatosis.

(b) Patellofemoral joint — chondromalacia patellae; patellar instability; osteoarthritis; osteochondral injuries; lesions of the infrapatellar mechanism.

Soft-tissue lesions

Ligament injuries

A sprain of the knee ligaments is one of the most common of all soft-tissue injuries. These ligaments are designed to prevent abnormal movement of the knee joint. The knee is normally stable in extension and the ligaments are then important static stabilizers of the knee. The flexed knee is less stable and some degree of axial rotation is possible so that abnormal stresses are then most apt to cause ligamentous injury.

The degree of ligamentous injury is classified into first-, second- or third-degree sprains.

First-degree sprains

Only a few ligament fibres are torn and the diagnosis and assessment usually presents no great difficulty. The patient's pain is reproduced by stressing the ligament. For sprains of the medial ligament this is achieved by applying a valgus strain to the joint; for sprains of the lateral ligament by a varus strain to the joint. Tenderness is localized over the site of the injury, which may be either over the joint line or at its upper or lower attachments. The knee joint is stable and there is no synovial effusion, although some swelling over the site of the injury may be present.

Management—The sprained ligament needs to be protected from further damage by resting the knee for 24–36 hours after the injury and ice is applied to minimize haemorrhage and swelling. Isometric quadriceps and hip exercises are com-

menced during this time. Subsequently, complete rest is neither justified nor necessary and the patient should continue the isometric quadriceps and hip exercises. Active exercises can be commenced as pain and discomfort settles, and the patient should continue isometric quadriceps then jog. Heat or ice may be applied before the exercise regimen. Full activity can be resumed when there is a full painless range of movement, usually within 3 weeks.

Second-degree sprains

These may be more difficult to assess as there is usually a synovial effusion within the joint and it may be difficult to determine whether any other intra-articular structure is damaged. Pain and disability is greater than in first-degree sprains, a mild degree of instability may be present and there may be a haemarthrosis.

Management—The early treatment of this injury is similar to that described above. In addition to rest and ice a compression bandage should also be applied to the knee to control swelling. A large effusion, if present, should be drained. The patient should rest and avoid weight-bearing on the injured leg for 24–48 hours and the degree of injury should then be reassessed. If the knee is stable in full extension and there is no evidence of damage to other knee ligaments, management by an active exercise programme, with special attention to the quadriceps muscle, can be instituted. In most patients with second-degree sprains a gradual return to weight-bearing activity is then possible. Since conservative therapy produces satisfactory results, surgery is not indicated (Elsasser, Reynolds and Omohundro, 1974). However, if pain is severe and the quadriceps development is poor the leg may need to be immobilized in a plaster cylinder or a cast brace with the knee in a slight degree of flexion for approximately 2 weeks. Isometric exercises for the quadriceps and hip are commenced immediately and should be supervised by a physiotherapist. After the plaster is removed more active exercises, including knee flexion, can be commenced.

O'Donoghue (1973) stressed that this degree of injury takes up to 8 weeks to heal, even though the original symptoms have subsided after a few weeks, and so full sporting activity should not be resumed for this period of time. If return to full activity is too early pain and effusion may result and the ligament may be further injured.

Third-degree sprains

These are due to a complete rupture of the ligament. The medial collateral ligament is usually torn from its upper femoral attachment; the lateral ligament is usually torn from its lower fibular attachment. In either case, a fragment of bone may also be avulsed which may be visible on X-ray. Immediate pain and disability is usually severe and the diagnosis can usually be readily made if the patient is seen immediately. The diagnosis can be easily missed subsequently as pain may not be marked and the patient may be able to walk into the surgery. Moreover, a synovial effusion may be absent as fluid and blood can escape from the synovial cavity through the capsular tear. Clinical tests to stress the ligament, which are described below, are necessary to demonstrate instability with subluxation of the tibiofemoral joint. X-rays may be useful in confirming the diagnosis; these may demonstrate an avulsion of bone (Woods, Stanley and Tullos, 1979) or the use of stress films may show that the side of the joint where the ligament has been completely ruptured will open under stress (Jacobsen, 1977). The original injury is apt to injure other structures in the tibiofemoral joint and these must also be tested.

Management—The management of a patient with an acute rupture of the medial ligament may be conservative or surgical. Prolonged conservative treatment in a plaster cast has been advocated but surgical repair of a recent injury is the treatment of choice. Surgery also permits the other knee structures damaged in the same injury to be inspected. In the medial compartment this involves especially the cruciate ligaments and the medial meniscus. The medial ligament is reconstructed and surrounding structures, especially in the posteromedial corner, tightened (Ginsburg and Elsasser, 1978). In chronic cases, O'Donoghue (1973) advised reattachment of the distal end of the ligament more anteriorly.

An acute rupture of the lateral collateral ligament and the surrounding musculotendinous structures should be repaired. In late cases, Nicholas (1977) recommends reattaching the iliotibial tract to the posterolateral capsule.

Anterior cruciate ligament

An isolated rupture of the anterior cruciate ligament may occur (Feagin, Abbot and Roukous, 1972), but it is much more common for this ligament to be damaged with other ligaments of the knee and/or the posterior horns of the meniscus. It may also rupture as the result of attritional stretching (Smillie, 1974). After a tear of the anterior cruciate ligament additional stress is placed on other soft-tissue supports, which may then give way. This then leads to an antero-lateral rotational instability with associated damage to the posterolateral capsular ligaments (Cabaud and Slocum, 1977).

The mechanism of anterior cruciate ligament injury involves hyperextension of the knee, such as a direct blow to the front of the femur with the foot and tibia fixed to the ground; or a deceleration injury that also involves rotation of the knee, such as in changing direction while running. The patient is usually conscious of something 'giving way' within the knee and is unable to continue playing. A tense effusion usually develops in the knee within the first 24 hours. Arthroscopy or arthrography may be necessary to confirm the diagnosis (Feagin, 1979).

Management requires considerable clinical judgement and depends on several factors:

(1) If the knee remains clinically stable management should consist of an active rehabilitation programme for the quadriceps and hamstring muscles.
(2) If the diagnosis is made during arthrotomy a primary repair of the ligament may be possible if it is torn or avulsed from its bony attachments. This is rarely possible if the tear involves the middle portion of the ligament.
(3) If primary repair is not possible the ligament may be reconstituted using a strip of fascia lata, iliotibial, tract or the patellar tendon.
(4) For management of late rotatory instability see page 143.

Ligamentous instability

Ligamentous instability of the knee is a common and often underdiagnosed condition associated with a considerable loss of function. There is usually previous trauma to the knee but, in late cases, a history of such trauma cannot always be obtained as the patient may have forgotten the incident.

The terminology used to describe ligamentous instability is confusing. For example, medial instability refers to the injury sustained by the medial ligamentous structures which become unstable. This then allows the tibia to sublux in a valgus, or lateral, direction of the femur. Thus the direction of the resultant subluxation, which is the important clinical finding, differs from the commonly used descriptive title. Similarly, an anteromedial instability results from an injury to the medial capsular ligament. The test for it depends, however, on demonstrating a subluxation of the anteromedial tibial condyle in an anterior and a lateral direction. Instability of the knee may be classified as being either straight, non-rotary; or rotary (Hughston *et al.*, 1976).

Straight, non-rotary instability is classified into four groups: medial, lateral, anterior and posterior (*see Figures 10.19–10.21*).

Rotary instability is classified into anteromedial, anterolateral, posterolateral and combined instabilities (*see Figures 10.22–10.24*).

STRAIGHT INSTABILITY
Medial instability   This is due to disruption of the

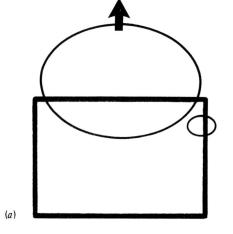

(a)

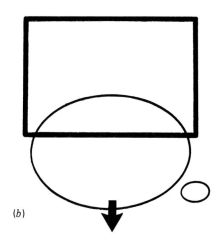

(b)

Figure 10.21 (*a*) Anterior instability. (*b*) Posterior instability; key as in *Figure 10.20*

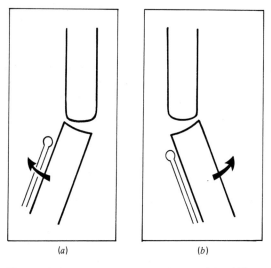

(a)   (b)

Figure 10.19 (*a*) Medial instability. (*b*) Lateral instability

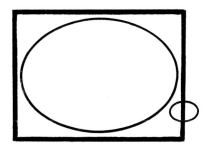

Figure 10.20 Diagrammatic representation of the normal relationship of the femoral condyles (square) to the tibial condyles (large oval) and fibula (small oval), viewed from above

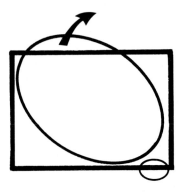

Figure 10.22 Anteromedial rotary instability; key as in *Figure 10.20*

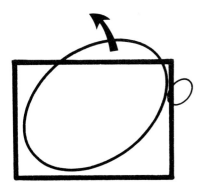

Figure 10.23 Anterolateral rotary instability; key as in *Figure 10.20*

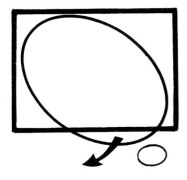

Figure 10.24 Posterolateral rotary instability; key as in *Figure 10.20*

ligaments of the medial tibiofemoral compartment and results in a valgus subluxation of the tibia on the femur (*see Figure 10.19(a)*). It is diagnosed by the presence of a positive abduction stress test. This is performed in two positions, first with the knee in 30 degrees of flexion and then with the knee straight. The normal knee is tested first to assess the degree of laxity normally present.

Initial position—The patient lies supine with the

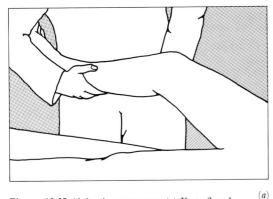

Figure 10.25 Abduction stress test. (*a*) Knee flexed. (*b*) Knee extended

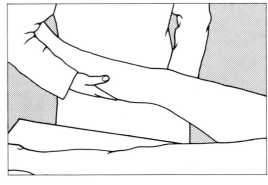

(*b*)

hip slightly abducted. The knee is flexed to 30 degrees over the side of the couch. The examiner hugs the patient's lower leg under his right arm and uses his right hand to steady the lower leg. The examiner's left hand is placed over the lateral aspect of the patient's knee (*see Figure 10.25(a)*).

Method—The knee is gently moved into abduction until pain is produced over the medial compartment or subluxation and gapping of the medial joint line is shown. This test is then repeated with the knee straight (*see Figure 10.25(b)*).

Interpretation—If this test is positive with the knee flexed to 30 degrees but negative with the knee fully extended it implies that the medial collateral ligament has been damaged. If the test is positive with the knee both at 30 degrees of flexion and in full extension it also implies damage to the cruciate and the medial capsular ligaments.

Lateral instability This is due to disruption of the ligaments of the lateral compartment and results in a varus subluxation of the tibia on the femur (*see Figure 10.19(b)*). It is less common than medial instability since the mechanism of injury requires adduction of the knee. It is diagnosed by the presence of a positive adduction stress test. The initial position is similar to that for the abduction stress test but the hands are changed over to apply an adduction stress to the knee.

Interpretation—If the test is positive with the knee flexed to 30 degrees but negative with the knee fully extended it implies that the lateral collateral ligament has been damaged. If it is positive also in extension it implies damage also to the cruciate and lateral capsular ligaments.

Anterior instability This is diagnosed if both tibial condyles can be displaced anteriorly in relation to the femur while the tibia is maintained in the neutral position. It is diagnosed by the presence of a positive anterior drawer test.

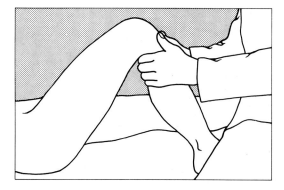

Figure 10.26 Test for anteroposterior instability

Starting position—The patient lies supine with the hip flexed to 45 degrees and the knee to 90 degrees; the examiner sits on the dorsum of the foot to stabilize it. The unaffected leg is examined first to determine the degree of normal laxity. The examiner's hands grasp around the patient's upper tibia and the fingers are used to palpate the hamstring tendons to ensure that they are relaxed (*see Figure 10.26*).

Method—The tibia is gently and repeatedly pulled and pushed to and fro to determine the degree of anterior movement. Great care must be taken to ensure that the knee is kept in a neutral position during this test, as a rotary instability may be present if this test is positive when performed in some degree of rotation.

Interpretation—A positive anterior drawer test is traditionally attributed to a rupture of the anterior cruciate ligament. This is no longer tenable, since patients with a positive anterior drawer test may be found to have an intact ligament at operation. Conversely, patients with a negative test may be found at operation to have a ruptured cruciate ligament. The usual mechanism for the production of this test is a tear of the medial and lateral capsular ligaments, which produces a combined anteromedial and anterolateral rotational instability. However, the degree of subluxation is increased if the anterior cruciate is also ruptured. Hence the anterior cruciate ligament may be regarded as the second line of defence against this instability (Norwood and Cross, 1979).

Variations—The anterior drawer test must be performed at three separate angles of rotation. It is first of all performed in neutral rotation as outlined above; then with the foot and leg externally rotated by approximately 30 degrees; and finally with the foot and leg internally rotated by approximately 15 degrees.

External rotation of the tibia tightens the medial capsular ligament and internal rotation of the tibia tightens the lateral capsular ligament. Excessive movement in either of these two positions indicates a rotary instability, as discussed below.

Posterior instability   This implies that the tibia can be displaced posteriorly on the femur while maintained in the neutral position (*see Figure 10.21(b)*). It is diagnosed by a positive posterior drawer test; the starting position is similar to the anterior drawer test.

Method—The tibia is again pushed and pulled to and fro to disclose any backwards movements of the tibia on the femur.

Interpretation—This test is positive after disruption of the posterior cruciate ligament together with a tear of the posterior capsular ligaments. This test can, at times, be very difficult to differentiate from the anterior drawer test, since the injured knee is originally subluxed posteriorly (*see Figure 10.27*) and the test movements will then draw the tibial plateau forwards.

ROTARY INSTABILITY

Rotary instability of the knee that is due to a ligamentous injury results in an excessive degree of rotation of the tibia on the femur. This may be either an inwards rotation or, more commonly, an outwards rotation. The patient usually presents with a history of the knee suddenly giving way, usually without any warning or pain but often with a feeling that one bone in the knee has moved or slipped on the other. This tends to occur on walking down stairs or over uneven ground when the leg is supporting body weight. It is particularly common when a runner suddenly changes direction or steps off the involved leg. There may be a history of pain and swelling of the knee after

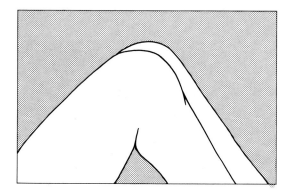

Figure 10.27 Ruptured posterior cruciate ligament of the right knee

trauma, when the patient may have been conscious of a sudden snapping sensation in the knee.

Anteromedial rotary instability   This is an anterior subluxation of the medial tibial condyle that also moves into external rotation on the femur (*see Figure 10.22*). It follows a tear of the capsular ligament of the medial joint compartment, which is then unable to limit the degree of external rotation of the tibia on the femur. This may occur as an isolated lesion but the degree of instability is accentuated if the medial collateral or cruciate ligaments are also ruptured.

Anteromedial instability is diagnosed in the presence of a positive anterior drawer test, which is performed while the tibia is held in external rotation.

Anterolateral rotary instability   This is an anterior subluxation of the lateral tibial condyle that also moves into internal rotation on the femur (*see Figure 10.23*). It is caused by insufficiency of the anterior cruciate ligament (Slocum, James and Singer, 1976; Galway, Beaupre and McIntosh, 1972). Rupture of the anterior cruciate was found in all of the 45 cases reported by Cabaud and Slocum (1977) but in only 13 of 21 cases reported by Andrews (1977). The degree of instability is increased if the lateral capsular ligament is also torn.

Several tests have been described to diagnose this condition:

(1) It is diagnosed by the presence of a positive anterior drawer test that is performed while the tibia is held in neutral rotation and the lateral tibial plateau can be seen to sublux forwards under the lateral femoral condyle (Hughston *et al.*, 1976).

(2) This test may be repeated with the tibia internally rotated by 15 degrees, when there will be anterior and internal subluxation of the lateral tibial condyle on the femur (Cabaud and James, 1977).

(3) The jerk test is performed with the patient supine with the hip flexed to 45 degrees and the knee at 90 degrees. The examiner grasps the patient's foot and fully internally rotates it so that the tibia is also fully internally rotated. A valgus stress is applied to the proximal end of the patient's tibia and fibula. The examiner then gradually straightens the knee (*see Figure 10.28*). At about 30 degrees of flexion the lateral tibiofemoral compartment may be seen to sublux or jerk forward suddenly. As the knee is further extended the tibia returns to its

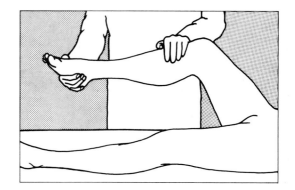

Figure 10.28 Jerk test for anterolateral rotary instability

former position (Hughston *et al.*, 1976). The method of production of this test has also been described as the lateral pivot shift (Galway, 1972).

Posterolateral rotary instability   This is a posterior subluxation of the lateral tibial condyle that also rotates internally (*see Figure 10.24*). It follows a tear of the arcuate complex and is diagnosed in the presence of an external rotation–hyperextension test.

Starting position—The patient lies supine with the knees straight and the examiner lifts the leg by the toes to produce hyperextension at the knee.

Method—As the knee is hyperextended, the tibia may be seen to rotate externally so that the knee develops a varus deformity. This test requires considerable experience to evaluate.

Complications of rotary instability   A tear may develop in the posterior horn of the meniscus. This is associated with degeneration of the meniscus as a result of its being repeatedly caught by the abnormal movement now possible between the femur and tibia. At times the blocking of knee movements by the torn meniscus can mask the presence of a rotary instability produced by the torn ligament.

After meniscectomy the rotary instability then becomes obvious and the patient complains of his knee letting him down. As a further complication of this injury degenerative changes may develop in the tibiofemoral joint (Slocum and Larson, 1968), or osteochondral injuries in the patellofemoral joint.

Management   Anteromedial instability may be controlled by transplanting the pes anserinus tendon, which converts the tendon from a primary flexor of the knee into a rotator of the knee. The tendon is removed from the medial aspect of the tibia and repositioned on the tibial tubercle. In this way the abnormal external rotation of the tibia is controlled. This operation may also be combined with a repair of the anterior cruciate or medial collateral ligaments (Slocum *et al.*, 1974). The late results in 51 patients who had undergone a pes anserinus transfer were found to be successful in 42 (D'Arcy, 1979).

Repair of anterolateral rotational instability may be possible by tightening or reattaching the complex of ligamentous and musculotendinous supports of the lateral compartment. A strap of fascia lata is used to provide additional support to the lateral ligament, thus maintaining the lateral tibial condyle under the femoral condyle in extension (Galway, Beaupre and McIntosh, 1972).

Pellegrini–Stieda lesion

This relatively common condition with ossification in the upper attachment of the tibial collateral ligament usually follows a direct injury with haematoma formation but may occasionally follow a first- or second-degree sprain. The patient, who is often involved in body-contact sports, presents with pain on the medial side of the knee, stiffness, or may be conscious of a tender lump. Examination reveals a tender swelling at the upper end of the attachment of the tibial collateral ligament and pain is reproduced by applying an abduction stress to the knee. X-rays confirm the ossification related to the medial femoral condyle.

MANAGEMENT
Treatment is with ultrasound and isometric quadriceps exercises at first, followed with mobilizing exercises. The painful area in the upper attachment usually responds well to an injection of local anaesthetic and corticosteroid which may be repeated a few times at monthly intervals. The pain usually settles but a slightly tender lump may persist for some months and the patient needs to be reassured about its benign nature. Surgery is not indicated.

Breast-stroke swimmer's knee

This is an overuse syndrome involving the medial collateral ligament of the knee. In breast-stroke swimmers the hips are first abducted with the knees internally rotated. The hips are then actively externally rotated, so placing considerable strain on the medial compartment of the knee and leading to an inflammatory change in the upper attachment of the ligament. The patient presents with pain well localized over the medial knee com-

partment and made worse by continuing activity. *Management* The patient needs to rest from breast-stroke swimming but other swimming strokes may be substituted. Ultrasound applied over the painful ligament helps to ease pain and localize the tender area, which should then be injected with 1 ml corticosteroid. The patient usually returns to full activity in 2–3 weeks.

Musculotendinous lesions at the knee

Late effects of quadriceps injury

In any injury to the quadriceps mechanism or after any knee-joint disorder, the quadriceps rapidly loses bulk and strength, especially the vastus medialis which is necessary to maintain balance in the quadriceps group. This, in turn, may lead to a self-perpetuating painful knee problem (Williams, 1971) which may then be confused with an intrinsic knee disorder or may lead to chondromalacia patellae. Treatment to strengthen the quadriceps by a full exercise programme is essential.

Quadriceps tendon

The quadriceps tendon at its insertion into the upper border of the patella may be partially or completely ruptured. It is a major injury since the quadriceps is unable to maintain stability of the knee on walking.

The tendon may tear if the patient actively flexes the knee while maintaining a maximum quadriceps contraction, as may happen during an unexpected fall or slip. It tends to occur more commonly in elderly male patients and may be associated with degenerative changes in the tendon. The tear in the tendon usually extends into the quadriceps expansion on either side of the patella. If untreated there may be some degree of repair but the patient will be unable to climb stairs or walk up hills without the knee giving way.

Major sign—The patient is unable to sustain an isometric contraction of the quadriceps muscle. This is best tested by having the patient sit over the edge of the couch with the knee fully extended. The examiner pushes above the ankle to flex the knee and the patient attempts to resist this movement but is unable to do so. A gap may be palpable in the tendon above the patella.

Management—Partial tears may be treated conservatively but treatment of a complete tear requires urgent surgery.

Gastrocnemius tendinitis

This little known, but relatively common, lesion involves the musculotendinous origin of the gastrocnemius, more commonly its medial head. It is due to an overuse injury, e.g. in distance runners. A typical history is that running has been modified, either by running at a faster rate or up hills, and it is common at the beginning of an athletic season. Pain is usually well localized above the joint line but when severe may radiate down the leg. The underlying bursa may also be inflamed.

Major sign—The patient lies prone and pain is reproduced by the examiner fully resisting knee flexion.

Confirmatory sign—Tenderness is well localized over the gastrocnemius head. This may be best felt if the patient lies supine and the examiner places one finger over the gastrocnemius origin and then fully flexes the knee with his other hand.

Bicipital tendinitis

The biceps tendon is inserted into the fibular head. Tendinitis follows an overuse injury usually from running and may be associated with a bursitis.

Major sign—Pain is reproduced by resisting flexion of the knee.

Confirmatory sign—Tenderness is well localized on palpation over the tendon insertion.

Popliteal tendinitis

The popliteus muscle runs from the posterior surface of the tibia and is attached by its tendon into the lateral surface of the lower femur. Pain is felt at the posterolateral corner of the knee joint and may be extreme for the first 24 hours after running but then usually improves. At times, the tendon may slip in and out of its groove on the femoral condyle, which produces a painful click (Mayfield, 1977).

Major sign—Pain may be reproduced on contraction of the muscle. This is best tested with the patient lying supine, the hip flexed, abducted and laterally rotated and the knee at right angles. The examiner then fully resists active flexion of the knee with one hand while palpating the tendon just posterior to the lateral collateral ligament with the other (*see Figure 10.29*).

Confirmatory sign—Tenderness may be felt just

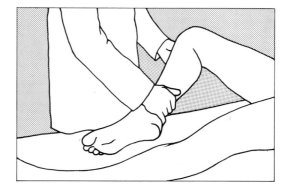

Figure 10.29 Test for popliteal tendinitis

above the joint line in the posterolateral corner of the knee joint.

Iliotibial tract

An overuse syndrome involving the iliotibial tract is a relatively common and well-described condition, especially in distance runners (Orova, 1978). The patient presents with pain over the lateral compartment of the knee where the iliotibial band passes over the lateral femoral epicondyle to which some of its fibres are attached. Pain is characteristically brought on after running a few miles along a flat surface or on running downhill but may also occur after the completion of a run and then becomes worse. Pain may radiate either distally or proximally and the patient may complain of a clicking hip.

Major signs—Compression over the iliotibial band while flexing and extending the knee should reproduce the patient's pain (Noble, 1979). The patient's knee is first flexed to 90 degrees and the examiner places this thumb over the iliotibial band just proximal to the lateral epicondyle. The knee is then gradually extended and at approximately 30 degrees of flexion pain is reproduced.

Confirmatory signs—The diagnosis may be confirmed on palpation; there will be a localized area of tenderness over the lateral femoral epicondyle approximately 3 cm proximal to the joint line. This may also be associated with a sensation of crepitus, creaking or clicking.

Management

(1) Rest. The patient usually needs to rest from distance running, especially if it involves hills, but other activities are usually possible.

(2) Anti-inflammatories and analgesics are prescribed.

(3) Physical methods including heat or ice are

usually of some benefit. Stretching the iliotibial band is also necessary.

(4) Injections of local anaesthetic and corticosteroid into the tender area usually produces
marked relief and may be repeated at
approximately two-weekly intervals, if necessary.

(5) Correction of training errors, biomechanical
disorders of the foot or running mechanics
such as overstriding is usually necessary.

(6) Surgery. If the conservative methods fail, or if
it is recurrent, surgery to free the posterior
fibres of iliotibial tract over the lateral
epicondyle may be very successful (Noble,
1979).

Chondromalacia fabellae

The fabella, a sesamoid bone in the lateral head of
the gastrocnemius, articulates with the femoral
condyle; its articular cartilage may develop similar
changes as the patella, which is its anterior
counterpart. Pain may be reproduced on full passive flexion or extension of the knee and tenderness is localized over the fabella. An X-ray is necessary to confirm the presence of a fabella and
degenerative changes may also be evident. If
symptoms are sufficiently severe the fabella should
be removed.

Bursitis

Prepatellar bursitis

This bursa lies between the anterior surface of the
patella and the skin. It is commonly involved by
direct trauma, often of a chronic repetitious nature
producing the 'housemaid's knee'. Examination
shows a distinctive prominent swelling in front of
the patella, which can grow to a large size.
Acute bursitis may also be caused by infections or
gout.

Infrapatellar bursitis

This bursa lies between the patellar tendon and
the infrapatellar fat pad. Bursitis is produced by
the same mechanism as patellar tendinitis. Pain
may be reproduced on full extension or full passive
flexion of the knee. The distended bursa is best
seen with the knee fully extended bulging on either
side of the patellar tendon and cross-fluctuation
between the two sides may be demonstrated.

Superficial infrapatellar bursitis

The superficial infrapatellar bursa lies between the
tibial tubercle and the skin. Bursitis is not common
and is produced by overuse of the patellar tendon.
In young people it needs to be differentiated from
Osgood–Schlatter's disease.

Anserine bursitis

This bursa lies between the tibial collateral ligament, and its attachment to the tibia, and the
overlying pes anserinus tendinous insertion. Bursitis may be produced by direct trauma but is more
common after an overuse injury or as a complication of osteoarthritis of the knee. Pain tends
to be well localized and may be made worse by
resisting knee flexion.

Semimembranosis bursitis

This bursa is found on the medial side of the
popliteal fossa between the medial head of the
gastrocnemius and the semimembranosis tendon.
It usually communicates with the knee joint and
also with another bursa between the posterior
capsule of the knee. Swelling due to bursitis is best
seen and felt with the knee in extension. In adults
it commonly results from a synovitis of the knee
and in children it usually presents as a large cystic
swelling in the popliteal fossa.

Bicipital bursitis

The bicipital bursa lies between the insertion of the
biceps tendon and fibular collateral ligament into
the head of the fibula. Bursitis may develop as a
complication of an overuse injury of the biceps
tendon or a sprain of a ligament. It presents as a
small swelling that can be made more obvious by
resisted flexion of the knee, and needs to be differentiated from a cyst of the lateral meniscus
which lies over the joint line.

Joints

Lesions of the tibiofemoral joint

The menisci

The medial and lateral compartments of the knee
each contain a fibrocartilaginous meniscus (*see
Figure 10.30*).

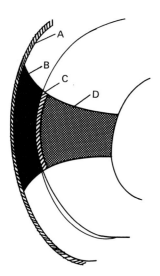

Figure 10.30 Peripheral attachments of the medial meniscus: (A) the joint capsule; (B) the vascular parameniscal zone; (C) a fibrous zone; and (D) avascular fibrocartilage

FUNCTION

One function of the menisci appears to be that they act as an intra-articular fibrocartilaginous washer (Radin, 1973). The convex femoral condyles are rounded to allow rotation as well as flexion and extension of the knee. The lack of bony symmetry between the femur and tibia produces a space, which is filled in by the menisci.

They also play an important role in stabilizing the knee and also aid in the control of rotary stability. This function may be confirmed clinically in patients who have had a previous injury of the knee ligaments but then develop a rotary instability after undergoing meniscectomy (Wang and Walker, 1974).

The menisci help to absorb the compressive forces developed as body weight is transmitted through the legs. Thus during compression of the knee joint the menisci may carry a substantial proportion of the applied load, which may be a primary function of the menisci (Wright and Dowson, 1975). Because of their elastic properties, they act as shock absorbers to protect the articular cartilage of the knee.

The menisci form a functional unit with the surrounding ligaments and move with movement of the knee joint, which allows the femur to glide on the tibia. During knee extension the menisci move anteriorly and during flexion they move posteriorly. They also move during axial rotation

so that on external rotation of the lower leg, the lateral meniscus moves anteriorly and the medial meniscus posteriorly. Similarly, on internal rotation the medial meniscus moves forward and the lateral meniscus backwards.

The menisci are commonly considered to aid joint lubrication and the even distribution of pressure within the joint (Highton, 1972).

MENISCAL TEARS: AETIOLOGICAL FACTORS

Age—The peak age for patients to present with a torn meniscus is in the 20–30 age group, and below the age of 16 this injury in a normally developed meniscus is quite rare.

Sex—The medial meniscus is more commonly torn than the lateral meniscus. Smillie (1974) gives the ratio as 3:1 but higher ratios are reported by other authors.

Occupation—This is a common sporting injury; it may occur in any type of sport but soccer is the most common and skiing a relatively uncommon cause. People whose occupations involve prolonged squatting or kneeling, such as miners or floor-carpeters, are particularly liable to develop cartilage damage.

Degenerative changes occur with age and play a role in cartilage tears in the more elderly age group. However, in younger sportsmen the cartilages are usually structurally normal.

History of trauma—There may be a history of a sprained ligament in the knee or of a fracture of the tibial plateau.

Mechanism of injury—The knee held in full extension is firmly locked and stable and so the cartilage is immobile but the meniscus may be torn during knee movements. The usual combination of events is to have the knee in some degree of flexion while weight-bearing so that the tibia is held fixed, usually in a position of external rotation. The medial meniscus can then be drawn into the centre of the joint space, where it is firmly held between the condyles of the femur and the tibia. As the patient then straightens up by extending the knee, the femur is forced into internal rotation; the meniscus is caught in the centre of the joint and torn.

Injuries of the lateral meniscus are less common than those of its medial counterpart since injuries of the lateral compartment are less common than of the medial compartment and the lateral meniscus is not attached to its collateral ligament and so is more mobile.

ASSOCIATED INJURIES

(1) The forces that produce a tear of the

meniscus with flexion, rotation and abduction or adduction are also the same forces that produce a sprain of either the collateral, capsular or cruciate ligaments. Thus the same type of injury may damage the ligaments or mensicus or both and meniscal tears may be associated with a sprain of the middle capsular ligament.

(2) Ligamentous injury resulting in instability of the knee may ultimately result in a meniscal tear, especially of the lateral meniscus.

(3) Chondral lesions. The articular cartilage lining the surface of the femoral condyle may also be damaged. This relatively common complication is found usually on the femoral surface opposite the site of the meniscal tear. It usually involves the chondral surface only, but an osteochondritis dissecans involving bone and cartilage may result.

(4) Patellofemoral lesions. Chondromalacia patellae may be associated with a torn meniscus, probably because normal patellofemoral rhythm is disturbed. Moreover, some cases of recurrent subluxation of the patella may also be complicated by the presence of meniscal tears.

(5) Osteoarthritis may develop as a late complication, especially if there has been any chondral injury.

TYPES OF TEAR

The cartilage may tear in either a longitudinal or a horizontal direction. Longitudinal tears are the more common and may involve either the anterior or the posterior horn or the cartilage substance. The longitudinal tear may involve only a small area of the meniscus and this torn section can then become displaced. A longitudinal tear sufficiently long to pass from the anterior to the posterior horn produces a 'bucket-handle tear' and the detached inner fragment can become displaced into the centre of the joint, where it may produce locking of the joint. At times the entire meniscus may be detached from its peripheral attachments.

Transverse tears occur more commonly in the lateral meniscus and then usually commence at the junction of the anterior and middle thirds of the cartilage. The tear commences on the concave edge and extends backwards and laterally into the mid zone. Owing to its appearance it is called a parrot-beak tear and may be associated with a cyst of the meniscus. Only rarely does a transverse tear become complete.

DIAGNOSIS

Taking the history is of paramount importance and should be designed to disclose the exact mechanism of injury and the subsequent history of the knee disability. The diagnosis of a torn meniscus can usually be readily made on clinical grounds but in some cases a prolonged period of observation and a high index of suspicion may be necessary before the diagnosis can be confirmed. In the doubtful cases, double-contrast arthrography and/or arthroscopy may be used to provide additional information.

SYMPTOMS

Pain   A meniscus tear produces pain that is usually sudden in onset, severe and located over the involved joint compartment or felt 'somewhere inside the knee'. It may be associated with a tearing sensation or an audible click and the pain is such that the patient is unable to continue with his activities. Although the type or degree of this pain cannot be differentiated clinically from that due to ligament sprain, the history may be of some assistance in that it is nearly always impossible for a patient with a torn meniscus to continue his activity, but with a ligament sprain he may be able to continue for a short time. However, the degree of pain produced by a torn meniscus can vary and it may be only a mild one at first and tends to disappear.

Different symptoms are produced in more elderly patients in whom a tear is associated with degeneration in the meniscus. The history is usually one of pain in the knee that increases over a period of time, tends to be worse with activity and is often present at night—when it may disturb sleep, especially if the affected knee is twisted or if one knee rests on the other. A knee effusion usually develops, especially after activity, and may gradually resolve only to return later after another period of prolonged use. Walking up stairs may be painful. They usually also report that previous attempts at conservative treatment have been unsuccessful.

Swelling   An effusion in the knee is nearly always present and starts to form several hours after the injury. This contrasts with a haemarthrosis of the knee, in which a painful swelling appears within the first hour.

Locking   A history of locking and unlocking of the knee is of considerable importance (*see page 131*). It indicates that a fragment of the meniscus is trapped between the femoral and tibial condyles, so preventing full extension but not flexion. A history of locking of the knee is more likely if the tear involves the anterior two-thirds of the meniscus. With a bucket-handle tear only the last few degrees of extension may be lost and if the displaced fragment lies within the intercondylar space no locking may occur.

Clicking There may be a history of recurrent, painful, often audible clicks or a snapping sensation in the knee.

Instability The patient may be conscious of a sudden giving way and instability of the knee, or that something slips in the joint. This symptom needs to be differentiated from ligamentous laxity or from the effects of quadriceps weakness.

EXAMINATION

Examination usually reveals the presence of a synovial effusion. Since the bulk of the quadriceps muscle, especially of the vastus medialis, is rapidly lost after a meniscus injury, quadriceps atrophy should be looked for.

Normal knee movement is usually lost, either as a loss of hyperextension or of the last few degrees of full knee extension, or loss of the last 10 degrees of full knee flexion. A meniscal injury may be suspected if pain is also reproduced with these knee movements. A meniscal tear also results in a loss of the range of passive axial rotation. Lesions of the anterior half of either meniscus produce a block to external rotation of the lower leg, and lesions of the posterior half of the meniscus produce a block to full passive internal rotation (Helfet, 1974).

SPECIAL TESTS

Various manoeuvres have been described to reproduce the patient's symptoms by manipulating the meniscus between the bony condyles. However, they may be negative in the presence of a torn meniscus and so this does not necessarily exclude the diagnosis of a torn meniscus.

Rotation

Starting position—The patient lies supine with the hip flexed. The examiner passively flexes the knee by grasping the patient's heel with one hand and palpates over the joint line with the fingers of his other hand:

Method—The lower leg is internally and then externally rotated rapidly while the examiner palpates over the joint line. Pain and tenderness over the involved cartilage may then become apparent. This test should be repeated with the knee in varying degrees of flexion.

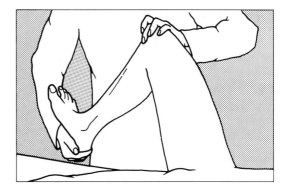

Figure 10.31 McMurray's test

McMurray's test

Starting position—The patient lies supine with the hip and knee flexed. In patients with a suspected tear of the medial meniscus, the lower leg is externally rotated and abducted (*see Figure 10.31*).

Method—While this position is forcefully maintained, the knee is slowly extended. As the knee is extended from 90 degrees of flexion, a painful click, which may be palpable or audible, indicates a positive test. In cases of suspected lateral meniscus tear the knee is internally rotated and then slowly extended while the examiner palpates over the lateral joint line.

Interpretation—This a useful test for tears in the posterior or middle thirds of the meniscus, but not for the anterior third.

Apley's test

Starting position—The patient lies prone with the hip extended and the knee flexed to 90 degrees. The examiner may also need to place his knee across the back of the patient's thigh to stabilize it.

Method—The lower leg is rotated internally and externally while at the same time applying first

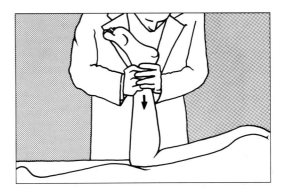

Figure 10.32 Apley's test: downwards compression

a downwards compression (*see Figure 10.32*) and then upwards traction.

Interpretation—If rotation of the knee with downwards compression produces pain or a painful clicking a tear of the meniscus is indicated. Pain reproduced on rotation with upwards traction indicates a ligament sprain.

Shearing strain

Starting position—The patient lies supine with the knee flexed to a right angle. The examiner places the heel of one hand over the lower femur and the heel of his other hand over the upper tibia (*see Figure 10.33*).

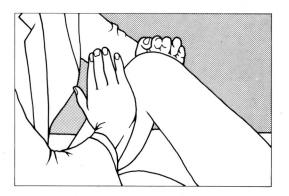

Figure 10.33 Shearing strain being produced across the knee joint

Method—The examiner forces his hands together, so producing a shearing strain across the joint. The position of the hands is then reversed and the shearing strain imposed from the opposite direction.

Steinmann's test

Starting position—The patient lies supine with the hip and the knee flexed.

Method—A point of maximum tenderness is found in the meniscus over the joint line. The knee is first more fully flexed and is then extended.

Interpretation—As the meniscus moves backwards and forwards the site of maximum tenderness will vary; however, in patients with a ligament sprain or osteoarthritis the point of tenderness remains fixed.

Hyperflexion test

Starting position—With the patient lying prone, the examiner grasps the foot and passively flexes the knee to 90 degrees.

Method—The lower leg is rotated externally and internally while the knee is forced further into flexion. A painful clicking may be elicited over the joint line in a positive test.

CONFIRMATORY TESTS

The patient lies supine with the hip and knee flexed while the examiner palpates the joint line with his index finger. Tenderness over the anterior or posterior thirds of the joint tends to confirm a meniscus tear, but tenderness over the middle third may indicate a meniscus or ligament injury.

Routine X-rays should always be taken to exclude bony injury or the presence of a loose body. Double-contrast arthrography is a useful technique performed using strict aseptic precautions in the X-ray theatre after the knee is first aspirated. 40 ml of air is first injected, followed by 4 ml of contrast medium and the knee fully moved. Special X-ray equipment is needed to take multiple views of each meniscus from the anterior to the posterior horn. Double-contrast arthrography produces a sharp outline of the borders of the meniscus, allowing it to be well outlined. The normal meniscus has a wedge-shaped appearance with its thin edge pointing towards the inside of the joint and its broad base on the outer side of the joint. A meniscal tear is recognized by the presence of air and contrast medium within the substance of the meniscus (Kaye and Freiberger, 1975). In the medial compartment this technique is accurate in 95 per cent of cases but in the lateral compartment it has an accuracy of only 80 per cent (Nicholas, Freiberger and Killorian, 1970).

Arthroscopy is a most useful, relatively simple technique, which can be used to inspect the menisci and other joint structures (Jackson and Abe, 1972). It may also be used by experienced operators to remove a partial tear of the meniscus.

MANAGEMENT

Tears of the meniscus vary greatly in extent, and it is also important to recognize the degree of any concomitant soft-tissue injury or underlying degenerative changes in the knee. Meniscectomy should never be undertaken lightly and many menisci that would have been operated on are now spared (Di Stefano, 1980).

Meniscectomy should be performed in younger patients in whom an extensively torn meniscus is diagnosed. The whole of the meniscus is removed if it also shows evidence of degenerative changes, but in younger athletes with only a partial tear partial resection often suffices (McGinty, 1977). Meniscoplasty in patients with a peripheral disruption is possible (Price and Allen, 1978). It is essential to commence quadriceps exercises once the tear is first diagnosed, and before operation is performed, to obtain a satisfactory postoperative result.

However, surgery should be deferred if the diagnosis is only suspected and no locking of the knee or loss of extension is present. A trial of conservative treatment should be instituted, with periodic reassessment of the patient's symptoms and signs. Postponement of operation in these circumstances is unlikely to cause any deterioration in the knee, and healing may take place if the tear is through the vascular peripheral attachment of the meniscus. Treatment is given to increase power in the quadriceps, hip flexors, and abductors; this should be combined with exercises to stretch the posterior structures, such as the hamstring and calf muscles. If symptoms are recurrent meniscectomy must be considered, as repeated attacks of locking may lead to osteoarthritis in later life.

A patient with a locked knee should be treated as soon as possible by manipulation. The following technique is described for the medial meniscus as it is the more commonly involved.

Starting position   The patient lies supine and as relaxed as possible. The therapist passively fully flexes the patient's knee with the hip at a right angle, places the left hand over the knee to stabilize it and grasps the patient's heel with his right hand. The medial compartment of the patient's knee is then opened up by fully abducting and laterally rotating the lower leg (*see Figure 10.34(a)*).

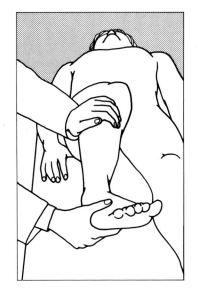

(*b*)

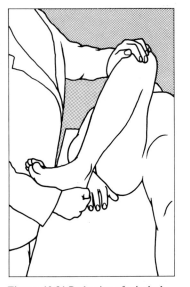

(*a*)

Figure 10.34 Reduction of a locked knee. (*a*) Starting position. (*b*) Final position

Method   While the leg is maintained in abduction and lateral rotation the knee is suddenly extended with a snap and then turned into medial rotation (*see Figure 10.34(b)*). The cartilage can usually be felt or heard to click, and after the knee is unlocked the patient can then extend the knee without pain. If this manoeuvre is not successful on the first attempt it may be repeated several times. However, if still not successful it is preferable to repeat the manipulation with the patient anaesthetized rather than to traumatize the knee further. Occasionally, full manipulation is not necessary because the displaced fragment can be felt to reduce while the knees are either flexing or rotating.

For the lateral meniscus the technique is similar except that the lateral compartment of the joint is opened by adduction and internal rotation of the lower leg.

If locking is recurrent the patient should undergo meniscectomy. However, there is often no further recurrence and it is presumed that the original locking of the knee may have been caused by a hypermobile meniscus.

More elderly patients with a degenerated meniscus may have only minor symptoms, often related to a loss of some power in the knee or a loss of some degree of movement. Hence, if these patients are not actively exercising, these symptoms may not be troublesome. Degenerative tears should be removed only if they cause mechanical symptoms and then as much of the meniscus as possible should be preserved (Jones, Smith and

Reisch, 1978). Treatment to increase the strength of the surrounding muscles and to increase joint mobility in these patients may produce sufficient improvement to allow the knee to function satisfactorily.

The presence of an associated ligamentous instability will usually lead to a poor surgical result. The instability is often not diagnosed preoperatively, especially if the torn meniscus blocks the knee and prevents adequate testing. Instability may become evident only at operation after removal of the meniscus or postoperatively and may then require a reconstructive repair.

POSTOPERATIVE DEGENERATION

Meniscectomy is not a benign procedure and should never be undertaken without good reasons. Several reports have recently detailed an increased incidence of osteoarthritis in knees after meniscectomy. The published figures vary, depending on the diagnostic methods, from 23 to 85 per cent (Jackson, 1968; Tapper and Hoover, 1969; Appel, 1970; Johnson, 1974). Assessment of the post-meniscectomy knee by arthroscopy showed degenerative changes in most cases (Glinz, 1978). In addition, degenerative changes may be more pronounced in lateral meniscectomy (Yocum *et al.*, 1979), in children (Medlar *et al.*, 1979), in the elderly (Jones, Smith and Reisch, 1978) and in total rather than partial meniscectomy (McGinty *et al.*, 1977). Experimental evidence in dogs was provided by Cox *et al.* (1975).
Reasons for degeneration include:

(1) The original injury may also damage the articular cartilage.
(2) Meniscectomy itself may injure the articular cartilage.
(3) The meniscus normally has important functions, described above.

After bilateral meniscectomy there is an average increase of 14 per cent in rotational instability (Wang and Walker, 1974).

CYSTS OF THE MENISCUS

A cyst of the meniscus involves the lateral much more commonly than the medial meniscus, the ratio being approximately 9:1. They are usually traumatic in origin and a parrot-beak tear can usually be demonstrated in the outer zone of the meniscus. Synovial cells may be displaced into the vascular area at the attachment of the meniscus, where they can multiply. They resemble a multilocular ganglion, filled with thick gelatinous material.

Symptoms are usually highly characteristic. The patient is usually a young male who presents with knee pain and may also be conscious of a swelling. Pain may be intermittent and occurs especially during running or climbing stairs, with a sudden severe painful 'catch' in the knee so that it gives way. Pain is usually dull and aching, made worse by activity and is often present at night, when it will disturb sleep. A tender lump is usually present which varies in size over a period of time and is visible and palpable over the joint line, usually in the middle third. This swelling is most obvious over the joint line when the patient sits with the legs over a couch and the knee is held at about 45 degrees of flexion. Synovial effusion is usually absent.

DISCOID MENISCUS

In this condition the meniscus is discoid in shape and not semilunar. It is considered to be a congenital variation showing persistence of the fetal state. It usually involves the lateral meniscus, may be present in both knees and was present in 5 per cent of meniscectomies reported by Smillie (1974). It is more liable to damage and minor trauma may result in a tear, most commonly of the parrot-beak variety.

The patient usually presents during his teens complaining of a painful snapping or clicking on knee movement, usually with the joint a few degrees short of full extension. This snapping can be easily palpated over the joint line. Surgical removal is the treatment of choice

Traumatic synovitis

Trauma may result in a haemarthrosis or acute synovitis of the knee. Haemarthrosis usually comes on more rapidly after an injury than does synovitis so that its onset is measured in minutes rather than hours. The knee is usually extremely painful, warm, tender and held in some degree of flexion. Haemarthrosis may follow a tear of the capsule associated with ligament sprains, a torn meniscus, or an intra-articular fracture. Non-traumatic causes of haemarthrosis are rare and include blood dyscrasias, anticoagulant therapy, pigmented villonodular synovitis or neoplasms.

Haemarthrosis may need to be differentiated from crystal deposition disease, inflammatory arthritis and septic arthritis. The definitive diagnosis of the underlying condition should be made by aspirating the knee and examining the synovial fluid.

CHRONIC TRAUMATIC SYNOVITIS

Finding an effusion in the knee without a history of recent trauma is not uncommon in sportsmen who present with 'water on the knee'. It must be recognized as a symptom, not a diagnosis, and its underlying mechanism should be established. Pain is not often a feature and the main clinical findings are a synovial effusion, which may be large, and wasting of the quadriceps muscle.

The main step in the diagnostic process is to obtain an adequate history, which includes the type of onset and relationship to any trauma. It is important to assess the degree of the original trauma to determine whether it is sufficient to cause long-continued trouble, since the patient may sometimes remember some minor trauma that is blamed as the cause of the trouble. A general examination is necessary to detect synovitis or arthritis in any other joints. In body-contact sports, knee synovitis may be caused by a direct contusion blow to the quadriceps. A routine examination of the knee movements and special tests to determine the presence of any ligamentous instability, meniscal damage or abnormalities of the patellofemoral joint should then be made. The knee is palpated for the presence of any localized areas of tenderness. Routine X-rays are taken and the knee should be aspirated and synovial fluid examined. Arthroscopy or double-contrast arthrography may provide additional information.

Osteoarthritis of the knee

The knee is a very common site of osteoarthritis, possibly because it is often subjected to trauma. Previous tears of the meniscus, fractures of the joint surfaces or ligamentous instability may all be complicated by subsequent degenerative changes. These may involve either the medial or lateral tibiofemoral compartment, the patellofemoral joint or any combination of these. Osteoarthritis usually commences in one compartment and in the tibiofemoral compartment may be related to the articular cartilage damage that follows meniscal tears (Helfet, 1974). One compartment is usually involved if there is any knee deformity present—e.g. the lateral compartment with valgus deformity—whereas with varus deformity the medial compartment is involved. As the disease progresses the degenerative changes in either compartment tend to increase the degree of the existing deformity. If there is any disparity in leg lengths the knee on the longer side is involved (Dixon, 1965).

In the tibiofemoral compartment the meniscus is also usually involved in the degenerative process; as the joint space narrows increased pressure is carried by the weight-bearing surface of the meniscus, which develops increased degenerative changes and a horizontal cleavage type of tear may occur. The meniscus is slowly ground away and the anterior part of the meniscus may disappear (Smillie, 1974).

MANAGEMENT

The general management of patients with osteoarthritis of the knee is similar to that previously outlined for osteoarthritis of the hip and includes rest, weight loss, aids, supports, anti-inflammatory drugs and physical therapy, especially quadriceps exercises.

Mobilization techniques aid in easing knee pain and stiffness. Small-amplitude stretching movements used at the limit of range are of most value. For example, if knee flexion is most limited treatment is commenced using anteroposterior pressures into extension. As the range of flexion improves so usually does the range of extension.

Surgery is indicated in patients in whom pain and stiffness are severe. The choice of operation lies between a total knee replacement or an osteotomy in patients with unicompartmental disease and a marked deformity.

Bony lesions

OSTEOCHONDRAL INJURIES

Chondral injuries, involving the articular cartilage alone, or osteochondral injuries, involving both the articular cartilage and subchondral bone, are common injuries that may involve the femoral condyle or patella. The presence of an osteochondral lesion is confirmed on X-ray but a chondral injury, being radiolucent, is more difficult to diagnose.

Osteochondritis dissecans is probably a variety of this type of injury in which a fragment of cartilage and subchondral bone separate partially or completely from the underlying bone. It tends to occur on the convex surfaces of joints and in the knee.

Eighty-five per cent of cases involve the medial femoral condyle (Aichroth, 1971), usually its lateral border. In 15 per cent of cases the lateral femoral condyle is involved, usually on its inferior surface.

There is considerable speculation about its aetiology and it may be due to more than one cause, although the most likely single cause is trauma. The site of the lesion is consistent with a traumatic origin. Aichroth found that more than 60 per cent of 200 cases were better class athletes and that its incidence parallels the degree of sport participation. It may be produced by the medial tibial spine, which impinges against the lateral surface of the medial femoral condyle. This can occur especially when the lower leg is in a position of abduction and external rotation with the knee held slightly flexed, e.g. when pivoting on one leg.

A juvenile form of osteochondritis dissecans also occurs from about the age of 4–15 years. Hereditary factors may play a role in this lesion, although minor degrees of trauma are still probably responsible for the production of symptoms.

Symptoms of osteochondritis dissecans   The adult form occurs more often in males and symptoms are determined according to whether the osteochondral fragment becomes separated. If the fragment remains unseparated the patient usually presents with pain which tends to be of insidious onset, dull and aching in character, poorly localized within the knee, made worse by activity and may be present at night. The knee may be swollen especially after activity.

A loose fragment may also produce locking or giving way of the knee, usually associated with a synovial effusion and may be difficult to distinguish clinically from a torn meniscus. X-rays, including intercondylar views, are necessary to confirm the diagnosis and the presence or absence of a loose bony fragment.

Management   If the diagnosis is made early and the osteochondral fragment is still in position treatment consists of rest to the knee and avoidance of weight-bearing activities. Extra rest may be obtained by use of a plaster cast with the knee flexed to reduce pressure on the involved area and weight-bearing can then be allowed. The plaster should be worn for only 4–6 weeks until the acute symptoms have settled as prolonged immobilization is unwise. X-rays are not a good guide to the stage of healing. However, if symptoms persist or if the fragment appears to be separating, further investigation by arthrography or arthroscopy is necessary. If the fragment is small and loose it may be possible to remove it through the arthroscope. If not, arthrotomy is necessary to remove the fragment of bone and cartilage. The crater that is left is smoothed out and its base drilled to promote healing with fibrocartilage. Pinning of the fragment has also been

advocated but is probably necessary only if a large segment of bone is involved.

OSTEONECROSIS

Spontaneous osteonecrosis of the femoral condyle (Ahlback, Bauer and Bohne, 1968) is relatively common. It involves the weight-bearing surface of the medial femoral condyle in elderly patients (*see Figure 10.35*). The aetiology is unknown but it appears that the original lesion may be an occlusion of the arterial supply to this area. It is more common in females, usually over the age of 65, in whom the knee is often previously normal. The onset of pain is usually sudden and severe, so that the patient can often remember the exact time it started. Pain usually becomes persistent, is often worse at night and is accompanied by swelling and stiffness of the knee.

The diagnosis may be suspected with the typical history and the finding of marked bony tenderness localized over the medial femoral condyle. Diagnosis needs to be confirmed by X-ray which may be normal at first, typical changes possibly taking several months to become evident. The first radiological change is a flattening of the condyle (Cleland *et al.*, 1976) followed later by a radiolucent defect in the condyle, which is subsequently surrounded by a sclerotic margin. Additional information may be obtained from tomography, double-contrast arthrography or a bone scan, which may be positive before radiological changes become evident. Synovial-fluid examination will show non-inflammatory fluid.

The subsequent history of osteonecrosis may depend on the amount of rest from weight-bearing that the patient can take, but degenerative changes often develop in the medial joint compartment and result in a genu varum.

Management—Management in the initial stages depends on the patient not bearing weight on the affected knee, and in some cases pain may settle at this stage. However, degenerative changes in the medial compartment often develop rapidly and surgery is then necessary.

Loose-body formation

Intra-articular loose bodies in the knee may be formed from cartilage, bone or osteochondral fragments. They occur in osteochondritis dissecans, osteochondral fractures, chondromalacia patellae, osteoarthritis or synovial osteochondromatosis. In general, small loose bodies cause more trouble than larger ones and in osteoarthritic joints

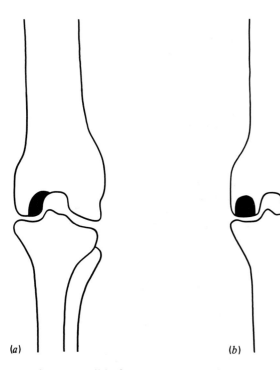

Figure 10.35 Usual site of involvement in osteochondritis dissecans (*a*) and in osteonecrosis (*b*)

may be responsible for recurrent attacks of synovitis. Clinically, loose bodies present as recurrent attacks of knee pain with locking and swelling. Diagnosis can be made by X-ray if the fragment contains bone.

OSTEOCHONDROMATOSIS

This is a benign tumour of the synovial tissue in which the synovium becomes proliferated and hyperplastic. Cartilage forms in the ends of the synovial fronds, which are invaded by the blood vessels in the synovial villus, and bone is also formed. These large osteochondral bones become detached from their synovial tissue and may produce locking of the joint and ultimately osteoarthritis.

Lesions of the patellofemoral joint

Patellofemoral pain

Retropatellar pain is an extremely common symptom, the characteristics of which have been described. In older age groups the most likely cause is osteoarthritis, but diagnosis and assessment is often more difficult in younger age groups. Chondromalacia of the patella is commonly diagnosed clinically as the cause of all such pain but it is really a pathological diagnosis caused by alter-

ations in the articular cartilage. Hence some patients have retropatellar pain without having chondromalacia and alternatively chondromalacia may be present but not necessarily be the primary cause of the patient's symptoms. The patellofemoral joint should be regarded as part of the link system of joints in the lower limb, which may be subjected to great pressure (Ficat and Hungerford, 1977). Pressures may be increased by knee flexion (*see Figure 10.36*) and also by many structural abnormalities or rotational deformities in the leg that lead to increased loading on the patellofemoral joint. Common examples are varus deformity of the rear foot, tibial torsion, genu valgum and anteversion of the femoral neck.

Similarly, a flexion deformity of the hip or tight hamstrings alter the components of this link system. Any of these conditions may themselves lead to chondromalacia, and all patients diagnosed as having chondromalacia must undergo a full examination of the whole of the lower limb.

CHONDROMALACIA PATELLAE

This common disorder of the patellar articular cartilage is responsible for a considerable degree of knee pain and disability. The cartilage lesion is due to premature degeneration with softening, fibrillation and roughening—somewhat similar pathological changes to those in osteoarthritis although there are important differences.

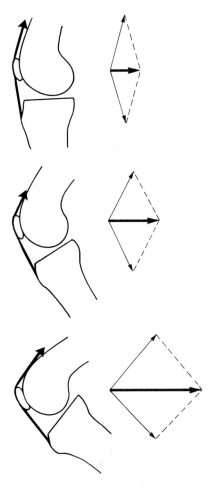

Figure 10.36 The resultant of the parallelogram of forces on the patellofemoral joint is increased as the knee is progressively flexed

Aetiology This condition may be due to trauma, be associated with a disturbance of the normal patellofemoral rhythm or occur as a primary condition.

Trauma—Direct trauma to the patella by a blow or a fall may result in chondral damage. These cases are usually unilateral. However, even if there is a history of trauma its role may be difficult to evaluate since it may not have resulted in any chondral damage and the patient may be recalling a minor traumatic incident that has been the precipitating factor in rendering an underlying chondromalacia symptomatic. Chondromalacia is also a common complication in patients who have recurrent subluxation or dislocation of the patella (Dandy and Poirier, 1975). This condition, which may be diagnosed on the history and examination,

should be carefully looked for in all cases but especially in young women.

Chondromalacia patellae can be associated with any condition that interferes with normal patellofemoral movements, which may be due to anatomical variations involving the patella, the femur, the suprapatellar pouch, the tibiofemoral joint, the surrounding muscles, or foot abnormalities:

(1) In the patella, anatomical variations include a high-riding patella (patella alta), a small patella, laterally orientated patella or abnormally angled patellar facet.

(2) In the femur, a ridge may normally be found at the superior margin of the articular surface of the medial condyle of the femur. This can then abut against the patellar cartilage during the first 30 degrees of knee flexion as the patella descends in its groove (Outerbridge and Dunlop, 1975).

(3) Normally, a wide communication forms between the synovium lining the knee and that of the suprapatellar bursa, so that they form a single cavity. However, in up to 20 per cent of people a remnant of their original division remains, known as the suprapatellar plica. This band may become thickened and fibrotic, especially with synovitis of the knee. If so it can then impede normal patellar movements as the knee moves from full flexion towards extension. Diagnosis may be made by palpation (when the band can be felt as a thickened cord), by arthroscopy, or by double-contrast arthrography.

(4) Chondromalacia patellae may be associated with any disorder that interferes with the normal rhythm of tibiofemoral movements, and so may occur as a complication of an intra-articular meniscus tear or synovitis of the knee. When knee movement is impeded normal patellofemoral rhythm is also lost so that the patella may be forced against the femur.

(5) Muscular abnormalities include tight hamstrings, which also cause a disturbed patellofemoral rhythm.

(6) Deformities of the foot, especially abnormal degrees of pronation, may occur and result in an abnormal degree of rotation in the transverse plane of the lower leg. Abnormal seating and movement in the patellofemoral joint can then occur.

In some cases no definite underlying cause may

be demonstrated and an overuse syndrome may be responsible. Most sporting activities involve movement of the knee and a full range of normal patellofemoral movement is necessary. The load on the patellofemoral joint on placing the weight on one leg while running has been estimated at being approximately 20 times the body weight (Williams, 1976). Since the load borne by this joint is large and is being constantly applied during sporting activities, any abnormality in the normal patellofemoral-joint relationship can then lead to local friction and cartilage damage. Goodfellow, Hungerford and Zindel (1976), for example, found that the lesion in chondromalacia most often affects the ridge that divides the medial patellar facet from the odd facet. This area may be subjected to increased loads or a shearing force during patellar movements.

Clinical features Chondromalacia patellae is more common in females than males, usually occurring in the late teens and often in certain occupations or sports—such as ballet dancing, long-distance running and bicycle riding. In recurrent subluxation of the patella the lateral patellar surface is usually involved, but in other cases the medial surface is more commonly involved.

Before it can be diagnosed clinically, chondromalacia must be symptomatic. Pain is usually described as a deep-seated ache, localized around the retropatellar area. It may be felt on going up or down stairs, on prolonged activity or after sitting for a prolonged time with the knees flexed —as in a car or at the theatre, or on squatting. Some patients complain that they need to get an aisle seat in a theatre so as to keep their knee extended or else that they have to get up and walk around during the show. The timing of the onset of pain may be a clue to the diagnosis: for example, in long-distance runners pain may often come on only after a run of a certain distance, usually 1 or 2 miles. Pain is normally not present in the morning or after rest. Associated symptoms include stiffness, catching, locking, swelling or a sensation of insecurity or giving way of the knee. The degree of the underlying pathological change correlates well with the frequency of locking (O'Donoghue, 1984). Synovitis is not common but may be caused by synovial irritation produced by the cartilage flakes.

EXAMINATION
The lower limb should first of all be examined for the presence of any of the conditions described above, e.g. patellar abnormalities or hamstring tightness, which are known to be associated with chondromalacia.

MAJOR SIGNS
The essential clinical finding is that the patient's pain can be reproduced by moving the undersurface of the patella against the femur. Three tests may be used:

(1) The patient lies supine with the knee relaxed and the patella is pushed distally by the examiner's hand. The patient then actively contracts the quadriceps muscle while the examiner maintains the pressure from his hand, inhibiting upwards patellar movement so that the patella is pulled over the femoral condyle (*see Figure 10.37*). A positive test is indicated by a sudden onset of pain and the patient being unable to maintain the contraction. However, interpretation of the pain response needs to be balanced against Gaughwon's (1982) findings wherein 78 per

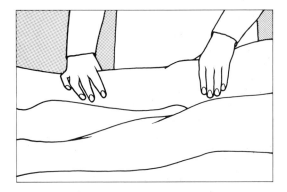

Figure 10.37 Testing for chondromalacia patellae: the patella is held while the quadriceps are contracted

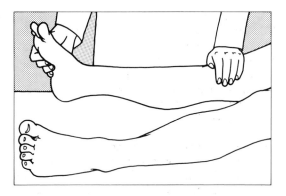

Figure 10.38 Chondromalacia patellae: compression of the patella while hyperextending the knee

cent of 12–13-year-olds had a painful response to the test.

(2) The patient lies supine and the examiner holds the patella down against the patient's femur with his left hand while passively hyper-extending the patient's knee with his right hand by lifting the leg upwards at the ankle (*see Figure 10.38*). If these tests are negative with the knee in extension they should be repeated with the knee held relaxed in 60 degrees of flexion.

(3) The patient lies supine and the examiner places his right hand over the parella to compress it against the tibia with his left hand placed on the superior border of the patella he pushes the patella caudad. The cephelad movement is produced with a slight distal movement of the hands to enable the left hand to apply the compression and the right hand to produce the cephelad movement of the patella (*see Figure 10.39*).

OTHER SIGNS

Retropatellar crepitus may be felt or heard. Retropatellar tenderness may be elicited with the patient lying supine with the knee relaxed so that the patella may be displaced to either side as far as possible, and the examiner can palpate the retropatellar surface with his finger. Tenderness is more commonly found under the medial surface. Rarely there may be a synovial effusion or a painful arc of movement during passive extension of the knee from the fully flexed position. Wasting of the vastus medialis muscle is found in nearly all cases. X-rays usually remain normal throughout the course of the disease, although minor degenerative changes in the subchondral bone have been described.

MANAGEMENT

The patient should first be examined for the presence of any leg or foot abnormality that may be associated with this condition; appropriate treatment, such as shoe orthotics, is given if these are found. Conservative therapy is always used first and may need to be continued for a prolonged time. This consists of:

(1) Rest. Activities that bring on patellar pain, such as running, and exercises that involve knee flexion, such as bicycling, should be avoided. It is only very rarely that pain is sufficiently severe to warrant the use of a plaster cylinder.

(2) Exercises to strengthen the quadriceps muscle, especially the vastus medialis, are essential and form the basis of conservative management (Dehaven, Dolan and Mayer, 1979). Isometric quadriceps exercises should be given, supervised by a physiotherapist, since they involve only minimal movement of the patella, do not exacerbate pain and strengthen the vastus medialis. Exercises that include knee flexion using progressive resistive exercises or squats are commonly ordered but place a greatly increased load on the patello-femoral joint and result in an exacerbation of the patient's symptoms. Exercise routines are also needed to strengthen the hip flexors and abductors and to stretch and strengthen the hamstring muscles.

(3) Anti-inflammatory drugs may be used to help ease pain.

(4) Physical measures such as heat have a very limited role but may be used to help settle any exacerbation in the patient's symptoms or before exercise therapy.

(5) Injections of local anaesthetic and steroid can be infiltrated around the attachments of the capsule to the border of the patella and under the tender patellar articular surface. They have only a limited effect in easing pain and should never be repeated at frequent intervals.

(6) Mobilization techniques may be useful. The first treatment session must be performed gently so as not to provoke pain and to allow an assessment of the irritability of the condition. If the disorder is very painful or irritable gentle passive movements are performed with distraction of the patella from the femur (*see Figure 10.39*). As pain improves, passive movements are increased with movements of the patella in more than one direc-

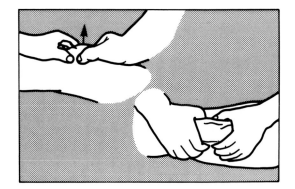

Figure 10.39 Patellofemoral distraction

tion and with varying degrees of compression of the patella, and by varying the angles of knee flexion while performing the movements against different surfaces of the femur.

(7) Aftercare. Conservative management usually produces satisfactory results and the patient can then be gradually remobilized but should continue to perform at a progressively increasing pace on a good surface. He should also continue to perform the isometric quadriceps exercises. Using conservative treatment, Dehaven, Dolan and Mayer (1979) reported an 82 per cent successful return to normal activity and Williams (1976) reported a 97 per cent success rate.

(8) Surgery may be necessary if symptoms are recurrent but careful patient selection is necessary and arthroscopy is advisable to confirm the diagnosis. Many operations have been devised and include:

(a) That described by Hughston (1972) in which the lateral retinacular fibres are released and may be combined with a reefing of the capsule on the medial side. This procedure appears to be the best.

(b) Operations to relocate the insertion of the patellar tendon into the tibial tubercle include an anterior advancement of the tibial tubercle (Maquet, 1976) or Hauser's procedure, which releases the extensor insertion and transfers it medially. This procedure may, however, produce subsequent problems due to an abnormal tibial rotation.

(c) Shaving of the patellar surface or the ridge on the medial femoral condyle.

(d) Total excision of the affected area of articular cartilage (Goodfellow, Hungerford and Zindel, 1976).

(e) Patellectomy. This seriously weakens the knee and should rarely be contemplated, but O'Donoghue (1984) reported 'gratifying' results from removal of a patellar facet.

Recurrent subluxation of the patella

Recurrent subluxation of the patella is common and tends to occur in knock-kneed teenage girls or more commonly in athletes (Hughston, 1969). The patient usually presents with a history of pain, locking and a sensation of instability in the knee. These symptoms can be most difficult to distinguish from those of a torn meniscus.

EXAMINATION
Examination may reveal postural abnormalities such as genu valgum or wasting of the vastus medialis muscle (*see Figure 10.40*). With the patient sitting with knees over the edge of the couch, the patella may be shown to be abnormally seated, e.g. either high or directed laterally. The patella is excessively mobile, best tested by the examiner sitting with the patient's knee flexed to 30 degrees and lying across his thigh. This relaxes the quadriceps muscle and it then becomes easier to apply

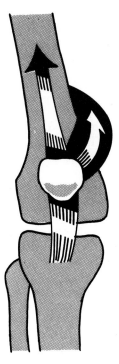

Figure 10.40 The action of the vastus medialis muscle (shown in black) in stabilizing the patella

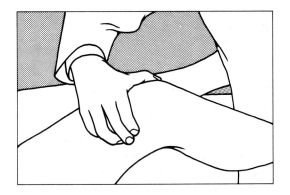

Figure 10.41a The apprehension test: as the knee is flexed the patella is pushed laterally

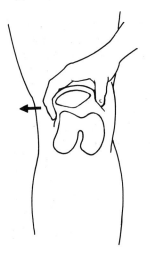

Figure 10.41b The apprehension test: as the knee is flexed the patella is pushed laterally

pressure to the medial aspect of the patella to assess the degree of hypermobility as the patella slips over the lateral femoral condyle.

MAJOR SIGN: THE APPREHENSION TEST
The examiner pushes outwards against the medial border of the patella while flexing the knee with his other hand (*see Figure 10.41a and b*). As the patella begins to subluxate laterally, the patient feels pain and becomes acutely aware that the patella is about to dislocate. He actively resists any further attempt to move the patella by contracting the quadriceps.

CONFIRMATORY SIGNS
The patella is examined for crepitus, retropatellar tenderness, or evidence of chondromalacia. X-rays should be taken and the retropatellar view (Hughston, 1969) may reveal a subluxed or abnormally seated patella or an avulsion injury of the patella.

MANAGEMENT
Conservative treatment consists mainly of an isometric exercise regimen to strengthen the quadriceps and the hip flexors and abductors. Bracing with a horseshoe-shaped felt pad in an elastic knee bandage may also be used for sporting activities. These measures may produce excellent results (Henry and Crosland, 1979).

If symptoms are recurrent surgery is necessary, and the type of operation depends on the underlying pathology. The capsule and extensor retinaculum on the lateral side of the joint usually needs to be released and the medial structures tightened. Other procedures include realignment of the patellar tendon insertion.

Infrapatellar pain

Pain in the infrapatellar region is most commonly due to patellar tendinitis, which may be complicated by a partial or complete rupture or by a peritendintis. Other causes include lesions of the patella, e.g. osteochondritis, a stress fracture or a prominent, elongated lower pole; hypertrophy of the infrapatellar fat pad; bursitis and Osgood–Schlatter's disease. Some of these conditions may also be associated with chondromalacia of the patella; patellar abnormalities, such as hypermobility or patella alta; or knee deformities, especially genu recurvatum or genu valgum.

Patellar tendinitis

The quadriceps forms into the patellar tendon, which runs from the lower pole of the patella to its insertion into the tibial tubercle. Tendinitis occurs in active sportsmen after the apophysis of the tibial tubercle has fused as an overuse injury, particularly in runners, fast bowlers, and ballet dancers. Degenerative changes may occur in the patellar tendon, which will show a central-core degeneration similar to that seen in the Achilles tendon (*see page 167*).

JUMPER'S KNEE
Blazina, Fox and Carlson (1974) noted that this occurred most commonly in people whose activity involves repeated jumping off one leg. It is associated with a small area of degeneration at the tendon attachment at the lower pole of the patella, characterized by pain and extreme local tenderness. In patients with patellar tendinitis, pain may be present at first only after activity, but in severe cases pain begins during activity and severely limits athletic performance. The patient may report an occasional sensation of weakness or 'giving way' of the knee.

Clinical signs   Pain is reproduced on resisting active knee extension. Crepitus may be present on passive movement of the patellar tendon. In jumper's knee, tenderness—usually severe—is found on palpation of the lower pole of the patella, especially if the patella is pushed distally. X-rays are normal but are necessary to exclude any patellar abnormality. In particular, a stress fracture or an elongated lower pole of the patella may cause similar symptoms.

Complications   The patellar tendon may undergo partial or complete rupture. Complete rupture is rare and occurs mainly in patients who have had tendinitis for a considerable period of time. An incomplete tear also occurs but is difficult to distinguish from tendinitis alone. Its presence may be confirmed by the use of xeroradiography to outline the soft tissues.

MANAGEMENT OF PATELLAR TENDINITIS

(1) Rest. Symptoms are usually brought on by activity—e.g. running, jumping or kicking—and these should be curtailed. In younger patients other activities can be substituted, but in professional sportsmen this is extremely difficult.

(2) Anti-inflammatory drugs are given.

(3) Physical measures such as heat or ice may help to relieve symptoms. Exercises should first be given to the hip flexors and abductors; as the symptoms subside, isometric quadriceps exercises may be added. Progressive resistive exercises with the knee flexed are contra-indicated.

(4) The patella should be mobilized using the techniques described above.

(5) Injections of 1 ml of corticosteroid may be given around the tender area in the tendon but never into the tendon substance. Extra rest is advised after the injection, which should be given as infrequently as possible and with at least 1 month between each injection. If symptoms do not improve significantly injections should be stopped.

(6) Surgery is indicated if conservative measures fail or if tendinitis is recurrent and prevents full participation in sport. Surgical treatment consists of decompression of the tendon and removal of any area of focal degeneration, adhesions around the tendon or an area of chondromalacia. Operation is followed by an intensive programme of rehabilitation and the patient can usually return to full activity.

OSGOOD–SCHLATTER'S DISEASE

This form of osteochondritis is associated with a partial avulsion of the patellar tendon at its insertion into the tibial tubercle before this apophysis unites. It occurs mainly in active boys aged 9–14 years, who present with a gradual onset of pain and a tender lump over the tibial tubercle. It tends to run a protracted course over several years before gradually settling.

Major signs A tender swelling is present over the tibial tubercle and pain is reproduced on resisting active quadriceps extension. X-rays will confirm the changes produced by separation of the tendon from the tibial tubercle but these changes take some time to develop.

Management This is often difficult since the patient is young and active, and symptoms may not fully resolve until the apophysis is fully united.

Pain is usually such that participation in activities requiring running or jumping is not possible, but complete immobilization of the knee is neither necessary nor practical. Isometric quadriceps exercises with the knee straight are essential.

Gentle, carefully controlled passive-movement techniques may reduce pain. This condition usually settles after a prolonged time without any additional active therapy, but is apt to recur on return to activity and then requires a careful balance between rest and activity.

OSTEOCHONDRITIS OF THE PATELLA

This relatively uncommon condition occurs mainly in active young boys and may be bilateral. The patient presents with an aching pain, made worse by activity and localized to the lower pole of the patella. X-rays show fragmentation of this pole of the patella.

11 The lower leg

The superior tibiofibular joint

The two bones of the lower leg, the tibia and fibula, are joined proximally at the superior tibiofibular joint and distally at the inferior tibiofibular joint. These two joints form a functional unit that is involved in movements of the ankle joint.

On plantar flexion of the foot, the narrower posterior part of the trochlear surface of the talus moves forwards in the ankle mortise. To maintain stability the lateral malleolus of the fibula needs to move inwards and downwards. Similarly, on dorsiflexion of the foot, the broader anterior part of the trochlear surface of the talus presents in the ankle mortise and to accommodate it the lateral malleolus of the fibula must move outwards and upwards.

These movements are also reflected in the superior tibiofibular joint, so that on dorsiflexion of the foot the superior tibiofibular joint moves upwards and inwards and on plantar flexion of the foot the superior tibiofibular joint moves downwards and outwards. The range of these movements is only small but can be readily felt by palpating over the head of the fibula with the knee flexed and then plantar and dorsiflexing the ankle.

Two other movements produce movement in the superior tibiofibular joint. These are inversion and eversion of the foot, and passive rotation of the talus in the ankle mortise.

Accessory movements

There are five accessory movements in the superior tibiofibular joint:

(1) Anteroposterior movement, which is produced by pressure from the thumbs over the anterior surface of the fibular head (*see Figure 11.1*).

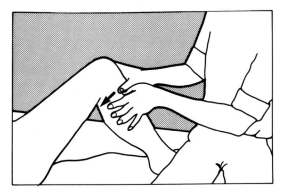

Figure 11.1 Anteroposterior accessory movement

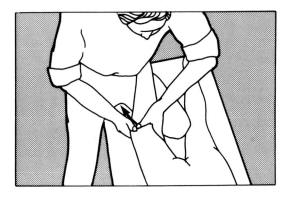

Figure 11.2 Posteroanterior accessory movement

(2) Posteroanterior movement is produced by pressure over the posterior surface of the fibular head (*see Figure 11.2*).

(3) Longitudinal cephalad movement is produced by eversion of the heel.

(4) Longitudinal caudad movement is produced by strongly inverting the patient's heel.

(5) Compression. These movements should be repeated with the fibular head compressed against the tibia with the heel of the hand.

Lesions of the superior tibiofibular joint

These include direct trauma, subluxation, and instability.

Direct trauma

This joint may be injured by direct trauma, which will cause haematoma formation and may result in calcification of the joint capsule. Joint movements are then restricted and pain is reproduced especially on ankle movements. X-rays reveal the calcified haematoma, usually on the inferior joint surface.

Subluxation

The superior tibiofibular joint may be subluxed or dislocated after an inversion sprain of the ankle. This may follow a fall onto the leg in which the inversion strain is applied to the ankle while the knee is held flexed and in a varus position. The force is transmitted through the fibular shaft to the posterior tibiofibular ligament, which is ruptured

and so allows the fibular head to sublux forwards. This injury has also been described in footballers and parachute jumpers (Muckle, 1973). The diagnosis is confirmed on X-ray, which shows an undue prominence of the fibular head.

Instability

This uncommon condition occurs as the result of injury or rheumatoid arthritis. The patient presents with pain over the lateral compartment of the knee, radiating down the leg. The superior tibiofibular joint clicks out of place on walking and so this condition is often mistaken for a tear of the lateral meniscus.

Major sign—Pain is reproduced on movement of the joint.

Compartmental syndromes of the lower leg

The opposed interosseous surfaces of the tibia and fibula are joined together by the interosseous membrane and, in addition, the bones and the muscles of the lower leg are invested by a layer of deep fascia, from which three extensions pass to the tibia and fibula (*see Figure 11.3*). In this way, the muscles of the lower leg are enclosed within four fascial compartments, which are known as the anterior, medial, lateral, and posterior compartments.

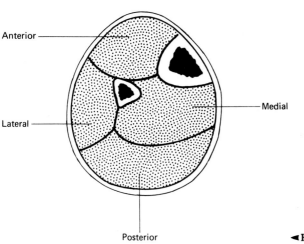

Anterior

Lateral

Medial

Posterior

◀**Figure 11.3** Fascial compartments of the lower leg

The anterior compartment

The anterior compartment lies anterolaterally between the tibia and fibula and is bounded deeply by the interosseous membrane and superficially by the deep fascia of the leg. It contains the tibialis anterior muscle and the extensors of the toes, the deep peroneal nerve and the anterior tibial artery. The deep peroneal nerve supplies the muscles in this compartment and forms a sensory nerve supplying the dorsal surface of adjacent sides of the first and second toes.

Any swelling in this compartment may compromise the arterial supply and produce symptoms of anterior tibial compartment syndrome. Swelling may follow muscular activity with resultant muscular oedema, which may cause an increase of 20 per cent in the weight of an exercising muscle (Wright, 1961). In this tight inelastic space, oedema produces an increase in the compartmental pressure which may then lead to obstruction of the fine intramuscular arterial vessels (*British Medical Journal*, 1979). Either an acute or chronic type of syndrome may result, determined by the degree of swelling and the distensibility of the fascial walls.

Acute anterior tibial syndrome

An acute anterior tibial compartment syndrome is a medical emergency that is fortunately rare. It usually follows sudden, severe or unusual running activity but it may also occur after moderate degrees of activity in people who have only recently taken up running.

The patient presents with a history of pain in the anterior compartment of the leg that rapidly becomes severe. Pain is made worse either by passive plantar flexion of the ankle joint or by isometric contraction of the dorsiflexors of the ankle. The overlying skin may be reddened, warm and oedematous. If the compression is unrelieved necrosis of the muscle and a compression neuropathy of the deep peroneal nerve, with a resultant foot drop and sensory change in the first interdigital cleft, may be produced.

Management

The patient is admitted immediately to hospital and completely rested in bed. If symptoms are severe or do not resolve quickly within a few hours an emergency fasciotomy must be undertaken to decompress the compartment. This entails a wide splitting of the entire fascial sheath to permit all the muscles within this compartment to bulge outwards.

Chronic anterior tibial syndrome

In chronic anterior tibial compartment syndrome symptoms similar to those of arterial insufficiency may develop. Pain comes on with exercise, usually becoming so severe that the patient is unable to continue his activity, and is relieved by rest. When the patient is seen in a clinic, signs are usually absent and the differential diagnosis includes arterial insufficiency. However, some swelling and diffuse tenderness over the anterior tibial compartment may be evident after exercise and the patient's pain is reproduced on passive dorsiflexion of the toes or ankle. If the patient continues to exercise muscle necrosis, or compression of the deep peroneal nerve with foot drop, may develop.

Management

The patient is advised to modify his activities so that symptoms abate, otherwise an acute syndrome may be produced. However, if symptoms persist fasciotomy may be performed; this usually produces excellent results (Bradley, 1973).

Tendinitis of tibialis anterior muscle

This overuse condition involves the musculotendinous junction of the tibialis anterior muscle in the lower third of the leg. The anterior tibial muscle is the principal decelerator of the foot at heel strike when running. If the runner is unaccustomed to a forceful heel strike during the early stage of vigorous training, or after changing to running on a hard surface, overuse of the muscle may occur. The patient complains of pain made worse by ankle movements, and a marked crepitus is palpable or even audible over the involved area of muscle.

Management

This condition usually responds well to a regimen of rest, local application of ultrasound or ice, anti-inflammatory drugs and injection of corticosteroid into the anterior aspect of the lower third of the tibialis anterior muscle.

Medial compartment

The medial compartment of the lower leg is enclosed between the deep fascia of the medial side of the leg, the interosseous membrane and a deep transverse intermuscular septum which separates if from the posterior compartment. It contains the tibialis posterior, the flexor hallucis longus and the flexor digitorum longus muscles, together with the posterior tibial artery and nerve.

Medial tibial compartment syndrome

This syndrome is similar in aetiology to the anterior tibial syndrome, in that exercise produces a swelling of the muscle fibres in a tight medial compartment (Puranen, 1974). It is the most common of the compartmental syndromes and may be bilateral. In 2750 overuse injuries in athletes presenting with pain in the lower leg, 58 per cent suffered from a medial compartment syndrome (Orava and Puranen, 1979). Its chronic form with pain and tenderness over the medial tibial border, known as shin soreness and shin splints, if produced by traction on the origin of the tibialis posterior. It usually occurs during the early part of a training season, especially after running on hard surfaces, and may follow a change of running shoe.

The patient presents with pain over the lower third of the medial border of the tibia, which is at first dull and aching, comes on with running, and is relieved by rest. Pain gradually increases so to continue running the patient may have to alter his action by shortening the running stride and running flat footed. If he does continue to run pain will be present at night and usually becomes so intense that ultimately even walking becomes difficult.

Pain may be reproduced by either passive plantar flexion of the ankle, active dorsiflexion of the ankle or isometric contraction of the tibialis posterior muscle. Marked tenderness is found along the posteromedial border of the tibia over its middle and lower thirds. A mild degree of warmth and a tender thickening is usually found along the medial tibial border.

Oblique X-ray views may be necessary to differentiate this condition from a stress fracture of the tibia.

MANAGEMENT
This condition is often difficult to treat. The methods used include:

(1) Rest. The patient needs to rest from all activities that include running. Strapping may be applied from the lower third of the leg to pass under the heel to restrict the range of plantar flexion of the ankle and produce some inversion of the foot.
(2) Anti-inflammatory drugs are usually prescribed but rarely produce any substantial benefit. Analgesics are often necessary, especially to allow the patient to sleep.
(3) Physical methods. Ultrasound given over the painful tender area is of some value in this condition, especially to help localize the painful area. Short-wave diathermy or ice are rarely of value.
(4) Stretching of the medial compartment muscles, even if it provokes some degree of discomfort, is essential; this should also be combined with stretching of the posterior calf muscles. Mobilization of the locally tender area with the therapist's thumbs may also be useful.
(5) Injections. The locally tender area around the tenoperiosteal origin of the tibialis posterior muscle may be injected with corticosteroid. When the patient is first seen, the involved area is usually too diffuse to justify such an injection but after treatment the tender area becomes more localized and can then be injected using a 25-gauge needle.
(6) As the patient's condition improves attention must be given to the type of running style, and hard running surfaces should be avoided. Correction of any postural faults in the leg should also be made.
(7) Surgery. In patients who have a tight fascial compartment management consists of dividing the thickened fascia over the medial compartment for a distance of approximately 10 cm. Orava and Puranen (1979) reported on 70 patients who underwent this operation with great success.

Lateral compartment

This compartment contains the peroneus longus and brevis muscles and the lateral popliteal nerve. An acute peroneal compartment swelling is rare but may occur several hours after strenuous exercise (Reneman, 1975).

Pain is made worse by active and passive inversion of the foot. Swelling may also compress the lateral popliteal nerve and result in sensory changes followed by a footdrop with inversion of the foot. This surgical emergency usually requires urgent decompression of the fascial compartment.

Posterior compartment

This compartment of the leg contains the gastrocnemius, the soleus and the plantaris muscles, which form the Achilles tendon. Lesions of this compartment include:

(1) A tear of the gastrocnemius.
(2) Acute posterior compartment syndrome.
(3) Chronic posterior compartment syndrome.
(4) Achilles tendon injuries.

Tear of the gastrocnemius

A tear of the gastrocnemius muscle is a common injury which occurs especially in middle-aged men, usually while jogging or playing tennis, hence its popular name of 'tennis leg'. However, minor degrees of this injury can also occur in the elderly while walking, especially on an uneven surface. The typical history is that a sudden severe pain in the calf is experienced during activity and the patient looks around to see if someone has hit him in the leg with a stone or other object. The degree of damage can vary from a slight tear with little resultant disability, to a moderate degree in which the patient can walk only by limping painfully on his toes, or to a severe degree of damage so that the patient is unable to walk. The mechanism of production of this injury usually occurs with the ankle in full dorsiflexion and with knee in extension; this stretches the gastrocnemius so that as it contracts while in this position it is liable to tear.

It is also quite common for the patient to report that a day or two beforehand there had been a slight aching or stiffness in the calf, which may have been associated with some loss of extensibility in the muscle. Stiffness and loss of extensibility also probably explains why this injury is much more common in middle-aged patients.

The site of this injury was formerly attributed to a ruptured plantaris muscle. It is now recognized to be a tear of the gastrocnemius, almost always in the medial belly or at the medial musculotendinous junction. It may occur rarely in the lateral belly of the muscle in patients with a genu varus deformity.

Major signs

Pain in the calf is reproduced on stretching the gastrocnemius, which is achieved by the examiner passively dorsiflexing the ankle. The range of this ankle movement is also usually restricted because of the associated muscle spasm in the gastrocnemius. Pain can also be reproduced on actively contracting this muscle by having the patient attempt to stand up on the toes, or by the examiner testing resisted plantar flexion of the ankle.

Other signs

These vary according to the site of involvement and the degree of the tear. In the calf the muscle belly may be swollen and bruising may be apparent over the site of the tear and the lower leg may be oedematous. In a severe degree of tear, a gap may be palpable in the muscle. In minor degrees or in the latter stages of a severe tear an area of tender thickening is palpable in the muscle. Swelling is uncommon with tears at the musculotendinous junction but localized pain and tenderness on palpation is often severe and prolonged. Blood may extravasate at the site of the tear, track down beneath the deep fascia, and appear as bruising around the ankle.

This injury may occasionally be complicated by pressure on the deep veins of the calf resulting in a venous thrombosis. If this is suspected, because the degree of ankle oedema is marked, venography should be carried out.

Management

INITIAL MANAGEMENT
The patient needs to rest, ice is applied to the painful area and the leg should be elevated to prevent swelling.

SUBSEQUENT MANAGEMENT
This depends on the degree of the original injury. With severe degrees of tear the patient is usually unable to walk freely and may need to use crutches for a few days. An elastic stocking or possibly a crêpe bandage is used to control ankle oedema.

With moderate or minor degrees of injury the patient can walk around, but a raise of 2.5 cm should be inserted in the shoe under the patient's heel. This reduces the strain on the muscle, which lacks extensibility due to the tear, and facilitates walking.

It is important to emphasize to the patient that he should use the leg as normally as the pain will allow. Crutches or a stick can usually be discarded within a few days and the heel raise after approximately 2 weeks.

Physical methods of treatment include ultrasound or ice and both active and passive stretching exercises. As the tear heals, exercises are progressed and the patient can increase the amount of walking or running at a slow pace. A rubber heel should be inserted in the running shoe. Commonly, the tear heals with a small area of fibrosis in the muscle fibres that prevents full extensibility of the muscle and is apt to cause recurrent tears. This area can be readily felt on palpation as a tender thickening. It is best treated with an injection of local anaesthetic and corticosteroid, deep-friction massage and stretching.

AFTERCARE

The patient must not return to active sport until all pain and tenderness has subsided and the muscle has regained full painless strength and extensibility. A gradual return to full activity is advisable and for approximately 3–4 weeks a 2-cm heel raise should be worn in the sandshoe or running shoe.

Acute posterior compartment syndrome

An acute posterior compartment syndrome is rare. Exercise produces an acute ischaemia of the soleus muscle in the tight fascial confines of this compartment (Kirby, 1970). Treatment consists of splitting the deep fascia over the medial side of the soleus muscle.

Chronic posterior compartment syndrome

This posterior compartment syndrome (Matsen and Clawson, 1975) may follow an overuse syndrome or a previous fracture of tibia and fibula. It is characterized by pain in the calf on activity and may be associated with altered sensation on the plantar surface of the foot and weakness of ankle flexion.

MAJOR SIGN

Pain is reproduced on passive dorsiflexion of the foot, so stretching the structures in the posterior compartment.

Lesions of the Achilles tendon

The Achilles tendon is formed from an aponeurosis at the musculotendinous junction of the gastrocnemius which is joined more distally by the soleus muscle and the plantaris tendon, which is an unimportant vestigial remnant. The Achilles tendon curves around the concave posterior surface of the calcaneus, from which it is separated by a bursa, to be inserted into the lower part of the posterior surface of the calcaneus. The tendon does not have a surrounding tenosynovial layer but is invested by relatively rigid fibrous tissue that forms a paratenon and contains the major part of the blood supply to the tendon in thin-walled blood vessels.

The action of the Achilles tendon is to plantar flex the ankle joint, and so the foot. This action is most efficient with the knee extended, as in the push-off phase of walking. When the foot is dorsiflexed, the first point of contact of the tendon lies proximally on the posterior surface of the calcaneus, but with the foot plantarflexed the tendon uncoils from around the curved posterior surface of the calcaneus so that its efficiency is increased (Kapandji, 1974). As the Achilles tendon plantar flexes the ankle joint it also acts on the subtalar joint to produce supination and adduction of the foot.

The Achilles tendon is the strongest tendon in the body and can withstand forces up to 5–10 kg. mm^{-2}, or approximately 1000 kg in the average adult (Burry, 1978). In the push-off phase of running the foot and ankle function as a second-class lever with body weight distributed between the fulcrum of the Achilles tendon and force applied at the end of the foot. The effect of this lever arrangement is such that a 100-kg man may require a force of 300 kg to push off from the ground. Degenerative changes, similar to those described in other tendons, are commonly found in the Achilles tendon. Burry and Pool (1973) described a central-core degeneration in which an area of degenerated, damaged fibres of approximately 10 mm^2 is found within an area of normal tendon. Its cause is unknown but is presumably due to vascular changes. At operation the tendon may appear to be dull and lustreless and, on incision of the tendon, a central area of granulation tissue is found, often with cystic softening which may be filled with blood.

Lesions of the Achilles tendon include:

(1) Acute tendinitis and peritendinitis.

(2) Chronic thickening of the paratenon.
(3) Achilles bursitis.
(4) Rupture:
    (a) Complete.
    (b) Partial.
(5) Avulsion of the attachment of the calcaneus.
(6) Osteochondritis of the calcaneus.
(7) Ossification of the tendon.

Achilles tendinitis

Achilles tendinitis occurs as a combination of degenerative and/or inflammatory changes due to overuse, which involve the tendon or its paratenon. Anatomical considerations may also play a role as the tendon may undergo attrition as it coils around the posterior surface of the calcaneus, and this tendency is increased if a retrocalcaneal exostosis is present. It also occurs more often if there is an associated restriction in the range of movement at either the subtalar or ankle joints. Acute inflammatory changes may occur either in the tendon itself or in the surrounding paratenon; but as the tendon has no surrounding synonium tenosynovitis is an incorrect description. The inflammatory swelling in the paratenon may be visible on inspection on either side of the tendon.

The onset is related to overuse of the tendon and so the patient should be asked about the number of miles run each week and the type of surface run on. The patient's history is often one of having run on hard surfaces or of having recently changed from running on soft surfaces to a hard surface, or changing from cross-country running to track running. Enquiries should also be made about the type of shoe worn, since many modern running shoes lack an adequate heel.

The patient is usually an active young or middle-aged male who presents with pain related to the Achilles tendon that is made worse by activity. If he continues to run the pain usually becomes severe and may then be made worse by walking. The patient complains that the tendon feels stiff, especially when he first gets out of bed. On examination the tendon may appear thickened, oedematous and tender, and pain and crepitus may be produced on movements of the tendon.

Management

(1) Rest. The tendinitis is usually of such a degree that rest from sporting activities is essential. However, if the tendinitis is only of a mild degree it may be sufficient merely to curtail the amount of running.
(2) A raise is worn in the shoe to elevate the heel and take strain off the tendon. An orthotic device may be worn in the shoe if any rearfoot deformity is present.
(3) Anti-inflammatory agents are prescribed.
(4) Physical methods. Ultrasound over the inflamed tendon is an important part of treatment. It may be used in conjunction with ice or short-wave diathermy. Deep-friction massage may be incorporated once the severe pain has subsided.
(5) Mobilization and stretching of the tendon by full-amplitude dorsiflexion and plantar flexion of the ankle should form part of the treatment, as should medial and lateral movements of the ankle.
(6) Injections. In most patients, tendinitis gradually settles over a few weeks. Injections of corticosteroid should never be given in the early stages of this condition, when the lesion is diffuse, and never into the tendon substance itself. However, a small residual area of tenderness can not infrequently be palpated around the medial or lateral (or both) borders of the tendon, which usually settles well with 1–3 injections of corticosteroid around the tendon using a 25-gauge needle.
(7) Aftercare. In all patients the return to activity must be gradual, so that a sudden application of the load normally applied in training is avoided. The patient is advised to walk at first and then jog so that the distance and the pace of running is progressed gradually and the tendon stretched.
(8) Surgery. In those patients who do not fully respond to this regimen or who suffer repeated attacks of tendinitis, the possibility of chronic thickening of the paratenon, central-core degeneration or else a partial rupture of the tendon should be considered and may require surgery.

Chronic thickening of the paratenon

This condition, described by Williams (1973), is produced by chronic inflammatory changes in the paratenon. It probably occurs as a complication of acute peritendinitis as the result of continued overuse. The paratenon becomes thickened and adherent to the Achilles tendon, restricting tendon movement and producing recurrent attacks of

Achilles tendinitis. It may also be found in association with a central-core degeneration of the tendon.

Management

If mobilization techniques and ultrasound do not produce any improvement chronic thickening of the paratenon is best treated by an operation to strip the thickened paratenon from around the tendon. The results of this operation are usually excellent (Williams and Sperryn, 1976).

Bursitis

Two bursae, one deep and the other superficial, are found in relation to the Achilles tendon. The superficial posterior calcaneal bursa lies between the skin and the tendon; bursitis is usually produced by friction due to shoes, especially high-heeled shoes. The deep retrocalcaneal bursa lies between the tendon and the calcaneus, sitting like a cap over the posterosuperior angle of the bone. Retrocalcaneal bursitis, which may be associated with an Achilles tendinitis, produces swelling that may be seen bulging on either side of the tendon. Tenderness may be present and is elicited by squeezing in front of the tendon with the thumb and index finger.

Management

Management of retrocalcaneal bursitis is similar to that of Achilles tendinitis. An injection of steroid into the bursa itself can be easily given with a 25-gauge needle and produces rapid relief of symptoms.

Rupture of the tendon

This may be complete or partial. Complete rupture of the tendon is uncommon in younger patients and occurs more commonly with increasing age. In a series of 33 cases reported from the Mayo Clinic, the average age was 40 and the oldest patient was 70 years old (Goldman, Linscheid and Bickel, 1969). The site of rupture occurs usually at about 5 cm from the tendon insertion, and underlying degenerative changes, which can usually be observed at operation (Arner, Lindholm and Orell, 1958), are considered to be the predisposing cause (Burry, 1978). The role of previously injected corticosteroids in the aetiology of rupture remains controversial. In theory, injections into the tendon itself could lead to a weakening of the tendon collagen fibres, or produce compression of blood vessels in the paratenon with loss of blood supply to the tendon. However, in practice, local corticosteroid injections do not appear to be commonly associated with such a rupture, which often occurs in tendons that have never received injections. Lundquist (1968), in his classic monograph describing tendon rupture, found no evidence to support the view that these injections were an important predisposing cause. Nevertheless, when injections are indicated they must always be given around, and not into, the tendon.

Most cases occur during sporting activities and, in the middle-aged patient, there is often a history of having recently taken up jogging. Rupture may occur during running, jumping and hurrying up stairs, when the tendon is suddenly stretched, or in a skiing accident, when the skier suddenly falls forward so that the ankle is dorsiflexed with the foot anchored in the ski. As the tendon ruptures suddenly and dramatically, the patient experiences severe pain and usually falls over. Walking becomes difficult at first because of weakness of ankle plantar flexion, but subsequently the patient may be able to walk with some limp.

Clinical findings

The proximal part of the ruptured tendon rolls upwards, leaving a gap between the ends of the torn tendon that is visible and palpable. Subsequently the gap is filled with blood clot and may not be so readily appreciated. The correct diagnosis is then often not made for a considerable time and the injury is mistaken for a sprain of the ankle. On inspection the tendon is seen to be grossly thickened and the normal gutters on either side of the tendon are obliterated. After a few days, bruising appears around the ankle.

Major sign

The patient lies prone with both feet over the edge of the couch. The calf muscles on the normal leg are squeezed by the examiner's hand and the patient's foot can be observed to plantar flex. In the affected leg, squeezing the calf fails to flex the foot as the tendon is disrupted (*see Figure 11.4*).

Confirmatory signs

With complete rupture the range of passive dorsiflexion of the ankle is increased in the affected leg.

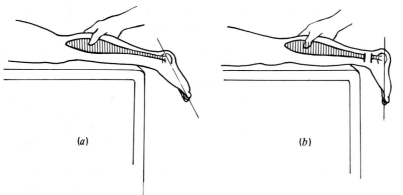

Figure 11.4 Test for ruptured Achilles tendon: (*a*) normal foot movement if the tendon is intact; (*b*) with a ruptured tendon the foot remains stationary

There is marked weakness of plantar flexion of the ankle, best appreciated by asking the patient to stand on tiptoe, which is then virtually impossible on the affected side.

A tender gap in the tendon may be palpable in the middle of the tendon, and is often better appreciated by having the patient lie supine with the knee flexed rather than prone.

Management

The treatment of choice is surgery, which needs to be undertaken within 3 weeks of the rupture. The divided ends of the tendon are sutured and the lower leg is then immobilized in a plaster cast with the ankle in plantar flexion for 6 weeks. After the plaster is removed active rehabilitation is essential to allow full recovery of function.

Partial rupture

Partial rupture of the Achilles tendon (Lundquist, 1968) is a condition that is becoming increasingly recognized. The patient suffers a sudden sharp pain in the tendon, usually while running, and pain is then experienced, especially when stepping off the affected leg. Subsequently the patient usually complains of chronic tendon pain. The site of rupture usually occurs a few centimetres above the tendon insertion and palpation reveals a small, tender thickening within the tendon itself. At times, a small gap within the tendon and immediately above this a small, tender, rolled-up segment of the tendon may be palpated.

Clinically, differentiation between chronic thickening of the paratenon, central-core degeneration and partial rupture of the tendon may be extremely difficult and they may occur together.

Surgical exploration may be necessary to distinguish between them and provide definitive treatment.

Management

Conservative treatment is similar to that outlined for Achilles tendinitis. However, results are not generally satisfactory and the patient often suffers recurrent pain and disability. Surgical exploration is then preferable (Williams and Sperryn, 1976), and the tendon is debrided and repaired.

Avulsion of the Achilles tendon

This serious injury is rare and occurs in an elderly patient when a portion of the calcaneus is avulsed with the attachment of the Achilles tendon. Treatment is surgical.

Ossification

Ossification in the tendon may occur as a rare complication of Achilles tendinitis and the diagnosis is confirmed on X-ray. Rarely this area of bone may fracture (Lotke, 1970), which produces severe pain, and the tendon itself may also rupture at the same time.

Pathological conditions

The Achilles tendon and bursa may be involved in a number of generalized conditions. Spondyloarthritis may produce, or present with, tendinitis or bursitis. Rheumatoid involvement of the bursa may produce erosive changes in the calcaneus and

X-ray of the heel may also reveal a thickened Achilles tendon that has been displaced posteriorly (Weston and Palmer, 1978). The tendon may also be thickened due to the presence of a rheumatoid nodule, tophus, xanthoma or, rarely, a neurofibroma.

Osteochondritis of the calcaneus

This condition occurs most often in young males, aged from 7 to 14. It is due to traction by the Achilles tendon on the un-united calcaneal apophysis. Sever (1912) described this form of osteochondritis in which X-rays revealed fragmentation and sclerosis of the calcanean apophysis, although these X-ray findings may be non-specific (Ferguson and Gingrich, 1957). The child is nearly always engaged in sporting activities that involve much running, and he usually presents during the middle of the athletics or football season.

Clinical findings

The patient is usually a young boy who presents with pain and stiffness in the heel. Pain is at first related to activity and is relieved by rest but usually increases so that he is unable to continue running.

Clinical examination localizes the site of the lesion to the insertion of the Achilles tendon into the posterior aspect of the calcaneus, where there may be some degree of swelling or thickening and tenderness. This condition is often associated with a mechanically inefficient action of the Achilles tendon and loss of full passive ankle dorsiflexion. A varus hind-foot deformity is a commonly associated finding. An X-ray may show the changes in apophysis described above and also a prominent posterosuperior angle of the calcaneus (Ferguson and Gingrich, 1957).

Management

Management consists of rest from running and the use of a pad to elevate the heel. Physical methods of treatment usually produce only temporary relief but should be given a trial.

12 The ankle joint

The ankle is a modified hinge joint in which the surrounding bones form a mortise and tenon arrangement. The mortise is formed by the medial malleolus of the lower end of the tibia and the lateral malleolus of the fibula, all lined by articular cartilage. The tenon is formed by the superior, or trochlear, surface of the body of the talus (*see Figure 12.1*).

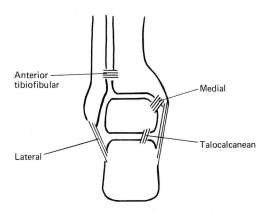

Figure 12.1 The ligaments stabilizing the ankle mortise

Only two active movements occur at the ankle joint: extension and flexion. The axis of this movement runs through the body of the talus—passing from the medial surface (distal to the medial malleolus) to its lateral surface, where it runs through the tip of the lateral malleolus. When the foot is plantar flexed, the narrower posterior part of the body of the talus moves forwards into the mortise and the talus can be passively moved laterally to and fro between the malleoli. With the foot dorsiflexed, the broader anterior part of the body

moves backwards into the mortise. When the ankle joint moves from dorsiflexion to plantar flexion the articular surfaces glide and are at first compressed and then distracted.

During active plantar flexion of the joint the talus can also internally rotate a few degrees; this is accompanied by movement in the lateral malleolus, which also rotates internally and downwards.

Examination

(1) Inspection—with the patient standing, walking and lying down.
   (a) Gait.
   (b) Deformities.
   (c) Swelling.
(2) Movements:
   (a) Active.
   (b) Passive.
   (c) Accessory.
   (d) Isometric.
(3) Palpation:
   (a) Warmth.
   (b) Synovial thickening.
   (c) Tenderness.

Inspection

Examination of the ankle forms an integral part of foot examination, and some abnormalities—such as deformities and gait disturbances—will be discussed later.

The ankle should be inspected both from the front and behind with the patient first standing, then walking, and finally lying down. The presence of an effusion into the ankle joint can best be appreciated by inspection of the ankle with the patient standing. The ankle is inspected both from the front and rear. Anteriorly, the effusion may be seen to bulge into the synovial space, which follows the line of the reflection of the synovium proximally up over the anterior surface of the tibia (*see Figure 12.2*). Posteriorly, an effusion in the ankle joint may be seen bulging out behind the malleoli so that it fills in the normal gutter between the malleolus and the Achilles tendon. Effusions into the tendon sheaths crossing the ankle are readily visible. The tibialis posterior and peroneal tendons run behind their respective malleoli, and effusions in their tendon sheath produce a crescent-shaped swelling along the line of the tendon.

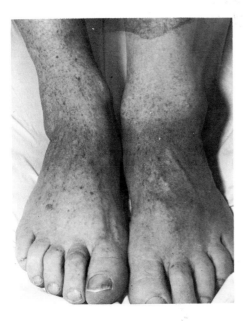

Figure 12.2 Synovial effusion into the left ankle joint

These synovial swellings need to be differentiated from oedema which, because of dependency of the leg or inflammatory changes in surrounding soft tissue, may complicate ankle lesions. Bruising and swelling around the ankle may be evident after recent ligament sprains.

Movements

Active

The only active movements at the ankle joint are dorsiflexion and plantar flexion. The active range is measured with the ankle in the neutral position; that is, with the foot at 90 degrees to the leg. The active range is 20 degrees of dorsiflexion and 30 degrees of plantar flexion. However, movement in the transverse tarsal joints also contributes to the range of these movements. The range of ankle movements varies widely with age and physical training. The range may be restricted due to an arthritis, a sprain of the collateral ligament or swelling around the ankle. Decreased range is also associated with an equinus deformity of the ankle and may be due to a contracture of the gastrocnemius-soleus muscle and Achilles tendon complex.

Passive

DORSIFLEXION
Full passive ankle dorsiflexion, greater in range than active dorsiflexion, is usually to about 30 degrees. However, much of this movement takes place in the transverse tarsal joint. To test the passive range at the ankle joint accurately, therefore, the transverse tarsal joint needs to be immobilized by one of two methods. Firstly, the transverse tarsal joint is locked by the examiner fully passively inverting the foot; secondly, the examiner may grasp the patient's foot proximal to the transverse tarsal joints with one hand (*see Figure 12.3*). With either of these methods the examiner places his left hand behind the patient's calf to stabilize the ankle and uses his right hand to move the ankle joint into full passive dorsiflexion.

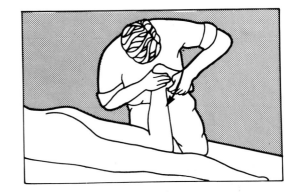

Figure 12.3 Passive dorsiflexion of the ankle

Clinical measurement of this range is important, as it reflects the range of dorsiflexion that can be produced at the ankle during locomotion. A decrease in this range is known as an equinus of the ankle and is due either to a contracture of the gastrocnemius-soleus muscle and Achilles tendon complex or to a lesion of the ankle joint itself.

PLANTAR FLEXION

The passive range of plantar flexion is also normally greater than the active range. The range of passive movement may be found to be restricted and painless or restricted and painful. A painful restriction of this movement is most commonly due to a sprain of the lateral ligament of the ankle joint.

Accessory

Accessory movements need to be tested first in the inferior tibiofibular joint and then in the ankle joint.

INFERIOR TIBIOFIBULAR JOINT

There are six accessory movements in the inferior tibiofibular joint:

(1) Posteroanterior. An oscillatory pressure is produced by pressure against the posterior border of the lateral malleolus (*see Figure 12.4*).
(2) Anteroposterior, which is produced by pressure against the anterior border of the lateral malleolus (*see Figure 12.5*).

(3) Longitudinal caudad movement is produced by inversion of the calcaneus.
(4) Longitudinal cephalad movement is produced by eversion of the calcaneus.
(5) Separation of the fibula relative to the tibia occurs mainly on full dorsiflexion of the ankle.
(6) Compression is produced by pressure over both malleoli (*see Figure 12.6*).

ANKLE JOINT

There are six accessory movements at the ankle joint:

(1) Posteroanterior movement, which is produced by pushing the calcaneus forwards (*see Figure 12.7*).

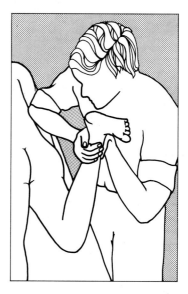

Figure 12.5 Anteroposterior accessory movement—inferior tibiofibular joint

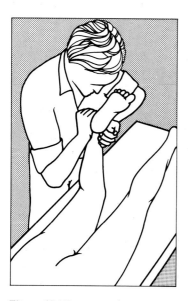

Figure 12.4 Posteroanterior accessory movement—inferior tibiofibular joint

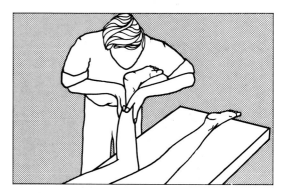

Figure 12.6 Inferior tibiofibular joint: compression

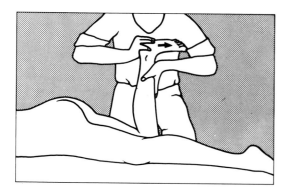

Figure 12.7 Posteroanterior accessory movement: ankle joint

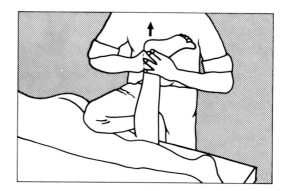

Figure 12.10 Longitudinal caudad accessory movement

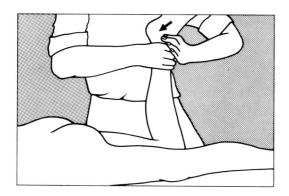

Figure 12.8 Anteroposterior accessory movement: ankle joint

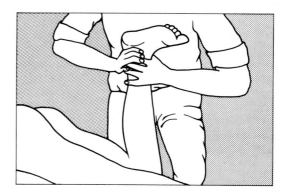

Figure 12.11 Rotation of the ankle joint

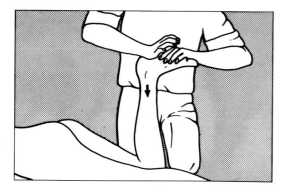

Figure 12.9 Longitudinal cephalad accessory movement: ankle joint

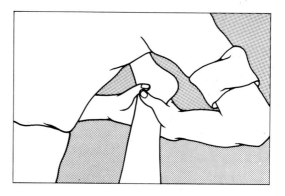

Figure 12.12 Ankle joint; lateral rotation

(2) Anteroposterior movement is produced by gripping over the talus and pushing it posteriorly (*see Figure 12.8*).

(3) Longitudinal cephalad movement is produced by compression through the calcaneus (*see Figure 12.9*).

(4) Longitudinal caudad movement is produced by distraction of the ankle (*see Figure 12.10*).

(5) Medial rotation is produced by movement of the talus and heel in the mortice (*see Figure 12.11*).

(6) Lateral rotation is produced by an opposite movement of talus and heel in the mortice (*see Figure 12.12*).

Isometric tests

Dorsiflexion of the ankle is produced mainly by the anterior tibialis muscle, which is inserted into the medial aspect of the first cuneiform and the base of the first metatarsal bones. It is tested with the foot fully inverted and the ankle fully dorsiflexed; the patient resists the examiner's attempt to force the foot into plantar flexion. The tendon may then be seen and palpated on the medial side of the ankle joint.

Pain may be due either to tendinitis of the muscle in the lower third of the leg, in which case there is associated crepitus; or to a tendinitis at its insertion. A painless weakness is associated with a foot drop, which may be due to a lesion of the L5 nerve root or the lateral popliteal nerve.

Plantar flexion of the ankle is produced mainly by the gastrocnemius and soleus muscles. It is usually very difficult for the examiner to detect any weakness in these muscles by resisting plantar flexion of the foot. A better method of reproducing pain is to have the patient stand up and down ten times on the toes of one foot. Pain may be due to a tear in the gastrocnemius or a lesion in the Achilles tendon. A painless weakness may be due to S1 nerve-root pressure or a long-standing rupture of the Achilles tendon.

Palpation

The bony outlines of the malleoli and the anterior margin of the lower end of the tibia are subcutaneous and easily palpated. The joint line can also be palpated posteriorly behind the medial malleolus by having the patient actively dorsiflex and plantar flex the ankle.

The ankle is palpated for any increase in warmth by comparing it with the opposite ankle. Palpation may reveal or confirm the presence of synovitis in the ankle. The patient lies supine and the examiner holds the back of the ankle behind the malleoli with one hand to squeeze fluid into the more extensive anterior part of the joint. With his other hand the examiner palpates the area around the anterior joint line using either the fingers or thumb. Tenderness is sought especially over the joint line and the attachments of the collateral ligaments.

Classification of ankle lesions

(1) Soft tissue:
  (a) Ligament sprains.

(b) Recurrent instability of the ankle.
  (c) Tendon lesions.
(2) Bone:
  (a) Talotibial exostoses.
  (b) Osteochondritis dissecans.

Ligament sprains

Lateral collateral ligament sprain

The three bands of fibres that make up the lateral ligament are injured by different mechanisms, determined by the function of the ligament and direction in which the fibres run (*see Figure 12.13*).

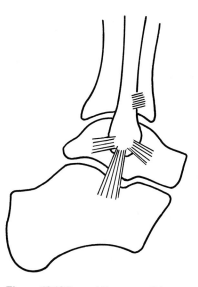

Figure 12.13 Lateral ligaments of the ankle joint

The anterior talofibular ligament runs from the anterior border of the lateral malleolus, passes medially to the neck of the talus, and fuses with the anterior capsule of the ankle joint. It is taut during plantar flexion of the foot and so may be damaged by a sudden forced or excessive degree of plantar flexion. Since this is the position of the foot in which most injuries occur, the anterior bundle is the most commonly involved of the fibres that make up the lateral ligament.

The ligament may be damaged at either its upper or lower attachments, more commonly the former. This history given by the patient is often one of having fallen over while running, walking or jumping, especially on a rough surface.

The middle band of the lateral ligament, the fibulocalcaneal ligament, runs vertically downwards from the tip of the lateral malleolus to the lateral surface of the calcaneus. It is taut with the ankle at a right angle and so tends to be injured with the ankle in this position.

The posterior band of the lateral ligament runs from the lateral malleolus medially to the talus, strengthening the posterior aspect of the ankle capsule. It is only rarely injured and the underlying mechanism occurs, for example, in long-jumpers, who after having landed on their feet have their body weight suddenly carried forward, forcibly dorsiflexing the ankle.

Anterior tibiofibular ligament sprain

A sprain of the anterior tibiofibular ligament is a relatively common ankle injury and may occur as the result of the usual type of inversion strain. It may also follow either an eversion or a dorsiflexion injury. In an eversion injury of the ankle the talus is forced against the medial malleolus, which produces a widening of the ankle mortise so that fibres of the anterior tibiofibular ligament may be torn. After a severe degree of injury this ligament may be ruptured and produce a diastasis, or widening, of the inferior tibiofibular joint, with disruption of the normal ankle-joint mortise. Sprain of this ligament may also follow forced dorsiflexion of the ankle in which the anterior part of the body talus is forced into the ankle joint, disrupting the ligament fibres. This injury may also produce a rupture of the Achilles tendon, or a malleolar fracture.

Medial ligament sprain

Sprains of the medial ligament do not often occur because the ligament is strong and eversion injuries are relatively uncommon.

Diagnosis of ligament sprains

Diagnosis depends on an accurate history of the mechanism of the injury, a history of previous sprains, the site of pain and clinical examination. At the time of injury there may be an audible crack or snap, even in minor sprains. It is always useful to examine the ankle movements as soon as possible after the injury, before any swelling develops. The site of the ligament sprain should be accurately localized and an assessment made of the degree of injury, which may require repeated examination over a few days. The normal leg is examined first to determine the normal range and degree of ligamentous laxity. The affected ankle is inspected for oedema, bruising, deformity or synovitis.

Second-degree sprains involving mainly the outer fibres of the ligament may be associated with a large haematoma formation and soft-tissue oedema. Second-degree sprains with a capsular sprain usually present a less dramatic clinical picture but are associated with a synovitis of the ankle, which may be blood stained, and can lead to more prolonged disability if not properly treated. However, if the capsule is completely torn an effusion is usually absent.

Pain is reproduced on ankle movement by stretching or compressing the injured ligament, by moving the foot into inversion, eversion, plantar and dorsiflexion. In sprains of the lateral ligament, pain may be reproduced either on inversion of the foot or on full passive eversion of the foot, since the painful area in the ligament is apparently compressed between the fibular malleolus and calcaneus. In sprains of the anterior tibiofibular ligament pain may be produced on plantar or dorsiflexion of the ankle, but especially on plantar flexion with inversion of the foot. Tenderness is sought by careful palpation over the ligamentous attachments and the surrounding soft-tissue structures.

Management

Ankle sprains are often poorly managed; if X-rays are normal the patient is usually advised that 'it is only a sprain' and further treatment may not be undertaken—hence the common statement that ankle sprains are a worse injury than a fracture, since the period of disability is prolonged. The management that was previously advocated consisted of prolonged immobilization even for minor sprains but this produced subsequent muscle weakness, joint stiffness and pain. This led to the popular concept of 'once a sprain, always a sprain', a negative outlook that should never be allowed to prevent a patient's return to full activity.

INITIAL TREATMENT
Treatment in the first 48 hours after injury is designed to minimize swelling by using ice, compression and elevation to prevent oedema formation and so limit subsequent adhesion formation and stiffness. A useful adjunct in patients with a sprain of the lateral ligament if seen soon after injury is to strap the ankle in eversion. The lower leg is first

shaved and Friar's Balsam is applied to the skin. A Gibney basket-weave adhesive-tape strapping gives the most effective support and when properly applied limits inversion, eversion and rotation of the ankle. The strapping is applied from the medial side of the leg, passed under the heel with the foot held in eversion and extended up the lateral side of the leg. A piece of foam rubber may be incorporated over the ligament to prevent haematoma formation. The foam rubber is cut in the shape of a horseshoe and bevelled so that it can be applied around the malleolus. The foam rubber is then kept in place by compressing it with the strapping. The foot and lower leg may need to be supported by a crêpe bandage to control swelling. The patient is advised to rest for 1–2 days and the crêpe bandage is removed at periodic intervals so that ice can be applied over the adhesive-tape strapping, which is left undisturbed. The strapping is then removed and the degree of ligament injury is reassessed; bruising and oedematous swelling should be minimal.

SUBSEQUENT TREATMENT

Most injuries are first-degree or second-degree sprains without any joint effusion. The aim with these is to exercise and stretch the ankle within the limits of pain to mobilize it as rapidly as possible:

(1) The patient is encouraged to walk as normally as possible with a heel-to-toe gait within the limits of pain, and may be assisted in this by the use of crêpe bandage to support the ankle.
(2) Anti-inflammatory drugs may also be given for pain relief.
(3) Physical methods are of benefit and consist of heat or ice, the latter usually being preferred.
(4) Active exercises and postural re-education with the use of a wobble board are given daily. The reason for this treatment is that articular nerve fibres and their mechanoreceptors which are involved in reflex stabilization of the ankle joint (Freeman and Wyke, 1967) are disrupted. Exercises are designed to increase neuromuscular co-ordination by having the patient balance on a board that moves at first in one plane and, having accomplished that, on a board that moves in all planes. This exercise leads to increased proprioceptive control (Freeman, Dean and Hanham, 1965).
(5) Mobilization by passive movement to restore both accessory and physiological movements to a full pain-free range is also important. Without pain-free movements the use of act-

ive exercises and the wobble board will be limited in their extent to restore muscle power and co-ordination.
(6) Local injections and massage are not necessary and are contraindicated during this early stage.
(7) As pain and tenderness resolve, the patient can begin to run at half pace and then be rehabilitated by the use of functional activities to full activity.

TREATMENT OF COMPLICATIONS

By these methods the ligament usually returns to full strength. In some patients, particularly those who initially have been treated inadequately, the lateral ligament may remain tender and painful on movement, especially with full passive inversion of the foot. Pain is felt on running, often when there is a need to change direction suddenly. The site of tenderness is usually found around the attachment of the lateral ligament to the lateral malleolus. The pathological basis of this lesion has never been determined and has been assumed to be due to adhesion formation. It is more likely to be due to an area of chronic granulation scar tissue, similar to that found in tenoperiosteal lesions, e.g. lateral epicondylitis of the elbow.

This ankle lesion may be treated by:

(1) An injection of 1 ml of local anaesthetic and 1 ml of corticosteroid given into the tender area in the ligament on one or two occasions.
(2) Mobilization techniques to the ankle.

If pain is the predominant problem manual therapy techniques are commenced using large-amplitude rocking movements, taking care not to produce any discomfort. The principal technique used is rotation with the patient lying prone and the knee flexed to 90 degrees. Rotation is produced by holding around the patient's foot and rocking

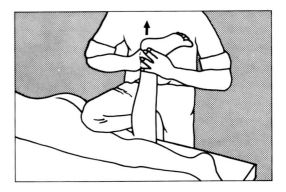

Figure 12.14 Distraction

it. As the degree of pain decreases, this same treatment is used at the limit of the range (*see Figure 12.11*), so producing stretching and some discomfort; distraction (*see Figure 12.14*) with slow oscillatory stretching is also used. In patients with pain and stiffness of the ankle the amount of treatment given varies depending on the degree of joint irritability. Physiological movements, usually dorsiflexion of the ankle, are used first. Accessory movements are then added at the limit of the available range of dorsiflexion, using posteroanterior movements (*see Figure 12.7*), anteroposterior movements (*see Figure 12.8*) and inversion of the heel (*see Figure 12.15*).

If stiffness is the predominant problem dorsiflexion is again used as the first treatment method

but it is now taken further into the range (*see Figure 12.16*). Additional physiological movements are used strongly in other directions and accessory movements are then added at the limit of each range. As the pain settles, active exercises are recommended.

A similar lesion may also involve the anterior tibiofibular ligament. Pain then occurs especially when running with sudden acceleration or sudden stopping. Tenderness is localized over the ligament and treatment is with local corticosteroid injection.

Finally, a similar type of lesion may involve the anterior capsule of the ankle joint and leads to a loss of ankle movement. Pain may not be reproduced on testing active ankle plantar flexion but is present on testing passive movements. The range of full passive plantar flexion of the ankle is decreased and over-pressure then reproduces the patient's pain. In football players this lesion leads to considerable disability as the foot needs to be fully plantar flexed to kick a ball and sudden stretching of the capsule produces quite severe pain. Treatment consists of stretching the ankle, best performed by a forced manipulation of the ankle under a general anaesthetic, to restore the full passive range of plantar flexion.

Third-degree sprain

Third-degree sprains with complete rupture of the ligament produce ankle instability. Ankle stability is normally dependent upon the integrity of the joint surfaces, as the talus is locked into the tibiofibular mortise with the malleoli on either side

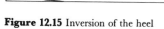

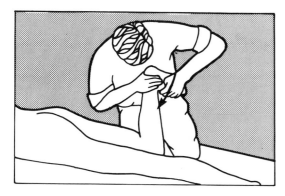

Figure 12.15 Inversion of the heel

Figure 12.16 Ankle-joint dorsiflexion

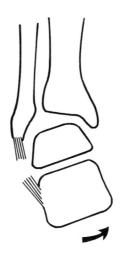

Figure 12.17 Talar tilt on inversion stress

exerting a pincer-like effect. Its integrity also depends on the ligamentous support provided by the anterior tibiofibular ligament superiorly and the two collateral ligaments on either side of the ankle joint.

Lateral instability of the ankle follows rupture of the lateral collateral ligament (*see Figure 12.17*), especially the calcaneofibular ligament, and may also be associated with a rupture of the anterior talofibular ligament. It is tested for with the ankle in plantar flexion. The examiner grasps the calcaneus and fully passively inverts the foot. Normally a small range of movement is present but if the ligament is ruptured a greater degree of inversion is possible as the talus rocks in the ankle mortise.

The diagnosis needs to be confirmed by X-ray with stress inversion of the ankle to demonstrate the presence of any tilting of the talus (*see Figure 12.17*). This first stresses the anterior talofibular ligament and the joint capsule. Should they be torn the talus will tilt medially. Further inversion then stresses the calcaneofibular ligament so that gross tilting of the talus indicates a tear of this ligament also. The film is taken with the foot in plantar flexion and inversion. The normal degree of talar tilt is from 0 to 5 degrees but varies according to age (St. Jacques and Laurin, 1965) and may be increased in patients with ligamentous laxity. If a minor degree of tilt is found and its significance is uncertain a similar view of the other ankle should be taken for comparison.

Anterior instability is also caused by a rupture of the anterior talofibular ligament so that the talus becomes loose in its mortise. It is tested clinically by the anterior drawer sign.

STARTING POSITION
The patient sits over the edge of the couch with the legs hanging down and the foot in a slight degree of plantar flexion. The examiner places one hand over the anterior aspect of the lower tibia and grasps the patient's calcaneus with the other.

METHOD
The tibia is pushed posteriorly by one hand and the calcaneus and talus are pushed anteriorly with the other hand. Normally no anterior movement is possible but if the anterior talofibular ligament is ruptured the talus may be felt to move anteriorly, often producing a 'clunking' noise.

X-rays are also used to demonstrate this instability. A lateral X-ray may show a forward displacement of the talus greater than 3 mm.

Medial instability due to a tear of the medial ligament is tested clinically in a similar manner to a lateral ligament tear but the examiner now everts the foot and the talus may be felt to tilt in the ankle mortise. The diagnosis may be confirmed on X-ray, which shows a widening of the space in the medial compartment of the ankle between the medial malleolus and the talus. This injury is also commonly associated with a diastasis of the inferior tibiofibular joint (*see Figure 12.18*).

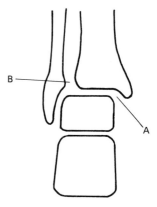

Figure 12.18 Rupture of the medial ligament showing (A) widening of the medial joint space; and (B) diastasis of the inferior tibiofibular joint

MANAGEMENT
Management of these injuries remains controversial. Surgical repair, immobilization and active exercises have each been advocated. In complete ruptures of ankle ligaments with talar instability, it might appear logical to attempt surgical repair of the disrupted ligament. Nevertheless, these injuries can be treated successfully by active exercises and postural re-education of the ankle (Freeman, 1965). However, if pain is severe and causes difficulty in walking, immobilization first in a cast brace or a plaster may be preferable. The former consists of a Litecast upper section worn below the knee into which is incorporated a polyethylene plastic shoe insert (Henning and Legge, 1977). This allows plantar and dorsiflexion of the ankle but prevents inversion or eversion strains. Alternatively, the ankle may be immobilized in a plaster cast with the ankle held in eversion. This is worn for 4–6 weeks and active exercises are then instituted.

For patients with chronic recurrent instability

a late operation for reconstruction of the lateral ligament may be performed using a modified Evans repair (Ottosson, 1978).

A complete rupture of the deltoid and tibiofibular ligaments may be treated similarly with plaster immobilization and compression of the plaster to approximate the malleoli and reconstitute the ankle mortise arrangement. If this fails the tibia and fibula may need to have an internal fixation with a screw to approximate the separated joint surfaces.

Recurrent instability of the ankle

The patient with recurrent ankle instability may complain of recurrent ankle sprains, that the ankle turns over easily or that the ankle feels insecure and often lets him down. The ankle is often painful and stiff and there may be recurrent swelling. These symptoms may be present while walking or running, particularly over rough ground, and the patient usually can often feel or hear a click in the ankle. Recurrent instability may be due to:

(1) Functional instability.
(2) Complete ligamentous rupture.
(3) Inadequately treated ligament sprains.
(4) Foot deformities.
(5) Undiagnosed causes.

Functional instability

This is common after a ligamentous injury in the ankle and has generally been considered to be the result of a mechanical derangement of the joint. However, Freeman (1965) produced evidence that what he termed a functional instability of the foot was the most common cause. This follows an injury of the joint and capsule and ligaments with loss of the sensory proprioceptive nerve fibres. These fibres subserve the reflex arc that stabilizes the foot and ankle during locomotion and so when they are lost, reflex stabilization is impaired and the foot tends to give way.

MAJOR SIGNS

The presence of functional instability is tested for by a modified Romberg's test (Freeman, Dean and Hanham, 1965). The patient first stands on the uninjured leg with his eyes open and then closed and then on the injured leg with his eyes open and then closed. Impaired stability may then become evident either to the examiner or to the patient.

Complete ligamentous rupture

This may involve the anterior talofibular or the calcaneofibular ligament or both so that the talus becomes loose in its mortise and can be recurrently subluxed. The clinical tests and X-ray findings in this condition have already been described but arthrography can also be used and may reveal a large pouch of synovium protruding through the capsule and bulging out onto the distal surface of the tibia.

Inadequately treated sprains

These may lead to pain and a sudden giving way of the ankle, especially with sprains of the lateral ligament. This is most likely to occur when the patient is running and suddenly changes direction, such as in swerving or turning quickly. The underlying pathological basis for this condition may be due to formation of chronic granulation tissue at the ligament origin or to formation of adhesions.

Careful examination of the foot and ankle will reveal excessive pain on stretching the inadequately treated area. The movements most often found to be still painful on stretching are: adduction of the heel, inversion of the foot, and a longitudinal caudad movement of the ankle. An area of marked tenderness can usually be palpated over the origin of the ligament from the lateral malleolus.

Foot deformities

Foot deformities, especially those due to a valgus deformity of the forefoot in which there is an alteration in the peroneus longus function, are often associated with recurrent pain and disability in the lateral compartment of the ankle joint.

Undiagnosed causes

In a small proportion of patients, particularly females, no obvious cause can be demonstrated, although it has been attributed to wearing inadequate shoes, such as high heels or with heels that wear unevenly. Management depends on the diagnosis of the underlying cause. Active exercises and proprioceptive retraining are usually necessary. Localized tender areas may be treated with corticosteroid injections, deep-friction massage or manipulations. A shoe-raise with a wedge and a float may also help. If a complete rupture of the lateral ligament can be demonstrated by a stress inversion film showing a talar tilt, reconstructive surgery may be necessary.

Tenosynovitis of the ankle tendons

Tenosynovitis commonly involves either the peroneal tendons over the lateral compartment of the ankle or the tibialis posterior tendon over the medial compartment. Tenosynovitis may follow trauma, such as a sprain of the collateral ligaments of the ankle joint; overuse of the ankle; or inflammatory conditions such as rheumatoid arthritis or spondyloarthritis in which tenosynovitis may, at times, be the presenting symptom. The patient complains of pain, swelling and/or restricted movement, and examination reveals swelling that has a characteristic linear appearance as it bulges out from behind and below the malleolus.

Peroneal tendons

Peroneal tenosynovitis may occur along the course of the tendon from behind the fibular malleolus to the outer side of the foot.

MAJOR SIGN
Pain is reproduced by the examiner either fully resisting eversion of the foot, or stretching the peroneal tendons by fully passively inverting the foot. At the same time as these manoeuvres are being carried out the examiner palpates for tenderness and crepitus over the peroneal tendons behind the lateral malleolus.

COMPLICATIONS
These are:

(1) Subluxation.
(2) Tendovaginitis.
(3) Rupture.
(4) Weakness.
(5) Ganglion formation.

Subluxation of the peroneal tendons occurs after an ankle injury that disrupts the peroneal retinaculum binding the peroneal tendons in their grooves at the back of the fibular malleolus. The tendons can then sublux over the fibular surface, usually during dorsiflexion of the foot, and are repositioned on plantar flexion of the foot. Treatment is surgical.

Tendovaginitis of the peroneal tendons occurs as localized thickening of the common peroneal tendon sheath, similar to a de Quervain's syndrome at the wrist. It occurs as an overuse injury and is particularly common in athletes and ballet dancers. The patient presents with pain localized over the peroneal tendons, and a thickened, tender swelling may be palpated below the lateral malleolus. Treatment consists of rest and a local corticosteroid injection but if pain persists the peroneal sheath may be excised.

Rupture of the peroneal tendon is a rare complication that needs to be differentiated from weakness of ankle eversion due to a neurological lesion, such as L5 nerve-root pressure.

Weakness of these tendons may be associated with a recurrent sprain of the ankle.

A ganglion may be formed around the peroneal tendons.

Tenosynovitis of the tibialis posterior tendon

In this condition tenosynovitis involves the tibialis posterior tendon behind or just below the medial malleolus. Apart from the causes described above, tenosynovitis may also occur as a complication of pes planus associated with valgus deformity of the rear foot, which produces a strain on the medial compartment structures.

MAJOR SIGNS
Pain is reproduced by the examiner either resisting active inversion of the foot or stretching the tendon by fully passively everting the foot. At the same time, tenderness and crepitus is sought by palpating along the course of the tendon behind the medial malleolus.

COMPLICATIONS
(1) A tarsal-tunnel syndrome may develop (*see* page 204).
(2) Tendovaginitis occurs as localized thickening in the tendon sheath.
(3) Rupture of the tibialis posterior tendon is a rare occurrence but is associated with marked loss of foot function.

Talotibial exostoses

This ankle lesion is characterized by the growth of bony exostoses on the surface of the talus and tibia around the ankle joint. Exostoses develop on the anterior margins of the ankle joint on the upper surface of the neck of the talus and the lower end of the tibia just above the joint margin. The tibial exostoses may reach large proportions and can develop anywhere along the anterior tibial margin, out to the malleolus. At times an exostosis develops only on the tibial surface and is associated with a large erosion in the neck of the talus. Occasionally the tibial exostosis may break off to form a loose bony body inside the joint.

It was originally believed that the bony outgrowths grew only around the anterior margins of the ankle joint. Similar changes were subsequently described around the posterior margins of the tibia and talus and were considered to be a separate condition. It is now evident that both anterior and posterior exostoses are due to the same fundamental mechanism and that both sites are commonly involved around the ankle joint.

The relationship of this condition to athletic training was investigated by O'Donoghue (1977), who showed that in the push-off phase of running direct bony apposition resulted between the anterior border of the tibia and the talus (*see Figure 12.19*). In full plantar flexion of the foot, as occurs during running, the posterior talus will hit the bony block of the lower posterior margin of the tibia (Kapandji, 1974) (*see Figure 12.20*). Anatomical considerations, such as a long posterior process of the talus or a separate os trigonum,

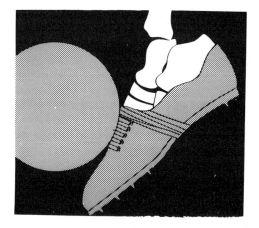

Figure 12.20 Diagrammatic representation of talotibial impingement on plantar flexion of the ankle

make these lesions about the posterior aspect of the joint more likely. A long posterior process of the talus may be compressed more readily by the calcaneus against the tibia.

Symptoms

Pain is the usual presenting symptom; it may be present on activity, especially running or going down stairs. A dull ache may be present after exercise. The ankle feels stiff and the patient may complain of a loss of speed when starting off to run. Locking of the ankle joint may occur if an exostosis is broken off to produce a loose bony foreign body.

Signs

This condition usually produces more symptoms than signs, which may be difficult to elicit. On inspection some swelling or fullness over the an-

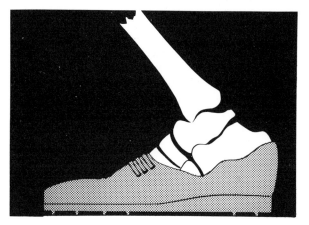

Figure 12.19 Diagrammatic representation of talotibial impingement on dorsiflexion of the ankle

terior aspect of the ankle may be apparent. Active ankle movements may be of full range.

MAJOR SIGNS

Pain may be reproduced on either full passive plantar or dorsiflexion of the ankle. Anterior exostoses tend to be associated with pain and restriction at the limit of ankle dorsiflexion; and posterior exostoses with a painful restriction at the limit of plantar flexion.

Over-pressure applied at the limit of either of these ranges can usually reproduce the patient's pain.

OTHER SIGNS

Tenderness should be sought by palpation over the ankle. Anteriorly it is found over the anterior border of the tibia or the neck of the talus. Posteriorly it is usually most marked just behind and above the medial malleolus; pressure over this site while the foot is fully plantar flexed may reproduce the patient's pain.

MANAGEMENT

(1) Rest. The patient needs to rest from those activities, such as running, that are associated with pain.
(2) Anti-inflammatory agents are used to control pain.
(3) Injections. The inflamed area around the anterior or posterior exostoses responds well to an injection of local anaesthetic and corticosteroid solution.
(4) Physical methods. Ultrasound may be used to ease pain and localize the tender area. Exercises and massage are contraindicated.
(5) Passive-mobilization techniques should be incorporated as part of the management when examination of the passive movements provokes pain. The techniques are used to restore the maximal pain-free range of ankle movement.
(6) Surgery is only rarely indicated; it should be used in those patients who either fail to respond to conservative measures or have recurrent troubles on resuming full activity. Treatment by bevelling off the exostosis produces excellent results and the patient can usually resume normal activities. In patients who have fractured the tibial exostosis and have symptoms of joint locking, operative removal of the loose fragment is necessary.

Osteochondritis dissecans

This osteochondral fracture occurs especially in adolescents. The usual site of involvement is the superior surface of the talus, more commonly on the fibular side (*see Figure 12.21*). It usually follows an inversion strain of the ankle, which may occur when the ankle is dorsiflexed and so presents the broader posterior area of the talus in the ankle mortise, where it is more readily impinged against the fibular malleolus. It may also occur if the patient lands on the foot after having jumped into the air.

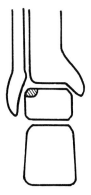

Figure 12.21 Usual site of osteochondritis dissecans of the talus

The patient presents with pain in the ankle, often associated with some swelling that may recur intermittently or after prolonged activity, and a limp. There may be a history of injury. There are no specific tests for this condition but two clinical signs may be present:

(1) Movement of the joint surface under compression may reproduce the patient's pain. This is obtained with the patient lying prone and the knee flexed to 90 degrees. The examiner compresses the talus by leaning on the sole of the foot and pushing it towards the patient's knee. While this compression is maintained the examiner rocks the ankle through a full range of dorsi- and plantar flexion.
(2) Tenderness may be found over the superolateral surface of the talus especially on plantar flexing and inverting the foot so that the involved area on the body of the talus be-

comes palpable. X-rays are necessary to confirm the diagnosis.

Management

Occasionally symptoms are mild or intermittent, and treatment with rest to the ankle may suffice. However, weight-bearing may need to be avoided for 6–12 months. When movements under compression provoke pain, passive-mobilization techniques may be used. Within the first few treatment sessions it will become apparent whether such movements are contraindicated and whether rest should be enforced.

If symptoms are persistent or there is locking of the joint, removal of the loose body with curetting of the cavity is indicated but can be a difficult operation as the fragment may extend under the tibia. If pain due to degenerative changes is present fusion of the ankle joint may be necessary.

13 The foot

The foot may conveniently be divided into three areas: the hind foot, the mid-tarsal region and the forefoot. The hind foot comprises two bones, the talus and the calcaneus. The mid-tarsal region is made up of five bones: the navicular, the cuboid and the three cuneiform bones. The seven bones that make up the hind foot and the mid-tarsal regions together are known as the tarsus. The forefoot comprises the five metatarsal bones and

their corresponding toes (*see Figures 13.1 and 13.2*).

The subtalar joint

The talus articulates with the calcaneus at two separate sites, one anterior and the other posterior,

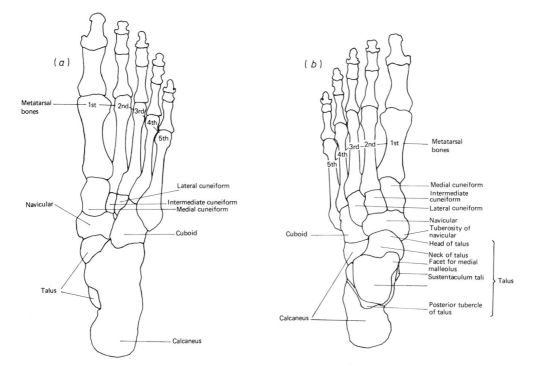

Figure 13.1 The bones of the left foot. (*a*) Plantar aspect; (*b*) dorsal aspect

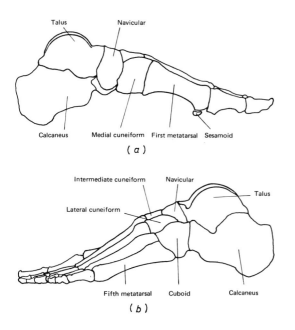

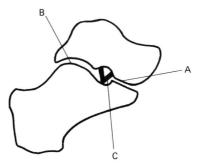

Figure 13.3 (A) Anterior talocalcanean joint; (B) posterior talocalcanean joint; and (C) tarsal tunnel, with V-shaped interosseous ligament

Figure 13.2 The bones of the left foot. (*a*) Medial aspect; (*b*) lateral aspect

to form the talocalcanean joints. These two synovial joints form a functional unit known as the subtalar joint (*see Figure 13.3*). The anterior talocalcanean joint is also continuous with the talonavicular joint formed between the head of the talus and the navicular. The talocalcaneonavicular joint so formed is the largest synovial joint in the foot. The talonavicular joint also forms part of a functional unit, the transverse tarsal joint, which comprises the talonavicular and calcaneocuboid joints.

The anterior and posterior talocalcanean joints are separated by a canal, the tarsal canal, formed by two grooves on the reciprocal surfaces of the talus and calcaneus. This canal contains the powerful interosseous ligament, which is as important for the stability and dynamic function of the subtalar joint as the cruciate ligaments are for the knee. It is involved in the transmission of body weight, which is normally directed a little behind and to the lateral side of the centre of the upper articular surface of the body of the talus and thence to the foot. The interosseous ligament assists in spreading much of this load to the calcaneus. The ligament is lax on pronation of the foot (*see Figure 13.4*) but becomes tense on supination, so that it then increases stability of the foot.

The subtalar axis

The curved anterior and posterior talocalcanean joints lie on an arc of two circles. The arc formed

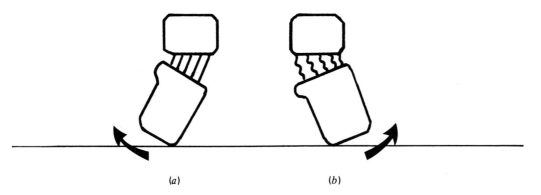

Figure 13.4 (*a*) On supination the interosseous ligament is tense and increases stability in the foot; on pronation it is lax

by the anterior talocalcanean joint has its centre at the upper border of the neck of the talus. The arc formed by the posterior talocalcanean joint has its centre in the tuberosity of the calcaneus. A line drawn through these two centres runs obliquely from the posterolateral plantar surface of the calcaneus to pass upwards, medially and forwards through the tarsal canal at right angles to the interosseous ligament to the neck of the talus. This line is called Henke's axis or the subtalar axis (*see Figure 13.5*).

It forms an angle of approximately 42 degrees with the floor (Inman, 1966) and an angle of 16 degrees medial to the long axis of the foot. The subtalar axis controls the three types of movements that occur in the subtalar and also talonavicular joints. When the foot is non-weight-bearing, movement in the subtalar joint in one direction will invert, adduct and plantar flex the calcaneus. Movement in the opposite direction will evert, abduct and dorsiflex the calcaneus (Root *et al.*, 1971).

Subtalar function

The subtalar joint forms the major key to normal and abnormal function of the foot. The normal functions of this joint are:

(1) To take part in the movement of inversion and eversion of the foot.
(2) To maintain body balance, since body weight is normally transmitted through this joint.
(3) To act as a shock-absorbing mechanism for the body weight.

(4) To allow the foot to adapt to the alterations in the ground contours so that the foot can be maintained flat on the ground.
(5) To allow the foot to be maintained flat on the ground with the leg in varying angular positions, such as when turning while running at speed.
(6) To rotate, which is important during ambulation. When the foot is planted firmly on the ground the calcaneus is fixed. Rotation in the subtalar joint then produces movement of the talus, which then imparts rotation to the lower leg. With supination of the subtalar joint the leg externally rotates on the foot; with pronation of the subtalar joint the leg internally rotates on the foot.

The total range of movement in the subtalar joint is approximately 30 degrees. Since supination of this joint can invert the calcaneus by twice the range of eversion, the normal subtalar joint has 20 degrees of inversion and 10 degrees of eversion. The minimum range of movement necessary for proper functioning of the subtalar joint is considered to be 8–12 degrees for locomation (Root *et al.*, 1971). A greater range is apparently necessary in athletes. Dysfunction of this joint plays a major role in most of the types of foot deformities described later.

Movements of the transverse tarsal joint

The transverse tarsal joint has two common axes of motion (Hicks, 1953), which allow the talo-

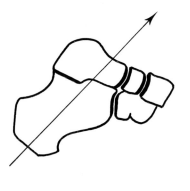
(a)

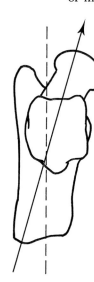
(b)

Figure 13.5 The subtalar axis of Henke (arrow): (*a*) from the side; (*b*) from above. It runs at an angle to the long axis of the foot (dotted line)

navicular and calcaneocuboid joints to function together. One axis allows supination and pronation, as described above. Other hinge movements produce adduction–abduction and flexion–extension as the navicular and cuboid bones move inferiorly and medially or superiorly and laterally. With the foot in the neutral position—that is, with the calcaneus directly under the talus and perpendicular to the floor—the axis of the calcaneocuboid joint lies parallel with the ground. In this position the axis of the talonavicular joint lies slightly oblique to that of the calcaneocuboid joint (*see Figure 13.6*).

With pronation of the subtalar joint the axes of the talonavicular and calcaneocuboid joints lie parallel with each other so that free movement at the mid-tarsal level is possible (*see Figure 13.7a*). This is called unlocking of the transverse tarsal joint. On pronation it allows the hind foot to adapt to the underlying surface during weight-bearing and brings the forefoot flat on to the ground.

During supination of the subtalar joint the axes of the talonavicular and calcaneocuboid joints lie at an increased angle to each other (*see Figure 13.7(b)*). Movement in the mid-tarsal region is restricted; this restriction is called locking of the transverse tarsal joint and is also associated with

tightening of the interosseous ligament of the subtalar joint. The foot is converted into a rigid support so that it forms a more efficient lever for propulsion.

Inversion and eversion of the foot

During inversion the sole of the foot is turned inwards so that its medial border is elevated; during eversion the sole of the foot is turned outwards so that its medial border is depressed. Movement occurs mainly in the tarsal joints, with some movement in the more distal foot joints. Inversion is a combined movement comprising: supination (a medial rotation about an antero-posterior axis); adduction, in which the front of the foot moves inwards; and plantar flexion. Eversion is a combined movement made up of pronation, abduction and dorsiflexion. Much of these active movements are controlled by the subtalar and transverse tarsal joints, which work as a functional unit. The movement of the subtalar joint can take place in three separate planes around the subtalar axis. The talus remains fixed in the ankle mortise

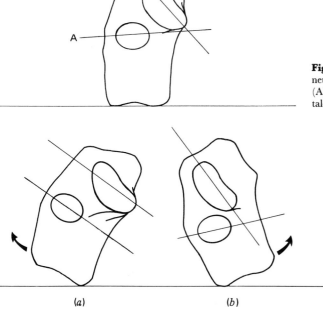

Figure 13.6 The transverse tarsal joint. In the neutral position, the axis of the calcaneocuboid joint (A) is parallel with the ground. The axis of the talonavicular joint (B) crosses it at an oblique angle

(a)   *(b)*

Figure 13.7 (*a*) With pronation of the subtalar joint the axes of the talonavicular and calcaneocuboid joints are parallel and the transverse tarsal joint is unlocked. (*b*) With supination of the subtalar joint the transverse tarsal joint is locked

and the calcaneus moves under it. Movements in the subtalar joint are well described by Kapandji (1974), who compares movements in the calcaneus to that of a ship that can roll (rotate from side to side), turn (move from one side to the other) and pitch (move up and down).

Inversion is controlled by the tibialis anterior and posterior muscles, which are attached medially to the subtalar axis. The navicular is then pulled medially and inferiorly under the talus and so the cuboid can also move medially. Eversion is controlled by the peroneal muscles attached lateral to the subtalar axis. The cuboid and navicular are then pulled laterally.

Intercuneiform movements

Intercuneiform movements are of a gliding nature in a plantar and a dorsal direction and take place during plantar flexion and dorsiflexion. Movements are limited by strong dorsal and plantar ligaments, so that only a small degree of movement can be detected.

Tarsometatarsal joints

The tarsometatarsal joints form part of the transverse arch of the foot, which has the second cuneiform bone as its keystone. The transverse arch is supported by the peroneus longus tendon, which runs transversely from the lateral to the medial side of the foot to be inserted into the base of the first metatarsal and also into the medial cuneiform and the second metatarsal bones. The metatarsal bone with its corresponding toe and tarsometatarsal joint form a functional unit, or ray. In the medial three rays one metatarsal articulates with a corresponding cuneiform bone; in the lateral two rays the metatarsal articulates with the cuboid bone.

Arches of the foot

The foot is formed into two longitudinal arches, the medial and the lateral, and a transverse arch. On the medial side the longitudinal arch is formed by the bony configuration of the calcaneus, navi-

cular, the three cuneiforms and the medial three metatarsal bones. On the lateral side the longitudinal arch is formed by the calcaneus, cuboid and the lateral two metatarsal bones. The shape of the medial arch on the undersurface of the foot has been likened to one half of an inverted bowl. When someone is standing with the weight distributed evenly on the two feet the two halves complement one another to form a complete bowl, which is a stable structure for the transmission of body weight. The outer margin of each foot is made up of the lateral longitudinal arch, which lies flat on the ground and forms a static weight-bearing support, and the raised dome of the medial longitudinal arches provides a flexible lever-like arrangement from which the body is propelled on locomotion.

The integrity of the medial longitudinal arch is dependent on bones, ligaments and muscles. The shape of the arch is formed by the interlocking bones but stability is not dependent on the bony configuration, and the arch is supported mainly by ligaments, which receive additional support from the muscles. The main ligamentous support is provided by the short and long plantar ligaments and the strong plantar fascia. Last (1978) states that the arch is supported mainly by the tendons of the tibialis posterior muscle and the flexor hallucis longus, which has a bow-string action across the sole of the foot. However, Basmajian and Stecko (1963) demonstrated that muscular activity in the normal foot does not contribute to stability.

The transverse arch runs from the undersurface of the cuboid and navicular to the anterior metatarsal heads and will be considered later.

Foot function

The normal foot is ideally adapted to its functions of weight-bearing and locomotion. The lateral border of the foot is buttressed by bone and the inner border is formed into a longitudinal arch that functions as an ideal elastic shock absorber but can also become a rigid weight-bearing system for forward propulsion of the foot. Body weight is normally transmitted through the ankle to the body of the talus and is then distributed to the heel and metatarsal heads and borne by the flexible medial longitudinal arch. The joints of the foot need to be flexible to allow this function of the arches of the foot and at the same time allow the foot to adapt to irregularities in the ground. The foot must be correctly presented to the ground and the position it needs to adopt varies according to the angle or position of the leg and alterations in the slope of the ground.

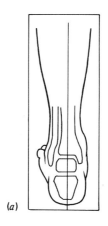

Examination of the foot

(1) Inspection, with the patient standing, sitting, walking and lying down:
  (a) Deformities.
  (b) Skin changes.
  (c) Swellings.
  (d) Muscle wasting.
  (e) Shoes.
  (f) Gait.
(2) Movements:
  (a) Active.
  (b) Passive.
  (c) Accessory.
  (d) Isometric.
(3) Palpation.
(4) General examination.

Inspection

The foot is examined with the patient standing, walking, sitting with the feet over the edge of the couch, lying supine and then prone. When the patient stands he should look straight ahead; the foot should be inspected from the front, the side, and then from behind. It should also be inspected first of all with the patient adopting as natural posture as possible, and then standing with the feet together. The normal posture of the foot with the patient standing should reveal that the calcaneus lies vertical to the floor, the subtalar joint is in a neutral position, and the five metatarsal heads lie in contact with the ground. The general conformation of the foot is noted, including the relative length of the toes.

DEFORMITIES
These may be present in the hind foot, mid-tarsal region and the forefoot.

The hind foot may show either a valgus or a varus deformity. A valgus deformity is manifested by an eversion of the calcaneus relative

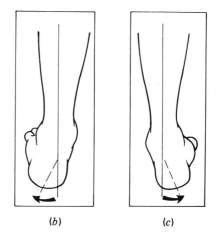

Figure 13.8 (*a*) Normal alignment of the talus and calcaneus. (*b*) Valgus deformity of the left hind foot. (*c*) Varus deformity of the left hind foot

to the weight-bearing surface. A varus deformity is manifested by an inversion of the calcaneus relative to the weight-bearing surface (*see Figure 13.8*).

In the mid-tarsal region the medial longitudinal arch may be either depressed (pes planus) or elevated (pes cavus). A deformity of the forefoot relative to the hind foot may be of either a varus or valgus type.

The toes may be laterally deviated into valgus deformity, which most commonly involves the great toe (hallux valgus). Other toe deformities include:

(1) A cock-up deformity, or claw toe, in which the proximal phalanx is subluxed dorsally on to the metatarsal head, which is depressed into the sole of the foot. The proximal inter-

phalangeal (PIP) joint develops a flexion deformity and the terminal interphalangeal (TIP) joint is hyperextended (*see Figure 13.9*).

(2) Hammer toe, in which a hyperextension deformity of the metatarsophalangeal (MTP) joint is associated with a flexion deformity of the interphalangeal (IP) joints.

(3) Mallet toe, in which there is a flexion deformity of the TIP joint.

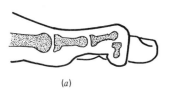

(a)

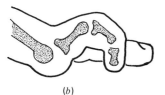

(b)

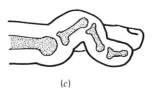

(c)

Figure 13.9 (*a*) Mallet toe; (*b*) claw toe; (*c*) hammer toe

SKIN CHANGES

The skin is inspected for any rashes, colour changes, nodules, ulcers or nail changes. A callus is an area of thickened skin in the sole of the foot that results from abnormal friction or pressure. They are commonly found under the metatarsal heads or in the heel and are produced because of abnormal foot mechanics. Hard corns are areas of hyperkeratosis developing in the thin skin over deformed toes as the result of abnormal pressure from the shoe. They normally have a painful central core, which is evident when the outer layers of skin are removed. Soft corns occur in the moistened surfaces between the toes, especially in the fourth interdigital cleft, and also result from abnormal pressure.

SWELLING

Soft-tissue swelling is usually evident on inspection. Synovitis of the subtalar joint usually causes a bulge laterally through the sinus tarsi, and synovitis of the mid-tarsal joints a bulge onto the dorsum of the foot. Tendon-sheath swelling usually occurs either in the retromalleolar areas as a linear swelling or over the dorsum of the foot. Swelling in the bursa over the first or fifth MTP joint may be evident on inspection. A generalized swelling of the toes in patients with spondyloarthritis produces a typical 'sausage-shaped' deformity.

WASTING

Wasting of the small muscles is not easily detected in the foot, although wasting of the extensor digitorum brevis may be evident over the sinus tarsi in patients with L5 nerve-root compression.

SHOES

These are inspected to see whether they conform to the shape of the patient's foot. Unequal wearing of a part of the shoe may correspond to the presence of any foot deformity. For example, with an equinus deformity of the ankle the tips of the soles are excessively worn; with a valgus deformity of the rear foot the inner side of the heel is worn and the medial counter is broken; prominent displaced metatarsal heads will indent the anterior part of the sole. In patients with a toe-out gait excessive shoe wear is produced on the lateral aspect of the heel and the medial part of the forefoot. In patients with a toe-in gait wear is most prominent on the medial aspect of the heel and the lateral part of the forefoot.

GAIT

The angle of gait is the position adopted by the feet during locomotion. Normally the foot forms an angle of 7–10 degrees of abduction—that is, toe-out—relative to the line of progression. However, the position of the foot varies from person to person and even in the same person from step to step. The angle tends to increase with age but should not exceed 15 degrees of abduction. It may be altered by structural changes in the foot, especially in the subtalar joint, or in the lower limb so that the angle is decreased (toe-in gait) or increased (toe-out gait).

Movements

Active and passive movements

Active and passive movements tested routinely include:

(1) Inversion and eversion of the whole foot.
(2) Subtalar joint inversion and eversion.
(3) Transverse tarsal joints:

    (a) Adduction and abduction.
    (b) Plantar flexion and dorsiflexion.
    (c) Rotation.

(4) Tarsometatarsal joints—adduction and abduction.
(5) First tarsometatarsal joint—plantar flexion, dorsiflexion, and rotation.
(6) Metatarsophalangeal joints—flexion and extension.
(7) Proximal interphalangeal joints—flexion and extension.
(8) Terminal interphalangeal joints—flexion and extension.

INVERSION AND EVERSION OF THE FOOT

The patient lies supine with the knee extended and the foot aligned with the leg so that the long axis of the tibia, if extended, would fall along the second metatarsal. The patient actively turns the sole of the foot inwards into inversion and then outwards into eversion. The normal range is approximately 30 degrees of inversion and 20 degrees of eversion.

These movements are then repeated passively by the examiner grasping above the ankle with one hand and grasping the forefoot with his other (*see Figure 13.10*). The range of passive inversion and eversion is normally a few degrees greater than the active range.

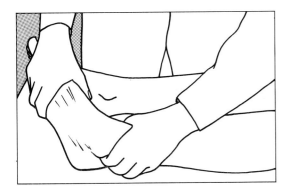

Figure 13.10 Test for passive inversion of the foot

SUBTALAR JOINT MOVEMENTS

These may be tested by a combination of active and passive movements. The patient lies supine with the knee flexed to 90 degrees and the ankle fully dorsiflexed to fix the talus in its mortise. The examiner grasps the heel and moves the heel first inwards and then outwards (*see Figure 13.11*). The patient co-operates in this movement by simultaneously moving the heel inwards and outwards. The normal range is approximately 20 degrees of inversion and 10 degrees of eversion.

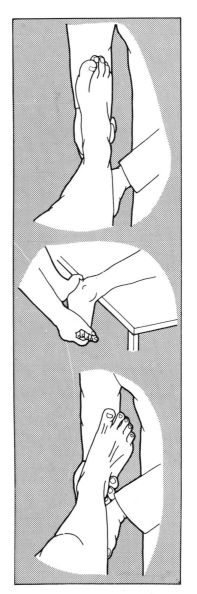

Figure 13.11 Test for movement in the subtalar joint

ADDUCTION AND ABDUCTION OF THE TRANSVERSE TARSAL JOINT

These are tested passively with the patient lying prone with the knee flexed to a right angle.

Abduction of the forefoot on the hind foot is tested by the examiner holding the heel stabilized in the neutral position with his right hand with the thumb over the lateral border of the calcaneus (*see Figure 13.12*). The left hand holds over the lateral border of the foot with the thumb over the cuboid. Movement is produced through the examiner's arms by approximating the elbows, not by pressure from the thumbs, and the forefoot is moved laterally without producing any rotation. The normal range is approximately 10 degrees.

Adduction of the forefoot on the hind foot is tested by the examiner holding the medial border of the foot with both hands, the left thumb over the talus and the right thumb over the navicular (*see Figure 13.13*). Movement is produced by the arms and not by the thumbs, and the forefoot is moved medially without producing any rotation. The normal range is approximately 20 degrees.

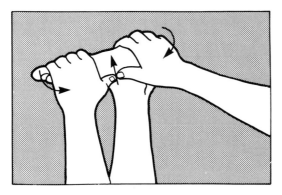

Figure 13.12 Abduction of the forefoot on the hind foot

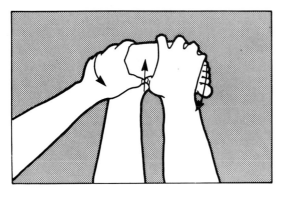

Figure 13.13 Adduction of the forefoot on the hind foot

Abduction and adduction of the tarsometatarsal joints are tested in a similar manner. For abduction the thumbs are placed over the cuboid and the tuberosity of the fifth metatarsal bone, respectively. For adduction the thumbs are placed over the medial cuneiform and the base of the first metatarsal bone, respectively.

PASSIVE MOVEMENT OF THE FIRST TARSOMETATARSAL JOINT

This is tested by the examiner fixing the patient's first cuneiform bone with his left hand and holding the head of the first metatarsal with his other (*see Figure 13.14*). The first metatarsal is then moved in a plantar and then in a dorsal direction. The normal range is about 10 degrees in each direction. Rotation can also be tested in this joint by holding the cuneiform with one hand and rotating the metatarsal by gripping the phalanx.

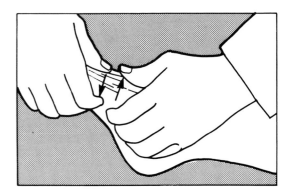

Figure 13.14 Test for passive movement at the first tarsometatarsal joint

The range of MTP joint movement is best tested passively. The MTP joint of the great toe normally extends passively to approximately 90 degrees and flexes to about 35 degrees. In the lateral four joints the range is approximately 40 degrees flexion and 40 degrees extension.

The PIP joints can be actively flexed to about 50 degrees but there is no active extension of these joints.

The TIP joints are tested passively. They can normally be flexed to about 60 degrees and extended by about 30 degrees.

Accessory movements

SUBTALAR JOINT

There are 10 accessory movements in the subtalar joint:

(1) Medial gliding of the calcaneus under the talus.
(2) Lateral gliding of the calcaneus under the talus.
(3) Adduction of the calcaneus under the talus.
(4) Abduction of the calcaneus under the talus.
(5) Anteroposterior gliding of the calcaneus.
(6) Posteroanterior gliding of the calcaneus.
(7) Medial rotation of the subtalar joint around the axis of the tibia.
(8) Lateral rotation of the subtalar joint around the axis of the tibia.
(9) Longitudinal caudad.
(10) Longitudinal cephalad.

TRANSVERSE JOINT
There are 10 accessory movements in this joint. Similar types of movements take place in the talonavicular and the calcaneocuboid joints, which are tested separately.
Talonavicular joint   The ten accessory movements in this joint are:

(1) Superoinferior gliding movement of the navicular in a plantar direction on the talus.
(2) Inferosuperior gliding movement of the navicular in a dorsal direction on the talus.
(3) Medial gliding of the navicular on the talus.
(4) Lateral gliding of the navicular on the talus.
(5) Supination around the axis of the foot.
(6) Pronation around the axis of the foot.
(7) Longitudinal caudad.
(8) Longitudinal cephalad.
(9) Adduction.
(10) Abduction.

Calcaneocuboid joint   There are 10 accessory movements in this joint which are similar to those in the talonavicular joint except that the cuboid is moved relative to the calcaneus.
Cuneiform–navicular joint   Ten accessory movements take place in this joint. These are similar to those in the transverse tarsal joint.
Intercuneiform joints   There are four accessory movements in these joints:

(1) Superoinferior gliding.
(2) Inferosuperior gliding.
(3) Supination.
(4) Pronation.

Tarsometatarsal joints   Testing of the five accessory movements in the tarsometatarsal joints consists of tests for:

(1) Posteroanterior movement. The base of a metatarsal bone is moved posteroanteriorly on

its adjacent tarsal bone by the tips of the examiner's thumbs placed over the plantar surface of the metatarsal.
(2) Anteroposterior movement. The base of the metatarsal is moved anteroposteriorly on its adjacent tarsal bone by the tips of the examiner's thumbs placed over the dorsal surface of the metatarsal.
(3) Gliding. A gliding movement is produced by holding the bone of a metatarsal in one hand and the corresponding tarsal bone in the other and moving the adjacent bones in opposite directions in line with the joint surface.
(4) Rotation. The examiner passively flexes the toe at its metatarsophalangeal and interphalangeal joints and rotates the appropriate metatarsal bone.
(5) A small transverse movement. Small medial and lateral gliding movements are produced by the examiner applying pressure with the thumbs against the anterolateral or anteromedial surfaces of the bases of the metatarsal to push it either medially or laterally.

Isometric tests

Five isometric movements are tested routinely in the foot. These are:

(1) Inversion.
(2) Eversion.
(3) Dorsiflexion of the great toe.
(4) Dorsiflexion of the toes.
(5) Flexion of the great toe.

INVERSION OF THE FOOT
This is tested by the examiner first fully passively everting the patient's foot and then fully resisting the patient's attempt to move the foot back into inversion. This movement is controlled mainly by the tibialis posterior muscle, and its tendon is palpated behind the medial malleolus while the test is being carried out. A painful weakness of inversion usually indicates tendinitis or tenosynovitis of the tibialis posterior muscle. A painful weakness occurs with rupture of the tendon or with L4 nerve-root compression.

EVERSION OF THE FOOT
This is tested by the examiner first fully passively inverting the foot and then fully resisting the patient's attempt to move the foot back into eversion. This movement is controlled mainly by the

peroneus longus muscle and its tendon, which should be palpated behind the lateral malleolus while this test is being carried out. A painful weakness usually indicates a lesion of the peroneus longus. A painless weakness occurs either with rupture of the tendon or with an L4 or L5 nerve-root compression.

THE EXTENSOR HALLUCIS LONGUS MUSCLE

This is tested by the examiner fully resisting the patient's attempt to actively dorsiflex the great toe. A painful weakness occurs with tenosynovitis of the tendon. A painless weakness indicates the presence of an L5 nerve-root compression.

THE EXTENSORS OF THE TOES

These are tested by the examiner fully resisting the patient's attempt to dorsiflex the toes. A painful weakness of this movement indicates a tenosynovitis of the extensor digitorum longus and a painless weakness occurs in an L5 nerve-root lesion.

THE FLEXOR HALLUCIS LONGUS

This is tested by the examiner resisting the patient's attempts to flex the great toe. A painful weakness indicates tenosynovitis of this tendon and a painless weakness may occur with rupture of the tendon or in patients with a tarsal-tunnel syndrome.

Palpation

Many of the foot structures lie subcutaneously and are identifiable on palpation. On the lateral side of the foot the lateral malleolus of the fibula is easily identified and the peroneal tendons may be palpated as they run at first behind and then below it. The opening of the sinus tarsi may be palpated one finger-breadth in front of the anterior border of the lateral malleolus; this is covered by the fleshy belly of the extensor hallucis brevis, which is the only intrinsic muscle on the dorsum of the foot. The sinus tarsi may be felt to open up when the foot is inverted. The peroneal tubercle can be felt a finger-breadth below as a bony swelling on the lateral aspect of the calcaneus. It separates the two peroneal tendons and the peroneus longus tendon passes under it. Three finger-breadths anteriorly lies the styloid process at the base of the fifth metatarsal bone into which the peroneus brevis is inserted. The calcaneocuboid joint may be felt to open and close halfway between the lateral malleolus and the styloid

process during inversion and eversion of the foot. The shaft of the fifth metatarsal runs distally from the styloid process and ends in the rather prominent metatarsal head of the fifth MTP joint.

On the medial side of the foot, the medial malleolus is easily palpable, as is the tibialis posterior which runs behind and then under it. A thumb's breadth anteriorly lies the sustentaculum tali, which supports the head of the talus. A further two finger-breadths anteriorly lies the tuberosity of the navicular, which becomes more prominent on the inversion of the foot. The line of the talonavicular joint lies between these two bony prominences, and the movement of the joint is easily appreciated during inversion and eversion of the foot. The head and neck of the talus can easily be grasped between the finger and thumb just below the ankle joint and the head can be brought into prominence by extension of the foot. A finger-breadth distal to the tuberosity of the navicular, the base of the first metatarsal bone can be palpated where it flares out slightly. The first metatarsocuneiform joint lies at this level. The first metatarsal can be palpated along its length as far as the first MTP joint.

To palpate the dorsum of the foot, the medial and lateral malleoli are again identified. Three tendons cross the front of the ankle joint. The most medial and easily recognized is the tibialis anterior tendon as it passes to its insertion into the medial cuneiform and base of the first metatarsal bone. The tendon of the extensor hallucis longus and the dorsalis pedis artery may be palpable between this tendon and the tendons of the extensor digitorum longus. In the heel the tuberosity of the calcaneus is subcutaneous and the Achilles tendon may be felt as its insertion. The medial tubercle of the calcaneus can be palpated on the plantar surface of the hind foot.

Palpation of the foot for swelling or tenderness will be described according to the area involved.

The IP joints

These are palpated by the examiner placing his thumb and forefinger between the toes and feeling over the joints for any swelling or tenderness.

The MTP joints

These should always be examined carefully as they are a common source of disability and accurate assessment requires considerable experience. However, careful palpation will often provide a clue to the clinical diagnosis. Two methods for palpating this joint are described.

In the first method synovitis of the MTP joint should be sought by the examiner placing both thumbs under the plantar surface of the joint and palpating with the index finger of both hands first over the dorsal surface of the joint and then between adjacent metatarsal heads to detect the presence of any soft-tissue swelling or thickening (*see Figure 13.15*).

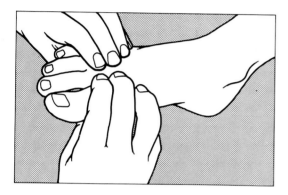

Figure 13.15 Palpation of the second MTP joint

In the second method the examiner places his thumb over the dorsal aspect of the joint and his index finger under its plantar aspect. Since the plantar surface of this joint extends slightly more distally than the dorsal surface, the finger on the plantar surface should be placed a few millimetres more distally (*see Figure 13.16*). The joint is then moved up and down between the examiner's finger and thumb.

The alignment of the bones forming the joint can also be palpated and plantar deviation of the metatarsal head or dorsal displacement of the

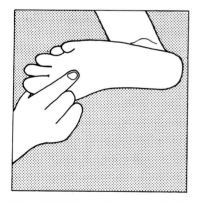

Figure 13.16 Alternative method of palpating the second MTP joint

proximal phalanx may be palpable. In Freiberg's disease the enlarged metatarsal head is usually easily palpable. Stress fracture of the metatarsal can usually be accurately localized over the site of involvement in the shaft of the bone. Palpation between the metatarsal heads may reveal the site of a digital entrapment neuropathy (Morton's metatarsalgia). Any painful condition in the region of the metatarsal head may be exacerbated by squeezing together the metatarsal heads.

The mid-tarsal region

Swelling is usually visible on the dorsum of the foot in this region; and tenderness, swelling or warmth may also be appreciated by palpation. Localized bony tenderness over the navicular is present in patients with Köhler's disease or a stress fracture.

The heel

In the heel, the tuberosity of the calcaneus and the retrocalcanean areas are palpated for any soft-tissue or bony tenderness.

General examination

The arterial supply of the foot is always assessed by palpating the dorsalis pedis and posterior tibial arteries; a full neurological testing is also necessary.

Classification of foot disorders

Foot pain and disability due to musculoskeletal disorders are divided into generalized and localized conditions. Neurological, vascular, traumatic, metabolic and skin disorders need to be differentiated but will not be considered here. The classification is thus:

(1) Generalized conditions:
   (a) Deformities.
   (b) Arthritis.
   (c) Sudeck's atrophy.
   (d) Entrapment neuropathies.

(2) Localized regional conditions:
   (a) Pain in the toes.
   (b) Pain in the anterior metatarsal region.
   (c) Pain in the mid-tarsal region.
   (d) Pain in the heel.
   (e) Pain in the plantar region.

Generalized conditions

Foot deformities include:

(1) Pes planus.
(2) Pes cavus.
(3) Varus deformity of the hind foot.
(4) Ankle equinus.
(5) Varus deformity of the forefoot.
(6) Valgus deformity of the forefoot.

Pes planus

Pes planus is a descriptive title for lowering of the medial longitudinal arch of the foot. It is also known by many other synonyms, including pes valgus, pronated feet, subtalar valgus and pes valgoplanus. Confusion arises because some of the terms used describe anatomical components of this condition. Flattening of the medial arch should be regarded as a clinical finding, the cause of which needs to be determined and which may not be the cause of the patient's symptoms.

Body weight is normally transmitted a little behind and to the lateral side of the upper articular surface of the talus and then through the talocalcanean joint. If body weight falls to the medial side of this line it will be applied to the medial longitudinal arch, which will tend to flatten out; this needs to be balanced by soft-tissue structures such as the interosseous ligament of the subtalar joint, the spring ligament and muscles in the medial compartment of the ankle. Should these compensatory mechanisms fail, the normal distribution of weight is altered and ligamentous pain is produced.

Pes planus may be associated with causes outside the foot. These include genu valgum, external rotation of the limb, shortening of the Achilles tendon with a valgus deformity of the hind foot and hypermobility syndromes. In the foot, pes planus may be caused by congenital lesions, e.g. a congenital vertical talus.

STATIC DEFORMITY
In this type there is depression of the medial longitudinal arch, which remains flexible, associated with a valgus deformity of the hind foot and abduction of the forefoot. The most common cause of this deformity is an excessive pronation of the subtalar joint. Hereditary factors may be responsible, with derangement of the subtalar joint surfaces and laxity of its interosseous ligament (Kapandji, 1974). It may also follow a deficiency in bony supports of the neck of the talus (Harris and Beath, 1948).

As a consequence of the subtalar joint pronation:

(1) The hind foot is carried into valgus.
(2) The axis of the talonavicular and calcaneocuboid joints become parallel so that the normal locking mechanism of the transverse tarsal joint is lost. The foot becomes hypermobile during the propulsive phase of gait and the forefoot becomes dorsiflexed on the hind foot.
(3) There is a shortening of the Achilles tendon, which increases the valgus deformity of the hind foot.
(4) Depression of the medial arch occurs about its keystone, the navicular, so that the head of the talus—lacking its normal bony support—turns medially and becomes plantar flexed.
(5) There is weakening of the normal ligamentous supports.
(6) There is failure of the muscular support, which is normally provided by the peroneus longus and tibialis posterior tendons. When the peroneus longus acts on the pronated foot it tends to pull the first metatarsal into abduction, leading to instability of the first metatarsal ray.
(7) The plantar fascia shifts laterally and loses its normal supportive bowstring effect on the medial longitudinal arch.
(8) The line of the body weight falls over the medial side of the subtalar joint and the medial border of the foot from the medial malleolus to the tubercle of the navicular becomes increasingly more prominent.
(9) Pronation in the hind foot is compensated by a supination and abduction of the forefoot, which is turned outwards.

Clinical features Symptoms do not correlate with the degree of these structural alterations and symptoms may be absent while the foot remains supple. Even if this deformity is present it is not necessarily the cause of the patient's foot pain and the presence of pain may indicate that the compensatory mechanisms, which maintain stability, are beginning to fail. In symptomatic cases foot pain, either in the mid-tarsal or anterior metatarsal regions, is usually the presenting symptom. Pain is usually exacerbated by activity and becomes worse as the day goes on. The patient may also complain of aching legs, or cramps in the calf and leg. Symptoms often commence during adolescence, often after sporting activities or starting a new occupation or possibly due to growth. In adults, symptoms may also be brought on or exacerbated by pregnancy, increasing weight, trauma, or after a period of prolonged bed rest. Heel pain may be due to a plantar fasciitis.

Signs In the foot, there is loss of the medial longitudinal arch on standing and a valgus deformity of the hind foot with lengthening of the inner border of the foot. The weight-bearing line of the lower leg no longer falls between the first and second toes but over the medial side of the foot, so that structures on the medial side of the foot are unduly prominent. The forefoot is usually in a position of abduction, supination and dorsiflexion. The shoes should be inspected for excessive wear along the inner border of the sole and heel.

In the leg the Achilles tendon may be seen to be displaced laterally and leads to loss of the range of passive ankle dorsiflexion. The gait is often awkward and lacking in its normal spring so that the patient seems to use the lower extremities as pedestals.

Management This condition requires treatment only if it is painful. Arch supports have been traditionally prescribed but should no longer be used since they do not form a system with the foot to provide sufficient biomechanical control. They apply a force under the navicular bone whereas the primary fault lies more proximally in the subtalar joint. Management should consist of:

(1) Orthotic supports. The valgus deformity of the hind foot may be controlled by orthotic supports, with a supinator wedge placed under the inner side of the calcaneus to return it to its vertical position. A thinner pronator wedge may be placed under the base of the fifth metatarsal bone to lift the lateral border of the foot, combined with a support under the navicular if pain is severe.
(2) The shoe should be made with a reinforced heel counter to stabilize the hind foot and the waist made tight over the instep.
(3) Exercises designed to strengthen the intrinsic muscles of the foot to restore the medial arch. An exercise for the plantar flexors of the toes

include picking up objects such as marbles or a piece of cloth. Stretching exercises to correct a tightened Achilles tendon are usually necessary, combined with exercises to increase the range of internal rotation of the lower leg. Heel-to-toe walking with the weight on the outer border of the foot is encouraged. The patient often commences these exercises enthusiastically but in many enthusiasm soon wanes and only rarely are they carried out as long as necessary.

(4) Mobilization techniques. These should be used to improve joint stiffness or pain and allow exercises and postural control to be more effective.
(5) Operations. Surgery may be indicated if pain is severe and unresponsive to conservative therapy and if a severe degree of deformity is present. Many operations have been devised. Young (1939) described a soft-tissue operation designed to correct the anatomical abnormalities with lengthening of the Achilles tendon and repositioning of the tibialis anterior tendon insertion proximally on the navicular. Surgery is also indicated in patients with a congenital vertical talus (Beck and McGlamry, 1973).

RIGID DEFORMITY
This is produced by degenerative changes in the foot at a late stage of this deformity. The foot is painful, stiff and fixed in valgus. X-rays show degenerative changes in the talonavicular and cuneonavicular joints. Strong mobilizing techniques may dramatically relieve the pain even if only a small improvement in range is achieved.

SPASTIC FLAT FOOT
This condition, also known as peroneal spastic flat foot, is not uncommon. It is associated with a marked spasm mainly of the peroneal muscles and also of the long extensors of the toes (Harris, 1965), the underlying cause of which appears to be synovitis of the subtalar joint. It may be associated with congenital tarsal bars, which alter the normal foot mechanics and render the subtalar joint liable to trauma or overuse, so producing a synovitis. Synovitis may also occur after trauma or in the early stages of degenerative arthritis of the subtalar joint. This condition occurs most commonly in adolescent boys and is usually unilateral. There is often a history of recent sprain or overuse of the ankle or of having recently started

work that entails prolonged standing or walking; this condition has also been called 'apprentice's foot'.

The patient complains of pain which is usually severe and may be felt over most of the foot, especially in the mid-tarsal region. It tends to worsen as the day goes on, is exacerbated by weight-bearing and is eased to some extent by rest. The patient usually walks with a limp.

Signs include a flattening of the medial longitudinal arch and marked muscle spasm in the peroneal and long extensors of the toes, and the foot is everted. The outer toes may be hyperextended at the MTP joints with a flexion deformity of the IP joints produced by the spasm in the long extensor muscles. Tenosynovitis may occur in the peroneal tendon sheath. Passive inversion of the foot is markedly restricted by pain and produces an increase in the degree of muscular spasm. Ankle movements are usually normal.

X-rays are necessary to determine the presence of a bony synostosis and an oblique or a posterior oblique view or tomograms may also be necessary. Degenerative changes may ultimately develop in the talonavicular or subtalar joints (Harris and Beath, 1948).

Management
(1) Rest to the foot is essential and weight-bearing may need to be avoided. If pain is severe the foot and ankle are immobilized in the neutral position in a plaster cast. A general anaesthetic may initially be required to overcome the muscular spasm and the foot is manipulated into the neutral position. The plaster is worn for 6–8 weeks, after which symptoms usually subside.
(2) Analgesics and anti-inflammatory drugs are given as required.
(3) Injection of the subtalar joint is a useful technique. The patient lies supine with the foot fully inverted to open up the site of injection through the lateral opening of the tarsal canal. The opening can be easily palpated at a point one finger-breadth below and one finger-breadth anterior to the tip of the lateral malleolus and can be felt to gape open as the foot is passively inverted. A 23-gauge needle is inserted into the canal opening and directed slightly anteriorly for a distance of approximately 4 cm. It normally meets no resistance as it slides along the tarsal canal. 1 ml of corticosteroid and 2 ml of local anaesthetic are injected into this site.

(4) Manipulation or mobilization of the painful joints does much to relieve pain and muscle spasm.
(5) Surgery may be required in patients with a congenital bony bar who do not respond to conservative therapy. A triple arthrodesis may be required if degenerative changes develop in the subtalar joint or in patients with a fixed valgus deformity of the foot.

Pes cavus

Pes cavus is a foot deformity associated with an increased elevation of the medial longitudinal arch, so that the forefoot lies at a lower level than the hind foot. The foot is foreshortened and in time the dorsal ligaments become contracted and the toes clawed. Either the posterior or anterior bony compartments of the medial arch may be primarily involved. The posterior type of deformity is associated with an equinus hind-foot deformity and the calcaneus is displaced so that it lies in a more vertical direction producing elevation of the medial arch. It may be due to tightness of the Achilles tendon, deformity of the hind foot, external tibial torsion or an imbalance of the muscles that lie anteriorly to the ankle.

The anterior type of deformity has an equinus deformity of the forefoot, which may be due to a muscular imbalance between the tibialis posterior and peroneus longus muscles and the intrinsic foot muscles. This may be associated with neurological disorders such as peroneal muscular atrophy, Freidrich's ataxia, spina bifida or poliomyelitis. When an underlying neurological disorder is suspected electromyography should be performed. Rarely, muscle imbalance may be considered to follow the wearing of inadequate shoes, which may be either too short or high-heeled shoes without an adequate platform under the heel. However, in most patients no underlying neurological disease can be demonstrated and this common foot deformity is classified as idiopathic.

In many cases the deformity may not be marked and may be asymptomatic. Claw toes are mechanically produced and may follow an imbalance between the long toe extensor and weak intrinsic muscles of the foot. Pain is usually caused by the excessive pressure borne under the second and third metatarsal, under which painful callosities develop. Pain may also result from pressure effects over the dorsal surface of the clawed toes. In the hind foot, pain may result from ankle instability and recurrent sprains of the ankle.

MANAGEMENT

Treatment is required only if the foot is symptomatic. Management then consists of:

(1) Orthotic supports, which are designed to redistribute pressure more evenly and to relieve pain, which is usually centred under the metatarsal head. An insole, made of moulded cork to increase the area of the foot in contact with the ground, consists of a support for the high arch and a support behind the metatarsal heads. A varus or valgus deformity of the hind foot is corrected by pronator or supinator wedge.

(2) Shoes need to be made with sufficient room to accommodate the insole and the clawed toes. They should also have a low heel and stout leather soles.

(3) Exercises are mainly designed to strengthen the intrinsic muscles of the foot. Faradic foot baths may also be used for this purpose.

(4) Mobilization techniques are used to relieve pain and improve movements.

(5) Operations are indicated only if the foot remains painful despite conservative management. Soft-tissue release and tendon transfers, either tenotomies of the extensor tendons or transfer of the flexor tendons into the extensor tendons, may be combined with arthrodesis of the IP joints of the toes. Steindler's operation, in which the soft tissues attached to the calcaneus are detached and allowed to slide forward, does not usually provide a satisfactory long-term result. An osteotomy of the calcaneus may be necessary to correct a varus deformity of the hind foot. In severe degrees of deformity an anterior wedge osteotomy of the tarsal bones to realign the forefoot may be necessary.

Varus deformity of the hind foot

This is a relatively common deformity in which the posterior surface of the calcaneus is inverted relative to the Achilles tendon (*see Figure 13.8*). It is not considered to be of functional significance unless the deformity is greater than 5 degrees in the adult or 8 degrees in children. It may be produced by a varus deformity of the tibia or by congenital or acquired lesions of the subtalar joint, in which the range of movement is reduced from the normal 30 degrees to about 20 degrees. As a result of the hind-foot varus deformity, the plantar surface of the foot becomes inverted and

the patient tends to walk on the lateral surface of the foot. To compensate for this deformity and to maintain the foot on the ground during walking, pronation occurs mainly at the mid-tarsal joint. The pronated foot in turn leads to hypermobility of the forefoot, which produces pain under the metatarsal heads (especially the second) with callus formation, and a shearing strain is imposed on the soft tissue under the metatarsal heads on walking. Posterior heel pain may be due to plantar fasciitis or to a retrocalcaneal exostosis that develops as a reactive hyperostosis to abnormal pressure at heel strike and causes stretching and inflammation in the overlying Achilles tendon. As the calcaneus needs to pronate excessively to bring the heel into contact with the ground, abnormal movement also occurs in the knee and may result in chondromalacia patellae. Finally, degenerative changes may ultimately develop in the subtalar and mid-tarsal joint.

MANAGEMENT

This consists of placing a pronator wedge under the lateral aspect of the heel to maintain the talus and calcaneus in the neutral position. Pain may be relieved by mobilization, using strong techniques at the limit of range and large-amplitude movements up to the limit of range. Surgery is rarely indicated, but if pain remains a problem an osteotomy of the calcaneus may be necessary (Dwyer, 1959).

Ankle equinus

A congenital equinus deformity is a flexion deformity of the ankle and in its most severe degree the calcaneus is unable to touch the floor. More commonly, an equinus deformity indicates a decreased range of dorsiflexion of the ankle joint. It is usually produced by shortening or tightness in the gastrocnemius–soleus and Achilles tendon complex or by restricted ankle-joint movement. The cause of the shortening in the gastrocnemius–soleus complex may be congenital or acquired, due to pes cavus, wearing high-heeled shoes or after prolonged bed rest. Limitation of the range of movement or dorsiflexion may be observed as a premature heel rise during ambulation. As a compensatory mechanism the subtalar joint may be excessively pronated, which allows unlocking of the transverse tarsal joint, and increased dorsiflexion can take place at the transverse tarsal joint.

Pain may be experienced in the mid-tarsal

region, particularly after prolonged walking or running, and may be associated with leg pain or pain under the metatarsal heads or heel. The patient may also complain of back pain, as excessive lumbar flexion may be necessary to bring the centre of gravity forwards over the feet during ambulation. Abnormal ankle movement can also lead to a flattening of the trochlear surface of the talus, because the ankle joint then requires a greater radius of curvature to increase its range during locomotion (Inman, 1976).

MANAGEMENT
(1) A raise may be worn under the heel of the shoe.
(2) Mobilizing techniques should be used to restore a pain-free range of ankle movement.
(3) The patient is taught stretching exercises to the calf muscles.
(4) Surgery to lengthen the Achilles tendon may sometimes be required.

Varus deformity of the forefoot

This common deformity, in which the forefoot is inverted relative to the hind foot, is also known as metatarsus adductus or varus (*see Figure 13.17*). The basic abnormality lies in the talus, in which the normal degree of valgus rotation in its head and neck fails to develop. Until the age of 2 years a varus deformity of up to 5 degrees is common and requires no treatment. However, deviation of the forefoot greater than 5 degrees will ultimately lead to foot pain and needs to be treated. The first metatarsal may become hypermobile due to

ligamentous stretching and pain results as excessive weight is taken by the second metatarsal head. To compensate and allow the forefoot to bear weight during walking, the subtalar and transverse tarsal joints must pronate and can ultimately lead to degenerative changes in these joints.

Examination of the foot with the patient standing shows that the forefoot is adducted and the medial metatarsal heads are raised relative to the outer ones. There is a convexity of the lateral border of the foot so that the base of the fifth metatarsal appears unduly prominent. The medial border of the foot is concave, with an increased medial angulation at the first metatarsotarsal joint and increased space between the first and second toe. The hind foot is usually in valgus. This condition needs to be differentiated from pes planus in which the forefoot is abducted. Measurement of the degree of forefoot varus is made with the patient lying prone and comparing the line of the metarsal heads to an imaginary line drawn to bisect the calcaneus. This angle may also be measured on X-ray by drawing a line to bisect the calcaneus and the line of the forefoot.

MANAGEMENT
In children this deformity may be corrected by a series of plaster casts applied while the foot is manipulated into a position of varus at the hind foot with the forefoot in abduction. In adults, a rigid type of orthotic device is made to accommodate the deformity with the subtalar joint in the neutral position. Numerous operations, including soft-tissue releases and osteotomy of the metatarsals or the first cuneiform, have been described.

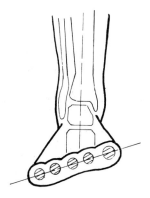

Figure 13.17 Varus deformity of the right forefoot relative to the hind foot

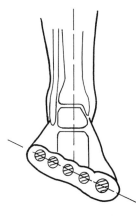

Figure 13.18 Valgus deformity of the forefoot relative to the hind foot

Valgus deformity of the forefoot

This condition, which occurs when the plane of the forefoot is everted relative to the calcaneus (*see Figure 13.18*), is caused by an increase in the degree of valgus torsion that takes place in the head and neck of the talus during normal development. It may involve all of the metatarsals; or only the first metatarsal, which is plantar flexed and will be described later. Compensatory mechanisms to overcome this valgus forefoot deformity take place by supination first in the transverse tarsal joints and then in the subtalar joints.

The patient may present with forefoot pain, which is usually below the second or fifth metatarsal heads, and with callus formation. The midtarsal joint is unable to develop full pronation during the push-off phase of walking, so excessive strain is placed on the first metatarsal ray, which becomes unstable. Pain is also experienced in the lateral compartment of the ankle and the patient may present with recurrent ankle sprains.

PLANTAR-FLEXED FIRST RAY
In this relatively uncommon condition the head of the first metatarsal lies below the transverse plane of the other metatarsal heads. It may be due to a congenital deformity or more commonly is associated with a valgus forefoot deformity. A fixed flexion deformity of the first metatarsal develops so that it is impossible to push its head up to the plane of the lateral metatarsals. On walking, the rigid first metatarsal strikes the ground first. The foot must then supinate quickly to bring the foot level with the floor and so the fifth metatarsal hits the ground forcibly. Pain and callus formation develop under the first and fifth metatarsal heads.

MANAGEMENT
(1) An orthotic device to control the biomechanics of this deformity should be made.
(2) In severe cases operation may be required to elevate the head of the first metatarsal. The peroneus longus tendon may be lengthened, or a vertical osteotomy through the base of the first metatarsal may be necessary.

Sudeck's atrophy

This disorder causes severe pain, swelling and disability in the foot. It may also occur in other joints of the lower limb and has been also known as reflex sympathetic dystrophy. Its aetiology is unknown but it probably represents a neurovascular disorder leading to an intense hyperaemia and osteoporosis of bone, similar to the shoulder–hand syndrome. It may be idiopathic or follow prolonged immobilization but commonly follows trauma, which may even be trivial. The natural history is one of prolonged pain and disability lasting for up to 2 years; the condition then resolves, usually without any joint deformity. At times it may resolve in the affected foot only to appear later in the other foot.

Clinical features

The patient, usually middle aged, presents with foot pain which may be of sudden onset. The pain becomes progressively worse, so that the patient is unable to walk on the foot, and may be present at night. The foot is swollen, often markedly, and the skin is usually red and hot. Stiffness and effusion in the ankle joint are common and movements in the foot joints are restricted. Any area in the foot may be involved, not necessarily the site of the original trauma, and changes may start in the anterior metatarsal bones and then spread proximally.

X-rays are necessary to confirm the diagnosis. Spotty decalcification of the bones of the foot, especially around the joint margins, appears after a variable length of time. Decalcification usually starts about the metatarsal heads and then may involve the whole of the foot and ankle. Osteoporosis may be severe but the joint spaces always remain well preserved, an important point in differentiating this condition from arthritis. Laboratory tests are usually normal.

MANAGEMENT
(1) The patient needs to be reassured that the ultimate prognosis is good, although the course of the disease may be prolonged and painful.
(2) Analgesic and anti-inflammatory drugs are given to control pain.
(3) The patient is encouraged to walk as much as possible even though pain is a problem, since prolonged rest will make this condition worse.
(4) Mobilization of individual joints in the foot should be used to relieve pain, thus assisting active movement and exercises.
(5) Physical methods used in an attempt to control pain and swelling include alternate

applications of heat and cold, interferential therapy and active exercises performed in a warm bath.

(6) A translumbar sympathetic nerve block may be given and repeated if it succeeds in relieving pain.

Entrapment neuropathies

Tarsal-tunnel syndrome

This is an entrapment neuropathy of the posterior tibial nerve as it passes in its neurovascular bundle behind and then below the medial malleolus to gain access into the foot. In this site the nerve runs in a fibro-osseous tarsal tunnel, which is roofed over by the flexor retinaculum; this is also termed the laciniate ligament, which runs from the medial malleolus to the calcaneus. Besides the posterior tibialis nerve the tarsal tunnel contains the tibialis posterior, flexor digitorum longus and flexor hallucis longus tendons, each surrounded by its own synovial sheath. As the posterior tibial nerve passes through the tarsal tunnel it divides into the medial and lateral plantar nerves. The medial plantar nerve supplies sensation to the skin of the heel and the medial three and a half toes; the lateral plantar nerve supplies the lateral one and a half toes through its superficial division.

Tarsal-tunnel syndrome may be caused by a tenosynovitis of the tendons in the tarsal tunnel, especially the posterior tibial tendon after trauma, overuse or inflammatory conditions. The tarsal tunnel overlies the medial ligament of the ankle joint and an entrapment neuropathy may follow sprain of this ligament. It may also follow a fall onto the feet, and cases of bilateral tarsal-tunnel compression have been described after this injury. Postural abnormalities of the foot, particularly the pronated foot, may be associated with this condition. Overuse may follow sporting activity or occupations involving excessive use of the ankle, e.g. by climbing ladders. Tarsal-tunnel syndrome may rarely complicate rheumatoid arthritis or even more rarely may be its presenting symptom.

The patient presents with pain, described as burning or throbbing and often severe, in the plantar aspect of the foot and toes. At first it may be brought on by prolonged standing or ankle movements but subsequently it may be present at rest or radiate up the leg. The patient may also complain of pins and needles or numbness in the plantar distribution of the nerve.

Examination usually reveals tenderness over the tarsal tunnel just posterior and distal to the tip of the medial malleolus. Pressure over this area for a few minutes should reproduce the patient's symptoms and a positive Tinel's sign may also be elicited. In the foot, sensory disturbances may be found in the distribution of the nerve and occasionally there is weakness of flexion of the interphalangeal joints. Evidence of tenosynovitis of the tibialis posterior tendon or of foot deformities such as pes planus may be present. Confirmatory evidence may be obtained by nerve-conduction studies to demonstrate sensory or motor disturbances in the branches of the plantar nerves.

MANAGEMENT
(1) A foot deformity, such as pes planus, should be corrected with the use of orthotic devices.
(2) Local injection of 1 ml of corticosteroid into the tarsal tunnel is often most successful in relieving symptoms. The patient lies supine with the affected leg externally rotated. A 25-gauge needle is used and is directed from above downwards into the hollow directly behind the medial malleolus to slide under the laciniate ligament.
(3) If these methods fail exploration and surgical decompression of the tarsal tunnel will be necessary.

Entrapment of the medial plantar nerve

The medial plantar nerve is a branch of the posterior tibial nerve and runs through an opening, where it may be entrapped, in the abductor hallucis muscle. Entrapment may follow a foot deformity, especially pes planus or pes cavus, in which the nerve is compressed against the fibrous opening in the abductor hallucis muscle. It may also follow trauma, either direct or secondary to wearing an ill-fitting arch support. Symptoms are similar to those of a tarsal-tunnel syndrome but tenderness is located in the sole of the foot over the anterior portion of the calcaneus. Pressure localized here should reproduce the patient's symptoms.

MANAGEMENT
(1) Orthotic control of any foot deformities that may be present.
(2) Injection of 1 ml of corticosteroid and 1 ml of local anaesthetic may be given into the tender area in the abductor hallucis muscle.

(3) If these methods fail exploration of the neuro-vascular bundle is indicated.

Digital nerves

An entrapment neuropathy in the course of a digital nerve between the metatarsal heads most commonly involves the third plantar digital nerve, which supplies sensation to adjacent surfaces of the third and fourth toes. The second interdigital space is the next most common site of involvement. The plantar nerves travel deep to the level of the metatarsal heads in a narrow fibrous tunnel which then angulates dorsally through the fibres of the intermetatarsal ligament. Entrapment may follow excessive dorsal angulation of the nerve due to overuse of the foot or alterations in the normal anatomical relationship.

Overuse may occur in walking or running, or with postures that involve excessive extension of the toes; for example, in occupations that involve squatting, such as carpet layers. It may also follow the wearing of high-heeled or tightly fitting shoes, which produce hyperextension of the toes, or foot deformities.

This condition occurs most commonly in females (often in those who are middle aged), may be bilateral and has characteristic symptoms. Pain is usually described as severe, burning or throbbing, sited at first in the region of the meta-tarsal heads and shooting up into the toes. The patient may at times localize the pain to the opposing surfaces of the involved toes and it may also radiate proximally into the foot. Pain is usually related to walking but may be persistent and present at night. A most characteristic symptom is that the patient often has to stop walking, sit down, remove his shoe and massage the foot to try to obtain relief. The patient may also complain of paraesthesias in the toes.

Examination reveals an extremely tender area in the soft tissues between but not over the meta-tarsal heads, and sustained pressure here should reproduce the patient's pain. Pain may also be reproduced by squeezing the metatarsal heads together for some minutes. Sensory disturbances may be elicited in the corresponding toes. A useful confirmatory test to reproduce pain is to press a pen or similar blunt instrument into the web space between the toes and roll it up and down while compressing the metatarsal heads with the other hand. Occasionally the swelling around the nerve may be palpable. The whole of the foot should be examined for the presence of any predisposing deformities.

MANAGEMENT
Conservative treatment should be instituted first since it often provides relief.

(1) The patient should avoid the use of high-heeled or tightly fitting shoes and try to avoid stresses that produce hyperextension of the MTP joints or excessive walking.
(2) It is not usually possible to design a support to alter the anatomical relationships of the nerve but a metatarsal support may occasionally provide some pain relief.
(3) Injections of local anaesthetic and corticosteroid into the affected intermetatarsal ligaments are easy to perform and produce pain relief for varying lengths of time.
(4) Mobilization of the intermetatarsal area may be valuable for the relief of pain. Four mobilization techniques may be used:

(a) Gliding of the metatarsal heads against one another (*see Figure 13.19*).

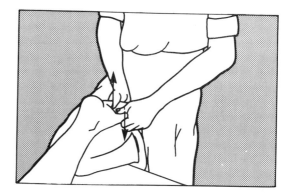

Figure 13.19 Gliding of the metatarsal heads

(b) Horizontal flexion.
(c) Horizontal extension.
(d) Flexion of the MTP joint.

(5) Surgery to divide the intermetatarsal ligament and remove the area of swollen nerve is indicated if symptoms are sufficiently severe or if conservative measures fail.

Deep peroneal nerve

The deep peroneal nerve crosses the dorsum of the ankle covered by the extensor retinaculum.

As it passes distal to the retinaculum it lies superficially over the tarsal bones and ends by supplying sensation to the lateral half of the great toe and medial half of the second toe. The nerve may be entrapped in front of the ankle as it lies beneath the extensor retinaculum, and because of its exposed position it may be damaged by direct trauma—such as wearing poorly designed lace-up shoes. The patient complains of sensory disturbances in the first interdigital cleft and rarely there may be weakness of the extensor hallucis longus.

Localized regional conditions

Pain in toes

Painful conditions of the toes may be due to:

(1) Hallux valgus.
(2) Hallux rigidus.
(3) Hammer toes.
(4) Mallet toes.
(5) Varus deformity of the fifth toe.
(6) A bunion of the fifth metatarsal head.
(7) Arthritis.

Hallux valgus

Hallux valgus, a lateral deviation of the proximal phalanx of the great toe on the first metatarsal, is easy to recognize clinically but its aetiology is much more complex. It becomes symptomatic most often in middle-aged women but symptoms may develop during the teens. Hereditary factors play a part in its aetiology but it may also complicate conditions with ligament laxity and muscular imbalance and produce lateral instability of the first MTP joint. These include metatarsus primus varus, a congenital shortening of the first metatarsal, varus deformity of the forefoot, pes planus and inflammatory arthritis.

The wearing of tight shoes, especially fashion shoes worn by women, remains a controversial cause, though they can be implicated in the production of symptoms. A survey of natives in St Helena found hallux valgus present in 25 per cent of the population who did not wear shoes and in 48 per cent of the women who had worn shoes (Shine, 1965).

The components of this deformity are well described and include:

(1) Valgus deformity of the great toe at the MTP joint.
(2) An imbalance between the adductor and abductor hallucis tendons.
(3) Rotation of the great toe around its longitudinal axis, which causes the plantar surface of the great toe to face the second toe.
(4) The extensor tendon comes to lie on the lateral side of the MTP joint, which increases the lateral deviation.
(5) The medial side of the metatarsal head becomes prominent so that its overlying bursa becomes inflamed, which produces a bunion.
(6) The sesamoid bones in the flexor tendons move laterally.
(7) The great toe crowds out the second toe, which is forced to lie either over or under the great toe. At times the second MTP joint may dislocate.
(8) Degenerative changes may develop in the first MTP joint.
(9) Corns develop at pressure sites, usually over the dorsal and plantar aspects of the toes.
(10) There may be valgus deformity of the IP joint of the great toe.

This condition is much more common in women than in men. Piggott (1960) studied the natural history of this condition in children and described two main types of abnormality. One was non-progressive and amounted to about 10 per cent of the total. Even though the lateral deviation was at times marked, the opposing joint surfaces between the hallux and the first metatarsal remained congruous. The other group showed divergent joint surfaces and became progressive with ultimate subluxation.

CLINICAL FEATURES
The patient may present with pain related to the first MTP joint or pain due to any of the changes listed above. Pain may be due to an inflamed bunion, which may become infected and break down forming a fistula. At times the only complaint may be painless deformity or swelling of the MTP joint of the great toe. Symptoms due to pain under the outer metatarsal heads may follow either unequal weight distribution or an entrapment neuropathy of a plantar digital nerve. The diagnosis is readily made on inspection and

the remainder of the foot is examined for any associated abnormalities.

X-rays may be performed to record the degree of deformity. The degree of metatarsus primus varus can be measured from the angle subtended by a line drawn through the centre of the first metatarsal with a line drawn through the centre of a second metatarsal. Normally this does not exceed 5 degrees.

MANAGEMENT

Conservative measures cannot correct this deformity but the patient's pain may be eased by his wearing a moulded, roomy shoe with protective pads. Mobilization of the MTP joint—with oscillatory movements in flexion–extension, abduction, adduction, rotation and compression —may provide pain relief.

Surgery is indicated for pain. It needs to be carefully planned if a satisfactory result is to be obtained. Four types of operation have been described.

(1) Soft-tissue operations include simple bunionectomy, which is not often of lasting value, and McBride's operation, which releases the adductor hallucis tendon from its insertion into the proximal phalanx and transfers it to the first metatarsal.
(2) Arthroplasty of the MTP joint is the most commonly performed procedure and three operations have been described. Keller's operation removes the proximal third of the proximal phalanx and the prominent medial part of the metatarsal head. Mayo's operation excises the metatarsal head but results in shortening of the first metatarsus with extra weight being taken under the other metatarsal heads. Swanson has described an arthroplasty of this joint using a silicone implant.
(3) Osteotomy of the first metatarsal either through its neck or near its base is sound in theory but difficult in practice. It may be combined with other operations, such as a Keller's procedure.
(4) Arthrodesis of the first MTP joint relieves pain but may give rise to subsequent degenerative changes in the IP joint.

Hallux rigidus

This descriptive title for osteoarthritis of the first MTP joint is not particularly apt, because restricted joint movement—the hallmark of the condition—rarely produces complete rigidity. It occurs most often in middle-aged men and is often bilateral. Dorsiflexion of the great toe is restricted and symptoms arise because in the push-off phase of walking the joint becomes traumatized. Prominent osteophytes develop on the dorsal or dorsomedial aspect of the joint, which becomes palpably thickened.

The patient usually presents with a gradual onset of pain and stiffness in the MTP joint of the great toe. Pain may become quite severe and persistent, especially after standing or walking for any length of time. The joint compensates by becoming hyperextended and may develop a painful callosity on its plantar surface. Pressure from the shoe may then result in pressure effects on the toenail, which becomes thickened. Pain under the outer metatarsal heads may also sometimes be the main complaint as the patient has to roll his foot to attain extension during propulsion.

The MTP joint becomes enlarged by osteophytes which may be palpable, and an adventitious bursa is often found over the dorsal surface of the joint. There is loss of the normal passive range of MTP movement, which is most marked in extension. In younger patients degenerative changes may be much less prominent and symptoms are related to synovitis of the joint, often of sudden onset, with a soft-tissue swelling palpable on the dorsum of the joint.

The diagnosis of degenerative changes in the MTP joint is confirmed by X-ray. In older patients the condition may by asymptomatic and a chance radiological finding but in younger patients symptoms may be in excess of the radiological changes.

MANAGEMENT

(1) Shoes and supports: shoes need to be roomy to avoid friction against the hyperextended IP joint. A thick pad may be made to fit under the sole with a gap cut in it to fit under the MTP joint of the great toe and allow some freedom of movement. A rocker bar placed under the first MTP joint may also allow pain-free gait.
(2) An injection of corticosteroid is useful to relieve symptoms of acute painful episodes. It is given on the dorsal surface directly into the synovium of the joint by directing a 25-gauge needle under the extensor tendon.

(3) Firm mobilization techniques can often assist in relieving pain.

(4) Surgery for the relief of pain is often necessary and two different procedures are available: arthroplasty or arthrodesis. Arthroplasty of the joint is a satisfactory procedure and may be combined with a silicone implant. Arthrodesis is also advocated to relieve pain and does not cause any major functional disability as the patient is accustomed to having a stiff joint.

Hammer toe

This common toe deformity is due to a fixed flexion contraction of the PIP joint, which may be congenital or acquired. One or more of the outer four toes may be involved but most commonly the second. In time the extensor hood, which extends from the MTP joint to the distal third of the proximal phalanx, may develop a contracture. The proximal phalanx becomes hyperextended and the head of the metatarsal may migrate plantarwards, with the formation of a painful callosity under the metatarsal head.

Pain results because of pressure from the shoe, which produces a painful callosity over the dorsum of the involved PIP joint.

Palliative treatment—such as strapping, pads, removal of the painful corns or wearing roomier shoes—is rarely successful. Surgical treatment includes resection of the head of the proximal phalanx, which may be combined with a soft-tissue release of the extensor hood, or removal of the proximal end of the middle phalanx. Arthrodesis of the proximal joint is a satisfactory alternative.

Mallet toe

A mallet toe is a flexion deformity of the TIP joint of one or more toes. Pain is caused by a callosity that develops under the pulp of the toe or over the dorsum of the joint. Treatment is surgical and may entail amputation of the terminal joint.

Varus deformity of the little toe

This is a congenital deformity in which the little toe comes to lie across the base of the fourth toe. It does not usually produce symptoms until adulthood when pressure effects may become an increasing problem. Pain is often due to a hard corn on the dorsal surface of the little toe and a soft corn between the 4th and 5th toes. Surgical treatment requires division of the extensor tendon and the capsule of the 5th MTP joint and a z-plasty of the overlying skin.

Bunion of the fifth metatarsal head

This is produced by inflammation in an adventitious bursa overlying the lateral aspect of the fifth metatarsal head. It may occur in patients with rheumatoid arthritis but is more commonly caused by an exostosis in the underlying bone. It has also been given the name of 'tailor's bunion' as it occurs in people such as tailors, who sit cross-legged. If surgery is indicated either the bony exostosis or the head of the fifth metatarsal may need to be resected.

Arthritis

In spondyloarthritis due to psoriasis or Reiter's disease, inflammatory changes in the IP joints and tendons of the dorsum of the toe are common. This leads to a reddened swelling of the digit, aptly named a 'sausage-shaped digit'. Examination may also reveal the presence of associated nail changes and X-rays may show joint changes and/or periostitis.

Anterior metatarsalgia

Pain in the forefoot is a common symptom, and when it arises in the musculoskeletal system it is given the descriptive title of anterior metatarsalgia. It needs to be differentiated from other causes of pain in this region, which may result from diabetes or vascular, neurological or skin diseases. Before we describe the common musculoskeletal causes the concept of the anterior transverse arch must be mentioned; this arch is described as spanning the heads of the first and the fifth metatarsal bones and as having the second metatarsal as its keystone. However, it is only an anatomical concept in the non-weight-bearing foot. The arch flattens out in the standing position and on walking so that body weight is taken by all five metatarsal heads. The amount of weight transmitted to each individual metatarsal head varies according to the different positions adopted by the leg and foot, and most is borne by the first and fifth metatarsals (Steindler, 1955).

It was previously considered that anterior metatarsalgia was caused by a dropped anterior arch, often due to ligamentous weakness. However, since the forepart of the foot does not function as an arch this concept must be incorrect. Clinically, it may be found that the line of the metatarsal heads may become convex and weight distribution is abnormal, but the causes for this and the reason for the patient's pain must be investigated further.

The common musculoskeletal causes of anterior metatarsalgia are:

(1) Foot deformities.
(2) Arthritis of the MTP joints.
(3) Trauma.
(4) Entrapment neuropathy (*see* page 205).
(5) Freiberg's disease.
(6) Morton's syndrome.
(7) Hypermobility of the first metatarsal.

Foot deformities

Most of the foot deformities described may be the underlying cause of anterior metatarsalgia. Symptoms usually arise from unequal distribution of body weight so that excess weight is carried under the metatarsal heads, which causes pain and callus formation under the MTP joints.

In pes planus the forefoot is abducted and the peroneus longus is weakened so that its tendon functions poorly in controlling movement of the first metatarsal, allowing excess weight to be taken on the more lateral metatarsal heads. The extensor tendons of the toes have an increased angle of pull on the phalanges, thus extending the toes and producing a plantar deviation of the metatarsal heads. Pes cavus, with claw toe formation, leads to excessive weight being borne on the metatarsal heads and eventual plantar subluxation of the MTP joints.

Arthritis of the MTP joints will not be considered here. Traumatic conditions to be considered include stress fracture, traumatic synovitis of a MTP joint and sesamoiditis.

Stress fracture

A stress fracture in the second metatarsal bone is common but the third or fourth bones may also be involved. The second metatarsal is perhaps most commonly involved because it is the longest and most fixed of the metatarsals. The stress fracture occurs usually as an overuse phenomenon in active young people engaged in running but it may also develop in middle-aged people, especially women, due to conditions that produce overloading of the second metatarsal, such as a short first metatarsal or hypermobility of the first ray. It may also occur as a complication of other foot disorders such as rheumatoid arthritis or deformities such as hallux valgus or an uncorrected talipes deformity.

The condition was first described in army recruits involved in unaccustomed heavy activity and was known as a march fracture. Any part of the shaft of the bone may be involved and it occurs most commonly in the neck, followed next by the middle third, and rarely at the base.

CLINICAL FINDINGS
The patient presents with an aching pain, which is usually of sudden onset and is made worse by activity. If the patient continues to exercise, pain becomes quite severe. There may be some oedema over the dorsum of the foot and tenderness can be accurately localized by palpation over the bone. As the fracture heals, periosteal new-bone formation may be formed in excess and a tender lump may be palpable.

The diagnosis must be confirmed by X-ray, although as with stress fracture in other sites the radiological signs can take some time to develop. Periosteal new bone is seen to be formed around the shaft and the fracture line may be visible.

Treatment at first consists of rest from weight-bearing combined with strapping around the foot. The patient can usually walk without producing an exacerbation of pain after a few days and can resume full activity in approximately 6 weeks. Rarely, pain may be so severe that a walking plaster needs to be applied for 3 weeks.

Traumatic synovitis of the metatarsophalangeal joint

This is a relatively uncommon condition, usually brought on by running. Predisposing factors include a plantar deviation of the metatarsal head, as occurs in a pes cavus or other foot deformities. On clinical examination, active and passive flexion and extension of the MTP joint may be restricted and painful and tenderness may be localized over the joint. Synovial swelling may be visible and palpable. This condition can be distinguished from a stress facture of the metatarsal bone or Freiberg's disease by X-rays.

Treatment consists of rest, a metatarsal pad behind the MTP joint and injection of corticosteroid into the dorsal aspect of the joint. Passive mobilization, gently in the initial stages but progressing to more vigorous techniques as pain recedes, is an important part of treatment.

Sesamoiditis

Pain arising from a lesion of the two sesamoid bones in the flexor tendon of the great toe is usually due to trauma. A fracture may result from direct trauma, which needs to be severe; or a stress fracture may result from overuse. The separated parts of the ossicle are evident on X-ray but must be distinguished from a developmental bipartite sesamoid, which should also be shown on an X-ray of the other foot. Pain may also occur at a later stage due to degenerative changes produced by the osteochondral damage.

TREATMENT
This consists of support with a sponge-rubber pad, which is placed behind the sesamoid bone. An injection of corticosteroid can be given using a 25-gauge needle around the flexor tendon. Occasionally, surgical excision of the sesamoid may become necessary.

A fracture of the sesamoid is immobilized in a plaster cast. If osteoarthritis develops and produces recurrent symptoms the sesamoid bone may be removed.

Freiberg's disease

Freiberg's disease involves the head of the second, or rarely the third, metatarsal bone during adolescence. It is usually classified as one of the osteochondritides, due to an avascular necrosis of the bone, but has also been considered as an osteochondritis dissecans due to an osteochondral fracture. At times a loose bony fragment may be found within the involved MTP joint.

It may be asymptomatic or the patient may present with pain, swelling, and tenderness localized over the second metatarsal head and made worse by weight-bearing. An enlargement of the metatarsal head may be palpable. X-rays taken after a few weeks show a typical deformity with broadening of the head and sometimes the neck of the metatarsal and the articular surface presents with an S-shaped deformity. The bone in the centre of the head is sclerotic and the joint space is widened. The natural history is for pain to resolve slowly over weeks or months but for the X-ray appearances to remain unaltered. In later years degenerative changes develop within the joint.

MANAGEMENT
If the diagnosis is made in its early stages management consists of a suitably placed metatarsal pad and rest to the foot. Smillie (1967) reported that an operation to increase the blood supply to the head of the metatarsal may be successful if carried out before the bone ends separate. In later years the metatarsal head may be restricted but symptoms of varying severity may persist after resection. More relief may be obtained from excision of the base of the proximal phalanx and remodelling the metatarsal head, similar to a Keller's operation for hallux valgus. Hoskinson (1974) reported good results from an operation to remove the loose bony fragments.

Morton's syndrome

This condition was described by Morton (1935), who believed that the configuration of the foot in this syndrome was similar to that of prehistoric man and considered it to be the most common cause of foot disability. There is congenital shortening of the first metatarsal with hypermobility of the first tarsometatarsal joint, which is also abducted (metatarsus primus varus).

The second metatarsal is longer than the others and since it has to take excessive weight becomes hypertrophied, which causes callus formation under the second metatarsal head. A similar clinical picture may result from an acquired deformity of the first metatarsal after surgical correction for hallux valgus. In athletes with this condition a stress fracture of the second metatarsal may develop.

A platform built under the head of the first metatarsal to redistribute the weight should relieve pressure on the second metatarsal.

Hypermobility of the first metatarsal bone

The fundamental cause of this condition is ligamentous laxity of the first tarsometatarsal joint leading to hypermobility of the first ray and it may develop as a complication of a varus deformity of the forefoot. It becomes symptomatic on weight-bearing as the first metatarsal does not take its share of the load, and the second MTP joint receives excessive weight causing pain and callus formation under the second metatarsal head.

Hypermobility may be tested for by the examiner placing one thumb under the plantar surface of the first MTP joint and the other thumb under the plantar surface of the second MTP joint. These two joints are then forced into passive dorsiflexion and the examiner notes whether an increased range is present in the first ray.

Mid-tarsal pain

Mid-tarsal pain is a common complaint and may be due to:

(1) Foot deformities.
(2) Joint lesions:

  (a) Arthritis.
  (b) Hypomobility.

(3) Bone:

  (a) Stress fracture of the navicular.
  (b) Osteochondritis of the navicular.
  (c) Dorsal exostosis.

(4) Soft-tissue lesions.

Foot deformities

These have already been considered; patients with either a pes planus or a pes cavus may present with mid-tarsal pain.

Joint lesions

Hypomobility lesions of the transverse tarsal joints are relatively common and may follow trauma with sprain of these joints. Pain may be felt diffusely in the mid-tarsal region but is most common on the plantar aspect of the foot in relation to the spring ligament. Preliminary examination usually reveals that inversion or eversion is painful and restricted; additional tests are then necessary to assess the individual joints of the tarsus to find the appropriate joint. For example, if inversion is painful and limited additional tests are required for the subtalar joint and then the transverse tarsal joints. In this condition accessory movements in the transverse tarsal joints are lost,

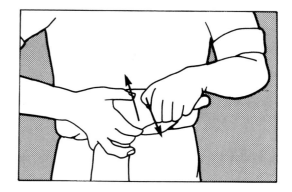

Figure 13.20 Intertarsal dorsiflexion

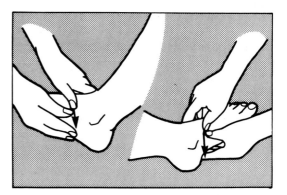

Figure 13.21 Intertarsal anteroposterior movement

and these movements should reproduce the patient's pain.

The treatment of choice is passive-mobilization techniques, which usually produce a rapid and marked improvement in symptoms. Mobilization techniques to treat the transverse tarsal joint use small-amplitude movements into the painful range at the limit of the restricted range. For example, if dorsiflexion is painful and limited, treatment consists of small-amplitude dorsiflexion movements with movement localized to this area by the therapist's thumbs (*see Figure 13.20*). An additional treatment using anteroposterior movements of the transverse tarsal joint with the patient supine and the foot in dorsiflexion is also helpful (*see Figure 13.21*).

Bone

Stress fractures of the *navicular* are rare and usually occur in sprinters. In most patients the condition heals with adequate rest, but occasionally surgery is required because of persistent pain and incapacity.

Osteochondritis of the navicular (Köhler's disease) is also rare. The patient is usually a child aged between 3 and 8 years, who presents with pain in the mid-tarsal area and walks with a limp on the lateral aspect of the foot. There may be some swelling over the navicular bone, which is the site of maximal tenderness.

The diagnosis is confirmed by X-ray, which shows which sclerosis of the navicular is reduced in size and has a squashed appearance. If the diagnosis is suspected in the early stages X-rays of both feet should be taken for comparison. X-ray changes gradually revert to normal over approximately 2 years but degenerative changes in the talonavicular joint may develop in later life.

Dorsal exostosis is an osteocartilaginous swelling over the dorsum of the first tarsometatarsal joint. It is often painless and may represent a response to pressure, as from the lacing of shoes too tightly, and an adventitious bursa may sometimes develop over it. X-rays usually show surprisingly little bony swelling. Treatment consists of preventing pressure on this area from the shoe and only rarely need surgery be contemplated.

Soft-tissue lesions

PERONEAL BREVIS TENDINITIS

The tendon of the peroneus brevis is inserted into the base of the fifth metatarsal and an overuse lesion of this tendon is not uncommon. The patient presents with pain around the base of the fifth metatarsal bone made worse by running. On clinical examination, isometric contraction of the muscle, caused by the examiner resisting eversion of the foot, reproduces the patient's pain. This injury needs to be differentiated from an avulsion fracture of the styloid process of the fifth metatarsal bone, which will be evident on X-ray.

Treatment consists of rest, anti-inflammatory drugs, mobilization and injection of the locally tender area around the styloid process with 1 ml local anaesthetic and 1 ml of corticosteroid.

Causes of heel pain

(1) Soft-tissue lesions:

  (a) Plantar fasciitis.
  (b) Bruised heel.
  (c) Lesions of the Achilles tendon.

(2) Bone:

  (a) Direct trauma, including fractures.

  (b) Indirect trauma, producing stress fractures.
  (c) Paget's disease.

(3) Joints:

  (a) Synovitis of the subtalar joint.
  (b) Hypomobility of the subtalar joint.

Plantar fasciitis

The plantar fascia originates from the tuberosity of the calcaneus and extends distally, covering the intrinsic foot muscles. Its bowstring effect plays an important role, together with the long and short plantar ligaments, in maintaining the integrity of the medial longitudinal arch and stabilizing the foot during toe-off. The plantar fascia becomes stretched either when the medial arch is flattened or on the take-off phase of walking when extension of the toes pulls the fascia more distally. Stretching produces traction on its calcaneal attachment (Hicks, 1961) and tension on the fascia may then increase to twice the body weight. Forces are obviously increased during running, especially on a hard surface. Inflammation of the plantar fasciitis occurs at its attachment into the periosteum.

Plantar fasciitis is a common cause of heel pain. It occurs in patients of either sex, usually over the age of 40, except in active sportsmen when the patient, usually a male, may be in his twenties. It is commonly found in people whose occupation involves prolonged standing or walking. Plantar fasciitis also occurs in some foot deformities and may be associated with restricted movement in the subtalar joint. It may also be associated with hallux rigidus.

Pain is accurately localized over the tuberosity of the calcaneus, nearly always on the medial side, but it may radiate along the sole of the foot. It may be severe and then usually interferes with function. Pain is made worse by activity, such as walking or climbing stairs, may be present at night and is often present when first getting out of bed in the morning. It tends to be relieved by rest. Pain may begin suddenly during activity, when it may be caused by a tearing of some of the fibres of the plantar fascia, or may follow direct trauma to this area.

Clinical examination usually localizes the site of the pain and tenderness accurately to the attachment of the plantar fascia into the calcaneus. Pain may be reproduced by stretching the fascia, e.g. on full dorsiflexion of the ankle.

X-rays may be normal or show a calcanean spur, which represents the process of repair; hypertrophic bone grows out along the lines of stress in the plantar fascia. The spur itself should not be regarded as the source of pain as it may be asymptomatic and a chance finding on X-ray of the feet for an unrelated condition. X-ray changes in patients with inflammatory arthritis may reveal erosive or periosteal changes. In addition a bursa is commonly found under the attachment of the plantar fascia and an inflammatory bursitis may occur in rheumatoid arthritis. Subcutaneous nodules may develop here and become painful and tender on walking. Gout does not often involve this area and should it do so the patient usually has long-standing clinical gout, so that the diagnosis is usually not difficult.

MANAGEMENT

Rest The patient is advised to rest from running until pain settles, which unfortunately often takes a considerable time.

Supports Standard treatment is with a pad made of sponge or Sorbo rubber placed under the heel to raise it approximately 1 cm and lessen the strain on the attachments of the plantar fascia. The pad should have a piece removed to correspond with the painful area in the heel and is worn at all times in shoes or slippers. Nevertheless, this type of support rarely provides much relief and the insole described by Rose (1955) usually gives much better results. He reasoned that, since the site of pain is nearly always over the medial attachment of the plantar fascia just medial to the vertical axis drawn through the subtalar joint it would be more logical to relieve the tension on the fascia by tilting the heel with a convexly wedged insole under the medial arch. It is easy to make, often starts to ease pain within a week and should be worn for some months. Also, in patients with a varus or valgus deformity of the hind foot, it may be necessary to insert a suitable wedge into the shoe. A further modification that may be used is a spring-loaded heel in the shoe.

Anti-inflammatory drugs These may be given for relief of pain.

Mobilization techniques These may relieve pain; those techniques that stretch the plantar fascia or mobilize the hind foot and subtalar joint are usually the most effective.

Corticosteroids Injections of these into the painful area in the heel are quite effective. The patient lies prone with the knee and ankle flexed to a right angle and with the tender area over the tuberosity of the calcaneus, which is found by palpation. A 21-gauge needle is used and directed through

the heel pad to the periosteum. This injection is usually quite painful and so 2 or 3 ml of local anaesthetic should be added to 1 ml of corticosteroid in the syringe. The area around the bone and the plantar fascial attachments must be widely infiltrated. The patient is advised to rest from weight-bearing for a day after the injection and warned that the pain may be severe after injection. The injection may be repeated several times at fortnightly intervals.

Physical methods These are not usually very successful, although daily application of ultrasound may lessen the pain and help to localize the tender area.

Surgery This is rarely indicated. Stripping of the plantar fascia from its origin on the calcaneus enjoys only moderate success. The spur is removed at the same time, but removal of a spur without stripping the fascia is not advisable.

Bruised heel

This is a relatively common condition in athletes or in elderly joggers. The normal structure of the fibro-fatty pad of the heel is shown in *Figure 13.22*. With age or repeated trauma the fibrous septa of this pad may be disrupted and the fat pad may

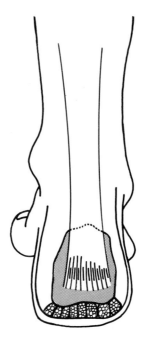

Figure 13.22 Structure of the fibro-fatty pad of the heel

be dispersed. The heel is painful and swollen and may feel tender and thickened on palpation.

Treatment is often difficult and may require prolonged rest. Heel pads are of little value and more relief can be obtained from a moulded cup to compress the sides of the calcaneus and prevent the fat pad from being dispersed.

Exostosis of the superior tuberosity of the calcaneus

A bony exostosis on the posterolateral surface of the calcaneus is usually found in young adults and is often associated with a varus deformity of the hind foot. In young females it may be caused by wearing high-heeled shoes and has been given the descriptive title of 'pump bump' (Dickinson *et al.*, 1966). The patient may present because of an unsightly swelling only, or there may be pain which is made worse by wearing shoes, or there may be an inflammation in the overlying Achilles tendon or bursa.

Treatment consists of correction of the varus deformity of the heel, if it is present. Shoes are worn with a high heel and pliable uppers with a sponge-rubber pad to cushion the back of the heel. Surgical removal of the exostosis is a very successful procedure if conservative measures fail.

Synovitis of the subtalar joint

Synovitis may follow trauma, such as hyperflexion of the foot or a sprain of the ankle joint. Pain, usually felt in the heel or the mid-tarsal region, persists after the original trauma has settled. On examination, movement in the subtalar joints is restricted and painful and a valgus hind-foot deformity may be found. If degenerative changes develop in the posterior talocalcanean joint pain and stiffness increase and the hind foot develops progressive valgus deformity.

MANAGEMENT

(1) The patient needs extra rest from weight-bearing and the joint may be supported by a posterior slab worn at night.
(2) Anti-inflammatory drugs are prescribed.
(3) Injection of local anaesthetic and corticosteroid may be given into the lateral opening of the tarsal canal.
(4) Mobilization techniques are used to ease joint pain and stiffness.
(5) If these measures fail the patient should be treated in a short leg plaster for up to 6 weeks.

(6) A triple arthrodesis may be necessary for persistent pain due to osteoarthritis.

Hypomobility of the subtalar joint

Restriction of movement in the subtalar joint may develop in patients who have had an ankle sprain, have spent a prolonged period of time in bed, or who have had a leg immobilized in plaster. Mobilization techniques are the treatment of choice.

Plantar pain

Pain in the plantar aspect of the foot involving the heel and the forefoot or due to a tarsal-tunnel syndrome has already been discussed. Other causes include:

(1) Soft-tissue lesion:

    (a) Tendinitis of the flexor hallucis longus.
    (b) Ledderhose's disease.

(2) Foot deformities.
(3) Joint disorders:

    (a) Arthritis.
    (b) Hypomobility lesions.
    (c) Acute strain of the medial longitudinal arch.

SOFT-TISSUE LESIONS
Tendinitis of the flexor hallucis longus tendon   This is not uncommon, especially as a sporting injury from running on an unaccustomed surface; for example, running barefoot in the sand.

Major sign—Pain is usually reproduced by the examiner fully resisting plantar flexion of the great toe or by stretching the flexor tendon.

Other signs—An area of tenderness may be found along the course of the tendon, usually proximal to the head of the first metatarsal.

Treatment consists of rest from running, ultrasound, mobilization, and injection of the tendon sheath with a ml of corticosteroid.

Ledderhose's disease   This is a fibromatous swelling occurring in the plantar fascia, most often in the medial aspect of the middle portion, and may be present in both feet. It is related to Dupuytren's contracture in the hand and Peyronie's disease of the penis, either or both of which may be present. It can be asymptomatic but may produce pain, especially on weight-bearing, and may cause a compression neuropathy of the medial plantar nerve.

This condition may be helped by wearing a sponge-rubber cushion or an insole in which a hole is cut to accommodate the tender nodule. If this fails a wide excision of the nodule and plantar fascia may be necessary, but this condition may still recur.

FOOT DEFORMITIES

Plantar pain may be the presenting symptom in patients with pes planus or pes cavus.

JOINT DISORDERS

Plantar pain may occur in patients who have any of the following:

(1) Inflammatory arthritis.
(2) A hypomobility lesion of the transverse tarsal joint, which most commonly involves the talonavicular joint with pain related to the spring ligament.
(3) Acute strain of the medial longitudinal arch. This occurs mainly as a result of running that produces a repetitive depression of the medial longitudinal arch. It is an overuse injury involving the tibialis posterior tendon, the spring ligament and occasionally the flexor hallux longus tendon. Pain is felt under the medial side of the foot and is made worse by activity.

14   The temporomandibular joint

This synovial joint is formed between the condyle of the mandible which articulates with the mandibular fossa and the articular eminence of the temporal bone (*see Figure 14.1*). The mandibular condyle is biconvex, and the temporal surface is saddle shaped. This joint has several distinctive features: a separate joint is formed on each side of the face, and these two function as a unit; it is lined by fibrous and not by hyaline cartilage; and it contains an intra-articular meniscus that divides the joint into two separate synovial cavities.

Movements of the jaw produce opening and closing of the mouth, protraction and retraction of the mandible, and a lateral side-to-side movement of the chin. The inferior portion of the joint acts as a hinge joint that allows opening and closing of the mouth. On opening of the mouth the meniscus rotates and translates forwards under the articular eminence. The superior portion of the joint acts as a gliding joint, which allows forward, backward and lateral movement of the joint. During lateral movement to one side the

articular meniscus in one joint remains in its position while a forward sliding movement occurs in the opposite temporomandibular joint.

Temporomandibular pain

Pain in the jaw is a common complaint and needs to be differentiated from the numerous conditions that cause facial pain. Pain in the jaw may be referred from an unerupted third molar tooth and, in the elderly, from carcinoma involving the tonsil, tongue or pharynx. Pain may also be referred to this area from upper cervical-spine lesions; it has also been reported after cases of traumatic cervical-spine syndrome (Roydhouse, 1973), which can cause some confusion if the jaw has been simultaneously traumatized.

Local causes of temporomandibular pain are most commonly due to the condition of joint dysfunction in the younger age group, and to

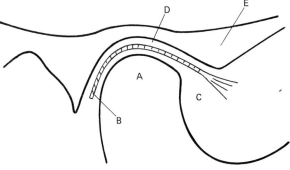

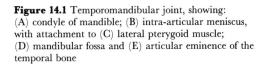

Figure 14.1 Temporomandibular joint, showing: (A) condyle of mandible; (B) intra-articular meniscus, with attachment to (C) lateral pterygoid muscle; (D) mandibular fossa and (E) articular eminence of the temporal bone

osteoarthritis in the elderly; in all age groups these may need to be differentiated from an inflammatory synovitis. The cause of pain in temporomandibular joint dysfunction is not known, and several theories have been propounded to explain it. One theory considered that pain arose from the surrounding muscles (Griffin and Harris, 1975), but Norris and Eakins (1974) injected local anaesthetic into the joint itself and relieved some or all of the symptoms within a few minutes. It appears that a likely cause of pain is a hypomobility lesion of the temporomandibular joint—which may also, of course, be associated with spasm of the surrounding muscles. This condition was first described by a dentist (Costen, 1934) and he attributed to it many other symptoms and signs, including occipital headache, a burning sensation in the throat, deafness, tinnitus, a sensation of fullness in the ear, vertigo and nystagmus.

Pain in the jaw may also occur in cranial or giant-cell arteritis. Pain occurs during eating and is caused by an intermittent claudication of the muscles in the jaw. Other features of this disease are usually present and the erythrocyte sedimentation rate is invariably elevated, often to 100 mm·h^{-1}. Diagnosis may be confirmed by a temporal artery biopsy, which shows the typical histological features of this condition.

Jaw pain of psychogenic origin is not common but may be suspected if a patient complains of a diffuse facial or head pain that is usually of sudden onset and is associated with inability or difficulty in opening the mouth.

Clinical examination

(1) Inspection:

  (a) Swelling.
  (b) Deformities.

(2) Movements:

  (a) Active.
  (b) Passive.
  (c) Accessory.

(3) Palpation:

  (a) Warmth.
  (b) Tenderness.
  (c) Swelling.
  (d) Crepitus.

Inspection

The face is inspected to detect the presence of any swelling, asymmetrical development, deviation of the chin, underdevelopment of the jaw (micrognathia) or an enlargement of the jaw (prognathism). In patients with condylar hyperplasia excessive growth in the mandibular condyle results in deviation of the chin to the opposite side, often with a bowing deformity of the mandible and a posterior open bite. Synovial swelling, which has to be marked before it becomes clinically obvious, presents just anterior to the external auditory meatus.

Movements

Active

Firstly, the patient is asked to open and close the mouth, move the mandible to the left and the right and then to protrude it forwards. Any deviation of the joint to either side during these movements is noted. The range of vertical and lateral movement is then measured. Vertical motion is tested by asking the patient to open the jaw maximally while slightly protruding the lower jaw. The distance between the upper and lower incisor teeth, usually between 3 and 6 cm, is measured. Lateral motion is tested by asking the patient to open the mouth partially, protrude the lower jaw and wriggle the joint from side to side. The normal range is approximately 2 cm.

Passive movements

All of these active movements are next carried out passively. Over-pressure is applied at the limit of each available range and is best performed by taking a firm grasp of the mandible with the thumb inside the patient's mouth. Over-pressure applied at the limit of passive movement allows the end-feel of the particular range to be appreciated and muscle spasm can be clearly differentiated from joint stiffness.

Accessory movements

Five accessory movements are tested:

(1) Transverse medial movement, which is produced by pressure over the head of the mandible (*see Figure 14.2*).

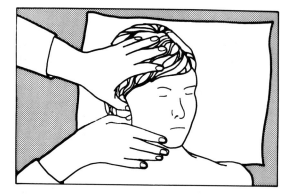

Figure 14.2 Transverse medial accessory movement

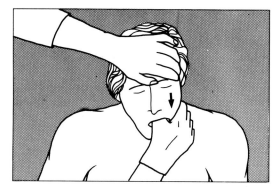

Figure 14.5 Longitudinal caudad movement

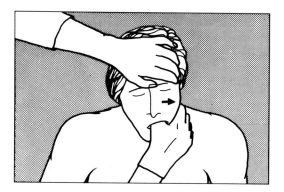

Figure 14.3 Transverse lateral accessory movements

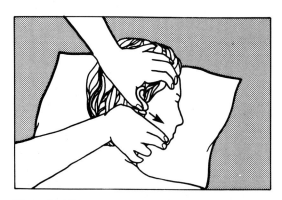

Figure 14.4 Posteroanterior accessory movement

(2) Transverse lateral movement, produced by placing the thumb in the patient's mouth and over the medial surface near the head of the mandible (*see Figure 14.3*).

(3) Posteroanterior movement, produced by pressure over the posterior surface of the mandible head (*see Figure 14.4*).

(4) Longitudinal caudad movement, produced by distracting the joint by pressure over the lower molars (*see Figure 14.5*).

(5) Longitudinal cephalad movement, produced by compression of the joint by pressure over the lower mandible.

Palpation

The joint is palpated first at rest to determine the relationship between the head of the mandible and the articular eminence of the temporal bone. Palpation over the joint confirms the presence of any warmth, local tenderness, soft-tissue swelling or thickening. Capsular thickening is palpable in chronic joint disorders and is more readily appreciated by comparison with the normal side. The joint is then palpated on movement while placing one finger in front of the patient's external auditory meatus. The movement and any crepitus in the joint can then be easily felt.

Lesions of the joint

(1) Temporomandibular joint dysfunction.
(2) Arthritis:

   (a) Osteoarthritis.
   (b) Ankylosis.

Temporomandibular joint dysfunction

This is the best term to describe a common disorder, characterized by facial pain and derangement of the temporomandibular joint. Both the terminology used to describe this condition and its underlying aetiology have been subject of controversy since the original description of this syndrome (Costen, 1934). It occurs much more commonly in females than males and is usually unilateral. Any age group may be affected but it tends to occur in two age groups: the main one consists of those in the early twenties who have their own teeth; and the other contains those who are middle aged and edentulous. Symptoms may be intermittent but can also be severe and widespread.

The presenting complaint is usually pain, which is felt either in the jaw or the ear but which often radiates widely into the face, temporal region or even the neck. The pain is often described as an aching, tight sensation and the patient usually has a history of clicking in the jaw. Pain may be related to the joint dysfunction and occur as the result of joint hypomobility with its associated muscle spasm. The patient is often conscious of a sensation of stiffness in the jaw, which may interfere with eating or be worse in the early morning. Locking of the jaw may occur, although this is usually a rare and late complication.

Major signs

Clinical examination reveals an abnormality of joint movement, which may be either a restriction of movement or a deviation of the jaw towards the painful side on opening the mouth. Clicking during jaw movement may be audible or palpable. Tenderness and thickening around the joint, appreciated by palpation over the joint with the patient's mouth both closed and open, are common.

Other signs

X-rays are usually normal, probably reflecting the fact that younger age groups are involved, although X-rays taken with the joint in the open and closed position may demonstrate a lack of the normal range of joint excursion. Cineradiography of both jaws (Ward *et al.*, 1963) has shown that the head of one mandible may move out of its fossa before the one on the other side. Arthrography may reveal abnormalities in the intra-articular meniscus (Katzberg *et al.*, 1979).

Aetiology

The aetiology is unknown but two major theories have been proposed to explain dysfunction of the joint and the surrounding muscles:

(1) That joint dysfunction is due to malocclusion, a very common condition caused by abnormalities of dental occlusion. This is often caused by loss of molar support (Griffin and Harris, 1975) and may be produced by abnormal or compulsive chewing habits, such as clenching or grinding the teeth, or excessive use of chewing gum. In a series of 586 patients with this condition, Griffin and Harris demonstrated malocclusion in all patients with full upper and lower dentures and in 91 per cent of those with their own teeth.

(2) That joint dysfunction follows muscular imbalance due to a psychosomatic disorder. According to this theory emotional stress causes tension and spasm in the muscles of mastication, which may lead to incoordination of movement, or it may be the underlying cause of teeth clenching and grinding and so lead to dental malocclusion. An electric apparatus for analysing mandibular movements with alternating magnetic fields was devised by Nakazawa and Takahashi (1974). They conducted a three-dimensional analysis of varying mandibular movements in patients with temporomandibular joint dysfunction and synchronously recorded noises and pain in the temporomandibular joint during movement. Their conclusion was that dysfunction of the muscles of mastication, especially the lateral pterygoid muscle, was responsible for this syndrome.

Management

(1) The patient needs to be reassured about the benign nature of this condition and the cause of the pain should be explained. Diazepam may be prescribed if muscle tension appears to be a major factor.

(2) Physical methods of treatment, such as heat or ice, have only a minor role to play in this condition.

(3) Exercises to stretch the tightened muscles and restore co-ordinated movement have been advocated by Schwartz and Chayes (1968). Of more value, especially since tension appears to play a large role in this condition, are relaxation exercises reinforced with biofeedback.

(4) Mobilization techniques: as with all mechanical joint disorders, mobilization techniques play an important part in restoration of pain-free movement. The techniques are of three basic kinds:

(a) When a jaw is locked a firm grasp is taken of the mandible with the thumb inside the patient's mouth and the head of the mandible is distracted from its opposing joint surface.

(b) Accessory movements applied externally to the head of the mandible are extremely valuable when pain is the patient's main complaint.

(c) Mobilization techniques involving stretching of the physiological movements and also applying accessory movements at the limit of the physiological ranges when joint stiffness prevents full function.

(5) Active exercises should be used as a follow-up to retain the increased range obtained.

(6) In chronic cases management should include a dental consultation to assess the degree of any malocclusion that may be present, if necessary with an articulated cast. Dental management includes occlusal grinding to alter the shape and grinding surfaces of the teeth to achieve a simultaneous bilateral contact of the molars and premolar teeth when the jaw is clenched. If these teeth have been removed dentures may be needed. A temporary bite-raising appliance may be used to modify the position of the condyle of the mandible in its glenoid fossa and allow muscle relaxation.

(7) Many surgical techniques, including meniscectomy, have been advocated but have not proved successful. Katzberg *et al.* (1979) consider that meniscoplasty may improve joint function.

(8) Acute episodes are best managed with analgesics, local heat, a soft diet, and intra-articular injections of 0.5 ml of local anaesthetic and 0.5 ml of corticosteroid. The patient sits on a chair with his mouth wide open. A 25-gauge needle is inserted into the depression above the condyle of the mandible, below the zygomatic arch and one finger-breadth anterior to the tragus of the ear. This lies anterior to the temporal artery. The needle is directed inwards and upwards and should lie freely within the joint cavity so that the injection is easily given.

If acute episodes are recurrent or common, mobilization techniques (as described above) may be useful as a prophylactic measure.

Osteoarthritis

Degenerative changes may involve the temporomandibular joint. Clinically, they may be asymptomatic (Toller, 1973) but Blackwood (1963), in a necropsy survey, found an incidence of 40 per cent in people over the age of 40. Osteoarthritis may follow previous trauma, such as an intracapsular fracture of the condylar head. It affects women much more commonly than men and is most common in the fifth decade.

Pain is present at rest or during joint movement, such as chewing or yawning, and is often described as a deep-seated, dull, aching type of pain felt in the preauricular region. Stiffness is often worse in the morning, making cleaning the teeth or eating breakfast difficult. Crepitus, tenderness and thickening are commonly present over the joint. X-ray changes are necessary to confirm the diagnosis, but the standard transcranial X-ray usually does not provide sufficient detail, and either tomography or a transpharyngeal projection may be more helpful.

Management

Treatment should consist first of conservative measures with anti-inflammatory drugs, the use of mobilization techniques, and intra-articular injections of corticosteroids. Correction of dental faults may be necessary. If symptoms persist mandibular condylectomy may be undertaken (Norman, 1975).

Ankylosis

Ankylosis of the joint may follow an inflammatory arthritis, trauma, septic arthritis and childhood infectious diseases. In the past ankylosis was often found as a complication of scarlet fever. In children, ankylosis of the joint leads to micrognathia and the appearance of a bird-like face. The diagnosis is confirmed radiologically but tomography should be used to confirm its presence. Treatment is by arthroplasty of the temporomandibular joint.

Part II—The spine

15 Classification

Spinal pain is the most common complaint of patients presenting with musculoskeletal disorders and this symptom is discussed in more detail in Chapter 19. Disorders of the vertebral column, called vertebrogenic disorders in The International Classification of Diseases, are the most common cause. Classification of these vertebrogenic disorders has always been difficult and the lack of a practical, widely accepted classification is one reason why their management remains so controversial. Classifications consist chiefly of lists, such as the anatomical structures involved and their lesions, but these are clearly of no practical clinical value.

Classifying spinal conditions would probably become straightforward if the underlying pathology was always known, but in a large proportion of patients this is unknown. However, an initial attempt is usually made clinically to diagnose those disorders in which pathology has been well described. This first category comprises specific orthopaedic and medical vertebral disorders, including various traumatic, degenerative, infective, metabolic, inflammatory and malignant spinal conditions. In this first category is also included a large group of patients in whom symptoms arise as the result of intervertebral-disc degeneration. Diagnosis in this first category can usually be made clinically from the symptoms and signs together with ancillary tests, such as X-rays and laboratory tests, although more extensive investigations may be necessary.

Nevertheless, after identifying all cases with a known pathological basis, there remain a considerable number of patients who present with spinal pain but in whom no demonstrable patho-logical basis for their symptoms can be identified. It is in this second category that classification remains a problem and can be made only on a clinical basis by describing certain clinical syndromes. Most of these patients have a mechanical derangement of the spinal intervertebral joint complex, which can be assessed clinically by detecting alterations in the normal pattern and range of spinal-joint movement.

Such an approach is still far from satisfactory but it does allow patients to be classified into recognizable clinical groups, and it would seem appropriate to accept this as a limitation to our present state of knowledge. These lesions of the spinal intervertebral joint complex can then be classified on the basis of an alteration in the range of movement, which may be either increased or decreased. The clinical syndrome associated with an increased spinal mobility is referred to as the hypermobility syndrome. The chronic lesion associated with a decreased range of intervertebral-joint movement is quite common, and hypomobility is the best title to describe this syndrome (Stoddard, 1969). It is capable of definition because of its constellation of symptoms and signs and details of these are described in Chapter 22. In addition, this descriptive title does not imply the presence of any basic pathological changes but refers to the essential clinical finding of restriction in the range of intervertebral-joint movement and its associated accessory movements. Accordingly, hypomobility may be diagnosed even though more than one cause for this syndrome is possible.

A common clinical situation might be described to illustrate a hypomobility lesion. A patient in his twenties presents with a dull aching pain in the right suprascapular area, which has been present for some months. Examination reveals a certain pattern of movements in the cervical spine. Active movements of extension, lateral flexion and rotation to the left side are of full and painless range; but neck flexion, lateral flexion and rotation to the right are restricted in range and reproduce pain. Testing of the passive spinal movements in the lower cervical spine reveals that movements of the C5–6 intervertebral joint are restricted and also reproduce the patient's pain. There are no neurological signs, and X-rays of the spine are normal.

Such conditions would be difficult to categorize under most existing classifications. It would appear highly unlikely that a prolapsed disc could be implicated as the underlying cause. What is more, that particular diagnosis could not be readily confirmed and the patient's prognosis and future management would be rendered more difficult by such a diagnostic label. It is more accurate to define such a mechanical derangement as a hypomobility lesion of the mobile intervertebral joint complex. The clinical signs of this lesion are reproducible and, with training, there is very little inter- or intra-observer discrepancy in eliciting them. It also has implications for patient management since, in the clinical example cited above, manipulative techniques are indicated and should relieve the symptoms.

The vertebrogenic disorders are classified under three main headings:

(1) Intervertebral-disc degeneration.
(2) Medical–orthopaedic disorders.
(3) Disorders of spinal movement.

This clinical classification encompasses most cases seen.

16 Spinal movement

The vertebral column has a considerable range of movement and is so constructed that it also functions as a rigid support and as a protection for enclosed neural tissue. The rigid support is required for the support of body weight and transmission of compressive and rotational forces and is achieved through the thick vertebral bodies, which are separated by the intervertebral discs. The neural arch, made up of two laminae and pedicles, provides a bony protection for the neural structures. These short bony processes enclose the spinal cord, the cauda equina and the nerve roots with their dural investments. Normal spinal function requires spinal movements to take place without any encroachment upon the vertebral canal or the numerous nerve fibres that pass with their blood supply into the intervertebral foramen. The active range of spinal movements, called here physiological movements, are flexion, extension, lateral flexion and rotation to either side. These physiological movements are a summation of the synchronized movements that take place at each individual intervertebral joint.

The mobile segment

At each spinal level below the second cervical vertebra the intervertebral joint is shaped as a three-pronged structure and comprises one anterior and two posterior joints, which act as

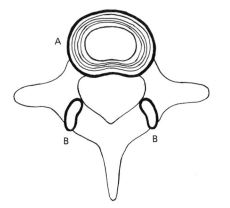

Figure 16.1 The mobile intervertebral joint, seen from above, is composed of the intervertebral disc (A) in front and the two apophyseal joints (B) behind

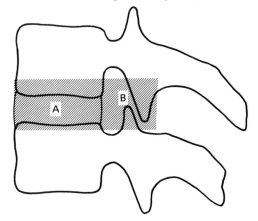

Figure 16.2 The mobile intervertebral joint (shaded) seen from the side, with the intervertebral disc (A) in front and the apophyseal joint (B) behind

a single unit (*see Figures 16.1 and 16.2*). Junghanns (1939) described this functional unit upon which the spinal column is built and referred to it as the 'mobile segment'. Accordingly, the spine may be considered as a complex, flexible system built up with successive layers of these mobile segmental joints.

The anterior joint between two vertebral bodies is formed by the fibrocartilaginous intervertebral disc, which has three components: the outer annulus fibrosus, the inner nucleus pulposus and the cartilaginous end-plates, the end-plates being attached to the bony end-plates of contiguous vertebrae. Anterior and posterior longitudinal ligaments are attached in front of and behind the annulus fibrosus. The two posterior elements of this joint complex are the synovial apophyseal joints which are formed by the bones of the articular processes, one of which descends from the superior vertebra, and the other ascends from the inferior vertebra. The joints are lined by articular cartilage and the synovial cavity is enclosed by a capsule. Tondury (1971) and Schmorl and Junghanns (1971) have described small menisci, which contain synovial tissue, within these joints.

Flexion in this three-pronged intervertebral joint involves a synchronized motion that takes place in both the anterior cartilaginous and the posterior synovial joints. In the anterior joint the vertebral bodies roll over the essentially incompressible gel structure of the disc nucleus, the function of which may be compared with that of a ball-bearing. The thickness of the normal disc varies in each of the three areas of the spine; it is thickest in the lumbar region and thinnest in the cervical region. Movement may also be accompanied by a movement of the nucleus of the disc in a posterior direction. This has been

disputed by Farfan (1973), but Shah, Hampson and Jayson (1978), using discography, showed that the nucleus so moves only when the intervertebral joint is loaded under compression. During extension the upper vertebral body rolls backwards in a posterior direction; this is accompanied by a movement of its inferior articular process in an inferior direction. Similar types of changes take place in the relationships of the intervertebral-joint structures during lateral flexion and rotation.

Apophyseal joints

The performance and range of spinal movements depend not only on disc function but also on the anatomical disposition of the apophyseal joints so that movement is controlled in its amplitude and direction primarily by a gliding motion between the two plane surfaces of the posterior joints. The size, shape and direction taken by the apophyseal joints differs in each of the three divisions of the spine.

The apophyseal joints of the upper four lumbar vertebrae lie mainly in the sagittal plain so that one facet faces medially and the other laterally. The facets in the thoracic spine are slightly convex and the superior facet faces posterior, superior and lateral, whereas the inferior facet faces anterior, inferior and medial. Hence they are set obliquely and so a greater range of rotation can occur here than in the lumbar spine. In the lower cervical spine the facets are placed obliquely. The facet on the superior articular process faces upwards and backwards and the facet on the

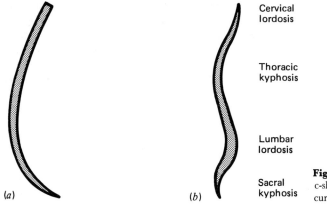

Cervical
lordosis

Thoracic
kyphosis

Lumbar
lordosis

Sacral
kyphosis

(a)   (b)

Figure 16.3 (*a*) In the fetus the spine has a simple c-shaped curve. (*b*) In the adult, compensatory curves are formed

inferior articular process faces downwards and forwards. Spinal movements are determined mainly by this anatomical arrangement, which gives a range of movement in each intervertebral joint complex. Movements are also influenced by the surrounding ligaments and muscles, the shape of the spinal curves and the accessory movements of the intervertebral joint.

Spinal curves

Before birth the spinal column is present as a single curvature with its concavity directed forward. The subsequent development of the three compensatory curves allows ease of movements, maintenance of the upright position and increases the inherent strength and ability to resist

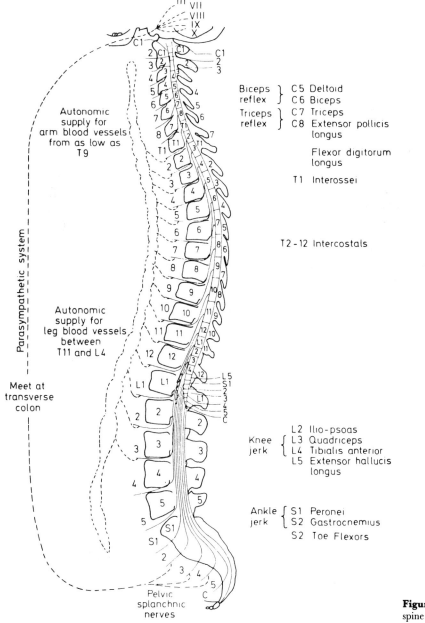

Figure 16.4 Nerve roots and the spine

axial compression by a factor of approximately 15 times. The cervical spine has an anterior convexity, the thoracic spine a posterior convexity, the lumbar spine an anterior convexity and the sacral region another posterior convexity. This cervical lordosis develops after the infant raises his head and the lumbar lordosis develops after he assumes the erect posture (*see Figure 16.3*).

Spinal nerves

The spinal cord with its dural investment lies within the confines of the vertebral canal and can normally adapt to the considerable alterations that take place during spinal movements. However, the emerging nerve roots in their course run in close proximity to the disc and bony structures before emerging through the intervertebral foramen (*see Figure 16.4*) and compression or irritation of the nerve root may result from lesions of these structures.

The ventral and dorsal nerve roots originating from the spinal cord are invested by funnel-shaped extensions of the spinal dura and arachnoid called 'root pouches'. These prevent angulation of the nerve roots at their exit from the dural sac and so protect them during spinal movement. A prolongation of the dura, the root sleeve, runs from the bottom of this pouch and attaches firmly to the nerve roots. The nerve root is capable of movement within the intervertebral foramen, and the lower lumbar nerve roots have been demonstrated to undergo an excursion of approximately 0.5 cm when the leg is passively elevated.

The intervertebral foramen is a short, funnel-shaped opening through which pass blood vessels and lymphatics, the spinal nerve which is formed by the union of the ventral and dorsal nerve roots, and the sinuvertebral nerve which courses back into the spinal canal. The foramen is bounded anteriorly by its adjacent vertebral bodies and disc, superiorly and inferiorly by pedicles, and posteriorly by the superior and inferior articular processes which have an apophyseal joint between them (*see Figure 16.5*).

Both the anterior and posterior joints of the mobile intervertebral joint complex help to form the boundaries of this foramen so that degenerative changes in either of these joints can reduce the foramen's cross-sectional area.

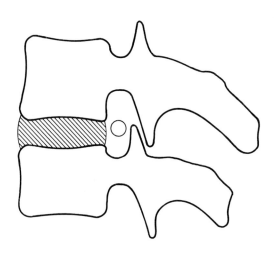

Figure 16.5 The intervertebral foramen with its nerve root is bounded in front by the intervertebral disc and vertebral bodies, above and below by the pedicles, and behind by the apophyseal joint

The ventral and dorsal nerve roots meet to form the spinal nerve from which the sinuvertebral nerve arises, just distal to the dorsal-root ganglia. This slender filament is joined by a branch from the sympathetic trunk and re-enters the spinal canal through the intervertebral foramen. It divides into a superior and inferior branch and ends as a fine, arborizing network of free nerve filaments (*see Figure 16.6*). These supply the dura, the posterior longitudinal ligament, blood vessels, periosteum (Stilwell, 1956) and possibly the outermost fibres of the annulus fibrosus. The nerve is also distributed to the superior and inferior spinal structures by anastomosing with the sinuvertebral nerve at these adjacent levels, and it also anastomoses with its contralateral nerve (*see Figure 16.7*).

The spinal nerve divides outside the foramen into anterior and posterior rami; the latter supplies the capsule of the apophyseal joints, interspinous ligaments and the fascia and muscles of the back. The posterior primary ramus travels approximately 5 mm from its origin and then divides into a medial and a lateral branch. The medial branch lies in close proximity to the bone between the transverse process and the superior articular process where it lies in a fibro-osseous tunnel. It supplies a branch to the apophyseal joint at the same segmental level and also to the joint above and below. The medial branch is then distributed to the medially arranged small muscles of the spine.

The lateral branch of the posterior primary

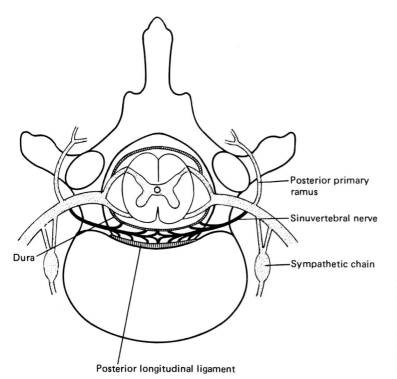

Posterior primary ramus

Sinuvertebral nerve

Dura

Sympathetic chain

Posterior longitudinal ligament

Figure 16.6 The sinuvertebral nerve arises from the spinal nerve and passes back through the intervertebral foramen to supply the dura and posterior longitudinal ligament. The posterior primary ramus is also shown dividing into a medial and a lateral branch

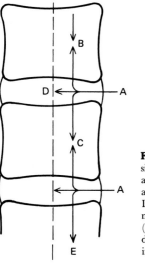

Figure 16.7 The sinuvertebral nerve (A) anastomoses with the nerve above (B) and below (C). It also anastomoses with the nerve from the opposite side (D). It may also pass downwards over several intervertebral segments (E)

ramus passes laterally close to the transverse process and penetrates the sacrospinalis muscle, which it supplies.

There are no pain fibres within the adult disc. They are to be found in the fetus but disappear by birth. The only pain fibres intimately related to the disc are found in the longitudinal ligaments, which are bound to the margins of the annulus. The innervation of spinal joints has been well described by Wyke (1970), who states that each joint has a dual nerve supply from specific articular nerves and from non-specific articular branches of nerves supplying related muscles.

17 The intervertebral disc

The vertebral bodies are united by 23 intervertebral discs, each of which is comprised of three structures: the annulus fibrosus, the nucleus pulposus and the cartilage end-plates. The annulus fibrosus forms an elastic fibrocartilaginous outer layer. In the adult it represents the largest portion of the disc and is formed into layers (or lamellae), which resemble the skin of an onion (see Figure 17.1). These lamellae are separated by loose connective tissue, and the fibres in each lamella run spirally from one vertebra to its neighbour. In each successive layer these fibres run obliquely in alternate directions and so criss-cross at angles to each other. In the lumbar region there are approximately 12 such lamellae; the deeper ones run from the cartilaginous end-plates and bone and the more superficial ones are firmly attached to the anterior margins of the vertebrae (see Figure 17.2). In the lumbar region the annulus is thicker anteriorly than posteriorly.

The nucleus pulposus, accounting for nearly half of the cross-sectional area of the adolescent disc, represents the adult remnant of the embryonic notochord. It has a dull semi-gelatinous appearance and in the lumbar spine lies towards the posterior region of the disc.

In childhood the vertebrae are covered by a thin plate of cartilage, which functions as an epiphysis. After puberty, secondary ossification centres appear in the peripheral areas of this cartilage (hence its title of a ring epiphysis), which then fuse with the vertebral bone after the age of 21. The central portion of the end-plate remains cartilaginous and forms the cartilage end-plate. Countersunk beneath its surface lie the vertebral end-plates, which contain numerous small perforations for vascular channels extend-

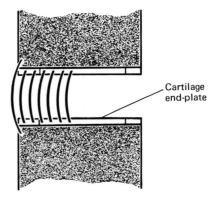

Figure 17.2 The fibres of the annulus are embedded in the cartilage end-plate and the vertebra. The anterior fibres are embedded in the anterior borders of the vertebra

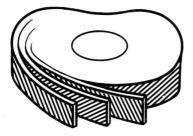

Figure 17.1 The annulus is composed of lamellae in which the fibres of each successive layer run at right angles to each other

ing from the cancellous bone of the vertebral body.

The disc, which lacks a blood supply, was considered to be an inert structure but is now recognized as possessing a system of fluid and nutrient exchange with high metabolic activity. These nutrients are derived from vascular channels, present in the spongy vertebral bone, via perforations in the adjacent cartilage end-plates.

Composition of the disc

The disc, like all other connective tissues, is composed of cells, collagen fibres, and proteoglycans; their relative proportions vary in the annulus and nucleus.

The cells in the adult disc are chondrocytes that are similar in structure and function to those in articular hyaline cartilage. The disc is metabolically active and the function of the chondrocytes consists of both synthesis and degradation. They are responsible for the production both of the collagen fibres and of the proteoglycans (Souter and Taylor, 1970); they also contain several lysosomal enzyme systems, the normal function of which appears to be to degrade proteoglycans in the ground substance (Naylor, 1971).

The collagen fibres arise from and are embedded in the cranial and caudal confines of the disc; that is, the cartilage end-plates and the vertebral bone. These fibres have a high tensile strength and are virtually inextensible. The annulus is composed mainly of collagen fibres and their orientation produces the previously described arrangement of the lamellae, which allows spinal flexibility. They also account for the tensile strength of the disc. These collagen fibrils are randomly orientated to form a three-dimensional lattice network in which the ground substance is immersed. The nucleus contains fewer, more irregular and delicate collagen fibres and so has a relatively larger content of proteoglycan.

The high proteoglycan content of the nucleus accounts for its gel structure and, because of its water-imbibing properties, allows fluid and metabolic exchange. It also accounts for its physical property of resilience—that is, of being able to recover from an applied pressure—and for disc turgescence which, in the young, will cause the

disc contents to bulge spontaneously if the disc surface is cut.

Function of the disc

The disc forms a cartilaginous joint between the two adjacent vertebrae. The normal disc is ideally adapted for its functions in that it can withstand large loads, is an efficient shock absorber in the otherwise rigid vertebral column, adapts to a wide range of spinal movements and distributes the mechanical stresses applied to it equally.

The functions of the normal disc have been well described by Armstrong (1967). He states that the nucleus has four functions:

(1) It acts as the fulcrum for intervertebral movement, the nucleus resembling a ball-bearing with the vertebral bodies rolling over its incompressible gel. The axis for the movement between two adjacent vertebrae runs through the nucleus.
(2) It distributes mechanical stresses equally by transmitting them radially in all planes so that they are absorbed by the surrounding annulus and cartilage end-plates (*see Figure 17.3*).

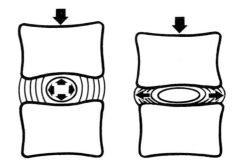

Figure 17.3 Mechanical stress is transmitted radially in all planes by the nucleus and is absorbed by the annulus

(3) It acts as a shock absorber. When pressure is applied to the nucleus it behaves as a viscid fluid and flattens out. When this pressure is released a marked elastic rebound occurs.
(4) It plays a major role in the fluid and nutritional exchange between the disc and vertebrae.

Armstrong ascribes five functions to the annulus:

(1) It plays a major role in vertebral stability by binding the vertebral bodies together.
(2) It allows normal movement between vertebrae as the spiral arrangement of its elastic fibres are altered in their direction.
(3) It acts as a check ligament to prevent excess spinal movement, especially hyperextension.
(4) It acts as an envelope to retain the nucleus.
(5) It acts as a shock absorber. Its normal elastic and tensile properties produce a spring-like action similar to a shock absorber.

There are three functions of the cartilage end-plate:

(1) It protects the vertebral bodies, having a similar function to hyaline cartilage in synovial joints.
(2) It allows fluid exchange between the discs and vertebral blood vessels.
(3) It serves as the growth-plate for the vertebra.

Age changes

The structure and chemical composition of the disc is different in infancy from that of old age. In youth the nucleus has a high water and proteoglycan content, mainly chondroitin sulphate. The collagen content is low. With increasing age the cell content gradually decreases, the water content falls and the proteoglycan composition also varies. The collagen content increases and becomes more hyalinized and fragmented. In old age it is not possible to determine the exact boundaries between the nucleus and the annulus. The nucleus appears as a more solid structure with loss of water content so that it appears dry and granular and loses its property of turgescence. The markedly reduced incidence of acute disc prolapse in the elderly may be explained by these age changes. The nucleus, devoid of its fluid content, is unable to fulfil its role of translating vertical pressure into horizontal pressure and so these pressures are not applied to an already weakened annulus.

Disc degeneration

In the early stages of disc degeneration the annulus becomes softened and fibrillated, and irregular tears and clefts are produced. The extent of the damage may be estimated pathologically by the number of lamellae involved. These annular tears begin in its inner aspect and involve particularly the posterior fibres. They develop radially, running backwards at first in the sagittal plane and may then branch laterally to form an inverted T shape when viewed from above (*see Figure 17.4*). These crescentic fissures between the lamellae may be filled with a brownish pigment, which may be derived from rupture of the cartilaginous end-plates and bleeding from the underlying spongiosa (Schmorl and Junghanns, 1971). As a consequence of annular degeneration its normal elastic properties are lost so that it can no longer fulfil its function of providing intervertebral stability. Moreover, nuclear material can now track through the perforations in the annulus.

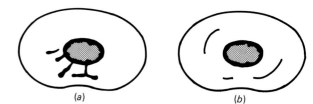

Figure 17.4 (*a*) Radial fissures in a degenerated annulus; and (*b*) concentric fissures

Disc prolapse

As the nuclear material of the disc escapes from the normal confines of the annulus it may prolapse in an anterior, superior, inferior or posterior direction (*see Figure 17.5*).

(1) Prolapse anteriorly is generally asymptomatic as no neural structures are involved.
(2) In adolescents prolapse in an anterosuperior direction through the developing epiphyseal ring is associated with Scheuermann's disease.
(3) A superior or inferior prolapse bulges through the vertebral end-plates into the vertebral body and produces a Schmorl's

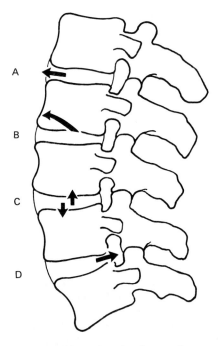

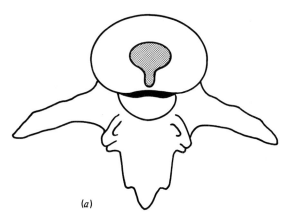

(a)

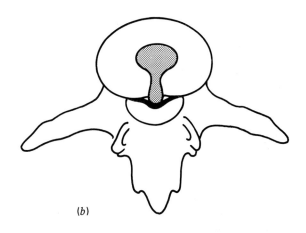

(b)

Figure 17.5 Direction taken by a nuclear prolapse. An anterior prolapse (A) does not impinge on any neural structures. (B) An anterosuperior prolapse associated with Scheuermann's disease. (C) A vertical prolapse producing Schmorl's nodes. A posterior prolapse (D) may produce neural compression

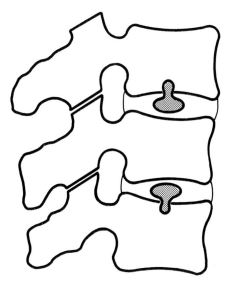

Figure 17.6 A Schmorl's node is formed by a prolapse of the nucleus into the superior or inferior vertebral body

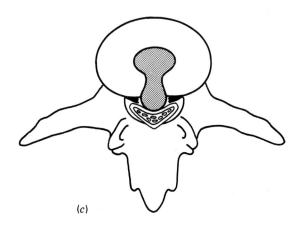

(c)

Figure 17.7 Lumbar-disc prolapse. (a) In the first stages of prolapse the nuclear material bulges posteriorly through defects in the annulus. (b) The prolapsed nuclear material is contained by the posterior longitudinal ligament. (c) Disruption of the posterior longitudinal ligament allows disc material to prolapse into the spinal canal

node. This mushroom-shaped prolapse is contained by a thin layer of compact bone, rendering it visible on X-ray. They are found commonly in the lower thoracic and upper lumbar spine (*see Figure 17.6*).

(4) The posterior aspect of the annulus is the thinnest and mechanically weakest and so is most easily disrupted. Nuclear material can prolapse until restrained posteriorly only by the integrity of the posterior longitudinal ligament, which determines to some extent the final direction taken by the prolapsed disc. If this ligament remains intact the disc may prolapse in a posterolateral direction; if the ligament is ruptured disc material may become sequestered within the spinal canal (*see Figure 17.7*). The prolapsed disc is not composed solely of nuclear material but of varying mixtures of nuclear, annular and separated cartilage end-plate. The prolapse usually stretches the nerve root but may compress it against the lamina or a thickened ligamentum flavum.

Spondylosis

If disc degeneration develops more gradually, reactive changes can take place in neighbouring structures, such as vertebral bodies, apophyseal joints, intervertebral foramina and spinous processes.

Vertebral bodies

As degenerative changes develop in the disc it loses height so that the annulus bulges beyond its normal confines. Ultimately osteophytes develop around the vertebral margins, most commonly on its anterolateral borders. They first grow outwards around the cartilaginous mass of the annulus but may then turn upwards or downwards and may eventually approximate osteophytes from adjacent vertebrae (*see Figure 17.8*). Anterior and lateral osteophytes are of little importance, but those that protrude posteriorly or posterolaterally may encroach on the neural canal and produce symptoms.

Osteophytes tend to develop where pressure changes are greatest and, by broadening the area between the disc surface and the vertebral body,

they may reduce the force per unit area. They are more common on concavities, such as the concave surface of a scoliotic spine. Posterior osteophytes are common in the cervical region and in this site are responsible for more clinical problems.

Changes develop in the vertebral bone. An area of sclerosis develops at first in the subchondral bone and later spreads to involve a large area of the vertebral body. Occasionally, vascular granulation tissue may invade the disc from the vertebral body and can then ultimately lead to an ankylosis. This is most commonly seen in the thoracic spine, where an ankylosis of the anterior margins of the vertebrae is produced.

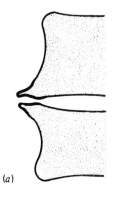

(a)

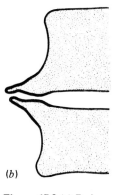

(b)

Figure 17.8 (*a*) Early stage of osteophyte formation, which grows outwards around the degenerated disc. (*b*) Later stage of osteophyte formation

Apophyseal joints

Degenerative changes in the disc result in a disturbance of the position and function of the apophyseal joint. The facets adopt the same relative position that they assume during spinal extension, and so this has been termed the stage of relative hyperextension (Macnab, 1973). The facet joints are then subjected to increasing strains during the course of daily activity which may result in degenerative changes, although these may differ from those described in the large weight-bearing joints (Vernon-Roberts and Pirie, 1977). Soft-tissue swelling, such as capsular thickening, is also present. With advanced changes the lower apophyseal facets may sublux, or impinge against the pedicle of the superior vertebra.

The intervertebral foramen

The diameter of the intervertebral foramen, with its emerging nerve roots, is reduced as a consequence of the diminished disc volume and of the osteophytic outgrowths that develop on the vertebral bodies and apophyseal joints. In the cervical spine degenerative changes in the joints of Luschka, which form part of the foramen boundary, also result in osteophytic outgrowths and produce a further reduction in its diameter.

The spinous processes

The alteration in the relative position of the vertebral bodies can result in approximation of the spinous processes. This is evident on X-ray and ultimately the contiguous borders of these processes become sclerotic, with formation of a false joint between the spinous processes which is known as 'kissing spines'. Clinically it is characterized by pain and restriction of movement on extension of the lumbar spine.

The aetiology of disc degeneration

Disc degeneration is initiated probably by an alteration in chondrocyte function, which may follow abnormal biomechanical forces (*see Figure 17.9*).

Altered chondrocyte function may then result in:

(1) Alteration in the collagen and proteoglycan composition of the ground substance. This leads to loss of the normal mechanical properties of the disc, which is then unable to withstand normal pressures.
(2) Release of lysosomal enzymes, which leads to an increased rate of matrix degeneration.

The net result of these changes is fibrillation and sequestra formation in the nucleus and the development of fissures in the annulus, and so sets the stage for a prolapse of disc material.

The role of abnormal spinal biomechanics is of fundamental importance and will now be considered.

Posture

It has been customary to blame man's upright stance and the fact that his spine has not evolved to an appropriate degree as the basic cause of disc degeneration. This is not the full story—as evidenced by the fact that some four-legged animals (including some breeds of dog, cat and rodent), whose discs have the same basic structure as the human disc, develop disc degeneration and subsequent disc prolapse. However, an increased load is imposed in certain areas of the spine and thus may contribute to the increased incidence of disc degeneration in these sites. This applies particularly to the lumbosacral junction, where the fixed sacrum articulates with the flexible lumbar spine so that, as body weight is transferred from the spine to the sacroiliac joints, a shearing force is applied across the lumbosacral joint.

Similarly, the effect of the lordotic curve in the cervical spine could result in an increased load on the C5 and C6 discs at the centre of the curve.

Besides these static loads, dynamic loads are imposed during movement and while lifting. The spine acts as a first-class lever system, and the intradisc pressure during such manoeuvres has been theoretically estimated. In lifting a 90-kg load with the hips and knees locked and the back arched, the effect of leverage on the lumbosacral disc was estimated to produce a load of approximately 1000 kg. However, subsequent bio-

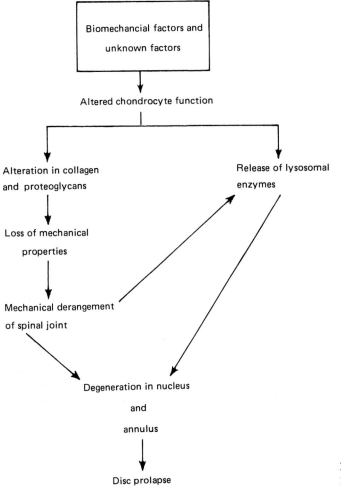

Figure 17.9 Proposed mechanism of disc prolapse

mechanical studies demonstrated that the spine could not withstand such great forces, hence some compensatory *in-vivo* mechanism must be present.

Nachemson and Morris (1964) conducted *in-vivo* experiments to measure the lower lumbar intradiscal pressures and found that these theoretical measurements were too high. Using 18 volunteers, a specially constructed discogram needle was inserted into one of the lower disc spaces. The needle had a pressure-sensitive membrane at its tip, so measurement could be made of the intradiscal pressure when the volunteers adopted certain standardized positions. These positions were:

(1) Sitting upright without support and with the arm hanging by the side.
(2) Sitting holding a 10-kg weight in each hand.
(3) Standing.

(4) Reclining.
(5) Standing but wearing an inflated corset, which allowed external pressure to be applied to the abdominal wall.

The intradiscal pressure and the total loading of the lumbar discs were then estimated in these positions. Pressure was found to be highest in the sitting position; the average intradiscal pressure varied from 10 to 15 $kg \cdot cm^{-2}$. This corresponded to a total load of from 100 to 175 kg.

The readings for the intradiscal pressure and total disc load in standing subjects were 30 per cent less than in the sitting subjects. This was presumably due to the effect of an increase in the intra-abdominal pressure, which turned the semi-fluid abdominal contents into a partially solid pillar and so protected the lumbar spine from some of the effects of weight-bearing. A similar mechanism operates during bending and

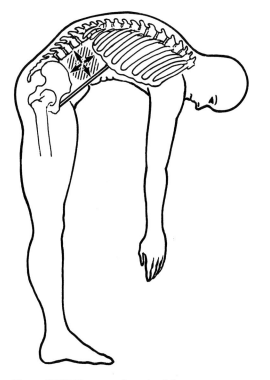

Figure 17.10 The protective role of the intra-abdominal contents in reducing pressure on the spine

lifting, when the rise in intra-abdominal pressure again plays a role in protecting the spine (*see Figure 17.10*). When the subjects were lying down the readings were 50 per cent less than when they were sitting. When the subjects wore an inflated abdominal corset the pressure on the discs was decreased by 25 per cent, which was probably due to the effect of increasing compression on the abdominal wall, so increasing this protective role.

Some occupations may produce added postural strains due to increased bending and lifting and these may be exacerbated if the methods of lifting are incorrect. Labourers are commonly considered to have an increased incidence of disc degeneration. Radiological surveys have tended to confirm this belief but the correlation between the degree of radiological abnormality and clinical symptoms is small.

The effect of torsional strain, rather than compressive load, was investigated by Farfan *et al.* (1970). They produced injury in a spinal joint with a slowly applied rotation within the usual range of normal lumbar movements and proposed that disc degeneration could result from torsional rather than compressive strain. They also believed that during torsional strains the posterior joints were responsible for normal spinal stability, and hence the presence of any apophyseal-joint defect could lead to an increased incidence of disc degeneration.

Pregnancy is associated with altered postural relationships. Kelsey (1975) suggested that it may have an aetiological role, possibly also associated with mechanical stress and the production of ligamentous laxity.

Intradiscal pressure is highest in the sitting position and this postural problem may be exacerbated by the poor design of most modern chairs. Car seats are often poorly adapted to the normal spinal mechanics (Keegan, 1953), and may be associated with the reported increased prevalence of back disorders in motor-vehicle drivers (Kelsey, 1975). Postural abnormalities due to an increased or a decreased lumbar lordosis, scoliosis, unequal leg length, hamstring tightness, weak abdominal and back musculature or use of incorrect footwear may all play some part in producing abnormal spinal mechanical stresses. Michele (1963) hypothesized that the iliopsoas muscle, ill adapted to the evolutionary changes in man's spine, is responsible for most spinal problems. He believed that if the length or strength of this muscle was reduced spinal deformities such as kyphosis, lordosis or pelvic obliquity may result. However, La Rocca and Macnab (1969) repudiated these theories. They took two groups of 150 people aged between 35 and 40 years who had been engaged in heavy work for all of their adult lives. One group had no back symptoms and the other was under treatment for low-back pain. The radiological anatomical variants, especially lordosis and the lumbosacral angle, were similar in both groups, so that there would seem to be no correlation between these anatomical variants and disc degeneration. Similarly, Hult (1954) was unable to demonstrate any correlation between the presence of lumbar lordosis and disc degeneration.

Congenital anomalies

Congenital anomalies in the lumbosacral spine are common (Tini, Wieser and Zinn, 1977); their relevance to degenerative disc disease remains controversial. Some conditions, such as spina bifida occulta or variations in the numbers of lumbar vertebrae, do not appear to be of any clinical significance. However, other anomalies, such as sacralization and lumbarization (particularly if there is fusion on one side and a false joint on the other side), or lumbosacral facet joint asymmetry, may lead to increased mechanical strains with consequent disc degeneration. There is a considerable degree of anatomical interchange possible between the last lumbar and first sacral segments, so that one may have the physical characteristics of the other. The majority of these anomalies are asymptomatic but symptoms may arise in two situations.

Firstly, the lower lumbar joints may be subjected to an increased and asymmetrical strain leading to accelerated disc degeneration. When the lower lumbar segment is completely sacralized disc degeneration may be found at the spinal level immediately above it. If sacralization is unilateral, disc degeneration tends to occur on the contralateral side at the same level. Secondly, the pseudarthrosis formed between the lumbar transverse process and the sacrum may undergo degenerative changes and may be associated with localized back pain.

The lumbosacral facet joints may lie in asymmetric planes, so that one or both lies in the sagittal rather than the coronal plane. This may produce a symptomatic ligamentous strain, or may predispose to a loss of normal rhythmical movement and ultimately to vertebral instability. Farfan and Sullivan (1967) found a very high correlation between asymmetrical facet joints and disc prolapse. This agrees with Farfan's theory, described above, of a rotational strain being the underlying cause of disc degeneration. The obliquely oriented facet is less capable of resisting a rotation strain and so maximum strain will be imposed on the posterolateral portion of the disc annulus.

Trauma

Trauma was originally assumed to be the sole cause of disc prolapse; a view later modified to its being considered the single most important factor. It is now apparent that trauma is implicated as the precipitating factor only in an already degenerated disc. The trauma necessary to produce a nuclear protrusion in the normal disc needs to be severe enough to fracture the vertebra, for discs can resist direct pressures of

up to 56 kg·cm^{-2}. In cases of aortic aneurysms it is the vertebrae, not the discs, that erode.

Racial characteristics

There are many reports of the rarity of disc disease in more primitive races, contrasting to the high and seemingly increasing incidence in Western races. For example, Lindblom (1948) found a higher incidence of lumbar-disc degeneration in Swedish men and women than in Eskimos and American Indians. Matheson (1966) reported that disc prolapse in the Bantu race was extremely rare and this was confirmed by Levy (1967). The basis for this finding is uncertain, and genetic factors could play a role, but Levy believed that the difference was due to the greater spinal mobility and physical activity in the Africans. Subsequently, it has been found that disc prolapse is more common in Africans who adopt a Western way of life.

Sedentary occupation

These above observations suggest that disc degeneration may be included in the group of hypokinetic diseases (Kraus and Raab, 1961) that afflict modern man. In the causation of disease processes, such as coronary heart disease, lack of activity and exercise appear to play an important role. The nutrition of the normal disc, which is dependent on fluid exchange, seems likely to be aided by the action of the surrounding muscles and spinal intervertebral joint motion. Lack of exercise results in a loss of these normal forces, so that disc nutrition could become disturbed and so produce degenerative changes.

Heredity

Hirsch and Schajowicz (1953), in their studies on disc degeneration, suggested the importance of hereditary factors but no adequate studies in humans have since been conducted to support this contention. However, it is not uncommon in practice to find some families with a high incidence of disc degeneration. Similarly, some breeds of animals (Berry, 1961)—especially certain breeds of dog (Ghosh *et al.*, 1975)—are more prone to disc degeneration than others.

18   Disorders of the vertebral column

The disorders of the vertebral column discussed in this chapter are mainly medical or rheumatological conditions. Some surgical conditions such as fracture, fracture–dislocations or structural scoliosis are therefore not included.

These vertebral disorders may be classified into:

(1) Inflammatory diseases:

   (a) Spondyloarthritis.
   (b) Rheumatoid arthritis.

(2) Metabolic diseases:

   (a) Metabolic bone disease.
   (b) Chondrocalcinosis.
   (c) Gout.
   (d) Acromegaly.
   (e) Ochronosis.

(3) Traumatic and degenerative conditions:

   (a) Spondylolysis.
   (b) Spondylolisthesis.
   (c) Ankylosing vertebral hyperostosis.
   (d) Scheuermann's disease.

(4) Infections.

(5) Tumours.

Inflammatory diseases

Spondyloarthritis

The group of diseases characterized by inflammatory lesions in spinal and peripheral joints are best classified as spondyloarthritis. They are also linked by inflammatory changes in the sacroiliac joints and frequent association with skin, mucous membrane, eye, bowel and urinary tract lesions. A further reason is their familial aggregation, related to the presence of the HLA B27 antigen, which can be demonstrated by tissue typing.

The diseases that are usually so classified include:

(1) Ankylosing spondylitis.
(2) Reiter's disease.
(3) Psoriatic arthritis.
(4) Arthritis associated with inflammatory bowel disorders, such as ulcerative colitis and regional enteritis.

Ankylosing spondylitis

This disease has as its essential feature the presence of bilateral sacroiliitis, and inflammatory changes also usually develop in the spinal joints. The earliest pathological lesion appears to be a lymphocytic infiltrate involving primarily cartilage, subchondral bone and the ligamentous and tendinous insertions into bone and periosteum (known as the enthesis). The resulting osteitis and/or chondritis especially involves central joints of the axial skeleton, such as the sacroiliac joint, symphysis pubis and the intervertebral joints of the spine. In the spine these changes result in an erosive lesion either anteriorly or posteriorly at the upper and lower surfaces of the vertebral body. This leads to the formation of granulation tissue, so that in the healing stage the outer fibres of the disc and vertebrae are replaced by a vascular fibrous tissue, which ultimately becomes ossified.

Synovitis also develops in the synovial apophyseal and peripheral joints and inflammation develops in the ¡usculotendinous attachments of the enthesis, especially around the pelvis and heel, with the production of an exuberant periostitis.

Early studies (Lawrence, 1963) suggested that this disease was rare and occurred in only four in 1000 males. However, a study by Calin and Fries (1975) of HLA B27 positive patients suggests that this figure may be a gross underestimation, and that 1.4 per cent of the population may have this disease.

The onset of this disease is usually in the late teens or early twenties; it is most uncommon for it to commence after the age of 40. It has generally been believed that ankylosing spondylitis is a disease of young males, and most earlier series have reported that at least 90 per cent of their cases have been in males. It has been apparent for some time that this figure is inaccurate and possibly a reflection of the fact that some of the series were reported from radiotherapy departments at which treatment was given predominantly to males. It now seems more likely that this disease occurs almost as often in females (Calin and Fries, 1975) in whom the disease may be more often atypical or run a milder clinical course. This disease is quite rare among black races, in whom the HLA B27 antigen does not occur, but occurs in up to 10 per cent of males in some tribes of American Indians.

AETIOLOGY

The aetiology is unknown. Mason (1958) found evidence of pelvic infection in 83 per cent of cases but the casual relationship remains uncertain. Ebringer *et al.* (1977) suggested that a Klebsiella infection may play a causative role, and cross-immunity between this organism in HLA B27 patients may occur (Seager *et al.*, 1979).

HISTORY

The typical history is one of pain in the lower back radiating to the buttocks, thighs and groin. Pain tends to be episodic and often alternates from one buttock to the other. Pain may radiate down the back of the leg to be confused with true sciatica but neurological symptoms are absent. The disease tends to come

in attacks at first, although later the pain tends to be more constant.

There is associated low-back stiffness, which is worse during the early hours of the morning or on awakening. It may be so severe that the patient needs to get up and walk about to obtain relief. The severity of the inflammatory process correlates well with the degree of stiffness, though most symptoms are exacerbated by immobility.

Calin *et al.* (1977) analysed the factors in the clinical history that may lead to a positive diagnosis of ankylosing spondylitis. The five most important factors were:

(1) Onset of back discomfort before the age of 40.
(2) An insidious rather than sudden onset.
(3) Persistence for more than 3 months.
(4) Association with early-morning stiffness.
(5) Improvement with exercise.

As a diagnostic screening procedure, the finding of four out of five factors appears to be highly accurate.

Peripheral joints may be involved, especially proximal joints (shoulders and hips) and lower limb joints such as knees, ankles, heels and feet. The small joints in the fingers are rarely involved.

SIGNS

A careful search may be required to detect any clinical signs in the early stages of this disease, for they are often then minimal. The early diagnosis of this disease depends on maintaining a high index of suspicion that it may be the cause of a patient's symptoms. Similarly, a diagnosis of psychogenic illness is often considered in the early stages of the disease when complaints of pain and stiffness are present without any obvious signs.

The overall range of lumbar-spine movements becomes reduced and is best appreciated by a limitation of lateral flexion. Forward flexion may also be reduced but, since most of this movement takes place at the hips, patients in the early stages of the disease may be able to touch the floor with their fingers. Muscle spasm is usually evident bilaterally, giving the spine a straightened or so-called 'ironed-out' appearance.

Clinical testing of the sacroiliac joints (*see* Chapter 29) is essential; it may reproduce the patient's low-back or buttock pain or produce pain over the sacroiliac joint. Chest expansion is limited if the costovertebral joints are involved and is an important and often early sign. Involvement of the cervical spine with pain and stiffness usually occurs later in the course of the disease.

Inflammatory changes occur at an early stage in the enthesis with involvement of musculotendinous insertions or tendons especially around the pelvis and Achilles tendon. Heel pain results from synovitis of the subtalar joint, Achilles tendinitis or plantar fasciitis. Changes similar to those in the sacroiliac joint are also found in the symphysis pubis and the manubriosternal joint, which produce local pain and tenderness. The costovertebral joints are often involved early, resulting in chest pain with restricted respiratory excursion. Temporomandibular-joint involvement and dysfunction may also occur (Davidson *et al.*, 1975).

OTHER PRESENTATIONS
(1) Ankylosing spondylitis may present first with peripheral-joint involvement in the lower limbs. The hip is commonly involved, but knee, ankle or foot pain may be present before spinal involvement is noted. In the upper limbs, proximal joints such as the sternoclavicular, acromioclavicular or shoulder joints are usually involved. Less often there is a generalized polyarthritis.
(2) It may present as spinal pain involving either the neck, chest or thoracolumbar junction or each of these areas simultaneously.
(3) It may commence as a generalized systemic illness with weight loss, fever and generalized aches and pains.
(4) Iritis may be the presenting complaint.
(5) Destructive lesions in the disc and vertebral bodies (Romanus and Yden, 1955) result from a granulomatous lesion of the disc that involves the cartilage end-plate or the vertebral rim. This spondylodiscitis occurs at any spinal level but is found usually around the thoracolumbar junction. X-rays show erosive, destructive bone changes with surrounding sclerosis, although tomography may be needed for adequate delineation. These lesions tend to be found in a mobile segment between ankylosed vertebrae and occur as the result of trauma and not of an inflammatory discitis (Cawley *et al.*, 1972).

CONFIRMATORY TESTS
X-ray evidence of sacroiliitis is essential before the diagnosis can be confirmed. Before these radiological signs are present the diagnosis can

only remain presumptive; but since it may take several years before the radiological signs become definite it may at times be necessary to organize treatment on the basis of such a presumptive diagnosis. The radiological changes in the sacroiliac joints are described in Chapter 29.

X-ray changes in the spine during the early stages include a squaring of the vertebrae, as filling in of the normal concavity with periosteal new bone formation results, with loss of the vertebral corners. Syndesmophytes, often seen at the thoracolumbar junction, are bony bridges formed between the outer fibres of the annulus fibrosus of the disc and the deep aspects of the anterior longitudinal ligament. Since they run from the margins of the vertebral bodies in a vertical direction syndesmophytes can be differentiated

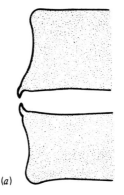

(a)

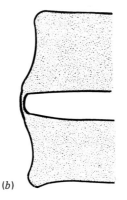

(b)

Figure 18.1
Syndesmophytes: (*a*) at an early stage, growing in the outer layers of the annulus; (*b*) at a more advanced stage

from osteophytes, which lie in a horizontal direction (*see Figure 18.1*).

Ossification subsequently develops in other areas of the spine such as the spinal ligaments and apophyseal joints. The X-ray picture of 'bamboo spine' is produced by symmetrical paravertebral ossification completely bridging across the disc space.

Laboratory tests are usually not of great assistance in diagnosis. There may be a mild normochromic anaemia, the erythrocyte sedimentation rate (ESR) is usually moderately elevated and serological tests for rheumatoid factor are negative. The presence of the HLA B27 antigen may be sought. Synovial-fluid analysis of involved peripheral joints shows moderately inflamed fluid with predominantly lymphocytic cell infiltration.

ROUTINE MEASUREMENTS

Continued assessment of the patient and his disease is essential. At approximately yearly intervals some basic measurements should be carried out. These include:

(1) Chest expansion, which measures change in thoracic joints such as the costovertebral joints.
(2) The distance the tips of the fingers reach from the floor on full forward flexion; this measures both hip and lumbar-spine flexion.
(3) When the patient stands upright against a wall the back of the head should touch the wall easily. If a flexion deformity of the neck is present the head is carried forward, and the distance from the back of the head to the wall should be recorded.

MANAGEMENT

Management involves three separate problems; control of pain, stiffness and deformity. Pain is due to inflammation; the greater the degree of inflammation, the greater the pain. For this symptom, anti-inflammatory drugs remain the treatment of choice. The patient needs to use appropriate anti-inflammatory agents in a sufficient dosage to maintain maximal mobility and activity. Deformity should be prevented by vigorous, organized exercise routines. In former years, management by deep X-ray therapy and immobilization by use of a plaster cast produced disastrous loss of function. During acute attacks most movements are painful and rest from such painful activities is then essential. However, as

the acute attack settles, the patient must be encouraged to resume exercise therapy.

General measures include use of a firm mattress with a bed-board, plus a small soft pillow. Postural care of the spine, including sitting with the back straight and supported to avoid long periods of spinal flexion, must be taught. The patient who becomes stiff easily while sitting for long periods is advised to get up periodically and walk around.

Proper patient management requires proper patient education. The implications and prognosis of the diagnosis must be explained, stressing that most patients lead an active life and that the mortality rate from this disease is extremely low. The advantages and limitations of therapy should also be carefully explained and the advantages of remaining as active as possible stressed.

DRUG THERAPY

The inflammatory changes in the spinal joints usually respond so well to anti-inflammatory agents such as phenylbutazone or indomethacin that they almost seem to be a specific therapy. The smallest dose compatible with clinical improvement is used, usually two or three tablets a day. Salicylates in doses up to 4 g daily may be first tried but are not quite as effective. Systemic corticosteroids are only rarely indicated but may occasionally be necessary to control an acute systemic reaction.

PHYSICAL THERAPY

(1) Exercises are essential in the management of this disease.

  (a) Isometric exercises are used especially for extensor groups of the spine and legs.
  (b) Breathing exercises are needed to maintain mobility in costovertebral joints.
  (c) Postural exercises are taught to enable the patient to control his posture while sitting or standing. The patient is also advised to sleep on a firm mattress with the use of only a small pillow. Long periods spent bending and stooping must be avoided.
  (d) Activities are encouraged so that the patient remains as mobile as possible. Body-contact sports present some difficulty but most other sports, especially swimming, are compatible with this disease.

(2) Heat may be of some advantage before an exercise programme is implemented.

(3) Traction and manipulation are contraindicated in these cases.

SURGERY

In peripheral joints operations such as synovectomy or joint replacement of the hip, knee and feet may be necessary. Spinal osteotomy is only rarely indicated to improve kyphosis but provides worthwhile results in those who otherwise would be condemned to a life spent looking at the ground.

Reiter's disease

Hans Reiter, a venereologist, described a triad of urethritis, conjunctivitis and arthritis in 1916. Since that time several other clinical features have been recognized, and the term Reiter's disease is now used to describe their varying combinations. The case that Reiter described followed an attack of dysentery, which may be an initiating factor. More commonly the disease follows a venereal infection due to non-specific urethritis, whose causative organism remains undetermined. Currently it is thought that a Chlamydia organism may be the causal agent.

CLINICAL FEATURES

Most cases occur in young adult males and it is very rare in females.

Any peripheral joint may be involved, usually joints of the lower limb, with a synovitis that is often intense and asymmetrical. Tendon sheath or tendon involvement, such as Achilles tendinitis, is common. This tendinitis may produce painful heels which may also be due to plantar fasciitis, periostitis or erosive changes in the calcaneus.

Sacroiliitis occurs ultimately in about one-third of patients with Reiter's disease. Spinal involvement may be asymmetrical at first but can progress to produce a clinical picture indistinguishable from ankylosing spondylitis.

TREATMENT

Rest for the affected joints is essential. Anti-inflammatory agents are given in a sufficient dosage to control symptoms but oral steroids are only rarely required. Large joints may be aspirated and injected with corticosteroids. Urethritis responds well to tetracyclines given as a 250-mg dose every 4 hours for up to 3 weeks.

Psoriasis

Psoriasis is a very common skin disease, which may be associated with a seronegative inflammatory polyarthritis. About 20 per cent of patients with psoriatic arthritis have spinal involvement, which is in some ways different from that in ankylosing spondylitis but has similar features to those in Reiter's disease (McEwen *et al.*, 1971). Sacroiliitis may be asymmetrical and spinal involvement may be unilateral. Syndesmophytes are present but may not arise at the vertebral margins as they do in ankylosing spondylitis, so tending to be separated from the outer margin of the disc. Any spinal segment may be involved but its progression tends to develop in a more random fashion than with ankylosing spondylitis.

Inflammatory bowel disease

Inflammatory bowel disease, due to granulomatous lesions in ulcerative colitis or Crohn's disease or to infections such as Yersinia, may be complicated by sacroiliitis, spondylitis and peripheral arthritis.

Rheumatoid arthritis

Rheumatoid arthritis commonly involves the cervical spine, possibly because of its mobility and the presence of some 29 synovial joints between the skull and the first thoracic vertebra.

Three factors determine classification of the cervical changes that may occur: firstly, the anatomical site of involvement; secondly, the underlying pathological process leads to erosive changes in the synovial joints and bursae, or to an extension of the synovitis from neurocentral joints into the disc substance; thirdly, the changes are classified according to the radiological findings present and occur as the end-result of these destructive processes (*see Table 18.1*).

Atlantoaxial joint

In the atlantoaxial joint, the odontoid process of the axis (or dens) is dependent for stability on the strong transverse ligament that runs between the lateral masses of the atlas. Synovial bursae may be found in three sites: one between the anterior arch of the atlas and the dens; one between the dens and the transverse ligament;

Table 18.1 Classification of spinal rheumatoid arthritis

Area	X-Ray changes
Upper cervical spine	Erosive changes in: (1) Dens (2) Atlanto-occipital joints (3) Lateral atlantoaxial joints Deformities: (1) Atlantoaxial subluxation, which may be: (i) Anterior—either 'slider' or 'tipper' (ii) Vertical (iii) Lateral (iv) Posterior (2) Collapse of lateral mass of atlas
Lower cervical spine:	Disc thinning without osteophytosis, vertebral end-plate erosions,
Discs and vertebral bodies	vertebral body erosions, osteoporosis and deformities—anterior subluxation of vertebra, and step deformities
Apophyseal joints	Erosive arthritis, blurring of joint space, and fusion
Spinous process	Cortical erosions and thinned-out spinous processes

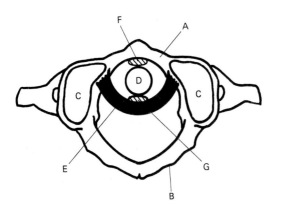

Figure 18.2 The atlas, showing: (A) anterior arch; (B) posterior arch; (C) atlanto-occipital joints; (D) odontoid process; (E) transverse ligament; (F) bursa between odontoid process and anterior arch of atlas; (G) bursa between odontoid process and transverse ligament

and one at the apex of the dens (*see Figures 18.2 and 30.3*). Inflammatory changes in these sites produce erosive changes, leading ultimately to attenuation and loosening of the transverse liga-

ment, which produces an anterior subluxation of the atlantoaxial joint.

Radiological changes in the upper cervical spine are produced by erosions or deformities. Erosive changes occur in the odontoid process, usually on its posterior aspect where a synovial bursa lies between it and the transverse ligament, but also on its anterior aspect in the joint between the dens and the anterior arch of the atlas. Erosive changes in the dens produce a number of different appearances. It may become pointed or have a steepled appearance; at times there may be a sclerotic or shiny appearance; and at times there may be deformity of the dens giving it an irregular or 'squeezed-out' appearance. The erosions may be so severe that they reduce the dens to a spicule of bone. As a result of these erosive changes the odontoid process may be so loosened that atlantoaxial subluxation may occur, even though the transverse ligament may be intact. A fracture of the odontoid through its base, which has to be differentiated radiologically from a congenital defect, may result in the odontoid process becoming loose and mobile. Erosive changes in the lateral atlantoaxial synovial joints of this region are best seen in the anteroposterior X-ray view.

As a result of these destructive changes the relationship of the atlas to the axis may be altered. Four types of deformity have been described:

(1) The most common deformity resulting from the progression of the destructive changes is an anterior subluxation of the atlantoaxial joint, diagnosed on X-ray by an increased gap between the anterior arch of the atlas and the odontoid process. Most commonly, the body of the atlas slides forwards on the axis. However, there may be another X-ray appearance as the atlas tips up on the axis.
(2) Severe erosive changes in lateral atlantoaxial joints may result in a lateral subluxation of the atlas on the axis.
(3) Softening and destruction of the lateral mass of the atlas allows the occipital condyles to descend onto the axis and to produce a vertical subluxation of the odontoid process, which may protrude through the foramen magnum. Similar bony changes result in an alteration of the relationship between the cervical spine and the base of the skull.
(4) A posterior atlantoaxial subluxation due to rheumatoid disease is very rare and can occur only if the odontoid process has been severely eroded.

Lower cervical spine

Rheumatoid granulation tissue growing in from the neurocentral joints may invade and destroy the intervertebral disc, which produces a discitis. This is usually associated with laxity of spinal ligaments and allows a forward subluxation of one vertebral body on the lower one. Multiple subluxations at C2, C3, C4 and sometimes C5 lead to a classic radiological finding of step-like deformities of the vertebral bodies. Rheumatoid discitis at C2–3 and C3–4 is diagnosed radiologically by a thinning of the disc without any accompanying osteophyte formation. Discitis also occurs at lower cervical levels but since degenerative changes there are also common in this age group interpretation of the radiological appearance can then be most difficult.

Erosive changes or osteoporosis may be seen in the vertebral bodies. Erosions occur either at the vertebral margins or more commonly through the cartilaginous end-plates. In apophyseal joints, erosions are seen usually at C2–C3.

Erosions may also be seen in neurocentral joints or as cortical erosions of the spinous process, usually at C7. Atrophic changes may lead to a thinning out of the spinous process.

SYMPTOMS

At times the cervical lesions may be asymptomatic and found by chance during X-ray examination. The main complaint in symptomatic cases is neck pain, usually associated with stiffness. Other common complaints include head pain, vertigo and a clicking or clunking sensation in the neck, which is usually associated with an exacerbation of severe pain.

Neurological symptoms do not occur as commonly as might be expected considering the severity of the X-ray changes, although transient blackouts, cord compression or sudden death has been described. Lower motor-neurone lesions of the upper limbs may occur in patients with anterior subluxation of the vertebral bodies below C4. Sudden head movements often produce paraesthesias or numbness in shock-like waves in the limbs. In the lower limb, evidence of upper motor-neurone lesions may be difficult to evaluate in the presence of the deformities resulting from the peripheral arthritis. Considering the severe radiological changes that may be present in the cervical spine, cord involvement can be uncommon. In a series of 130 patients with cervical subluxations who were followed up from 5 to 14 years, Smith,

Benn and Sharp (1972) described only four patients with definite cord compression and a further six with possible compression. However, 5 years after diagnosis, one-third of patients with anterior subluxation and half of those with downward luxation may have developed long tract signs (Mathews, 1974).

MANAGEMENT (*see Table 18.2*)

The most common complaint is of neck and/or head pain and in most of these patients pain relief is obtained by the use of a semi-rigid collar, analgesics and general management of their rheumatoid disease. Pain is usually relieved by these simple conservative measures, so surgery need be considered only in a very small percentage of cases. If the radiological changes are a chance finding and the patient is unaware of neck symptoms active treatment to the neck may not be required.

Table 18.2 Management of rheumatoid cervical lesions

Symptoms	Definitely indicated	Possibly indicated
Nil	Observation	
Pain	Collar	Surgery
Neurological complications:		
Lower motor-neurone lesions	Collar	Surgery
Upper motor-neurone lesions:		
(1) Minor	Observation Collar	Bed traction Surgery
(2) Major	Surgery	

The presence of neurological lesions requires greater judgement in management and each case must be assessed individually. In patients with evidence of a lower motor-neurone lesion in the upper limb, a collar is usually sufficient to relieve symptoms. Upper motor-neurone lesions of the lower limb vary in severity from the presence of a few signs only to definite evidence of cord compression. In the former the patient may only require a collar and periodic assessment to determine any progression of symptoms. If symptoms do progress the patient may then require a period of bed rest in hospital, possibly with neck traction. If there is evidence of any marked degree of cord compression surgery is indicated (Newman and Sweetnam, 1969; Brattstrom and Granholm, 1976).

Thoracic- and lumbar-spine involvement

Rheumatoid involvement of the thoracic and lumbar spines is rare. The essential lesion (Bywaters, 1981) is a rheumatoid discitis, spreading in from adjacent costovertebral or apophyseal joints. In the lumbar spine discitis may occur in an already degenerated disc and may be caused by vertebral instability, with the consequent chronic trauma producing discovertebral destruction. A similar mechanism has been proposed by Martel (1977) to explain the pathogenesis of rheumatoid discitis in the cervical spine.

Metabolic diseases

Four major metabolic bone diseases—osteoporosis, Paget's disease, hyperparathyroidism and osteomalacia—are found most commonly in elderly people. In patients over the age of 65, Leeming (1973) found a female prevalence of 25 per cent for osteoporosis and 6 per cent for Paget's disease. The prevalence of osteomalacia varies, being more common in poor communities because of dietary insufficiency.

Osteoporosis

In this condition the total amount of bone is reduced, the bone present being histologically normal but less dense.

Aetiology

This includes:

(1) Idiopathic.
(2) Disuse.
(3) Endocrine disorders:

  (a) Cushing syndrome.
  (b) Thyrotoxicosis.
  (c) Hypothyroidism.
  (d) Acromegaly.
  (e) Hypogonadism.
  (f) Steroid therapy.

(4) Malignancies—for example, secondary carcinoma or multiple myeloma.
(5) Genetic, such as osteogenesis imperfecta, or homocystinuria.
(6) A rare juvenile form.

Most cases of osteoporosis are idiopathic but have been considered to occur as the result of hormonal changes and so have been classified also as postmenopausal or senile osteoporosis.

The nature of this condition—whether due to disease or to the ageing process; whether due to decreased bone formation or increased bone resorption; and the role of calcium and diet—has caused considerable controversy. Osteoporosis should be regarded as a multifactorial process of diverse aetiology and it should be considered as a disease and not solely as part of the normal ageing process. This was shown by Adams, Davies and Sweetnam (1970) in a longitudinal study over 15 years in which 38 per cent of men and 22 per cent of women failed to show any bone loss.

Symptoms

Many cases are asymptomatic for long periods of time. Symptoms are produced as a result of the loss of cortical bone in areas, such as vertebrae or femoral neck, where the bone mass becomes insufficient to withstand the normally high stresses to which these tissues are subjected. The usual complaint is of pain in the thoracic or lumbar regions. This may be produced by vertebral fracture or collapse, in which case pain may come on spontaneously, follow sudden exertion such as shifting furniture, or follow minor trauma. The origin of the diffuse skeletal pain at other times is uncertain but it may be produced by postural alterations in supporting structures. The patient may be conscious of loss of height and the development of a kyphoscoliosis until, ultimately, the lower ribs approximate to the iliac crests. Neural complications due either to cord compression or sciatica are rare.

Investigations

X-rays are the most common method of investigation, although Lachmann (1955) has estimated that 30 per cent of the calcium in the bone needs to be lost before X-ray changes become definite. Changes occur most often at T12; the incidence decreases with increasing distance from this site, hence collapse above the T3 level is rarely due to osteoporosis.

Other investigations include bone biopsy to examine histologically decalcified sections, 24-hour urinary calcium excretion and bone mineral analysis.

Management

(1) Physical methods. The patient must be kept as active as possible, both to reduce the possibility of aggravating the problem by immobilization and to encourage the action of muscle in stimulating bone development. For these reasons isometric spinal exercises are taught, and belts and braces should be avoided. Manipulative techniques are contra-indicated.
(2) Analgesics may be needed for pain relief.
(3) The Jowsey regimen uses a combination of sodium fluoride, 40 mg per day, vitamin D, 50 000 units twice weekly, and calcium 1000 mg daily. Fluoride is used to promote osteoblastic activity to give new bone formation into which extra calcium needs to be incorporated. However, the value of this regimen has never been scientifically evaluated and it is of doubtful value.

Many other regimens advocated in the past are now no longer used. Controlled studies (*Medical Journal of Australia*, 1971) have shown that hormonal additives such as anabolic steroids are of little value. Calcium supplements on their own have produced disappointing results.

Paget's disease

Paget's disease of bone occurs in about 3 per cent of people over the age of 40; the pelvis and spine are the most common sites of involvement. Its aetiology is unknown. It occurs about twice as commonly in males as in females, is very rare before the age of 30, and a third of all cases occur after the age of 60. It is characterized by an excessive resorption of bone, followed by an attempt at healing with excessive and abnormal bone formation. This results in abnormal irregular trabecular surfaces with an increase in vascularity and fibrous tissue, and normal compact bone is replaced by a mosaic pattern with widening of the cortex. Since this bone is physically weaker, the normal stresses to which it is subjected lead to deformity.

The onset is insidious and may progress slowly. Many cases are asymptomatic for long periods. Paget's disease may be monostotic or polyostotic, with the lumbar spine the most common area involved. The patient may complain of pain, often made worse by movement. Pain may be deep, dull, aching, and is often worse at night. In a small percentage of patients pain is severe or intractable. Pain may also occur as the result of musculoskeletal complication—for example, bony deformity, kyphosis, nerve-root pain due to bony enlargement into the intervertebral foramen, fracture, basilar invagination, compression of the spinal cord, cauda equina or canal stenosis.

Diagnosis

Typical X-ray changes with increased bone density, disordered trabecular pattern and expanded cortex are necessary to confirm the diagnosis. X-ray changes need to be differentiated from secondary malignant deposits, especially of the prostate or breast, or haemangioma. The serum alkaline phosphatase levels are higher in this disorder than in most other conditions. An increase in urinary hydroxyproline excretion is also found.

Treatment

Specific treatment has only been available over the past few years and three groups of drugs are available. Calcitonin, which inhibits bone resorption; diphosphonates; and RNA inhibitors, such as mithramycin or actinomycin D. These treatments, none of which is completely satisfactory or completely evaluated, are used to relieve severe bone pain.

Osteomalacia

Osteomalacia results from defective calcification of normally produced osteoid tissue, thus producing weakening and structural alterations in adult bone. The disease results from an inadequate supply of calcium or vitamin D, which may result from dietary lack but is more commonly due to intestinal malabsorption or renal disease. Bone pain and tenderness is a common complaint, and radicular pain may occur as a further complication.

The diagnosis is confirmed by the radiological changes and alterations in blood tests. The early X-ray changes showing demineralization of bone are usually indistinguishable from those of osteoporosis, and the softening of bone later leads to the appearance of codfish vertebrae and compression fractures. X-ray of the pelvis may reveal the presence of pathological fractures, the so-called pseudofractures. Blood tests show a low serum calcium and/or phosphate concentration and a raised serum alkaline phosphatase.

Chondrocalcinosis

Chondrocalcinosis is a relatively common condition and is characterized by deposition of calcium pyrophosphate dihydrate crystals in articular cartilage. It occurs most commonly in the large peripheral joints but may also involve the intervertebral cartilage. In peripheral joints it is associated with a chronic form of arthritis and in 25 per cent with an acute attack of synovitis, termed pseudogout. Calcification in the spinal-disc cartilage involves the annulus fibrosus, leading to degenerative changes that may produce marked vertebral changes with a loss of the disc space, often asymmetrical, so that one side of a disc may be markedly narrowed whereas the opposite side of the superior disc may be uninvolved. These may be associated with large, often spoon-shaped osteophytes. A small proportion of patients present with attacks of acute spinal pain responding to anti-inflammatory drugs.

Investigations to confirm the diagnosis include the findings of calcium pyrophosphate crystals on aspiration of the peripheral joints, and X-ray evidence of cartilage calcification in peripheral joints. Investigations to exclude its known metabolic associates, including haemochromatosis and hyperparathyroidism, must be undertaken; these include tests for a serum iron, ferritin and total iron binding capacity, serum calcium and phosphorous, alkaline phosphatase and fasting blood sugar concentrations.

Gout

Gout is a metabolic disease associated with hyperuricaemia, and symptoms occur as the result of deposition of urate crystals in the tissues. The distal joints of the limbs are the site of predeliction for both acute and tophaceous gout and the spine is only rarely involved (Lichtenstein, 1956; Kersley, 1950; Koskoff, 1953; Vinstein and Cockerill, 1972). Despite the rarity of proved cases this is not an uncommonly made diagnosis. A major cause of confusion occurs when a patient with a degenerative condition, e.g. spondylosis, is found to be hyperuricaemic. The finding of

an asymptomatic hyperuricaemia is common (Fessel, 1975) and is insufficient evidence to diagnose gout.

Acromegaly

Acromegaly is caused by a pituitary adenoma, which produces excess growth hormone. This leads to gradual bony enlargement with enlargement of the hands and feet and joint changes due to synovial hypertrophy cartilage overgrowth and recurrent effusions. Spinal hypermobility and a dorsal kyphosis are common (Bluestone *et al.*, 1971). The width of the vertebrae is increased due to apposition of periosteal new bone on the anterior vertebral border and osteophytosis may lead to bony bridging across the vertebral bodies. The height of the discs is also increased.

Ochronosis

This rare genetic disorder of amino-acid metabolism is due to lack of the enzyme homogentisic acid oxidase. As a consequence, homogentisic acid is deposited in musculoskeletal structures, especially the spine (Lagier and Sitaj, 1974). It usually occurs in elderly males who complain of a stiff and aching spine. The typical X-ray findings are a marked narrowing of the intervertebral discs with relatively little osteophyte formation. The discs may be calcified owing to deposition of hydroxyapatite crystals (Bywaters, Dorling and Sutor, 1970). Pigmentation is found in the skin and ear; and the urine turns dark on standing, on alkalinization or on adding Clinitest tablets.

Traumatic and degenerative conditions

Spondylolysis

This is caused by a defect in the pars interarticularis, the narrow strip of bone lying between the lamina and the inferior articular process below and the pedicle and superior articular process above. Its aetiology has been the subject of debate for many years, and three theories have been proposed: that it is due to a congenital defect;

that direct trauma results in a fracture and ultimately non-union; or that indirect trauma results in a stress fracture.

Originally it was believed that spondylolysis was due to a congenital defect. However, this is most unlikely since the ossification centres in the vertebral body and neural arch for the development of the vertebrae do not correspond to the site of this defect. Also, spondylolysis does not appear to be present at birth: Willis (1931) found it in 4 per cent of adult skeletons but never in fetal skeletons. It is quite rare in children under the age of 1 year, although there is an increasing incidence with age up to the age of 50.

However, it appears likely that there is some inherent weakness in the pars, and familial or racial tendencies may play a role in its production. There is some evidence for an increased familial incidence, as it has been described in identical twins. It is also known that marked racial differences occur. In Americans and Europeans it has been reported in approximately 5 per cent of the population (Colcher and Hursh, 1952). Negroes have the lowest reported incidence (2 per cent) but it occurs in one-third of Eskimos aged 40 (Stewart, 1953).

Recent evidence supports the theory that spondylolysis is due to a stress fracture. The pars is subjected to extra stress since it is a pivot between the vertebral body and posterior apophyseal joints. The stress may be accentuated by man's erect stance and lumbar lordosis. In childhood this may occur when the child begins to stand and walk, so that the combination of a lumbar lordosis and the relative restriction in hip extension produces strain on the pars interarticularis.

Spondylolysis is not an uncommon sporting injury and may occur in weight lifters, rowers and fast bowlers. It occurs in right-hand fast bowlers in the pars interarticularis on the left side, and similarly the right pars in left-hand fast bowlers. This would seem to indicate that the stress fracture occurs on the side associated with rotation and extension of the back. Occasionally, no break in the bone is found but there is an elongation of the pars without any separation. This is attributed to repeated stress, which leads to microfractures; as they heal, these produce an elongated appearance of the bone. Spondylolysis also appears to be caused by a stress fracture in patients who have undergone spinal fusion; it then appears in the vertebra above the fused segment (de Palma and Marone, 1959).

Although this condition may be asymptomatic

the patient usually presents because of pain in the lower lumbar region or localized to one side of the spine. Pain may radiate out to the buttock or leg after continuous use of the back. Spondylolysis does not usually produce nerve-root pressure, so that in a patient with spondylolysis who presents with clinical evidence of nerve-root pressure an associated intervertebral-disc prolapse is probably present. Instability of the vertebral segment occurring secondary to the spondylolysis may have been responsible for the disc degenerative changes.

X-rays are necessary to confirm the diagnosis. The defect may be seen in a lateral view, but oblique views of the lumbar spine are usually required to show it clearly (*see Figure 18.3*). The area seen in the oblique view in the normal subject has been likened to the features of a Scotch terrier dog, in which the ears are represented by one superior articular process, the face by the transverse process, the eye by one pedicle seen end on and the forelegs by the inferior articular process. The body of the dog is formed by the lamina, and its tail and hind leg by the opposite articular processes. In spondylolysis the defect in the pars occurs in the region of the dog's neck and resembles a collar placed around the dog's neck.

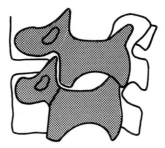

Figure 18.3 An oblique X-ray of the lumbar spine, which has the appearance of a Scotch terrier dog. In the lower segment a spondylolysis through the pars interarticularis appears as a collar around the dog's neck

Spondylolisthesis

Spondylolisthesis is defined as the forward displacement of one vertebral body on its lower neighbour. It was first described 200 years ago by obstetricians who recognized that, in its most severe form, it could lead to obstructed birth. Any vertebra may be involved but the fifth lumbar is the most commonly affected. The degree of spondylolisthesis, measured by the distance the slipped vertebra travels on its lower counterpart, is divided into four degrees: a first-degree slip is a displacement of one quarter of the anteroposterior vertebral body diameter and a fourth-degree slip results from a full-diameter displacement (*see Figure 18.4*).

A major factor in its production is the anatomical structure of the lumbosacral spine. In the standing position there is a constant downward and forward thrust on the lower lumbar vertebrae —especially at the lumbosacral junction, where a 30-degree slope is present—so that the weight of the body and normal movements can predispose to spondylolisthesis in the presence of any mechanical weakness. The potential slip is normally counteracted by a bony hook which consists of the pedicles, the interarticular portion of the neural arch, and the inferior facet; this hooks on the superior facet of the vertebra below. Forward slipping will not occur unless this bony hook becomes deficient. As these supporting structures stretch, the upper vertebral body with its pedicles and superior articular facets slip forward—away from the lower vertebra with its inferior articular facets, laminae and spinous process which remain in their original position. This accounts for the gap, which may be palpable above the affected level on clinical examination.

The five types of spondylolisthesis are: congenital; spondylolytic; traumatic; degenerative; and pathological (Newman, 1974).

Congenital spondylolisthesis

This is twice as common in girls than boys and symptoms usually become evident in the early teens. It occurs as a slip of L5 on S1 and may be associated with spina bifida or other evidence of a congenital dysplasia. These patients may develop a grade 4 spondylolisthesis and so may present with evidence of gross neurological deficit.

Taillard (1976) believed that a gap in the pars is due to a genetic disturbance in ossification. It presents in the years up to adolescence, increasing in incidence until 5 per cent of the population may have the defect at the end of the growth spurt. A familial history is common. Newman (1974) believed that spinal dysraphysim, as occurs in spina bifida, is a major factor. This is present in 10 per cent of the population and may be associated with other developmental abnormalities, such as inadequate development of the upper sacral facets. These cannot then withstand the force thrust on L5 by the body weight.

Spondylolytic spondylolisthesis

Spondylolisthesis may also be due to a bilateral spondylolysis. The L5 vertebra is most commonly involved. The mechanism of origin of spondylolysis has been considered above, and if the same forces continue to operate can lead to a spondylolisthesis. The resulting separation of the pars produces a moderate degree of slipping if it occurs in young adults but marked slipping may be present if it occurs in childhood.

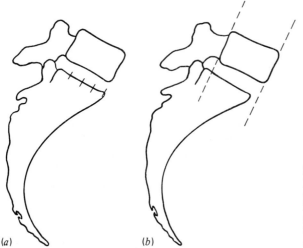

(a)   (b)

Figure 18.4 (*a*) Normally, the posterior margin of L5 is continuous with a line drawn from the posterior margin of the upper sacrum. The upper border of the sacrum is shown divided up into four equal segments. (*b*) Grade 1 spondylolisthesis. The body of L5 slips anteriorly as far as the first division on the sacrum

Traumatic spondylolisthesis

This is rare and may follow major trauma that results in a fracture of the pars interarticularis. It has been reported in parachute injuries or after falls from a roof. There are usually multiple fractures in the vertebral column, especially in the neural arch, which divide the bony hook so that forward slipping of the vertebra can result. The role of trauma in the causation of spondylolisthesis is, however, complicated by several factors. It is not uncommon for patients who have an asymptomatic spondylolisthesis to show symptoms only after injury. Trauma in a patient with a spondylolysis may also result in a spondylolisthesis or, in patients with a known spondylolisthesis, it may increase the degree of the existing slip.

Degenerative spondylolisthesis

This type occurs most commonly at the L4–5 level, is four times as common in women as in men and is not common below the age of 50 years. The degree of slip is usually grade one or two. Anatomical considerations are important in its production. The fourth lumbar vertebra is more mobile than the fifth lumbar vertebra, which tends to be wedged between the iliac bones. The L4–5 intervertebral joint is usually subjected to great stress with consequent degenerative changes in the disc leading to vertebral instability and degeneration in the apophyseal joints, which tend to sublux. Patients with this condition may stand with their lumbar spine in extension, placing further stress on the apophyseal joints.

Pathological spondylolisthesis

This can result from a local or generalized bone disease, which leads to a failure in the integrity of the bony hook in the neural arch. The causes include Paget's disease, tumours and infections.

Clinical findings

The patient presents with back and/or leg pain, which may be related to the effect of the spondylolisthesis on spinal mechanics. These effects vary with the degree of the slip, so that with minimal degrees of slip the effect on surrounding tissues may also be minimal. However, with increasing degrees of spondylolisthesis the soft tissues may be stretched and traumatized. When progres-

sion is gradual a buttress of bone may form at the anterior border of the first sacral segment, so reducing the tendency to slip. The hamstring and back extensor muscles tend to tighten, possibly in an attempt to stabilize the pelvis. Back pain may be due to vertebral instability or recurrent attacks of synovitis in the posterior joints. Sciatica is most commonly due to L5 nerve-root pressure which is usually unilateral, and may arise from:

(1) A pseudarthrosis at the site of the defect in the neural arch. This may produce a hypertrophied mass of fibrous tissue, which protrudes into the intervertebral foramen.
(2) A disc prolapse, either at the same or an adjacent level, may be found (Cyriax, 1976). However, a disc prolapse was found in only seven of 143 patients operated on at the Mayo Clinic (Sullivan, 1964).
(3) Spinal-canal stenosis.

Diagnosis

The diagnosis of spondylolisthesis may be suspected on clinical grounds from the patient's history of low-back pain that is made worse by standing and eased by sitting. On inspection an increased lumbar lordosis and bilateral extensor muscle spasm may be present. Examination may reveal a gap or dimple at one level and a step-like protuberance due to the spinous process of the lower level. The spinal movement most commonly altered is extension, which becomes painfully limited, and other movements are often of full range with pain experienced at the limit of the range. Passive intervertebral pressure applied to the spinous process over the affected level may also reproduce pain. X-rays are necessary to confirm the diagnosis and to assess the degree of the slip.

Management

Spondylolisthesis may at times be asymptomatic and if so requires no active treatment. In symptomatic patients treatment is designed to relieve symptoms, attempt to stabilize the spine and reduce the degree of lumbar lordosis. A radiological reassessment should be carried out periodically, especially in young children. Management also depends on the severity of the patient's symptoms. If pain is severe the patient may require a period of bed rest, with or without traction, local heat and analgesics. If pain is not so severe the patient may need to rest only from those activities known to exacerbate the pain, and the use of a corset may help to produce pain relief.

Treatment with passive-movement techniques are often helpful, especially lumbar traction and mobilization techniques using lumbar rotation. These are always applied gently at first but may be gradually increased in strength, provided that improvement is maintained. Forceful movements are always contraindicated. If symptoms improve exercises are given with a view to improving the patient's posture, together with isometric exercises to the abdominal and extensor muscles to increase the muscular control of the lumbar spine. The patient is instructed in the techniques of back care, described in Chapter 27, which includes avoidance of occupational and postural strains, care with lifting, and weight reduction if the patient is obese.

Surgery is indicated in patients who have a prolonged history of back pain or sciatica; evidence of a spinal-canal stenosis; evidence of cauda equina compression or a progressive lower motor-neurone lesion; or who show rapid progression to a grade 3 or 4 slip. Either an anterior or a posterior spinal fusion or a laminectomy with a decompression of the posterior structures and excision of the hypertrophied mass of fibrous tissue at the site of the defect may be indicated. In patients with spondylolitic spondylolisthesis the bilateral pars defects may be associated with a large pseudarthrosis, which is related to the emerging nerve root. The status of the disc above and below the level of the spondylolisthesis may also need to be assessed with myelography or discography. In patients with spinal-canal stenosis, decompression without fusion may be the operation of choice.

Ankylosing vertebral hyperostosis

This common degenerative condition was first described by Forestier and Rôtes-Querol (1950) as 'senile ankylosing hyperostosis of the spine'. Since then numerous reports have appeared showing that this condition is not confined to older age groups but may occur also in middle-aged patients. Resnick and Niwayama (1976) reported pathological changes in the spinal and extra-spinal structures in this disorder and suggested a more appropriate terminology to be 'diffuse idiopathic skeletal hyperostosis'. It is associated with a laying down of new bone on the anterio-lateral aspect of the vertebrae, which produces bony bridges across the disc space. This may occur in any area of the spine but is most common in the thoracic vertebrae. The sacroiliac joints are radiologically normal but degenerative changes may also occur in the weight-bearing joints.

The diagnosis is confirmed with X-rays, which show exuberant bony masses that have been likened to the flowing of hot wax poured over the anterolateral vertebral surface and which may proceed to complete bridging. These osteophytes occur almost exclusively on the right side of the thoracic vertebrae, the cause of which is unknown but is presumably that the aortic pulsation preserves the left side from similar changes. The vertebral changes occur in the absence of any gross X-ray changes in the disc spaces, apophyseal joints or sacroiliac joints, thus differentiating this condition from spondylosis and ankylosing spondylitis. Excessive bone formation and periostitis also occur around the insertions of extraspinal tendons and ligaments, especially in the pelvis and lower limb. Blood studies—such as a full blood count, ESR and biochemical profile—are normal.

The cause of this condition is unknown but it appears to be a disorder of ossification, since new bone formation is a prominent feature in spinal and extraspinal sites. It has also been suggested that it may be a form of degenerative disc disease with excessive bone production around the vertebral margins. Pathological findings (Vernon-Roberts, 1974) indicated that the original change may be an anterolateral extension of fibrous tissue from the disc, which then turns upwards and downwards underneath the periosteum. This in turn leads to a laying down of periosteal new bone, which produces the typical X-ray appearance.

Clinical findings

The patient presents with back pain and stiffness, although there is little correlation between the symptoms and the X-ray findings and it may be a chance X-ray finding in asymptomatic patients. Nevertheless, most patients are conscious of some degree of pain and stiffness, although it is only rarely severe. The marked degree of spinal stiffness seen in ankylosing spondylitis is not common and many patients with this condition have little loss of functional capacity.

Scheuermann's disease

This disease, of unknown aetiology, is produced by a vertebral epiphysitis. It is more common in males, and occurs in up to 6 per cent of the juvenile population, most commonly in the age group of 12–18 years. The most common site of involvement is the lower thoracic vertebrae, usually around T9, and it is extremely rare above T4. In the lumbar spine there is a decreasing incidence from L1, where changes are common, to L5, where they are rare. It is uncommon for only one vertebra to be involved and in about half of all patients there is involvement of more than five vertebrae.

Its aetiology is unknown. Scheuermann (1921) believed that trauma produced disturbances in the vertebral growth centres. Schmorl (1930) related the condition to fissures in the cartilage end-plate through which the nucleus pulposus herniated, which caused irregular ossification. Excessive use due to work or sport may produce a load beyond the normal capacity of the spine, which could be an initiating or extenuating factor. Persistence of vascular channels in the thoracic vertebrae, which normally disappear at about the age of 6 years, have also been considered to be a predisposing factor.

The relationship of Schmorl's nodes to Scheuermann's disease was investigated by Hilton, Ball and Benn (1976) in a post-mortem study. They suggested that Scheuermann's disease may be an unusually severe expression of Schmorl's nodes and that end-plate lesions arising in adolescence or at an earlier age may predispose the dorso-lumbar spine to disc degeneration in later life.

Clinical features

The condition may be asymptomatic and only a chance radiological finding. The usual complaint is of a mild or moderate degree of pain in the thoracic spine, although occasionally pain radiates to the lower lumbar region. Pain usually follows physical activity, especially if this involves overuse of the spine. It is unusual for a patient to present because of deformity alone.

The typical findings include:

(1) A smooth, rounded dorsal kyphosis that is most evident on forward flexion.
(2) Loss of spinal mobility. There may be a loss of the normal range of flexion and/or exten-

sion and of the passive intervertebral joint range.
(3) Tightness of the hamstring muscles.

Patients may present for the first time after adolescence, and the presumed basis for their pain is associated degenerative changes involving the spinal ligaments and the posterior joints. Stoddard (1972) found a marked association between Scheuermann's disease and later development of low-back pain with disc degeneration. Of 187 patients with vertebral osteochondritis, 102 also had evidence of lumbar-disc degeneration.

X-ray changes

X-ray changes are necessary to confirm the diagnosis; any three of the following changes must be present (*see Figure 18.5*):

(1) Wedging of the vertebral body.
(2) Kyphosis of the thoracic vertebrae or a loss of the normal lumbar curve.
(3) Irregular, narrowed intervertebral-disc spaces.
(4) Schmorl's nodes.

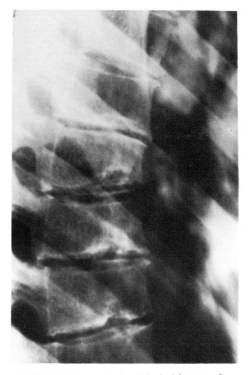

Figure 18.5 The typical radiological features of Scheuermann's disease of the thoracic spine

(5) Mottling and fragmentation of the ring epiphyses.
(6) Irregularity of the vertebral body surfaces.
(7) Disappearance of the upper and lower outer corners of the vertebral body.
(8) The epiphyses becoming dense but the vertebral bodies remaining wedged after repair.

Management

Management in patients who complain of pain consists of:

(1) Rest from activities, including most sports or work that involves bending and lifting if they provoke pain.
(2) Postural correction. This may require only the use of a firm bed and bed-boards. Support in a corset may also be required and, in patients with severe pain, a Milwaukee brace may be indicated; this should be worn for at least 6 months continuously and then intermittently until pain ceases.
(3) Exercises. Postural exercises cannot correct an existing deformity but can help prevent increase in the deformity. They consist of isometric and isotonic exercises, exercises to increase the degree of lumbar lordosis and exercises to stretch the hamstrings.

Spinal infections

The most common cause of infection is staphylococcal infection, which initially involves the disc and then spreads to involve the surrounding bone. This is reflected in the radiological findings in which the disc space is first lost, followed by destruction of the vertebral end-plates. The disease may occur at any age and its onset is often insidious. A primary source of infection, such as a skin or renal disease, may be present. Other causative organisms beside the staphylococcus include streptococcal and coliform organisms, such as salmonella. Chronic granulomatous spinal lesions may be produced by tuberculosis, brucellosis or fungal infections. The other site in the spinal column in which these infections occur is the sacroiliac joint.

Investigations in patients with suspected spinal infections include a full blood count, ESR, blood cultures, serum proteins and electrophoresis, aspiration biopsy of the disc space and specific serum agglutination tests. In staphylococcal infections the white cell count may be elevated or normal and the ESR is invariably high, up to 100 mm in one hour, but blood culture may sometimes be negative. X-rays are taken as a routine measure and tomography of the spine may also be useful.

Treatment consists of bed rest in hospital with adequate doses of suitable antibiotics, such as cloxacillin, 2 g orally five times daily combined with probenicid 500 mg three times daily. As healing becomes established over the succeeding months, the patient is mobilized in a spinal brace while antibiotics are continued for at least 6 months until healing is firm.

Tumours

Clinically, the presence of a spinal tumour may be suspected in several situations, for example:

(1) In a patient who is known to have had a malignancy and now presents with spinal pain. Pain at first is usually localized to the back but compression of nerve roots or the spinal cord may also occur and cause radiation of pain into the limbs.
(2) In a patient over the age of 50 who complains of back or limb pain without a history of a similar previous occurrence.
(3) In a patient with night-time exacerbation of spinal pain.
(4) In a patient whose symptoms are unremitting or progressively worse.

The tumour, either primary or secondary, occurs in the vertebrae more commonly than in the spinal canal. Secondary deposits, which are much more common than primary tumours, originate most commonly from the prostate, breast, kidney, lung and thyroid.

Benign primary bone tumours include haemangioma, aneurysmal bone cyst and osteoid osteoma. Primary malignant bone tumours are quite rare, although marrow tumours—including multiple myeloma or lymphoma—are more common.

Spinal tumours are classified as:

(1) Extradural, such as neuroma, fibroma, lipoma or angioma, which form about 20 per cent of spinal tumours.

(2) Intradural, which may be extramedullary, such as a neuroma, meningioma or sarcoma; intramedullary, such as angioma or glioma.

Neurofibroma may occur singly or multiply as part of Von Recklinghausen's disease. It originates in the spinal nerve root as a smooth or nodular encapsulated growth and is most often intradural but may be extradural or grow outside the spine and produce the so-called 'dumb-bell' tumour.

Investigations

Investigations include X-rays, full blood count, ESR and a biochemical profile that includes serum calcium and alkaline phosphatase levels. X-ray changes do not reveal any involvement of the disc and the vertebral body may collapse with the disc space still intact. This is in contrast to spinal infections, such as tuberculosis, in which a loss of the disc space is invariable. However, the X-ray changes of bone destruction are a late finding, so tomography, bone scanning, CAT scanning, bone biopsy or bone-marrow examination should be performed in doubtful cases. Tomography is especially helpful in the diagnosis of an osteoid osteoma.

19   Spinal pain

Pain felt in the spine may:

(1) Arise locally from spinal structures.
(2) Arise in visceral structures.
(3) Be vascular in origin.
(4) Be psychogenic in origin.

Local spine disease

Pain may be produced by lesions in the discs, bone, apophyseal joints, nerves, ligaments or surrounding soft tissues. These lesions may result from inflammatory, neoplastic, degenerative, traumatic or postural changes.

Pain in disc degeneration

The early stages of disc degeneration are asymptomatic, since no nerve fibres are found within the disc structure. As the disease progresses distortion of the posterior longitudinal ligament may stimulate pain-sensitive fibres of the sinu-vertebral nerve. Pain then is usually felt as a diffuse, dull aching in the lower back, which tends to be relieved by rest and is exacerbated by activity such as bending. Pain may radiate into the lower limbs but at this stage neurological symptoms are absent.

Using discography, Lindblom (1948) showed the posterior longitudinal ligament to be pain sensitive in normal subjects and that severe pain was experienced if the disc was abnormal. As the needle advanced into the disc there was no pain and injection of dye into a normal disc produced only mild back pain. However, injection into an abnormal disc reproduced the patient's back and leg pain. Disturbances of the intervertebral-joint mechanism, resulting in apophyseal-joint and muscular changes, may also be a source of pain.

Prolapse of disc material produces a space-occupying lesion in the spinal canal with pressure on the nerve roots and their dural sleeves. Pain—usually described as severe, sharp and having an unpleasant nagging quality—with sensory changes such as pins and needles or numbness, is distributed along the corresponding dermatome (*see Figure 19.1*). With L4 and L5 nerve-root pressure pain might be expected in theory to be felt predominantly in the distal part of the limb. This does occur clinically in patients whose pain starts distally or whose original back pain disappears to be replaced by distal limb pain. However, it is more common for patients to present with back pain that then radiates down the whole length of the limb and is not necessarily worse distally. A possible explanation is that pain is also referred into the upper leg as a result of pathological changes in the disc and contiguous structures, such as the posterior longitudinal ligament, dura or the dural prolongation along the nerve roots.

During spinal operations under local anaesthesia, traction or pinching—even on normal posterior roots—produces a sensation of severe 'shocking' pain of variable intensity. Indeed in spinal operations, rotation of the cord is limited by traction on posterior nerve roots. If a nerve compressed by a disc prolapse is even lightly touched by an instrument at operation, severe pain is felt in the dermatome and sclerotome distribution of the nerve. This occurs with compressed anterior and posterior nerve roots. Injection of local anaesthetic into the nerve abolishes this pain. When this anaesthetized nerve root is retracted the posterior longitudinal ligament and fibres of the annulus over the prolapsed disc are found to be quite tender and pressure over them still produces pain.

Inflammatory changes

Lindahl and Rexed (1951) reported that in patients with disc prolapse undergoing laminectomy the involved nerve root was often oedematous and severely inflamed even if the prolapse was small. Dilke *et al.* (1973) injected 10 ml of saline around the nerve root to reproduce this inflammatory change and found that all patients reported an exacerbation of pain. The successful use of extradural corticosteroid injections in cases of disc

prolapse may help to relieve this inflammatory oedema. Inflammation may follow chemical irritation from degraded disc material spilling into the extradural space (Marshall and Trethewie, 1973). They reasoned that some of the pain from disc prolapse results from the local chemical irritation of nerve roots from these substances at the site of disc injury. Lactic acid, which is produced under the anaerobic conditions of disc metabolism, may also be a source of chemical irritation (Nachemson, 1975).

Vascular changes

Vascular changes may also play a role in the pain of a disc prolapse. Arterial lesions may lead to ischaemia in the nerve root due to stretching of the nerve root and its dural investment. Alternatively, venous obstruction with dilatation of the epidural and subarachnoid venous plexuses that accompanies disc prolapse may be a cause. Veno-

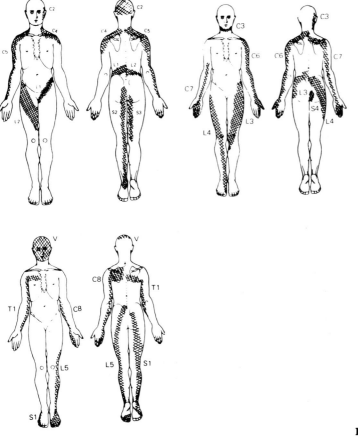

Figure 19.1 Dermatomes

grams of the vertebral plexus performed in these cases show abnormal patterns. This venous congestion may also partly explain the exacerbation of pain that is produced by coughing or straining.

Spondylosis

In spondylosis the spinal mechanics become altered and lead to degeneration and over-riding of the posterior facets. This may be experienced as a dull aching pain that is relieved or exacerbated by posturing the back. The role of the apophyseal joints in the production of pain has been investigated (Mooney and Robertson, 1976). Injections of hypertonic saline into these joints produced typical, diffuse low-back and leg pain. Injections of local anaesthetic relieved these symptoms. Finally, in some patients attacks of severe episodic back pain are produced, presumably by a mechanical derangement of the spinal movements or by a synovitis of the apophyseal joints.

A reflex protective paraspinal muscle spasm is usually found in association with a painful lesion of the intervertebral segment. This spasm itself could evoke painful stimuli by producing abnormal mechanical spinal forces or as the result of prolonged muscular action. There is, however, no direct evidence for this. One possible source of back pain not yet thoroughly investigated is an entrapment neuropathy involving some branches of the posterior primary ramus. It could be that this site of entrapment is in spinal muscles themselves, either as a primary event or after reflex muscle contraction, as described above. Neural plexuses around the blood vessels supplying the muscles could also be involved by a similar process (Wyke, 1970). This could be responsible for some back pain in the later stages of disc degeneration with posterior joint changes.

Pain in other spinal conditions

In inflammatory conditions, such as spondyloarthritis, pain associated with stiffness is typically worse early in the morning. With severe degrees of involvement it may disturb sleep so that the patient may have to get up and walk about. Stiffness eases after a variable period during the day, its duration being dependent on the degree of inflammation present. Although stiffness usually eases during the day it may return after a bout of heavy exercise. In patients with a spinal malignancy, pain is often severe, present by night, and may become progressively worse.

Pain may be aggravated or relieved in certain positions, thus offering a clue to diagnosis. Pain caused by intervertebral-disc prolapse is usually made worse by sitting or straining and is relieved by rest. Pain that intensifies on standing but eases when sitting is more characteristic of spondylolisthesis. Pain made worse by walking and eased by resting occurs in spinal-canal stenosis.

Nocturnal pain that prevents sleep occurs in two separate circumstances. It may indicate inflammatory changes associated with spondyloarthritis, disc prolapse, or tumours; but it is also common in depression. In patients with organic lesions there tends to be a lessening of pain with rest. Patients with psychogenic pain usually report that pain is constantly present and is unrelieved by most therapies, including rest.

Patients with back pain and a fever always require intensive investigations. Causes include infectious disease that produces a discitis or osteomyelitis; subacute bacterial endocarditis; tumours, particularly lymphoma; and a leaking aortic aneurysm. As well as fever, any of these may have an elevated erythrocyte sedimentation rate.

Sciatica

Sciatica is defined as pain in the distribution of the sciatic nerve or its branches that is caused by direct nerve pressure or irritation. It does not include leg pain referred from spinal joints, which has also been referred to by the meaningless phrase 'pseudosciatica'. Sciatica is a common symptom that may be due to pressure on the sciatic nerve anywhere along its course. The vast majority of cases follow an entrapment neuropathy of a nerve root either in the spinal canal or the intervertebral foramen, the most common cause being a prolapsed intervertebral disc. Less common forms of extradural space-occupying lesions include tumour, abscess or haematoma formation.

Some cases of sciatica follow disc degeneration in the absence of a disc prolapse (Macnab, 1973). Although not common, their recognition as a cause of sciatica is essential, if only to avoid operative failures. They include root lesions, which result from bone or ligamentous compression, and adhesive radiculitis. Bony entrapment may occur along the course of the nerve root as it traverses the inner border of the superior articular facet, where the nerve lies in a gutter before passing around the pedicle to emerge through the intervertebral foramen. Ligamentous compression may be produced by pressure from strong extraforaminal ligaments in the presence of the altered vertebral relationships after disc degeneration. Finally, adherent radiculitis may follow the inflammatory changes associated with disc prolapse so that the nerve adheres to the back of the disc.

Pain from visceral structures

In the lumbar area pain may be referred from retroperitoneal, pelvic and intra-abdominal structures. Retroperitoneal causes include disorders of the abdominal aorta or kidneys. Prostatic lesions in males or lesions in the pelvic organs in females are not a common source of back pain. Intra-abdominal lesions include peptic ulcer, pancreatitis and gall-bladder disease. In the thoracic region pleurisy, aortic aneurysm, coronary heart disease or bronchial carcinoma may produce back pain.

For a correct diagnosis an accurate history and general examination is necessary. Most cases of visceral pain will have associated features that should provide a clue, and pain from these lesions should not be made worse by spinal movements. However, it has been recognized for some time that in some patients with visceral disease, such as cholecystitis, an associated area of referred pain and muscle spasm may be found in paravertebral muscles. Indeed, some cases of visceral disease may present with an area of referred somatic pain and the pattern of referred pain from the viscera tends to be consistent, e.g. in cholecystitis. Pressure applied over this area may produce considerable pain. If local anaesthetic is injected into these locally tender areas pain may be relieved, sometimes for surprisingly long periods.

Vascular lesions

Back and buttock pain may occur in patients with an aneurysm of the abdominal aorta or a lesion of the abdominal aorta at its bifurcation, due to atherosclerosis or trauma. Pain may be either constant or of a typically claudicant variety that follows exertion and is relieved by rest. Diagnosis is made on the finding of alterations in the peripheral pulses in the lower limbs, together with a normal spinal examination. Vascular disorders need to be differentiated from spinal-canal stenosis, which may cause a claudicant-type pain.

Psychogenic factors

Psychogenic factors may be important in patients with spinal symptoms and either:

(1) The patient's symptoms may be psychogenically determined; or
(2) The patient with an organic spinal lesion may have a psychogenic overlay to his symptoms.

Their prevalence remains uncertain. Hench and Boland (1946) considered that up to 20 per cent of men attending a rheumatism centre were suffering from non-organic disease. Two subsequent studies on spinal pain have given conflicting results. Collette and Ludwig (1968) studied the specific personality characteristics of patients with backache but were unable to demonstrate any correlation between them. Westrin (1973) showed a high incidence of attacks of low-back pain in patients with psychological problems such as being unhappy in their work or domestic situations and considered that these were related.

It would appear that patients presenting with solely psychogenic low-back pain are uncommon but the influence of psychological factors, such as anxiety and tension, on the patient's reactions would appear to be quite common. Therefore, assessment of the patient with back pain is never completed by establishing a physical diagnosis; psychological and emotional reactions must also be assessed.

A person's body image is derived from the sensory input from the outside world, postural reactions and emotional and subconscious influences. The importance of the back in this image is reflected in many everyday expressions and in the patient's belief that the back is a complex, easily damaged structure.

Diagnosis

The accurate diagnosis of organic musculoskeletal disorders requires considerable expertise in assessing symptoms and signs. An accurate history of the site of pain, its quality, degree, rate of onset, periodicity and modification by such external factors as rest, movement, physical activities and diurnal variations help to establish an organic pattern to their symptoms. Musculoskeletal pain is usually described as being of a dull and aching quality made worse with movement; its site, radiation and behavioural patterns are also consistent. The detection of signs is based on a knowledge of anatomical relationships so that besides eliciting positive, confirmatory signs the recording of relevant negative findings is also important. Thus the presence of organic disease is confirmed by finding signs consistent with the symptoms and by the absence of inconsistent signs.

Psychogenic pain, on the other hand, is often described in terms such as throbbing, numbing, burning, pressure or knife-like; it is generalized or not localized to recognized anatomical sites; its site and radiation are often inconsistent, may be constantly present ('day and night') and unrelieved by most medications ('nothing works with me'). It is often only vaguely described, often with the use of the hands to indicate areas of involvement. The patient may be aware that symptoms are exacerbated at times of increased mental stress. At times they are content to rely on old X-rays or reports to justify their claims rather than on a detailed history of current problems.

Examination may then reveal a lack of consistently positive signs or there may be inconsistent signs, such as a discrepancy between the reported pain and the ability to move the affected parts, or complaints of marked tenderness.

Knowledge of psychological stresses or conflict, loss of a relative or recent domestic trauma can be of real benefit. The usual combination consists of a patient with a basically inadequate personality or with a psychoneurosis who is unable to formalize conflict after a stressful situation by appropriate action or expression. Many patients present a picture of smouldering resentment of their circumstances and it becomes much easier to blame a painful back as the cause of all their trouble.

Anxiety state

Tension associated with an underlying anxiety state is perhaps the most common psychogenic problem. Contributory factors include the patient's family or social situation and, at times, an underlying depression may be present. There is often a family history of arthritis or spondylosis and anxiety that they will eventually become crippled is very acute. Patients complain of musculoskeletal aches and pains, usually present over a long period of time, and have usually been given several non-specific diagnostic labels. Symptoms usually include stiffness, weakness and clicking in the spine; a feeling of exhaustion; lack of well-being; and, often, poor sleep patterns. Previous treatment has usually been with a wide variety of methods, all singularly unsuccessful.

These symptoms are the musculoskeletal expression of the underlying psychic tension and the proposed mechanism to explain them is a prolonged contraction of back muscles, ultimately leading to pain and fatigue. At any rate it is often valuable to give such an explanation to the patient to account for his symptomatology.

Depression

Depressed patients often present with somatic symptoms and musculoskeletal symptoms are common. Pain in the back and leg, often fleeting and accompanied by dysaesthesias, is a common presentation. Patients with neck pain or headache often also complain of strange sensations, usually of feeling as though they are going to faint.

If depression is overt it is usually easy to diagnose; in patients unaware of their depression the term 'masked depression' has been used (López-Ibor, 1972). Disturbances of the sleep pattern— either an inability to get to sleep or awakening early in the morning—aids in the diagnosis, although the patient often blames this on the presence of musculoskeletal pain. The patient may also present as being agitated or restless, and Basmajian (1974) has related this to a persistent hyperactivity in the motor units of their muscles, which may occur even when at rest.

Hysteria

Hysterical patients with back symptoms usually present with camptocormia, derived from the Greek word for 'bent trunk'. The complaint is of an exaggerated back stiffness, usually associated with diffuse lumbar pain and an acutely flexed back, with the arms hanging loosely and eyes directed downwards. This deformity often disappears when the patient adopts a different posture, such as lying down, or on distracting his attention, or on suggestion. Gait may also be bizarre. This condition often follows minor trauma, most often in young males such as army recruits or in workers seeking compensation for the trauma.

In these cases there is often a secondary gain to be obtained by the patient—either as a financial reward or as an emotional advantage in their interpersonal relationships, usually within the family. However, this secondary gain may not be readily obvious.

Malingering

Malingerers are conscious of the fact that their complaint of pain is untrue and are usually involved in medicolegal litigation. The condition is relatively rare and the diagnosis may be difficult to prove. There is often a great difference between the patient's description of pain and length of disability and the nature of the original injury.

Burn's test

The patient kneels on a chair and is asked to bend over to touch the floor with the fingers. In patients with sciatica this is almost always possible to do. If the patient is malingering he announces an inability to touch the floor, or else may tend to overbalance off the chair (*see Figure 19.2*).

Psychogenic overlay

Great difficulty may be experienced in assessing a patient who has, or has had, an organic back lesion but whose symptoms are exacerbated or prolonged by psychological factors. At times this may be more readily appreciated because of impending litigation proceedings, or because the patient uses symptoms to obtain financial or personal gain. Some are able to find the sympathy and attention of their family with complaints of backache, especially if the back needs to be visibly supported in a brace. For these patients, pain and suffering soon become a way of life. With other patients there may be a low pain tolerance, sometimes associated with an inability to accept any form of bodily discomfort. These patients often make excessive use of their hands, both in their description of pain and in the demonstration of its site.

Some problems may be iatrogenically determined, because of the lack of a firm medical diagnosis or prognosis or because of an incorrect use of diagnoses such as 'arthritis' or 'spondylitis'. These patients often present with aged X-rays on which minor osteophytic lipping has been highlighted with arrows drawn by the radiologist and are convinced that their ultimate fate is to be crippled in a wheel-chair.

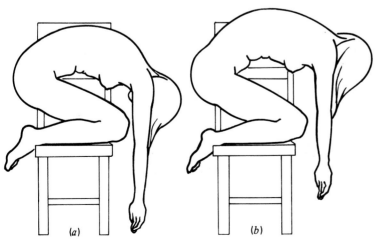

(a) (b)

Figure 19.2 Burn's test. (*a*) A patient with a lumbar-disc prolapse can still touch the fingers to the floor. (*b*) A patient who is malingering often cannot touch the floor or may overbalance

In patients with a psychogenic overlay symptoms are usually out of proportion to signs. Pain is often described as 'agonizing' without the patient exhibiting any obvious degree of suffering. They show inconsistency in either the anatomic relationship ('pain radiates up and down the spine'), its reaction to external factors or in a prolongation of normally expected rates of healing. However, interpretation also requires considerable expertise on the part of the examiner unless many patients with organic disease are to have a psychogenic label placed on them unfairly; examples abound of patients with organic disease, including secondary deposits, who are incorrectly diagnosed as having a psychosomatic disorder.

In testing patients with a psychogenic overlay the examiner utilizes his knowledge of anatomy to assess the consistency of the patient's responses of pain patterns with inconsistent joint findings and the finding of abnormal postures or gait. Some patients, who report that pain is produced during formal clinical testing, may not show such pain later during natural movements such as dressing. Alternatively, the examiner may perform another test without the patient realizing that the same joints and muscle groups are again being stressed. For example, while standing a patient may report that back pain is made worse by spinal extension, yet when the patient lies prone and the legs are extended pain may not be reproduced. In addition, tenderness is often diffuse so that even slight pressure on palpation can provoke an extreme reaction. It is also important to correlate the distribution of pain with inconsistent patterns of joint movements on examination, or any complaint of weakness with the presence or absence of any muscular atrophy.

Management

The management of a patient with psychogenically determined symptoms is often difficult. An accurate diagnosis to enable a firm reassurance of the origin of the patient's symptoms is the first requirement. Considerable time needs to be taken explaining the origin and significance of the symptoms, and the patient should never be told that there is nothing wrong or that the symptoms are imaginary. If symptoms are sufficiently intense a psychiatrist's help should be enlisted at an early stage. Anti-inflammatory drug therapy does not usually produce any great benefit, and physical methods of treatment are contraindicated as they tend to confirm the patient's fears of having an underlying organic basis while at the same time being most unlikely to provide any benefit.

20 Examination of the lumbar spine

The essential feature in the examination of a patient with musculoskeletal pain is that the affected parts should be moved to reproduce the patient's pain. In the peripheral joints tension is applied to the area by the use of active, passive and then resisted movements. In the examination of the spine, active spinal movements provide most information. Accessory movements can be tested directly in peripheral joints but in spinal joints indirect pressures must be applied. When pain can be reproduced during examination the exact degree of pain need not be evoked by these procedures, but it is essential that patients should recognize that the same type of pain is reproduced.

It is helpful to use a printed form with a diagram of the human figure to chart the site and radiation of symptoms. Pain from the spinal joints may be referred to other sites and so it is necessary to determine whether pain and/or restricted movement can be produced by the examination of the movement at the appropriate spinal level. For example, if a patient has buttock pain that is referred from the lumbar spinal joints then lumbar movements must reproduce the buttock pain. Alternatively, if lumbar movements do not reproduce buttock pain then the lumbar origin of the symptoms is unproved. Thus both positive information—of related movements that reproduce pain—and negative information—movements that do not reproduce the pain—are assessed. By these methods it should be possible to determine the site of origin of symptoms.

The nature of the underlying cause may be determined by other clinical findings, such as the history and the development of the disorder, together with ancillary tests, such as X-rays. Some points in the history of the pain that may help to provide a clue to the diagnosis include:

(1) The type of onset of pain, its severity, distribution and characteristics.
(2) Whether pain is constant, intermittent or progressive.
(3) Factors that aggravate or relieve pain—for example, rest, posture, exercise, coughing sneezing, straining and activity.
(4) Whether pain is present at night or only at certain times of the day.
(5) Whether movement is restricted, its relation to pain and any diurnal variation in stiffness.
(6) The presence of neurological symptoms, such as paraesthesias, and their distribution.

The patient's general history, especially of any past spinal symptoms or injury, should then be elicited, as should his type of occupation and the effect of his back trouble on this occupation; any sporting or unaccustomed activities; family history of spinal troubles; the effect of any treatments (such as medication or physiotherapy) and any side effects produced.

The whole of the spine and limbs need to be examined, but for ease of description examination will be divided into each of the three major spinal regions—lumbar, cervical and thoracic areas.

Lumbar spine

(1) Inspection. The patient's posture, build, gait and ability to move freely should be observed and the following assessed:

  (a) Pelvic level.
  (b) Spinal curves.
  (c) Deformities.
  (d) Muscle changes.

(2) Active movements test flexion, extension and lateral flexion. The following are observed:

  (a) Range.
  (b) Rhythm.
  (c) Reproduction and behaviour of pain.
  (d) Presence of an arc of pain.

(3) Auxiliary tests:

  (a) Over-pressure.
  (b) Rapid movements.
  (c) Sustained pressure.
  (d) Quadrant position.

(4) Passive movements:

  (a) Passive physiological range at each joint.
  (b) Accessory movements using pressures against spinous and transverse processes.

(5) Palpation.
(6) Neurological testing:

  (a) Power, sensation and reflexes.
  (b) Straight-leg raising and the femoral-nerve stretch tests.

(7) Sacroiliac joint tests.
(8) General medical examination.
(9) Ancillary tests.

  (a) X-rays.
  (b) Others.

Inspection

Inspection should begin as soon as the patient is met and considerable information may be gained by observing the patient's body build, gait and whether there is a limp. An assessment of whether spinal movements are free or restricted may be obtained by observing the patient getting into or out of a chair and the position that is adopted while sitting.

The patient should then be asked to stand with the back, shoulders and legs exposed for inspection. Good lighting is necessary so that features such as pelvic level, disturbances of spinal curves or other deformities, and intervertebral movements may be observed.

Pelvic level

The pelvic level is first estimated by the examiner standing behind the patient and noting any discrepancy between shoulder and scapular levels on each side or the level of skin creases in the back, buttock folds or posterior knee joints. The examiner's thumbs are then placed over the patient's posterior superior iliac spines with the fingers placed along the iliac crest to compare the relative heights of these two landmarks (*see Figure 20.1*). If any discrepancy between the two levels is noted wooden blocks, graduated in height from 0.5 cm, are placed under the heel of the

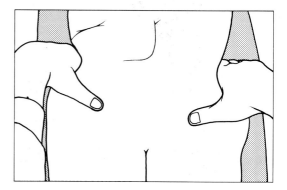

Figure 20.1 Determining the pelvic level in a patient with scoliosis. The fingers are placed along the iliac crests and the thumbs over the dimples of Venus

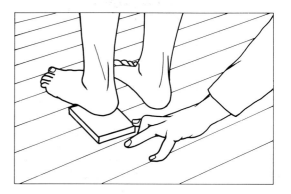

Figure 20.2 The use of blocks of varying sizes in a patient with a shortened left leg

shorter leg until the pelvis and the skin creases are on the same levels (*see Figure 20.2*). An antero-posterior X-ray may show that although the pelvis and leg length are normal the sacral table may not be horizontally level. This would then form the same basis for a scoliosis as would a short leg.

Leg length is measured from the anterior superior iliac spine to the tip of the medial malleolus of the ankle with the patient supine, the pelvis level and the hips in the neutral position. This may be inaccurate, especially in the presence of any pelvic rotation or asymmetry or hip deformity. The theoretically ideal measurement would be from the centre of the normal axis of hip movement. However, since this is sited in the centre of the acetabulum it is impractical, and so the nearby iliac spine is used. This site is lateral to the axis of movement, so any discrepancy in the angle between either of the legs and the pelvis will produce a difference in measurement. Hence the importance of first ensuring that the pelvis is level, with neither hip in an adducted or abducted position.

Normally, with the patient lying supine and both legs in line with the trunk, a line drawn across the two iliac crests is level and indicates that a line bisecting the hips would be at right angles to the pelvis. In addition, when the legs are extended the medial malleoli of both ankles should lie at the same level. These measurements can readily be made during inspection and palpation of the bony landmarks. If the pelvic level appears to be tilted an attempt should be made to set the pelvis square by moving the legs so that they lie in line with the trunk. The pelvis may then be seen to rotate. However, it is impossible to correct this pelvic tilt if a fixed adduction or abduction deformity of the hip is present. Accordingly, if one hip lies in a position of fixed adduction or abduction the other hip must then be placed at a similar angle before making the measurement. As an alternative method, apparent shortening may be estimated by measuring from the umbilicus to the medial malleolus of each ankle and noting the difference between these two distances.

Pelvic X-rays may provide the most accurate method of assessing leg length (Clarke, 1972), provided that scrupulous attention is paid to accurate positioning of the patient and the X-ray apparatus. The patient stands in front of a vertical Bucky diaphragm, weight taken equally on both feet 15 cm apart, and a plumbline of radio-opaque wire is suspended from a stand immediately in front of the patient to act as the vertical axis on the film. The pelvis is X-rayed so that the hip levels may then be assessed.

Leg shortening of 6 mm or less should not be regarded as a cause of symptoms; many asymptomatic patients have a difference of up to 12 mm in their leg lengths.

Spinal curves

The development of the normal curves in the lumbar, thoracic and cervical spines is observed with the patient standing. The degree of lumbar lordosis is determined by the lumbosacral angle, which is the angle of inclination that the upper border of the sacrum forms with the horizontal plane and is normally about 30 degrees (*see Figure 20.3(a)*). In the lumbar spine the lordosis may be increased, decreased or reversed (kyphosis).

An increased lordosis results from an increase in the normal lumbosacral angle to greater than 30 degrees. This causes the pelvis to tilt forwards, and to compensate the lumbar lordosis is increased (*see Figure 20.3(b)*).

A decrease in the normal lumbar lordosis is

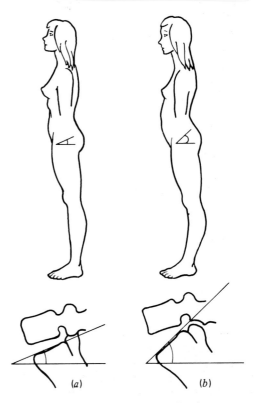

Figure 20.3 (*a*) The normal degree of lumbar lordosis is determined by the angle formed at the lumbosacral joint, the lumbosacral angle.
(*b*) Excessive lordosis is associated with an increase in the lumbosacral angle above 30 degrees

usually associated with the presence of marked paravertebral muscle spasm.

Lumbar kyphosis may be either localized or generalized. A localized lumbar kyphosis produces a posterior angular deformity, which is most often due to a localized bony abnormality such as a collapsed vertebra. A generalized lumbar kyphosis is usually associated with a protective muscle spasm and lumbar extension is then restricted. Scheuermann's disease is characterized by the presence of a smooth thoracic kyphosis, accentuated on forward flexion. In older patients a lumbar kyphosis may be due to spondylosis, ankylosing spondylitis, or metabolic bone diseases such as osteoporosis.

Scoliosis, a lateral curvature of the spinal column, is assessed by noting any lateral deviation from a line drawn between the spinous processes from T1 and the midline of the sacrum. Scoliosis may be either ipsilateral or contralateral, according to the relationship of the displacement of the patient's thorax to the painful side. An ipsilateral scoliosis is a lateral displacement of the patient's thorax towards the painful side. The cause of scoliosis may be structural, compensatory, or protective. With structural scoliosis the lateral curvature is associated with a vertebral rotation, and both the curve and the rotation become more accentuated on forward flexion. A compensatory scoliosis commonly develops in patients with a discrepancy in the pelvic level as the result of inequality of leg length (*see Figure 20.4*).

Scoliosis associated with a disc prolapse is protective in nature since it represents an attempt to decrease the tension on the nerve root. Other names for this protective scoliosis are antalgic or sciatic scoliosis. The term sciatic scoliosis is really a misnomer since a similar deformity may be present in a patient with central-back pain without leg pain. Its mechanism of production, however, is not clearly understood, as this finding may occur in patients with an acute mechanical derangement of an intervertebral joint without any definite evidence of a disc prolapse. For these reasons the term 'protective list' has also been used to describe this deformity. The relationship of these deformities to spinal movements will be considered later.

Other deformities

In advanced osteoporosis the patient loses height and the costal margins may impinge on the pelvic rim. A severe degree of spondylolisthesis may be suspected if any disparity in the skin creases, an increased lumbar lordosis or a palpable 'step' in the lumbar spine is found (*see Figure 20.5*).

Muscle changes

Paravertebral muscle spasm may be either unilateral or bilateral and is usually present due to a reflex protective mechanism. The spasm may be obvious on inspection, when it stands out as a prominent muscle band to the side of the spinous processes. Muscle spasm which is present on standing may increase, decrease or disappear during active spinal flexion or extension movements. At times spasm may become evident only during

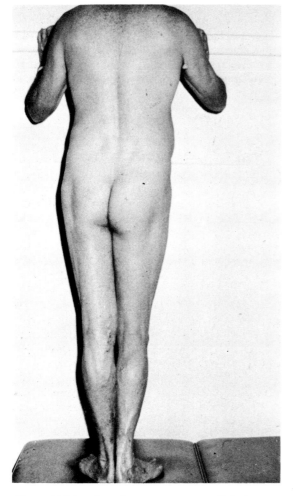

Figure 20.4 A patient with a compensatory scoliosis due to a short right leg. Note also the asymmetry of the buttock folds

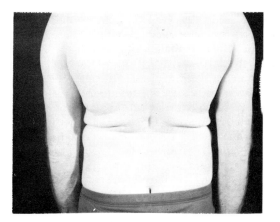

Figure 20.5 Abnormalities in the skin folds in a patient with spondylolisthesis

these movements. In patients with nerve-root pressure and lower motor-neurone lesions, muscle wasting and fasciculation may be seen in the buttock or leg.

Active movement

The patient, while standing as relaxed as possible with the feet together and the hands by the side, should first be asked whether any symptoms are felt in this position. Active lumbar spinal movements should then be performed to assess:

(1) The range of movement.
(2) Any disturbances of rhythm.
(3) Reproduction and behaviour of pain.
(4) The presence of an arc of pain.

These factors are usually assessed simultaneously as the patient moves. For example, while testing vertebral movements the examiner should also watch the body contours and spinous processes carefully to observe whether the spinal joints unroll rhythmically and evenly or whether there is any localized restriction of the movement in the spinous processes between two or three vertebrae. However, for ease of description these factors will be considered individually.

The patient is asked first to flex the spine by bending forwards to attempt to touch the toes with the knees kept straight and the feet together. However, much of this forward movement also takes place in the hips. Active movement into spinal extension is next tested followed by active lateral flexion to each side. Active rotation is not routinely tested in the lumbar spine, as most of this movement takes place in the thoracic spine.

Range of movement

The range of forward flexion may be assessed by measuring the distance that the patient's fingertips reach from the floor. Although a patient may be able to compensate for lumbar stiffness by flexion of the hips, the lumbar spine in this position will nevertheless have been flexed to the limit of its available range of flexion. The normal range of flexion shows wide individual variation but is usually taken to be 75–90 degrees.

Extension is tested next by asking the patient to arch the spine backwards, increasing the normal lumbar lordosis. The range of this movement is approximately 20 degrees.

The range of lateral flexion is assessed by asking the patient to slide the fingers down the leg and noting the position of the fingers to the knee. The examiner must be careful to ensure that the patient does not move the spine into slight flexion or extension during this manoeuvre. The normal range of this movement is approximately 25 degrees.

ALTERATION IN RANGE
The range of movement may be normal, decreased or increased. The normal range depends on the patient's age and build, so that it is always necessary to establish the usual distance the patient could flex before the onset of his disorder.

Restriction in range may be due to pain or stiffness and may be associated with muscle spasm. In intervertebral-disc prolapse, flexion (or less often extension) is usually painful and limited, whereas lateral flexion usually remains normal.

In lumbar spondylosis, ankylosing spondylitis or osteoporosis, movement may be diminished in all directions. Hypomobility syndromes may be suspected if there is limitation of movement in one or two directions only. Their usual pattern in the lumbar spine is of reduced lateral flexion, associated with limitation of either extension or flexion.

The range of movement may also be increased. In spinal hypermobility the patient may be able to flex sufficiently to place the back of the hands on the floor or the head on the knees.

Rhythm

These movements are again repeated while watching for any disturbance of the normal smooth rhythm. If the patient's pain is not severe repeated movements can also be used to detect any disturbance in their normal rhythm. This may be evidenced by a distortion or loss of intervertebral-joint movement, or else as a change in the normal contour.

The pattern of spinal movement in flexion and lateral flexion is best viewed by standing behind the patient. While observing lumbar extension it is preferable to kneel behind the patient and support the shoulders to prevent overbalancing (*see Figure 20.6*).

Normal rhythmical lumbar movement during forward flexion is comprised of a synchronous unrolling of each intervertebral level. At the same time

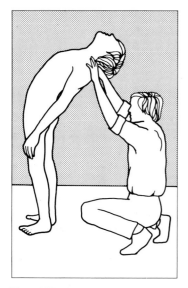

Figure 20.6 Observing lumbar extension

the normal lordosis becomes flattened until on full flexion there is a slight reversal of this curve, resulting in a continuous smooth convex lumbar and thoracic curve (*see Figure 20.7*). Simultaneously, a synchronous movement of the pelvis produces an increase in the lumbosacral angle, posterior displacement of the hips and rotation of the pelvis around the hips.

During lateral spinal flexion the normally mobile spine develops a C-shaped curve. Any restriction of intervertebral-joint movement sufficient to produce a flattening of this normal C-shaped curve may be of considerable significance, especially if it is associated with reproduction of the patient's pain (*see Figure 20.8*).

A scoliosis or kyphosis present on standing may have its contours altered on movement. Several different patterns of spinal deformity may now be produced and their presence can be detected by inspection during active spinal flexion and extension:

(1) Scoliosis present on standing may become more marked during the forward flexion movement.

(2) Scoliosis may only become evident during forward flexion.

(3) Scoliosis present on standing may disappear on forward flexion.

(4) Scoliosis that alternates from side to side may appear on forward flexion.

(5) There may be an arc in the middle range of forward flexion during which scoliosis appears, only to disappear on further movements.

(6) On forward flexion the extensor muscles on both sides may display marked reflex con-

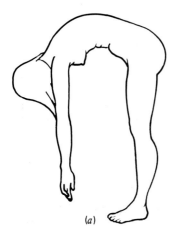

(a)

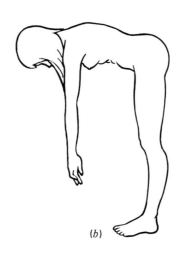

(b)

Figure 20.7 (*a*) Forward flexion is normally accompanied by a loss of the normal lumbar lordosis and a smooth curve between the lumbar and thoracic spines. (*b*) Forward flexion in a patient with restricted movement in the lumbar joints accompanied by persistence of the lumbar lordosis and loss of the normal smooth curve

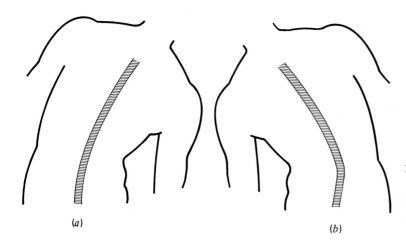

(a)

(b)

Figure 20.8 (*a*) Lateral flexion to the right is normal and accompanied by a smooth spinal curve. (*b*) Lateral flexion to the left is abnormal due to a limitation of movement at one lumbar spinal segment

traction, holding the spine rigid in a position of lordosis.

Reproduction of pain

If there is no pain while standing the patient is asked to move into the various directions being tested until pain is felt. If pain is present while standing at rest the patient should be asked to bend only until the pain begins to increase. The range of this movement is noted. If at this stage pain is not severe, or no distally referred pain is produced, the patient is asked to move further into the range and report any difference in severity, site or distribution of symptoms, such as an increase in severity of pain or an increased area of referral. Should pain become too severe or be referred distally the movement is stopped and the patient returned to the upright position. Otherwise, the patient continues to move to the limit of the available range and reports any changes in symptoms.

An arc of pain

Pain may be experienced only at one point in the range. One typical pattern is for the patient to stand without pain, but during forward flexion pain may be experienced at the mid range of the movement and then it disappears on further flexion. Alternatively, pain may be appreciated only on standing up straight from the forward-flexed position.

It is quite common to observe that a scoliosis develops at this same point in the range, although at times this may be painless for the patient. The presence of such a painful arc usually indicates an organic lesion of the intervertebral joint segment, such as vertebral instability.

Auxiliary tests

In most patients with symptoms arising from the lumbar spine, the tests described above are sufficient to reproduce symptoms. If not, and if it remains possible that the lumbar spine is the site of the symptoms, four additional manoeuvres should be used and assessed:

(1) Over-pressure is applied to the spine by the examiner at the end of the painless range. This is controlled by producing small oscillatory movements at this limit of range. Besides possibly reproducing the patient's symptoms, this movement also allows the examiner to determine the end-feel of the movement.
(2) Rapid movements: if pain is not provoked on normal spinal movement it may be helpful to repeat these test movements quickly. As an example, pain and muscular spasm may be reproduced only when the patient is directed to bend forwards quickly.
(3) Sustained pressure. This is applied for approximately 10 seconds with the lumbar spine first in extension and then in lateral flexion towards the painful side to determine if sustained pressure in this position can reproduce back or leg pain. This may also sometimes occur when the pressure is released.
(4) The quadrant position. This passive-movement test is designed to position the joint under maximum stress. For the lumbar spine it is found by passively moving the patient first into full lumbar extension, followed by lateral flexion and rotation towards the side

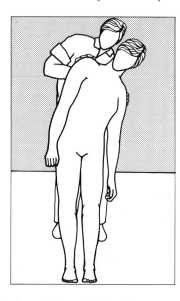

Figure 20.9 Quadrant test for the lumbar spine

of pain. This position results in maximal reduction in the size of the intervertebral foramen (Maitland, 1976).

The quadrant test: method (*see Figure 20.9*)

The examiner stands behind the patient and to one side. The patient is first moved to the limit of extension. This movement may be controlled by the examiner holding the patient's shoulder and having his shoulders positioned near the patient's occiput to take the weight of the head. Over-pressure is applied at the limit of this range and the patient guided into the quadrant position by laterally flexing and then rotating the spine towards the side of pain. This movement is continued until the limit of the range is reached, and the patient is asked whether pain is reproduced.

Passive movements

There are two distinct passive movements tested at each of the intervertebral joints.

(1) The passive range of physiological movements at each individual spinal joint is tested by the examiner producing the physiological spinal

movements with one hand and feeling the movement between adjacent bony spinous processes with the fingers of his other hand.

(2) The spinal accessory movements are tested by exerting pressure, first over the patient's spinous processes and then over the transverse processes.

These passive intervertebral movements can be used to assess the range of movement, reproduction of pain, the behaviour of the pain throughout the range of movement, the presence of any muscular spasm, and the end-feel of the movement.

Passive physiological movement

In the lumbar spine the physiological movements of flexion and extension, lateral flexion, and rotation are tested by passive movements and palpated to appreciate the passive movement of each individual joint. This is achieved by the examiner moving the intervertebral joint through a full range while palpating between adjacent bony prominences and comparing the movement obtained at each level. The ability to assess normal or abnormal movement by these means requires considerable practice to obtain a sense of 'feel' for this movement.

FLEXION–EXTENSION
These movements may be tested using either one or two legs of the patient but it is generally easier to use only a single leg, and this method will be described.
Starting position   The patient lies on the right side with the underneath right leg in a position of slight flexion at the hip and knee. The examiner stands in front of the patient's upper chest facing towards the hips. The left forearm is placed across the thorax so that the fingers of the left hand can palpate between the lumbar spinous processes, and the thorax is stabilized between the left arm and the left side. The patient's upper (i.e. left) leg is then grasped below the knee with the examiner's right hand (*see Figure 20.10*).
Method   Flexion and extension of the lumbar spine are produced by flexing and then releasing the flexion of the patient's left leg at the hip. The middle finger of the examiner's left hand in the interspinous space can feel the movement of flexion and extension as an opening and closing of the interspinous gap. The movements of flexion and extension should be stretched to their limits, and an opening and closing of the interspinous gap can

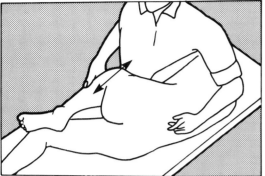

Figure 20.10 Passive testing of flexion–extension in the lumbar spine

be felt with the rocking of the patient's pelvis and leg.

LATERAL FLEXION

Starting position The patient lies on the right side with hips and knees flexed so that the lumbar spine is relaxed midway between flexion and extension. The examiner, standing in front of the patient, reaches across the patient's left side, his left forearm along the spine pointing towards the feet, and his right forearm grasping under the patient's ischial tuberosity. The pad of his left middle finger is placed facing upwards in the underside of the interspinous space to feel the bony margins of the adjacent vertebrae (*see Figure 20.11*).

Method By grasping the patient's pelvis and upper thigh with his right forearm and right side the examiner laterally flexes the patient's lumbar spine from below upwards by rocking the pelvis. This is achieved by pulling with the right forearm so that the patient's left ilium moves

cephalad. The pelvis is then returned to its mid position by the examiner pushing against the patient's upper left thigh with his right side. This oscillatory movement rocks the pelvis around the fulcrum of the underside hip and femur so that lateral flexion is easy to produce and palpate.

ROTATION

Although testing the active range of lumbar rotation does not provide much information, testing the small range of passive rotation is often of value.

Starting position This is similar to that used for testing lateral flexion and the examiner checks to make sure that the patient's top knee can slide freely forwards over the underneath knee. The examiner leans across the patient and places his left forearm along the back to palpate the interspinous space from underneath, while twisting slightly to face the patient's hips. He holds over the patient's left trochanter with his right hand, the heel of his hand anterior to the trochanter with all fingers spread out behind it (*see Figure 20.12*).

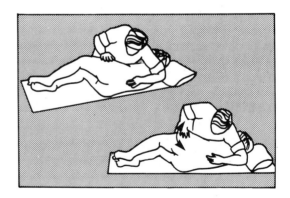

Figure 20.12 Passive testing of rotation in the lumbar spine

Method The examiner stabilizes the patient's thorax with his left arm. He then pulls the patient's pelvis towards him with his right hand so that the left side of the pelvis and lumbar spine rotate forwards. The palpating finger needs to keep pace with this movement so that the displacement of the distal spinous process from the proximal one can be easily felt. The pelvis is then returned to its original position by the heel of the examiner's right hand and forearm.

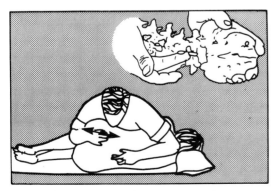

Figure 20.11 Passive testing of lateral flexion in the lumbar spine

Accessory movements

A passive movement may be produced at each intervertebral spinal joint when pressure is applied by the examiner against the patient's bony vertebral processes. The normal types of movement present can be appreciated after some practice and depend upon the presence of a normal range of spinal accessory movements. They are, therefore, an indirect method of testing these accessory movements. These tests are used not only to demonstrate a restriction in the accessory movements but also to determine the intervertebral-joint level that is at fault and responsible for the patient's symptoms by demonstrating the particular movement or movements that are painful or restricted.

Attention to detail is mandatory. To achieve the correct movement, posteroanterior and transverse pressures are applied by the examiner with the thumb or through the pisiform bone of the hand, firstly over the spinous and next the transverse processes. This pressure is used to produce an oscillatory movement, which needs to be applied at the correct speed to appreciate the movement of one vertebra in relation to the adjacent one. If the pressure is applied either too quickly or too slowly vertebral movement will not be clearly appreciated. Pressure need only be light and is applied and relaxed two or three times a second. At first the pressure is only applied extremely gently, two or three times. Provided that no pain is produced the amplitude and depth of this movement is increased further and repeated for another two or three times. This movement should then be repeated to a greater depth until either a painless normal range can be demonstrated, or else pain with or without any restriction of the movement is encountered.

METHOD

The patient lies prone, with his arms by his side and the head turned to one side. The three basic manoeuvres are:

(1) Posteroanterior pressure against the spinous process.
(2) Transverse pressure against the lateral surface of the spinous process.
(3) Posteroanterior pressure against the transverse process.

However, each of these can also be varied as follows:

(1) Posteroanterior pressure can be inclined either at the inferior margin of the spinous process towards the patient's head or at the superior margin towards the feet (*see Figure 20.13(a)*).
(2) Transverse pressure against the lateral surface of the spinous process can also be inclined towards the patient's head or feet (*see Figure 20.13(b)*). Similarly, the transverse direction can be inclined in varying directions and degrees until it becomes applied in a posteroanterior direction.
(3) Posteroanterior pressure over the transverse process may be varied either by directing the direction of the pressure towards the patient's head or feet, or else by directing it in a medial or lateral direction (*Figure 20.13(c)*).

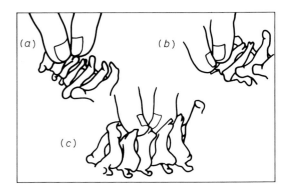

Figure 20.13 Passive intervertebral movement. (*a*) Posteroanterior pressure over the spinous process may be inclined in a cephalad or caudal direction. (*b*) Transverse pressure against the spinous process may be directed either laterally or inclined until it becomes a posteroanterior pressure. (*c*) Posteroanterior pressure over the transverse process may be inclined either medially or laterally

FINDINGS

Testing of these passive intervertebral-joint movements is essential in the assessment of painful spinal conditions. A lesion of the intervertebral joint complex is present if there is restriction of these movements associated with reproduction of the patient's symptoms or if local pain is produced at an appropriate joint. This is particularly relevant in hypomobility syndromes, where the essential clinical finding is a loss of such movement. In addition, the finding of a restricted movement will also indicate the type of mobilization therapy to be used.

These procedures may elicit pain, restricted movement and/or spasm. Pain may be felt at any stage in the range—it may be present at rest or at the limit of the range. Usually the intensity and distribution of pain increases with increasing movement; but it may vary also in that if it starts early in the range it may not worsen with increased movement. If the range of movement is limited the type of resistance, which is due to either a sense of tightness or of muscle spasm, is then assessed. Spasm may be such that little movement is possible, or it may be associated only with a slight limitation of the full range.

Palpation

The spinous processes are most readily palpable, especially on flexion of the spine; L1 and L2 are often the most readily identified because of their shape. The transverse processes can usually be palpated if the patient lies prone and relaxed, unless the overlying muscles are too thick. The body and spinous process of L4 usually lies in the line that joins the tops of each iliac crest. Palpation may detect any alteration in the bony alignments, such as spondylolisthesis.

The sacroiliac joint is not accessible throughout its extent to palpation, but its midpoint lies some two fingers lateral to the posterior superior iliac spine at approximately the second sacral segment level. On each side of the body the subcutaneous iliac crest ends at the posterior superior iliac spine and may be identified by an overlying skin dimple ('the dimple of Venus').

The presence of any muscle spasm may be felt, with the patient lying prone and relaxed, by a gentle transverse movement of the examiner's finger over the paraspinal muscles. Any areas of tenderness are usually felt over the interspinous ligament of the involved intervertebral joint or to one side of the joint. Thickening of soft tissue in the interspinous spaces is a regular finding in chronic disorders, the degree and quality of thickening being proportional to the duration of the disorder. Areas of tenderness in muscles or in relation to the iliac crest and posterior iliac spines are usually non-specific, and the area over the transverse process of L1 and L2 is often tender in normal patients. If each spinous process is tapped sharply with a tendon hammer or finger-tips pain may be provoked over the painful joint. Finally, the examiner palpates over the course of the sciatic nerve from the sciatic notch to the popliteal fossa.

Neurological testing

A thorough neurological examination to detect the presence of any sensory, motor and reflex change is necessary, not only because the patient may be unaware of any neurological deficit but also as a baseline for determining any future changes. Note is made of any gait disturbance, muscle wasting or fasciculation. Sensory disturbances are sought in the dermatome distribution of the lumbosacral nerves.

In general, isometric tests are used to test for any muscle weakness that may result from nerve-root compression. Although each nerve root supplies more than one muscle and most muscles have more than one nerve-root supply, none the less most muscles are supplied predominantly by one root. Those of clinical significance are listed in *Table 20.1*. However, plantar flexion of the foot cannot be adequately tested by an isometric contraction. Instead, weakness of plantar flexion will become evident if the patient stands on one leg and, with the knee in full extension, raises himself up onto the toes at least six times. Similarly, weakness of ankle dorsiflexion will become evident if the patient attempts to walk on his heels and then has difficulty in raising the foot or balancing. The girth of the limbs above and below the knee is measured by a tape measure to record any muscle wasting. Reflexes include the knee jerk (L3 and L4) and ankle jerk (S1 and S2), and plantar responses are tested for any evidence of an upper motor-neurone lesion.

Straight-leg raising and the femoral-nerve stretch are important tests and will be considered in detail.

The straight-leg raising test

The presence of a disc prolapse may produce stretching and pressure on the affected nerve root in its dural sleeve. While the patient is lying supine or if he raises the affected leg by flexing the hip and knee the nerve root is not subjected to any increase in tension. However, when the affected leg is elevated passively with the knee extended the inflamed nerve root is then put under increased tension as it moves in the invertebral foramen. In almost all patients with invertebral-disc prolapse producing L4, L5 or S1 nerve-root pressure, the range of straight-leg raising is reduced. It is, moreover, an objective sign, as the decrease in the range of the leg movement

Table 20.1   Isometric tests of the lumbar spine

Movement	Muscle	Nerve root	Isometric tests
Hip flexion	Iliopsoas	L2	The patient lies supine and holds the flexed hip and knee at 90 degrees while resistance is applied just above the knee
Knee extension	Quadriceps	L3	The examiner threads one arm under the patient's lower thigh to place his hand on the opposite thigh. While the patient holds the leg just short of the fully extended position resistance is applied against the front of the leg, just above the ankle
Ankle dorsiflexion and inversion	Tibialis anterior	L4	The patient holds the foot in dorsiflexion and inversion while the examiner applies resistance against the dorsomedial surface of the proximal end of the first metatarsal
Great toe extension	Extensor hallucis longus	L5	The patient holds the foot and toes dorsiflexed whilst resistance is placed against the nail of the big toe
Extension of toes	Extensor digitorum longus	L5 and S1	The patient holds the foot and toes dorsiflexed whilst resistance is applied against the dorsal surface of all toes
Ankle eversion	Peroneus longus and brevis	S1	The patient is asked to keep the heels together with the soles of the feet twisted away from each other. Resistance is applied against the lateral borders of the feet, pushing them together
Knee flexion	Hamstrings	L5 and S1	The patient holds the knee flexed to 90 degrees while resistance is applied behind the patient's heel
Hip extension	Gluteus maximus	L4 and L5 S1 and S2	The patient lies prone and holds the hip extended with the knee bent while the examiner applies a downwards resistance just above the knee with one hand, palpating the gluteal mass with the other hand to assess firmness
Plantar flexion	Gastrocnemius	S1	The patient stands on one leg and raises himself up onto the toes through a full range six times
Flexion of toes	Flexors digitorum and hallucis longus	S2	The patient holds his toes fully flexed whilst resistance is applied against the palmar surface of all toes.

correlates well with the degree of nerve-root involvement (Charnley, 1951). To be considered positive, it is also essential for this test to reproduce the patient's pain.

METHOD
A set clinical routine should always be followed, and at all times extreme gentleness is required.

(1) The patient lies supine and each leg is tested separately.
(2) To ensure that hip-joint movements are normal the hip should be passively flexed and rotated.
(3) The straight-leg raising test is initially performed on the painless side. The patient's hip is first placed in a slight degree of adduction and medial rotation. The leg is then passively lifted by the heel with one hand while the knee extension is maintained with the other hand. The range of movement of the normal side is estimated and may vary with age, joint

mobility and the degree of natural hamstring tightness. This range is usually 90 degrees but may vary from 70 to 120 degrees. The height of the leg raise is usually measured by estimating the angle that the leg forms with the horizontal; the distance of the malleolus from the bed may also be measured. This movement is normally painless, except for a possible sensation of tightness behind the thigh or knee. However, while this test is being carried out pain may at times be experienced in the affected leg (Woodhall and Hayes, 1950). Its mechanism will be discussed later.

(4) The leg on the affected side is then lifted by the heel while the knee is kept fully extended and the hip in slight adduction and slight medial rotation. The pelvis is not allowed to rise or rotate (*Figure 20.14 (a)*). The test movement is continued until pain and/or paraesthesias commence, and their distribution

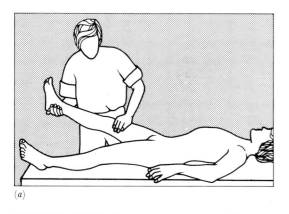

(a)

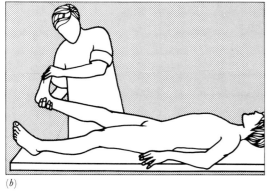

(b)

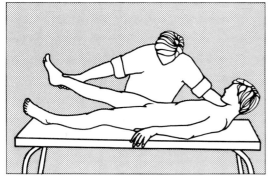

(c)

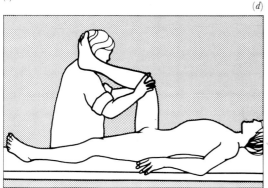

(d)

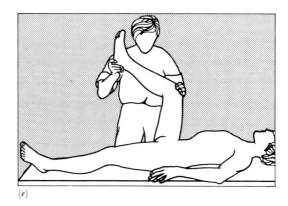

(e)

Figure 20.14 (*a*) The straight-leg raising test. Straight-leg raising is reduced in the right leg. (*b*) Pain is increased by passive dorsiflexion of the foot. (*c*) Pain may also be reproduced by lowering the leg and passively flexing the neck. (*d*) Popliteal compression test. (*e*) Lasègue's test

should conform to the patient's symptoms. The range of this movement is then estimated.
(5) If the foot of the affected leg is now passively dorsiflexed the patient's pain should be exacerbated as the nerve root is further stretched. This test confirms that pain is not being produced by ligamentous or muscle pull (*see Figure 20.14 (b)*).
(6) Other tests increasing tension on the nerve root and other pain-sensitive structures in the vertebral canal to reproduce the patient's pain include:

(a) Neck flexion: the affected limb is elevated, as described above, to a position just short of that producing pain. If the patient now flexes the neck the leg pain may be reproduced (*see Figure 20.14 (c)*).
(b) Popliteal fossa compression: the limb is elevated to an angle that is just short of producing pain. The knee is then slightly flexed and supported on the shoulder of the examiner, who then applies pressure over the popliteal fossa with both of his thumbs. The patient's pain should again be reproduced (*Figure 20.14 (d)*).
(c) Lasègue's sign: this test is performed with the patient supine and the hip and knee flexed to 90 degrees. The knee is then passively extended until pain is reproduced (*Figure 20.14 (e)*).

Straight-leg raising tests the free movement of the lower lumbar (L4 and L5) and the upper sacral (S1 and S2) nerve roots together with their dural sleeves within the spinal canal and their intervertebral foramen. While this test is being carried out, after the first few degrees of elevation of the leg, the sciatic nerve begins to move in the sciatic notch. During the first 30 degrees of movement the lumbosacral cord is moving but the nerve roots are still stationary. Beyond 30 degrees, the hip acts as a pulley to apply traction to the sciatic nerve and from about 35 to 70 degrees the nerve roots will move in the intervertebral foramen. The range of movement in the nerve roots was measured by Goddard and Reed (1965) as 1.5 mm in the fourth lumbar, 3 mm in the fifth lumbar and 4 mm in the first sacral root.

Accordingly, in patients with a disc prolapse that impinges on one of these nerve roots and their dural sleeve, traction on the nerve root during this test will reproduce their sciatic pain. On straight-leg raising the pelvis rotates slightly at first, followed by a movement in the lumbar joints. Hence lesions of these joints, as in cases of ankylosing spondylitis, may produce pain or limitation of the range of straight-leg raising. The restriction in the range of movement may be rendered even more pronounced by the hamstring spasm that usually accompanies these lesions. Furthermore, Fisk (1975) has demonstrated that straight-leg raising may be limited in patients who have back pain associated with marked back-muscle spasm alone.

Hakelius and Hindmarsh (1972) in a large series of surgical cases demonstrated an inverse relationship between the degree of restriction of leg movement and the degree of change present at operation. Edgar and Park (1972) demonstrated a relationship between the position of the disc prolapse and the site of pain felt at the limit of straight-leg raising test. Thus if back pain alone was produced at this limit then a central prolapse was liable to be found at operation. If leg pain alone was produced then a lateral disc prolapse was usually found. Should back and leg pain be produced the prolapse was found to be intermediate in position.

A negative straight-leg raising test is found only rarely in the presence of a lumbar intervertebral-disc prolapse. It may be found with a lateral-disc prolapse into the intervertebral foramen, canal stenosis, or root atrophy; or after migration of loose disc fragments into a different region of the neural canal.

The crossed straight-leg raising test

While testing straight-leg raising, pain may at times be exacerbated in the affected leg while the opposite non-painful leg is being lifted. This occurs when the stretch on the normal nerve root pulls on the dural sac, so increasing the tension on the affected nerve root and producing pain in the leg. This can occur in the presence of a large central disc prolapse. Hudgins (1977) described 351 patients with back pain who came to surgery. Of these, 58 had a positive 'well-leg raising test' of whom 56 were proved to have a prolapsed disc. A false-positive result has, however, been described by Vaz, Wadia and Gokhole (1978).

Femoral-nerve stretch test

In this test passive hip extension is used to place tension on the femoral nerve roots, especially of L3, and so reproduce the patient's pain.

The patient lies prone with the knee flexed to 90 degrees. The examiner places one hand under the thigh to extend the patient's hip while the other hand steadies the patient's pelvis. The normal leg is always tested first. If there is pressure on the femoral nerve roots the range of this hip movement is restricted and the patient's thigh pain is reproduced (*see Figure 20.15*).

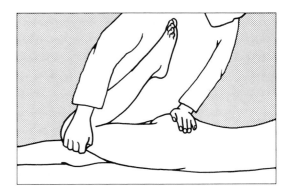

Figure 20.15 Normal femoral-nerve stretch test. The hip is passively extended with the knee flexed

As with the straight-leg raising test, the degree of nerve compression most often correlates with the degree of restriction in this movement. Thus in the most severe degrees of nerve-root involvement the patient will experience pain even when lying prone and fully extending the hip, or else on stretching the thigh by flexing the knee. If the patient can assume this position without pain the hip is then extended and, by comparing the degree of diminished movement with the affected leg as compared with the normal side, an estimation of the degree of nerve-root compression may be obtained.

As the patient's condition improves, the range of movement is correspondingly increased. It should be noted that this test reproduces pain derived from any of the structures being stretched; a similar result is found in a lesion of the quadriceps muscles, such as contusion injury or its complication, myositis ossificans. Clinically, these conditions are easily differentiated from nerve-root compression.

Sacroiliac tests

The sacroiliac joints are tested routinely in patients with back or leg pain; these tests are described in Chapter 29.

General examination

A general physical examination, including the abdomen and chest, is necessary. In cases of suspected pelvic lesions a rectal or vaginal examination is necessary, and no case of sciatica has been properly investigated until such an examination has been performed. Arterial supply to the legs is assessed by palpating the femoral, popliteal, posterior tibial and dorsalis pedis arteries.

Ancillary tests

Laboratory investigations

Laboratory tests to investigate spinal disease include a full blood count. The haemoglobin concentration may be low in inflammatory diseases or tumours; the white cell count may be increased in infections or discitis. The erythrocyte sedimentation rate (ESR) is a useful guide in inflammation or tissue destruction. It is always dangerous to ignore an unexplained elevated ESR, which may have resulted from inflammatory lesions or tumours. Very high levels may be associated with the presence of discitis, polymyalgia rheumatica, or multiple myeloma. A biochemical profile should include serum protein, creatinine, calcium, phosphorous and alkaline phosphatase levels and acid phosphatase activity if prostatic secondaries are suspected. Urine analysis should be performed routinely in all patients.

Radiology

X-rays need not be taken as a routine in all patients with back pain when they are seen for the first time and may have only a limited function, since demonstrating a particular radiological lesion does not necessarily prove that it is the source of the patient's pain. Moreover, some X-ray changes, e.g. congenital anomalies, may be of no clinical significance; and the early stage of many spinal conditions, such as tumours or osteoporosis, may not be evident on X-rays. They are often of most value in demonstrating that no abnormality is present in the bones or joints. However, X-rays are indicated especially if pain is severe, recurrent or persistent. They include anterior–posterior (AP), lateral and oblique views of the lumbar spine and an X-ray of the pelvis to show the sacroiliac joints.

The standard AP view is usually taken with the patient lying down and is centred on the body of L3. Lateral views are taken in two positions, one centred over L3 and the other over L5 to demonstrate the lumbosacral joint. Additional information may be obtained from a lateral view in full flexion and extension.

The vertebrae are inspected for any abnormalities in shape, size, texture, and their alignments. The shape of the bones is usually altered due to wedging—which indicates either a fracture after trauma, secondary deposits or osteoporosis, or Scheuermann's disease. The vertebral bodies may be biconcave due to softening and ballooning of the discs in osteoporosis or osteomalacia. The size of the vertebral body may be increased in Paget's disease and is associated with abnormalities of the trabecular pattern. This pattern is also altered with a haemangioma but the vertebral body is not increased in size.

Bony projections—such as the pedicles, transverse processes or spinous processes—are then inspected. They should be easily visible and equal; if one of them is missing a secondary malignant deposit is likely.

The intervertebral discs are radiolucent; the presence of disc disease may be determined radiologically but it usually takes some time for appropriate changes to develop. Narrowing may involve the whole or part of the disc; a partly narrowed disc shows a wedge-shaped disc deformity.

Oblique X-rays are useful for demonstrating a spondylolysis or degenerative changes in apophyseal joints. Lateral views taken in the upright position with the spine in flexion and extension may demonstrate vertebral instability. Normally in full flexion, the vertebral end-plates or adjacent vertebrae from T12 to L5 should remain parallel. X-rays may demonstrate a loss of this normal alignment and backwards or forwards vertebral movement. A pelvic X-ray should be part of the routine radiological assessment, particularly if malignancy, metabolic bone disease, Paget's disease or sacroiliitis is suspected.

MYELOGRAPHY

This technique carries a sufficient morbidity to ensure that it is never undertaken lightly, and is usually reserved for patients with suspected spinal-canal stenosis or spinal tumour, or is used to demonstrate the level of a prolapsed inter-vertebral disc. In these conditions it tends to be used as a confirmation that surgery is indicated. With disc prolapse the column of dye should be indented or distorted with evidence of compression or shortening of the nerve-root dural sheath. However, in cases of disc prolapse up to 25 per cent of results may be false negative, the major drawback being a failure to demonstrate a posterolateral disc prolapse. A further 10 per cent of results are false positive, which may be produced by benign tumours and vascular abnormalities. The iodized oil previously used often produced arachnoiditis but the incidence with the newer water-soluble media is minimal.

DISCOGRAPHY

This is only rarely indicated. The contrast medium, a water-soluble radio-opaque dye, is injected directly into the nucleus pulposus under X-ray control. The technique itself can provide some useful information, such as the volume and ease with which the injection is given, for degenerated discs admit a larger volume of dye more easily than do normal discs. The injection should reproduce the patient's pain before the test can be considered positive. However, discography may be more valuable in proving a disc to be normal and not the source of a patient's pain than it is in demonstrating the presence of an abnormality. Other techniques include radiculography, epidural myelography and venography.

Computerized axial tomography (CAT)

This technique uses a computerized display to re-create a three-dimensional image of the spine. It provides a non-invasive alternative to the techniques described above. Recent advances, such as the multiplanar display technique, have improved its capabilities to outline soft tissues (Glenn, Rhodes and Altschuler, 1979). CAT scanning is used to outline structural spinal problems involving both bony and soft tissues. These include lumbar-canal stenosis, vertebral diseases, disc prolapse and abnormalities in the facet joints (Carrera *et al.*, 1980).

If the diagnosis remains uncertain it may be combined with a metrizamide myelogram.

Bone scanning

This employs a radionuclide such as technetium-99m pyrophosphate, which is taken up by bone and bound to hydroxyapatite crystals. Thus it can show alterations in blood flow or metabolism, especially if a gammacamera is used. Its major role is in identifying pathological changes, especially infections, tumours (except multiple myeloma), inflammatory diseases or metabolic bone disease. It is a non-invasive, sensitive technique, which is usually more sensitive than conventional radiography (Harcke, 1978) but is not overly specific.

Other investigations

Electromyography may be used to localize the level of a spinal lesion with nerve-root pressure, and evidence of denervation may be found 2 weeks after the onset of nerve damage.

A lumbar puncture is not often indicated but should be performed if the diagnosis is in doubt and a spinal tumour is suspected. In lumbar-disc prolapse, the cerebrospinal protein concentration is usually normal, but a slight increase may occur and with a large prolapse the value may rise to $1 \text{ g} \cdot \ell^{-1}$ (11 mg· 100 ml^{-1}).

Bone-marrow examination may be indicated for the diagnosis of generalized disorders, especially myeloma or tuberculosis. Either a closed or open bone biopsy (Stahl and Jacobs, 1961) may then be necessary.

21 Lumbar intervertebral-disc syndromes

Several different clinical syndromes may occur as the result of disc degeneration.

Vertebral instability

This condition follows the early stages of disc degeneration; fissures appear with softening and bulging of the disc, which produce a mechanical spinal derangement (Morgan and King, 1957; Schmorl and Junghanns, 1971; Macnab, 1973). It occurs more commonly in males, usually in the third or fourth decades and usually involves the L4–5 disc. Instability produces an increased strain on surrounding soft tissues and ligamentous supports, thus forming the basis of the postural pain. With instability the spine is vulnerable to trauma, so that any forced or unguarded movements may result in apophyseal-joint synovitis or subluxation with consequent mechanical derangement (Macnab, 1973).

Pain—described as dull, aching, deep seated and usually constant—may be localized to the back, or radiate to one or both buttocks and legs. Only rarely does it radiate beyond the knees, and evidence of nerve-root pressure is usually absent. Pain is made worse by maintaining one posture for a long time, e.g. standing or sitting, and alteration in posture—such as lying down or arching the back—may relieve pain. This pattern is typically punctuated by attacks of severe pain associated with a sensation of 'locking'. These attacks may follow some traumatic incident, such as lifting a heavy weight or twisting.

Clinical signs may be difficult to elicit as the overall range of spinal movement tends to be normal, although at times it may be possible to find some loss of the expected range of flexion or extension. During testing of active movement, the mechanical instability may produce pain. This occurs typically as an arc of pain, which may occur either during forward flexion or else as the patient straightens up from the flexed position. Tenderness may be found locally over the involved segment of the spine.

Although the presence of vertebral instability may be suspected on clinical grounds, it needs to be confirmed by X-ray. However, it may be possible to demonstrate instability radiologically in 8 per cent of asymptomatic patients (Mensor and Duvall, 1959). The significant radiological findings include:

(1) The presence of gas within the disc. This implies disc degeneration with separation of its fibres so that gas can accumulate and is then evident on X-rays.

(2) A traction spur, which is found approximately 2 mm from the vertebral edge. The outermost fibres of the annulus arise from the anterior margins of the upper vertebral bodies and are inserted into the anterior margin of the lower vertebrae. The abnormal degree of vertebral movement produces traction on these fibres and so the traction spur develops by growing out horizontally (Macnab, 1971) (*see Figure 21.1*).

(3) Changes in lateral X-rays taken with the patient in full flexion and extension. With vertebral instability, abnormal movement

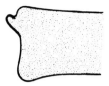

Figure 21.1
Vertebral instability.
A traction spur
develops a few
millimetres away
from the vertebral
margin in the line of
the outer fibres of
the annulus

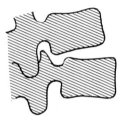

Figure 21.2 Vertebral
instability. The upper
lumbar vertebra is tilted
upwards and backwards
on the lower vertebra
with overriding of the
apophyseal-joint facets

with loss of the normal rolling mechanism may be detected. The superior vertebra may move forward on the lower one during flexion and may then be associated with a narrowing of the anterior part of the disc. Alternatively, on lumbar extension an excessive backwards sliding movement of the upper lumbar vertebra may occur (*see Figure 21.2*).

Discography may be used to provide confirmatory evidence but myelography does not provide additional evidence. Other causes of vertebral instability, such as spondylolisthesis, which have similar symptoms and signs may be differentiated by their X-ray appearances.

Intervertebral-disc prolapse

Some of the known clinical features associated with disc prolapse include:

(1) Age—The peak age is in the 20–45 age group. In patients below the age of 16 or over 50, with symptoms appearing for the first time, the diagnosis must be critically reviewed because other diagnoses are more common at these ages.
(2) Sex—Males are more commonly affected than females, by approximately 3:2.
(3) Site—Armstrong (1967), in 1000 cases of lumbar-disc operation, found that 46.8 per cent occurred at the lumbrosacral disc; 40.4 per cent at the L4–5 disc; 2.1 per cent at the upper three discs; and in 10.7 per cent of cases double lesions were present.

The clinical picture depends on the interrelationship between anatomical and pathological features involving the disc, the spinal canal and the neural elements.

The disc

The clinical presentation depends on the size of the disc prolapse; the direction it takes, which may be into a central, posterolateral or intraforaminal position (*see Figure 21.3*); and its relation to the nerve root, which may lie either medially, laterally or underneath the prolapse.

The spinal canal

The size and shape of the spinal canal varies. It may be congenitally narrowed or vary in shape

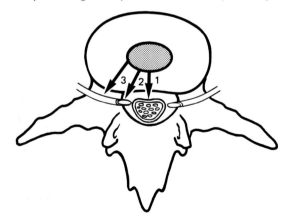

Figure 21.3 A disc prolapse may proceed (1) in the central midline and compress the dura; (2) posterolaterally and compress the nerve root; or (3) laterally and compress the nerve root in the intervertebral foramen

from oval, triangular or trefoil conformation. Congenital anomalies or acquired defects, such as spondylolisthesis or hypertrophic changes in apophyseal joints, may cause canal stenosis.

Spinal nerves

Anatomical considerations also determine which nerve root is involved. The nerve roots in the cauda equina run obliquely downwards across the superior disc before emerging through their intervertebral foramen (*see Figure 21.4*). At the L4–5 disc level, the L4 nerve root runs through its intervertebral foramen and the L5 and sacral nerve roots are contained within the dural sac. At the lumbosacral level the L5 nerve root is contained within its intervertebral foramen and the dural sac contains only the sacral nerve roots.

The nerve root compressed by the prolapse of the L4–5 intervertebral disc depends on the direction it takes. The L5 nerve root may be involved by a posterolateral disc prolapse, but with a lateral prolapse the L4 nerve root is involved in its intervertebral foramen, whereas a central disc prolapse may compress L5 or S1. Similarly, a posterolateral lumbosacral-disc prolapse usually compresses the S1 nerve root but a laterally directed prolapse may compromise the L5 nerve root in its intervertebral foramen. Other changes in the neurological presentation may occur because of anomalous spinal segmentation, the presence of a pre- or post-fixed plexus or because, in some 10 per cent of cases, multiple nerve roots are involved.

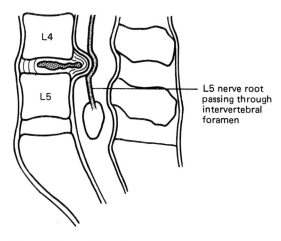

Figure 21.4 A prolapse of the L4–5 intervertebral disc may compress the L5 nerve root

Clinical findings

Back pain may occur for no apparent reason, but many patients tend to relate it to some minor traumatic incident or after a strain—such as bending, lifting or twisting—which may be associated with a tearing sensation. Pain—which is described as dull and aching or knife-like ('like a hot poker')—is felt in the low back, either in the midline or to one side. The onset of pain, usually confined initially to the lower back, may be sudden and severe or else may develop more gradually. Pain at first may be intermittent and relieved by rest or changes in position, but it is usually made worse by movement or sitting and sudden straining, such as coughing or sneezing. Pain is usually severe and may disturb sleep. There may be a history of attacks of back pain, sometimes associated with a sensation of back locking.

Back pain may be followed some later time by leg pain, which is almost always unilateral but is usually severe. The back pain may disappear when the leg pain begins. The distribution of the leg pain will vary according to the nerve root involved. Associated symptoms may include paraesthesias, numbness, hyperalgesia, leg cramps or weakness.

Examination

Signs consist of varying combinations and degrees of mechanical derangement of the lumbar spinal joints, and evidence of nerve-root involvement. Mechanical derangement is evidenced by alterations in posture, muscle spasm, alterations in the spinal contours and disturbance of movements.

ALTERATIONS IN POSTURE
The patients may be unable to bear any weight on the painful leg and so stands with hip and knee flexed and the back held rigid. The gait may also be antalgic, with as little weight as possible being transferred to the painful side.

MUSCLE SPASM
The paravertebral muscles are nearly always found to be in spasm due to a reflex muscular contraction. The underlying mechanism is a protective reflex that limits movements of the spine and the inflamed nerve root. The spasm may be bilateral or unilateral and usually extends over several lumbar spinal segments. It is usually easily

palpable, and should be assessed with the patient standing, moving and lying prone.

Alterations in spinal contour

Alterations in the normal lumbar curvature may be present either as scoliosis or loss of the normal lordosis. The scoliosis is protective in nature and is most commonly contralateral, being ipsilateral in approximately 15 per cent of cases. The mechanism to explain these findings is that the list is protective to alter the relationship of the nerve root to the prolapsed disc (*see Figure 21.5*). The presence of a scoliosis may be noted while the patient is standing, or while he is flexing or extending the lumbar spine. Scoliosis may be quite gross, most commonly after an L4–5 intervertebral-disc prolapse. In juvenile disc lesions a severe degree of scoliosis may occur with marked muscle spasm but relatively little pain.

Disturbance of movement

ACTIVE MOVEMENTS
The physiological movements of flexion, extension and lateral flexion are tested to determine their range, whether pain is reproduced, the behaviour of the pain with movement, the presence of any deformity, and whether an arc of pain is present. The patient is first asked whether any pain is felt while standing relaxed and, if so, to indicate its distribution. Then as the movements are carried out the patient is asked to report whether pain is altered or reproduced, to indicate the site of such pain and to cease the movement before pain becomes excessive.

Forward flexion is the movement most commonly reduced in range, and the degree of its loss usually reflects the severity of the disc prolapse. In a severe attack only a small range of forward flexion is possible before flexion is limited by pain and muscle spasm. If the attack is of a moderate degree the patient may be able to flex to approximately half the normal range. The forward movement may also be associated with a scoliosis.

Loss of extension is not as common as loss of flexion. However, in patients with a loss of their normal lumbar lordosis spinal extension will usually be markedly limited and associated with an increase in pain. Movement into lateral flexion varies. It may be of full and painless range to each side but may at times be painfully limited to one side. This occurs more commonly towards the side of pain; lateral flexion to the other side is then usually full and painless.

PASSIVE MOVEMENTS
The passive ranges of physiological and accessory movements are also found to be limited because of pain, stiffness and spasm.

Nerve-root involvement

Nerve-root involvement is indicated by the loss of freedom of movement of the nerve root in the

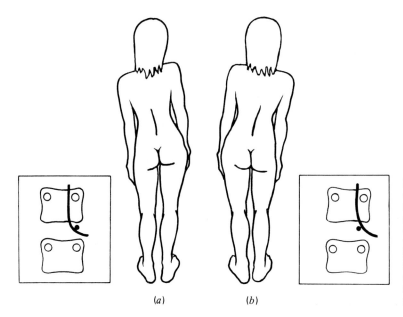

(a)   (b)

Figure 21.5 Relationship between a protective scoliosis and the site of nerve-root pressure. (*a*) A contralateral protective scoliosis is usually associated with a disc prolapse on the lateral side of the involved nerve root. (*b*) An ipsilateral scoliosis is usually associated with a disc prolapse on the medial side of the involved nerve root

spinal canal or its intervertebral foramen, and by the presence of any neurological deficit. The tests performed are straight-leg raising and the femoral-stretch test and neurological assessment.

Neurological assessment to determine the nerve root involved and its degree of compression is an essential part of the examination in all patients with disc prolapse. Motor changes include muscle weakness and wasting. Since the motor supply to muscle groups is supplied in the main by specific nerve roots, these tests provide a good indication of the involved neurological level. Muscles are tested by inspection, isometric contraction and functional movements. Sensation is tested by comparing both legs, and the knee and ankle jerks are also tested. The clinical findings are summarized in *Table 21.1*.

Palpation

The affected spinal level is usually tender to palpation in the midline or in the paravertebral area on the same side as the disc prolapse. The sciatic nerve may also be tender, particularly over the sciatic notch or in the popliteal fossa.

CLINICAL VARIATIONS

The most common pain pattern is back pain followed by leg pain, but this may vary and the patient may present with back pain or leg pain alone, or back and leg pain that occur simul-taneously. Variations in the pattern of neurological involvement are also possible.

(1) Back pain alone. Low-back pain, which may be intermittent or constant, is usually described by the patient as 'aching', is related to posture and activity and is usually relieved by rest. Pain may be felt only in the midline, may spread symmetrically across the back, or may be felt as a sacral or buttock pain. Attacks of sudden mechanical derangement may also produce lumbar pain and a sensation of 'locking' in the back.

(2) Sciatic pain alone. Leg pain, usually gradual in onset, either radiates distally from the buttock region or is felt in any part of the dermatomal distribution. The distance that the pain radiates is usually dependent on the degree of pressure on the nerve root and on pain-sensitive structures in the vertebral canal or intervertebral foramen. When the pain is felt below the knee or in the foot and is combined with numbness it is necessary to differentiate it from a peripheral-nerve entrapment.

(3) Simultaneous sciatic and back pain is a less common form of presentation.

(4) There may be sudden sciatic pain of such severity that the patient is unable to lie still. This usually indicates that a large piece of a disc has extruded through the posterior longitudinal ligament.

(5) Pain may radiate into both legs simul-

Table 21.1 Nerve-root involvement in intervertebral-disc prolapse

Involved root	Pain distribution	Sensory loss	Motor weakness	Reflex changes
S1	From buttock to back of thigh and leg, lateral aspect of ankle and foot	Lateral aspect of ankle, foot and posterior calf	Plantar flexion of ankle and toes, extension of hip and flexion of knee	Ankle jerk
L5	From buttock to the lateral aspect of leg and dorsum of foot and great toe	Dorsum of foot and great toe. Anterolateral aspect of lower leg	Dorsiflexion of great toe, dorsiflexion of other toes and dorsiflexion in eversion of ankle	Nil
L4	Lateral aspect of the thigh to the medial side of the calf	Medial aspect of calf and shin	Dorsiflexion and inversion of ankle and extension of knee	Knee jerk
L3	Anterior thigh to anterior region of knee	Lower inner aspect of thigh and knee	Flexion, adduction and internal rotation of hip	Knee jerk
L2	Anterior aspect of upper thigh	Upper outer aspect of thigh	Flexion and adduction of hip	Nil

taneously or consecutively. A large posterior prolapse may compress one root on either side of the midline or, rarely, a nuclear prolapse may occur on either side of the midline at one or different levels to implicate two nerve roots.

(6) There may be motor weakness alone without sensory changes; for example, this may present as a foot drop of sudden onset.

(7) A rare complication of severe nerve-root compression is atrophy or rupture of the nerve root. Pain will cease, but motor and sensory signs become more marked while straight-leg raising returns to normal.

(8) Neurological bladder disturbances may occur, even in the presence of minimal back or leg pain (Love and Emmett, 1967).

Lumbar spondylosis

Patients with this condition may complain of back or leg pain, either unilateral or bilateral, with or without neurological symptoms. The patient usually complains of a dull, aching lumbar pain associated with stiffness. Pain is typically sited in the lower lumbar midline but may radiate out to the groin or buttock. It usually tends to get worse as the day progresses but at times may be more pronounced after a night's rest, and then usually eases as the patient becomes more mobile.

Since degenerative changes involve both the anterior and posterior portions of the intervertebral joint complex it is not possible to implicate the exact mechanism of symptom production in any individual case. There may also be attacks of mechanical derangement of the lumbar joints. The most likely basis for these attacks is recurrent episodes of synovitis in the apophyseal joints after overuse, such as excessive bending or unaccustomed activities, with resultant strain of these joints.

Leg pain may be experienced in one or both legs, and three mechanisms may be involved:

(1) Pain may be referred into the leg. This may follow derangement in movement of the intervertebral joint complex, with stimulation of the sinuvertebral nerve.

(2) Sciatica may result from nerve-root pressure, for which there are three distinct causes. The first is an encroachment on the neural canal by the osteophytic outgrowths that arise from the vertebral and apophyseal joints. The

second mechanism results from the disturbance of the normal vertebral relationships that follows disc-space narrowing and approximation of the vertebral bodies. The nerve root may then be impinged upon either by the articular facets or by the pedicle of the superior vertebra. Finally, an acute intervertebral-disc prolapse may occur, although this is uncommon.

(3) Leg pain may be due to the presence of a canal stenosis.

Isolated disc resorption

In this condition severe progressive degenerative changes involve one intervertebral disc alone. Its importance lies in the fact that back and leg pain may develop due to altered spinal mechanics and not to disc prolapse. Crock (1970) described the pathological features in which the disc is virtually completely resorbed, leaving only a rim of annulus.

The principal radiological sign is a marked loss of disc space, usually associated with a vacuum phenomenon, sclerosis of vertebral margins and, often, a retrospondylolisthesis that leads to apophyseal-joint overriding and degenerative changes.

Spinal-canal stenosis

The term spinal stenosis is used to describe two conditions: one is the structural changes resulting in a narrowed spinal canal; the other is the associated clinical syndrome. The characteristic anatomical feature is a reduction in the anteroposterior (AP) and lateral diameters of the bony spinal canal. This abnormality in the canal's shape may be due either to a congenital defect or to a developmental change in the surrounding bones. In the normal spinal canal the neural structures lie between the vertebrae and discs anteriorly and the pedicles and laminae posteriorly, and there is ample space for movement. However, if the size and shape of the canal becomes narrowed the enclosed nerve roots may be compromised in the cauda equina, the lateral recess of the canal or in the intervertebral foramen (*see Figure 21.6*).

The causes of lumbar spinal-canal stenosis may be congenital or acquired. The congenital defect is

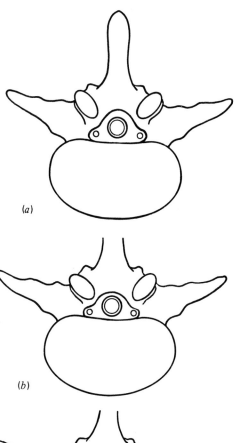

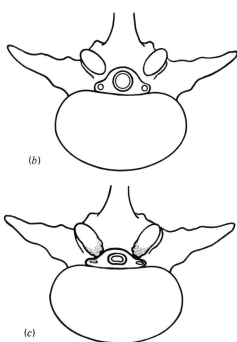

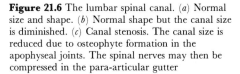

Figure 21.6 The lumbar spinal canal. (*a*) Normal size and shape. (*b*) Normal shape but the canal size is diminished. (*c*) Canal stenosis. The canal size is reduced due to osteophyte formation in the apophyseal joints. The spinal nerves may then be compressed in the para-articular gutter

associated with narrow AP and transverse diameters of the spinal canal and short pedicles, and it may be due to congenital conditions, such as achondroplasia. The most common acquired pathological changes occur as a result of degenerative changes in the disc and apophyseal joint and may also be associated with thickening of the ligamentum flavum. The disc lesion may be a nuclear prolapse, or more commonly a hard annular bulging with osteophyte formation. The hypertrophic apophyseal-joint changes, bulging into the spinal canal from its posterolateral angle, may produce a typical clover-leaf or trefoil shape when viewed from above.

Other causes of lumbar-canal stenosis include spondylolisthesis, spondylolysis, bone diseases (such as Paget's disease) and neoplasms; the condition may also occur after a laminectomy. Some patients suffer from a combination of a congenital narrowing, which is usually asymptomatic, with a pathological lesion, which causes a localized area of narrowing.

Clinical presentation

Symptoms of spinal-canal stenosis may be divided into three broad categories: claudicant, neurological and postural.

The patient's symptoms may be very similar to those produced by intermittent claudication due to arterial insufficiency. Pain in one or both legs comes on after walking a certain distance and may involve the whole leg. The pain may be associated with paraesthesias and/or leg weakness. Rest relieves the pain, and the patient may sometimes need to sit down immediately. Unlike the more rapid disappearance of pain in patients with peripheral vascular disease, relief of pain in patients with spinal-canal stenosis may require rest for a longer period; but it is often difficult to differentiate between these patients from the history alone.

Leg weakness may involve any part of the leg. At times the patient may give a dramatic account of suddenly losing all power in the legs and falling to the ground. Sensory impairment is often of a patchy distribution in the lower limb. Because these symptoms often tend to be vague or diffuse, the patient may be considered to be psychoneurotic.

Another type of neurological lesion is produced by involvement of the nerve root in the nerve-root canal. As the nerve root descends from the dural sac it passes obliquely across the pedicle and runs in a canal formed by the ligamentum flavum and the superior articular facet. Patients with stenosis of this root canal may present with leg pain. The L5 and S1 nerve roots are most commonly involved. Symptoms that are commonly experienced in disc prolapse, e.g. pain made worse by coughing or straining, do not usually occur in these patients.

Pain related to posture may involve the back and/or legs. The patient may report that certain postural changes in the back either exacerbate or relieve pain.

The exact mechanism of production of symptoms in canal stenosis is uncertain. The cauda equina nerve roots derive their blood supply from the radicular arteries. These end-arteries supply their respective nerve roots only and are not distributed to other structures. Actively conducting nerve roots require a large blood supply, and occlusion of a radicular artery leading to nerve-root ischaemia could readily occur in the stenosed spinal canal.

X-rays

Routine X-rays of the spine may lead to a suspicion of the correct diagnosis if gross degenerative changes involving disc, apophyseal joints or degenerative spondylolisthesis are present. Myelography may be used in suspected cases in order to outline the size and shape of the canal and to demonstrate any alteration in the dural sac, which may be present as an hour-glass constriction in the sac at the level of the stenosis (*see Figure 21.7*). CAT scanning is a useful non-invasive technique to outline the size and shape of the canal and its contents.

Cauda equina compression

This occurs after a sudden, massive extrusion of nuclear material through the posterior longitudinal ligament. In younger patients this may follow a sudden flexion strain. The patient usually complains of back pain with radiation into both legs and buttocks. Besides sensory and motor neurological defects in the legs, sensory changes in the sacral dermatomes involving scrotal and perianal areas are found. These are usually associated with urinary retention. Early recognition is imperative to allow early surgical decompression.

The juvenile disc syndrome

Disc prolapse, as has been discussed, usually occurs in patients over the age of 20. In adolescent patients the pathology and clinical presentation usually differs. Trauma appears to play a more important role in the production of this syndrome and may be caused either by direct trauma to the spine, or by indirect trauma which may follow a fall onto the buttocks. The patient may complain of varying degrees of pain, but marked spinal stiffness and muscle spasm are the predominant clinical characteristics. The lack of normal spinal movement may also be reflected by a rather peculiar, shuffling gait. There may also be an associated scoliosis, which may be present only on movement. A neurological deficit is more uncommon, but straight-leg raising is markedly restricted. Bulos (1973) reported similar clinical findings in eight adolescents, seven of whom were boys. Operation revealed the presence of a tightly bulging disc with an intact annulus but with no evidence of underlying disc degeneration.

The clinical course is usually prolonged and may persist for up to 2 years before it resolves. It is often difficult to influence it by conservative management.

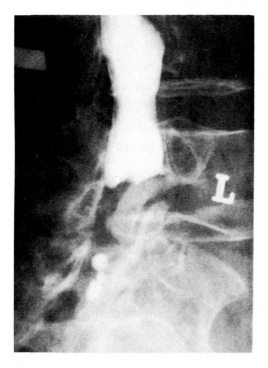

Figure 21.7 An oblique view of a myelogram showing obstruction to the flow of the dye in a patient with canal stenosis and degenerative apophyseal-joint changes at L4–5

22 Disorders of movement in the lumbar spine

The problem of classifying spinal disorders has already been discussed. After excluding those patients with pathological disorders of the intervertebral disc and of the vertebral column, a large proportion of patients still remain whose symptoms do not place them in either of these categories. Most of these patients may then be classified on clinical grounds according to any alteration in the range of spinal movement, which may be either increased or decreased.

The increase in the range of movement is known as hypermobility and is usually a generalized process involving all segments of the spine. It may sometimes occur, however, at one spinal level alone. A decrease in the range of movement usually involves a single segment of the intervertebral joint complex; this decrease is known as hypomobility. This is usually a chronic condition that produces a form of mechanical derangement of the joint complex. However, in the lumbar spine an acute form of mechanical derangement also occurs, which is known as acute lumbago.

Accordingly, in the lumbar spine, disorders of spinal movement may be classified into:

(1) Acute lumbago.
(2) Hypomobility lesions.
(3) Hypermobility.

Acute lumbago

The word lumbago means 'pain in the back' and so it could be used as a descriptive title for any type of back ache. It is used here in its more widely accepted sense to describe a lumbar spinal syndrome characterized by sudden onset of severe persistent pain, marked restriction of lumbar movements, and a sensation of 'locking' in the back. Attacks may vary in severity and range from severe and incapacitating to a more minor nature.

Clinical findings

If the attack is severe the patient presents with an onset of sudden, intense lower lumbar pain which may be bilateral. The pain and sensation of back locking may render the patient immobile with the back 'stuck' in one position, usually partly flexed. The patient may even fall down or have to lie down immediately and be unable to move, or may have to crawl to a bed.

The attack usually occurs after a forward flexion movement, which may have been slight—such as cleaning the teeth, standing up from a forward flexed position, sneezing, coughing, or bending and lifting a weight. There may be a combined twisting movement. A 'click' may be felt or heard. Pain is made worse by almost any back movement; straining, coughing or sneezing can produce incredibly intense pain, and even passing urine can become a problem.

Examination of the lumbar spine reveals that active movements are virtually impossible to perform. Marked bilateral paraspinal muscle spasm, often more prominent on one side than the other, is apparent on inspection.

Spinal deformity is present and, in severe cases, may be one of three types:

(1) In approximately half of the cases the patient has a scoliosis away from the more painful side and is unable to laterally flex the back towards the painful side.

(2) Not so commonly, the patient presents with a kyphosis or a reversal of the normal lumbar curve; he is stuck in forward flexion and unable to straighten up.

(3) A scoliosis towards the side of the pain is rarely found.

The patient has no alternative but to be at complete rest in bed. The severe pain usually eases in a few days to leave a dull, aching pain which in a typical attack gradually eases in the next few weeks and leaves no residual disability. At times pain may be quite dramatically relieved after a sudden movement, when the patient may again be conscious of something having clicked in the back.

Not all attacks are as severe. Sometimes a patient may experience a more minor degree of pain and then retains a limited degree of mobility. The onset is less dramatic and often the patient may awaken with back pain and experience difficulty in getting out of bed. There may be a history of some minor trauma to the back on the preceding day. There may be no obvious back deformity, but some degree of muscle spasm will be present.

Pathogenesis

Acute lumbago may be regarded as an acute form of mechanical derangement and locking of the intervertebral joint complex. Several theories have been proposed to account for its production. Some of these have been discarded but they include (*see Figure 22.1*): acute nuclear prolapse of the disc; acute hydrops of the disc (Charnley, 1951); annular tears (Cyriax, 1978); apophyseal-joint lesions, including subluxation, synovitis, an impacted synovial fringe or intra-articular structure, such as a meniscoid body; ligamentous tears; and a primary muscle lesion (Strange, 1966). A similar clinical picture also results from a fractured vertebra and, in the elderly, from a pathological fracture due to osteoporosis or secondary tumours. These can be differentiated by the history and X-ray changes.

Acute lumbago should be regarded as a syndrome in which more than one condition can produce a typical attack. However, in any patient

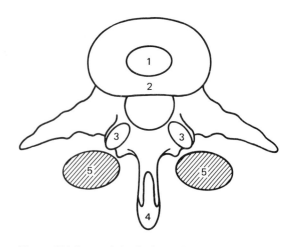

Figure 22.1 Proposed sites in the production of an acute lumbago: (1) the nucleus pulposus; (2) the annulus fibrosus; (3) the apophyseal joints; (4) the spinal ligaments; and (5) the muscles

during an attack it is usually impossible to diagnose a definite cause, and standard X-rays are normal. It is commonly believed that a disorder of the disc is responsible, but again there are no means of substantiating this diagnosis clinically during an attack. If a disc prolapse is responsible it can usually be confirmed only after a period of time; either the attack fails to settle over several weeks, or a subsequent attack of acute lumbago is associated with nerve-root compression. However, in a sizeable proportion of patients the natural history of this condition does not resemble that of disc degeneration. Attacks occur periodically until finally they cease with no evidence of disc degeneration. An unexplained feature is that it often recurs annually, and then often at about the same time of the year.

Hypomobility lesions

A hypomobility lesion with reduced range of joint movement is the chronic form of a mechanical derangement of the intervertebral joint complex. It is a common condition whose essential clinical features should include:

(1) Pain that is localized in the back or referred into the buttock, leg or abdominal regions.

(2) Pain that is reproduced on testing active spinal movements.

(3) A pattern in which these movements are restricted in certain directions only.

(4) A restricted range of accessory intervertebral movements.

(5) Possibly, other evidence of a mechanical derangement of spinal movements.

(6) X-rays that are normal for the patient's age.

The onset of pain may be sudden and the patient may relate it to bending, twisting or some other traumatic event. Pain varies in degree from minor to severe and is usually described as having a dull, aching quality. It tends to be localized but may at times be referred more widely into the buttock, abdomen, groin, coccyx or leg. Leg pain is rarely felt below the knee and is never associated with sensory disturbances. At times the distribution of pain may be atypical and hence the importance of a complete clinical assessment of movement at each lumbar joint in patients with pain of typical or atypical distribution. Finally, the patient may describe episodic attacks of pain but at other times a history of long-continued disability may be obtained.

Examination

(1) Testing the overall range of active physiological movement usually shows some evidence of restricted movement, although it should be noted that at times movements appear normal. When they are restricted they should also reproduce the patient's pain. In each area of the spine these restricted movements tend to fall into certain common patterns. For example, in a patient with unilateral lumbar pain, lateral flexion either towards or away from the painful side may be limited and may reproduce the patient's pain. This is then usually associated with pain either on flexion or on extension but only very rarely with both. The normal rhythmical pattern of lumbar movement may also be disturbed. This is best appreciated by standing behind the patient to observe the spinal movements. Restricted movement in the intervertebral segment usually results in an alteration in the rhythm of the spinal movements and in their contour.

(2) Should these tests fail to reproduce pain auxiliary tests (*see* page 269), such as rhythmical over-pressure at the end of the

range or the quadrant position, are used in an attempt to reproduce the pain or reveal joint signs at an appropriate level.

(3) Other evidence of deranged intervertebral-joint mechanics include the presence of a deformity, such as a scoliosis or loss of the normal lumbar lordosis.

(4) In all cases of hypomobility lesions there is a loss of the normal accessory intervertebral movements, which is assessed by applying rhythmical pressures against the vertebral bony processes. These pressures should also reproduce the patient's pain; this may occur at any stage within this limited range but occurs most often at the limit of the range, and is then often associated with a reflex muscle spasm that produces a characteristic 'springing' end-feel.

(5) Thickening of tissue in and around the relevant interspinous space may be palpable.

(6) Tenderness may be used as a confirmatory sign. It is usually felt over the affected joint, either over the supraspinous ligament or more laterally in the paravertebral area. Referred tenderness over the site of referred pain is also common.

(7) X-rays are normal for the patient's age.

Aetiology

The patient's symptoms and signs are caused by a loss of the normal intervertebral movements due to a minor mechanical derangement of the intervertebral joint. Thus a lesion in either the anterior or posterior portion of the spinal joint complex can produce the same clinical finding. Its aetiology seems likely to be related to minor traumatic or degenerative changes in either the disc or apophyseal joints, and many hypotheses have been presented to explain the syndrome on the basis of such changes. In apophyseal joints, these include nipping of synovial fringes, degenerative changes in articular cartilage, osteochondral lesions, intra-articular meniscoid structures, and finally adhesions.

An association with some recognized pathological or degenerative changes may also occur. A similar clinical presentation may be seen during the early stages of disc degeneration or in patients with spondylosis. In patients with a history of injury it may be possible to find tenderness localized over ligamentous structures, such as the iliolumbar ligament (Ingpen and Burry, 1970). Another form of a post-traumatic lesion follows manipulation, usually by un-qualified practitioners, that results in a mechanical spinal-joint derangement. Patients who have had a previous attack of acute back pain, especially if treated with prolonged rest, may also present with chronic symptoms due to a hypo-mobility lesion. Finally, it may be one cause of back pain in women after a confinement.

Nevertheless, most patients with hypomobility have no specific underlying pathological lesion that has been recognized; nor can the exact site of the derangement within the intervertebral joint complex be demonstrated. It is apparent that no single lesion is responsible for all cases of this joint derangement. If mobilization techniques designed to restore the normal range are success-ful it would appear that it is not always so important to determine their precise nature. The importance of this lesion should be thought of in terms of a reduction in function that results from the loss of normal joint range.

Site of involvement

Hypomobility lesions may be found in any of the spinal intervertebral joints. Similarly, they may be found either in the lower lumbar joints but also quite often in the upper lumbar levels. Lesions may be found at more than one level, when they are referred to as group lesions. It is also not infrequent to find a patient with disc degeneration at the lumbosacral joint and a hypomobility lesion at the thoracolumbar junction, and this latter may be associated with continuing symptoms.

Sacroiliac pain

A common site for referred pain and tenderness with hypomobility lesions of the lower lumbar spine is over the sacroiliac joint. For many years this led to the belief that the sacroiliac joint was responsible for most back problems, but as ex-plained in Chapter 29 it is now realized that this is not correct.

Coccydynia

In this condition the patient complains of pain experienced in the coccygeal area. Although this may arise at times from local trauma, the most common cause of pain is a referred pain from hypomobility lesions of the lumbosacral joint or even from higher lumbar joints. If so the patient's coccygeal pain must be reproduced by movement at one of these joints.

If treatment is directed to the lumbar joints the vast majority of patients will respond after a few treatments so that it is a most satisfactory condition to treat. Moreover, if the appropriate level is not treated the patient is often subjected to many therapies, including removal of the coccyx, all of which are usually to no avail.

Abdominal pain

Pain felt in the abdomen may be produced by a hypermobility lesion involving the lumbar spine. It may then closely mimic an intra-abdominal cause for pain. This likelihood is increased by the common finding of local abdominal-wall tender-ness, which is a referred tenderness. Perhaps the most common area of involvement is under the costal margin in either hypochondrium, which may be incorrectly diagnosed as gallbladder disease when the right side is involved. This can lead to claims by unqualified practitioners of their being able to cure visceral disease.

Fibrositis

Spinal pain and stiffness are extremely common symptoms, yet in a large group of patients with complaints of back pain evidence of any under-lying pathology is lacking. Of the many names given to this clinical condition the most common are non-articular rheumatism or fibrositis.

The clinical features of fibrositis—which usually runs a benign, intermittently recurrent and protracted course—are well described.

The patient complains of pain and stiffness in-volving mainly paraspinal muscle groups. Com-mon sites of involvement include the trapezius, the interscapular area and muscle groups related to the iliac crest. The pain of fibrositis tends to be worse with prolonged inactivity or after a period of exercise. Attacks tend to be episodic and are often related to weather changes or stress.

On palpation, examination reveals localized areas of tenderness in the involved muscle groups associated with palpably thickened areas known as trigger spots. Pressure over these areas often reproduces the patient's pain and also may induce more distal radiation. Local anaesthetic injected into the trigger zone abolishes this localized area of pain and tenderness.

All ancillary investigations, including X-rays and blood tests, are always normal. Other organic diseases should be excluded before the diagnosis is confirmed, and psychogenic symptoms are often difficult to differentiate.

Because a definite pathological basis for this condition had not been established, the concept of fibrositis as a disease has been consistently challenged. Nevertheless, it is common practice to see a large number of patients who fit this clinical description. Fibrositis would seem to be the best term to describe their condition and allows its benign nature to be explained. It would also appear that this condition may have more than one cause (Smythe and Moldofsky, 1978). However, in many patients with fibrositis involving paraspinal muscles it is possible to demonstrate a hypomobility lesion in a corresponding spinal segment. The neural basis is presumed to follow stimulation of the sinuvertebral nerve, resulting in referred pain and tenderness, which is experienced peripherally in the sclerotome distribution as a 'trigger spot'.

Mobilization techniques applied to the affected spinal segment in these patients may be expected to relieve pain, stiffness and also the trigger zone of referred tenderness.

The hypermobility syndrome

Hypermobility may involve spinal or peripheral joints and is defined as a range of joint movement in excess of the usually accepted range. It should be noted that throughout the hypermobile range this movement can be controlled by muscle activity. This needs to be differentiated from joint instability, which has an abnormal range of movement and may also at times be excessive but which cannot be controlled by voluntary muscular activity.

Descriptions of spinal hypermobility in the lit-erature tend to be confused with two other separate conditions. One is vertebral instability due to the early stages of the disc degeneration and not usually produced by or associated with generalized hypermobility. The other is found in patients with disc degeneration at one spinal level, when the adjacent level may demonstrate a hypermobile range of movement which may be asymptomatic.

Joint hypermobility may be found in:

(1) An idiopathic form, which is often familial or racial and occurs predominantly in females.
(2) Hereditary connective-tissue disorders, including Marfan's syndrome and Ehlers–Danlos syndrome.
(3) Metabolic disorders, such as homocystinuria.

Clinical features

The patients are usually young females. Hypermobility may affect spinal and peripheral joints or the spinal joints only. The features of hypermobility syndromes that affected peripheral joints were described by Kirk, Ansell and Bywaters (1967). In a series of 24 patients presenting with musculoskeletal pain, examination revealed no abnormality other than joint hypermobility.

In the spine, clinical features of this syndrome include:

(1) Back pain, either continuous or recurrent.
(2) A generalized increase in spinal mobility and the range of passive intervertebral movements (*see Figure 22.2*).
(3) An associated hypermobility of peripheral joints.
(4) Other investigations, including X-rays, are normal.

Back pain was first described by Howes and Isdale (1971), who used the term the 'loose back syndrome'. In a series of 102 patients with back pain (59 men and 43 women), a diagnosis of an organic back lesion was possible in virtually all the men. However, in 20 of the women no definite diagnosis could be made, except that 17 showed hypermobility.

In hypermobile conditions the spine and peripheral joints are more likely to be traumatized during everyday activities, which is the presumed basis for the production of their symptoms. However, there is one clinical finding in spinal hypermobility that has not been widely

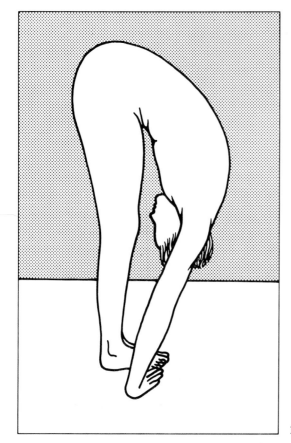

Figure 22.2 Spinal hypermobility

publicized but that may occasionally provoke pain. Although there may be an increased overall range of physiological movements, there may also be a reduction in the range of passive inter-vertebral movement at one spinal level. Testing this spinal level by passive-movement techniques may reveal this relatively hypomobile area and also reproduce the patient's pain.

23 Management

The management of a patient who has recurrent or chronic low-back pain is often complex. It is never as simple as prescribing a single therapy and expecting a satisfactory result on every occasion. The first requirement is diagnosis and an attempt should be made to categorize the patient's condition into one of the clinical syndromes described previously. A detailed history taking is essential and should also lead to an overall assessment of the degree of physical disability and loss of function present in each patient. It includes an overall view of the patient, his reaction to his clinical disability, and how it affects his daily routine, at home, at work or during recreational activities. The presence of any psychogenic overlay, expectations of treatment, fears for the future and ability to accept or live within any limitations should also be assessed.

While it is true that treatment remains largely empirical, relating the clinical diagnosis and its severity to the varying treatments available should provide the patient with an orderly treatment programme. The patient needs to be reassured and to have the biomechanics of low-back problems explained. Each patient then requires a programme of management outlined on an individual basis according to the degree of restriction and incapacity. Treatment should also be organized in the knowledge that an acute attack of low-back pain tends to be self-limiting and in the light of Newman's (1973) estimate that only one patient in every 100 who consults his general practitioner will come to surgery. Since no single therapeutic modality will suffice to treat each of the different clinical syndromes and since few satisfactorily controlled scientific trials exist the

treatment regimens in the following chapters are based on experience in the types of therapy likely to improve the underlying condition.

The different types of treatment available are:

(1) Rest:

    (a) Bed rest.
    (b) Supports—corset, brace, and plaster.

(2) Physical therapy:

    (a) Manual therapy—mobilization, traction, and manipulation.
    (b) Other therapies—heat, cold, transcutaneous nerve stimulation, interferential therapy, and exercises.

(3) Medication:

    (a) Analgesics.
    (b) Non-steroidal anti-inflammatory drugs.

(4) Injection therapy:

    (a) Local infiltrations.
    (b) Epidural injections.

(5) Surgery.
(6) Aftercare and prophylaxis.

These will be described in more detail in subsequent chapters. Manipulation, mobilization and traction techniques are then discussed at some length (Chapters 24–26). The use of these available methods in the management of the clinical syndromes that have been previously described is presented in Chapter 27. The different therapeutic modalities will be divided into three categories. Firstly, those producing the best results; secondly, those treatments that are of limited or doubtful value; and thirdly, those that are contraindicated. Finally, the role of manual therapy techniques in treating the lumbar spine is considered in Chapter 28.

24 Manipulation

Joint manipulation is a passive-movement technique that occurs when the joint is moved with a sudden movement or thrust at the normal limits of its range by the therapist. This movement is of short duration and amplitude but is performed so quickly that the patient is unable to prevent it.

Application of manipulation
Peripheral joints

In peripheral joints the clinical indications for manipulation include:

(1) Replacement of a dislocation or subluxation.
(2) Breaking down or stretching of adhesions.
(3) Reduction of an internal derangement of the joint, such as that produced by a cartilaginous body.
(4) Hypomobility lesions.

Manipulation is necessary to reduce a dislocation, as in the shoulder, or a subluxation, as in a 'pulled elbow'.

Joint stiffness after a sprain—associated with ligamentous pain, tenderness, and loss of joint function—responds well to manipulation. Manipulation in capsulitis of the shoulder, when used to break down the periarticular adhesions, usually results in increased mobility.

A locked knee joint, with a mechanical block to full extension produced by a cartilaginous displacement, may be freed with one manipulation.

Hypomobility lesions, lacking a precise pathological basis but associated with loss of joint accessory movements, also occur. One example is foot pain from hypomobile mid-tarsal joints which usually respond readily to manipulation, often with a 'snapping' sensation.

Spinal joints

It would be satisfying to be able to translate these examples of peripheral-joint lesions to the spinal joints, but the necessary evidence to diagnose a similar type of underlying lesion amenable to manipulation is lacking. Various theories to explain the success of manipulation have been formulated. In the apophyseal joints a subluxation or an internal derangement due to meniscoid bodies, loose cartilaginous bodies, nipped synovial fringes or 'joint lock' have been considered. Disc pathology has also been considered and includes annular tears or a nuclear prolapse, either bulging into the spinal canal or blocked between vertebral bodies.

Adhesion formation is a popular concept but it has not been demonstrated around the spinal joints. It seems highly unlikely that a breakdown of adhesions is a common mechanism. Finally, a hypomobility lesion with loss of the normal accessory movements is the main indication for spinal manipulation.

Main effects of spinal manipulation

The principal benefit obtained is an increased mobility due to an increased range of movement of an intervertebral-joint segment, with restoration of physiological and accessory movements.

Relief of pain: whatever the underlying lesion producing a reduced spinal mobility may be, it may also result in stimulation of the sinu-vertebral nerves and produce spinal pain. Hence restoration of spinal mobility will also relieve this source of neural irritation.

Possible benefits

There is usually a reduction in muscular spasm, which may help circumvent a pain–spasm–pain cycle.

There is an improvement in disc nutrition. Disc nutrition, dependent on fluid exchange between vascular channels in the vertebrae and the disc, may be aided by normal joint movement and impeded by loss of normal mobility. Hence restoration of normal joint movements may aid in preventing disc degeneration.

There are psychological benefits. No one would deny the psychological effects produced by the personalized care and 'laying on of hands' implicit in manipulative practice, nor that the patient receives very positive treatment without having to do anything himself.

Unlikely effects

It would appear extremely unlikely that spinal manipulation can regularly effect the reduction of a subluxation, reposition a piece of prolapsed disc material or break down adhesions. At times a single manipulation does produce a 'click' and give immediate relief of pain, though such an occurrence is uncommon; it would then appear that a loose cartilaginous body within the inter-vertebral joint complex may have been moved.

Precautions

(1) A careful overall assessment of the patient and his musculoskeletal problem is undertaken before any treatment is commenced.

(2) Those patients in whom manipulation is contraindicated should be excluded. This necessitates, besides the history and physical examination, an X-ray examination.

(3) Repeated testing is made to assess the response of symptoms and signs to the treatment technique used. Considerable practice in these techniques permits the recognition of patterns of joint behaviour. A patient with a certain degree of pain and stiffness should improve in an orderly progression after a prescribed level of therapy. Failure to fit into this pattern is often an early-warning sign of the presence of serious organic disease or psychogenic disorder.

(4) Manipulation under general anaesthesia is only rarely indicated. General anaesthesia is usually best avoided, since it also prevents any meaningful reassessment of the patient's reaction to a technique. Also, the spine is much more readily traumatized when the patient is unconscious, and it is extremely rare for one manipulation alone to cure a patient's symptoms completely. However, there may be an indication for manipulation under anaesthesia in certain circumstances. At times a patient may not be improving with routine therapy and may then be helped with anaesthesia. Also, a patient's build—or more especially type of muscle spasm—may occasionally preclude adequate positioning without anaesthesia.

(5) Extreme gentleness in the initial stages of treatment is always necessary and so mobilization techniques are selected first in almost all cases before the manipulative techniques.

(6) A joint should never be forcibly thrust in a direction that is protected by muscle spasm. To do so invites trouble. A different direction of movement for the same joint, unprotected by spasm, should be chosen.

(7) The depth and strength of movements should be increased only after reassessing the patient's condition to verify that there is no adverse reaction.

(8) Treatment involving forced flexion of the lumbar spine or manipulation with the

patient in a flexed position is extremely dangerous. However, mobilization techniques may be carried out in this direction, particularly if performed in a non-weight-bearing position.

(9) Manipulation using strong manual traction is unnecessary. It neither increases the incidence of satisfactory results nor renders the techniques safe.

(10) Minor increases in the range of movement may be all that is required if the patient's symptoms are improving. It may not be necessary to restore the expected full range of mobility. A patient's subjective feeling of stiffness does not usually correspond with the objective loss of joint range, which is measured by comparing movements to either side.

(11) A plan is essential. All joints that could be responsible for a patient's symptoms must be examined; if any are considered to be responsible for symptoms a treatment plan should be devised (Maitland, 1973).

(12) Finally, special precaution needs to be taken during pregnancy. The problems associated with manipulation in pregnant patients with spinal pain are related mainly to the technical problems associated with adequate posturing of the patient. Most patients can be treated with suitable mobilizing techniques without any undue complication.

Mechanism of action

The mechanism of action of spinal manipulation is still speculative and its use remains empirical. Attempts to demonstrate its effect have been made with contrast radiography but this X-ray examination is subject to many sources of error. After myelography or epidurography in disc prolapse an increase, a decrease, or no alteration at all in the size of the prolapse has been reported. Chrisman, Mittnacht and Snook (1964) reported that a group of patients with no demonstrable myelographic defect did much better after manipulation than did those in whom such a defect was demonstrated.

Chrisman and co-workers also used a rotary manipulation on patients lying on their side during a laminectomy for disc prolapse. Inter-vertebral-joint movement was observed, with the laminae separated by approximately 5 mm and with stretching of the ligamentum flavum and of the apophyseal joint capsule. Other parts of the spinal-joint segment, such as the posterior surface of the vertebrae with the posterior longitudinal ligament and the apophyseal joint, could also be seen to move.

These findings are important for two reasons. Firstly, the presence of a disc prolapse does not explain the benefits of manipulation. Obviously, a disc prolapse can never be repositioned by manipulation any more than toothpaste can be squeezed back into its tube. Secondly, it appears most likely that the successful action of manipulation is related to stretching or moving the intervertebral joint complex with restoration of lost movement. Consequently, benefit may be derived from improving any loss of this normal range.

The cracking sound

Crack-like sounds coming from the manipulated spinal joints are well known as a common phenomenon accompanying movement in a synovial joint. A bioengineering study using gas analysis in peripheral joints by Unsworth, Dowson and Wright (1971) showed that tension on the joint produces a low-pressure system in the synovial fluid that allows vaporization of the gas, which is then liberated, so opening up the joint space. This bubble of gas forms and collapses again in 0.01 seconds, and it is the collapse of the vapour bubble, not its formation, that produces the crack.

About 20 minutes is required before a joint is again ready to produce a crack, which represents the time taken for the gas to return into solution. The gas formed is carbon dioxide, not nitrogen as is commonly believed. Not all peripheral joints can be made to crack, possibly because of the size of the joint space or because of differences in ligamentous function. Similar changes presumably occur in the synovial apophyseal joints.

There is one situation in which cracking represents a useful sign. Manipulation of stiff joints may at times produce little appreciable movement during the first few treatments; it is not until the range of movement has improved that manipulation is then apt to produce a crack. Joint range is then invariably found to be increased.

It may be safely assumed that spinal manipulation does not generally produce its effect through rupturing adhesions. The noise of stretching adhesions—as heard, for example, when manipulating a patient with capsulitis of the shoulder—is quite different from the crack-like sound on spinal manipulation.

Finally, movement at a joint may be produced without any accompanying cracking sound. However, if a crack is produced it indicates that the joint has been satisfactorily moved.

Complications

It is a sound axiom that 'the bad results of manipulation are due to bad manipulators'; and considering the many spinal manipulations performed throughout the world each year, the number of recorded complications are extraordinarily few. Serious complication should not occur if the precautions listed above are heeded. Nevertheless, deaths have been reported (Smith and Estridge, 1962) as well as various vascular, neurological and bony complications. It is well recognized that alterations in vertebral artery blood flow may follow rotation of the head. Vascular lesions resulting in brainstem dysfunction have been reported by Pratt-Thomas (1947) after chiropractic manipulation. Ford and Clark (1956) reported two cases of posterior inferior cerebellar artery occlusions, one of which was fatal, and similar reports have been made by Green and Joynt (1959).

More recently, Mueller and Sahs (1976) reported three cases of brain-stem dysfunction after manipulation of the neck. One patient had only mild disability but one had a dislocation of C2 on C3 with residual motor signs in the left leg, and the third patient had a cerebellar infarct.

Neurological complications include cauda equina lesions, cord compression, nerve-root compression and rupture of a nerve root. Kuhlendahl and Hensell (1958) described a case of cauda equina compression produced by a massive disc extrusion after manipulation under anaesthesia.

Bone damage due to fractures or joint subluxation have been reported mostly after chiropractic manipulation; damage often stems from a failure to recognize the presence of a bone lesion, such as a secondary malignant deposit.

Controlled trials

Acceptance of manipulative methods of treatment is hindered by the lack of an adequately conducted, controlled double-blind clinical trial. One reason for this is the problem of assuring that the trial is double blind, since both the doctor and the patient will usually be able to recognize what treatment regimen has been allocated. Another problem is tailoring the type and degree of manipulative therapy to the patient's clinical problem. Despite the problems associated with setting up such a trial it clearly remains a major need. Some trials have been published, but have been heavily criticized on the basis of selection of patients and treatment technique. Glover, Morris and Khosla (1974) reported a trial of 84 patients with back pain who worked in an engineering plant. They were divided into two treatment groups, one to have one only rotational manipulation of the spine and the other a control group. The patients were then assessed within 15 minutes, 3 days later and a further 4 days later. There was no statistical difference between these two groups—except at the 15-minute assessment, when the manipulated group fared better. However, this result is certainly not surprising when only one treatment was given on one occasion.

Doran and Newell (1975) reported a multicentre trial of 456 selected patients with low-back pain, each of whom was allocated at random to one of four treatment groups: manipulation, physiotherapy, corset, and analgesics. Patients were assessed clinically after 3 weeks' treatment, again after a further 3 weeks, and by questionnaire after 3 months and 1 year. The manipulated group were given a minimum of two treatments per week and an average of six treatments. Again, there were no statistical differences between the four treatment groups. This trial suffered from the defects of being a multicentre trial with problems in the selection of suitable candidates for manipulative therapy, and in the standardization of the manipulative technique used. These defects were possibly reflected by the finding in the trial that certain patients responded well and quickly to manipulation.

Sims-Williams, *et al.* (1978) reported a trial of mobilization and manipulation in general practice. They included 94 patients with low-back pain severe enough to have warranted referral for X-rays of the lumbar spine. They were randomly allocated for either mobilization and manipulation by the Maitland technique or placebo physiotherapy. Most patients improved within 1 month, were capable of at least light work and felt that treatment had helped. The actively treated group did better in all respects, and more so in work performance than in pain relief or opinion of treatment.

Improvement was maintained at later follow-up at 3 months and 1 year, although the differences between actively treated and control groups progressively disappeared. No prognostic factors could be identified, other than more common improvement in patients where pain had been present for less than 1 month. This trial, although confirming that there is a high rate of spontaneous remission, indicated that manipulation may hasten remission in some cases without affecting long-term prognosis.

25 Mobilization

In most patients with spinal pain requiring a passive-movement technique a full manipulation is not necessary to produce an improvement in signs and symptoms. The initial passive-movement technique is usually mobilization, in which the joint is moved rhythmically within its normal range and at a speed that the patient can voluntarily resist or prevent. It is often surprising how much improvement can be obtained by quite gentle mobilization.

Management of musculoskeletal disorders with mobilization consists of:

(1) Investigations. These are required to eliminate those patients in which such methods of treatment would be either contraindicated or unsatisfactory.

(2) If pain is reproduced on passive movement, treatment with passive movements would appear to be a logical extension.

(3) The particular joint at fault is located by clinical testing.

(4) The movements of that joint which are painful or restricted are defined.

(5) A suitable technique is chosen according to the clinical findings and the degree of anticipated improvement.

(6) The amplitude of the treatment is selected.

(7) Treatment must be gentle at first, using mobilization techniques that may then be progressed in strength or in their grade of movement.

(8) It is only if these are not producing satisfactory improvement that a formal manipulation would be indicated.

For mobilization to be effective a sense of 'feel'

of movement is required, likened to feeling the meshing of cogs in the gearbox on changing gears.

The movements taking place are often not seen but sensed. Until this feel is acquired, treatment by mobilization can never be fully effective. For example, if the oscillation involved in a technique is too quick or too slow it is impossible to gain the proper feel of movement in the joint, and the movement will feel like stretching or shaking. There is no fixed rate, but approximately two or three oscillations per second is usual.

For a joint to be most effectively moved in any direction it should first be positioned approximately midway between all of its other ranges. An example of this is found in the metacarpophalangeal joint of the index finger. To achieve maximum distraction with the least effort a starting position midway between the normal limits of flexion, extension, abduction, adduction and rotation is used. If the joint is positioned at the limit of any one of these ranges the range of distraction will be limited.

When the head and neck lie in their normal alignment the lowest cervical intervertebral joints are in a slightly extended position. Therefore, when these techniques are being used for the lower cervical intervertebral joints the neck should be moved towards flexion to gain this mid-position between the limits of flexion and extension. Similar principles apply to the techniques of traction, longitudinal movement and rotation in the lumbar spine. For lower lumbar movement, the spine is positioned towards flexion; for upper lumbar joint mobilization the lumbar spine is positioned towards extension.

Mobilization techniques using pressure against

some part of the vertebra also require attention to detail. Only the thumbs or the hands should be used to produce movement by transmitting body weight to the vertebra. If the instrinsic muscles of the hands are used to produce this pressure the technique becomes uncomfortable both to patient and to therapist, the hands become tense and all possibility of 'feeling' the movement is lost. In all techniques in which direct pressure is applied to the vertebrae, the supporting fingers are positioned with the arms and thumbs over the movement. The correct starting position is important as it allows the patient to relax and the therapist to work effectively with the minimum of effort and the hands relaxed. Passive movement may be used as either a unilateral or a bilateral technique.

Unilateral techniques

Although producing movement in the whole of the joint complex, these techniques affect one side of the joint more than the other. The patient is positioned so that during each technique the intervertebral foramen is opened on the painful side.

Lumbar rotation

This technique should initially be performed by rotating the patient's pelvis away from the painful side, but since the amount of foraminal narrowing produced during lumbar rotation is very small, rotation in the opposite direction can also be used.

Cervical rotation

The intervertebral foramina on the painful side are widened from C2 to C7 by rotating the head towards the opposite direction. Similarly, rotating the head towards the painful side produces considerable narrowing of the intervertebral foramen on that side. This does not apply in the occipitoatlantal and atlantoaxial joints.

Cervical lateral flexion

This technique is initially performed by tilting the patient's head and neck away from the side of pain to open the foramen on the painful side.

Transverse vertebral pressure

This should be performed by pushing the spinous process towards the side of pain so that the intervertebral foramen is opened on the painful side.

Posteroanterior unilateral vertebral pressure

This technique is performed with pressure applied downwards on the painful side to open the foramen on that painful side.

Bilateral techniques

Traction, longitudinal movement and posteroanterior central pressures affect movement on both sides of the intervertebral joint.

Treatment grades *(see page 28)*

The amount of movement used in mobilization treatment must be modified according to pain, restriction of movement and muscle spasm. Movements may be graded according to their amplitude and the position within the range they occupy.

Grade I is a small-amplitude movement performed at the starting position of the range.

Grade II is a large-amplitude movement that carries well into the range. It can occupy any part of the range but does not reach the limit of the range. Grade III is also a large-amplitude movement at the limit of the range.

Grade IV is a small-amplitude movement at the end of the range.

Selection of technique

The particular technique chosen depends on the site of pain, the disturbance in rhythm of spinal movements, and its reponse to treatment.

If pain or restricted movement is unilateral, unilateral techniques designed to open up or move the same side of the intervertebral joint complex should provide relief. Thus a patient with a right-side back pain may be found to have a restriction of lateral flexion to the right. The technique selected aims at opening the right-hand side of the intervertebral joint, e.g. by transverse pressures against the spinous process from left to right.

Depth of mobilization

At first gentle techniques only should be used so as not to produce any exacerbation of symptoms or signs. It is often surprising how much improvement can be gained by these gentle manoeuvres. Any alteration in the degree of pain, spasm and stiffness, or any change in their position within the range, must be constantly assessed both during the treatment session and before the next session.

The depth of the mobilization is guided by pain and spasm.

Pain

This is the most important guide in determining the depth to which a technique can be given. Pain is assessed according to its severity, whether it is localized or referred, and the site within the range of movement at which it is produced. Six factors need to be considered:

(1) For patients with severe pain, movements must be small; usually grade I.
(2) With localized spinal pain, mobilization should be performed initially in the pain-free range, the movement being carried up to the point where pain begins. When pain is felt at the beginning of the range the mobilization must be performed with very small rhythmical movements (grade I). As the range of pain-free movement increases the mobilization can be performed still further into the range (grade II).
(3) Greater care is necessary if a mobilizing technique reproduces distally referred pain. Any subsequent mobilizing technique must be performed in the painless range, its effect being assessed immediately after the treatment and again 24 hours later. Provided that symptoms or signs have not been aggravated, the technique may be increased

slightly to the point where discomfort in the referred area can be felt. If referred symptoms are exacerbated the amplitude of the mobilization and its position in the range must be reduced. Assessment over 24 hours will indicate whether this technique should be continued. It is often necessary to provoke some degree of pain in order to produce an improvement in movements.
(4) When either local or referred pain starts in the last quarter of the range the techniques are more commonly used at the limit of the normal range or until meeting physical resistance. When such a resistance can be felt, either a large grade III or a small grade IV amplitude should be used. The latter movement tends to produce more local soreness; the former is unlikely to produce soreness, although it may not be as efficient at increasing range.
(5) When the patient has a painful arc of movement, large-amplitude grade II or grade III mobilization should be performed.
(6) In patients presenting with little pain but restricted movement, grade IV movements are often the only successful treatment. If such treatment does produce any exacerbation of symptoms, grade II or gentle grade III movements can be used to relieve local soreness.

To summarize: pain represents the major guide to the depth of the mobilization technique used; muscle spasm, the other guide, is usually induced later in the range.

Spasm

This is a protective mechanism to splint a painful joint and is usually readily recognized on inspection and palpation. Treatment techniques must always be extremely gentle at first to avoid provoking any excessive or sudden protective muscular reaction. Moreover, a joint should never be forced beyond this limit.

As the patient improves, the depth of mobilization and the range of spasm-free movement should be increased.

Duration and frequency of treatment

Treatment is usually initially carried out daily. On the first day treatment by mobilization techniques is normally only of short duration, as the joint has been subjected to sufficient movement by the examination. The patient should be warned that some temporary increase in symptoms may be expected, and the degree of any such reaction produced is assessed the next day. The number of any mobilizations in one session depends on the assessment of the degree of the patient's symptoms. With moderate degrees, three or four mobilizations of a joint, lasting approximately 30–60 seconds each, are given. In patients whose symptoms are minimal this can be increased, and six mobilization treatments are given to the joint when pain is severe, although only two mobilizations can usually be given at each session. Provided that any reaction to these treatments is not excessive, treatment can be progressed in subsequent sessions.

Assessment of techniques

(1) The chosen technique must initially be used gently without provoking any pain.
(2) After this, the patient's symptoms and signs are reassessed; the range of movements and of pain are compared with those previously present.
(3) If the clinical findings are unaltered the same technique may be repeated more firmly.
(4) The patient is reassessed.
(5) If there is still no improvement an alternative technique is selected.
(6) If the patient's symptoms have been exacerbated that particular technique should be discarded.
(7) A good guide to the success of treatment in patients with diffuse spinal pain is whether the joint range subsequently retained is at least 50 per cent of the increase gained during treatment.

Reaction to treatment

Mobilization techniques should result in an improvement of symptoms over a few days. The patient may experience some degree of soreness for a time after treatment if strong techniques have been used but this should be only temporary and should have eased before the next treatment. The degree of reaction is more marked if very strong techniques are used. Manipulation differs from mobilization in its effect on a joint since it is more vigorous and potentially more traumatic. The patient may then expect more soreness, which should disappear before a further manipulation is undertaken.

Indications and contraindications for manual-therapy techniques

In nearly all cases the gentler mobilization techniques should be used first, as they usually provide sufficient improvement without the need to proceed to manipulation. It must be emphasized that the indications are predicated on a full clinical assessment of the diagnosis and of the whole patient.

Manual-therapy techniques may be considered in four groups:

(1) Those conditions in which these techniques may be expected to be successful in most cases, or at least form a major role in the therapeutic regimen. These will be referred to as major indications.
(2) Those conditions in which they may help in some but not all cases. In these conditions other methods of therapy take precedence and the role of manipulation often varies according to the skill or experience of the therapist. These will be referred to as relative indications.
(3) Those conditions in which they are not contraindicated but only rarely produce any improvement in the patient's condition.
(4) Those conditions in which they are contraindicated.

Further discussion on the use of these techniques is to be found in the relevant chapters.

Major indications

The major indication for manual-therapy techniques is a mechanical derangement of vertebral-joint movement that produces pain in the absence of any neurological lesion.

Examples include:

(1) Patients with a spinal hypomobility lesion or any of the pain syndromes that may be associated with it.

(2) Patients with spondylosis, especially in the cervical spine. Mobilization techniques usually produce a marked improvement in pain and stiffness. It is often possible for patients to achieve some extra movement and an improvement in function in the neck; for example, being able to turn their head to reverse a car.

(3) Patients with minor attacks of acute lumbago or when they are recovering from a severe attack.

Relative indications

Intervertebral-disc prolapse

The role of manipulative techniques in the management of intervertebral-disc prolapse remains controversial and the amount of improvement that may be expected to be gained from manipulation is uncertain. The use of these techniques will depend largely on the experience and expertise of the therapist. Gentle mobilization techniques may be expected to be of value in patients without severe degrees of pain and no neurological deficit. Moreover, in patients with non-progressive neurological symptoms and signs—for example, paraesthesias or an absent ankle jerk—gentler techniques may be used as part of overall management.

However, a patient with a large space-occupying disc prolapse that produces nerve-root compression and a neurological deficit should not be treated with manipulation. Nevertheless, as these patients improve treatment with mobilization techniques may be added, and provided that clinical improvement is maintained treatment may be increased in intensity. What is being achieved in patients who improve remains uncertain, since the prolapsed disc material is never replaced into

its original site. However, occasionally a sequestrum of disc material within the intervertebral joint may be moved, which results in the restoration of some degree of mobility with pain relief.

Spondylolisthesis

Patients with spondylolisthesis who present with either back or leg pain may be helped with mobilization techniques or traction. In a small proportion pain is made worse and in a similar proportion pain is unimproved, but some relief of symptoms may be expected in approximately 60 per cent of cases.

Hypermobility syndromes

Hypermobility syndromes with spinal pain usually respond poorly to most forms of therapy, and manipulative therapy would appear to be no exception. However, in some patients it may be possible to demonstrate a hypomobile lesion in one spinal segment, movement of which reproduces symptoms; treatment by mobilization of that segment is indicated.

Vertigo

The problem of vertigo in disorders of the cervical spine is considered in Chapter 32. A patient who complains of vertigo needs careful assessment before mobilizing techniques are used, and tests designed to assess the presence of any vertebral-artery compression are described later. However, mobilization techniques may be useful in patients with this symptom who have reduced cervical mobility and no evidence of vertebral-artery compression. It should also be realized that if any cervical technique ever produces vertigo subsequent manual-therapy technique is contraindicated.

Undiagnosed patients

As a general rule, patients in whom a firm clinical diagnosis has not been established should not be treated with manipulation. However, there are exceptions to this rule. Patients with undiagnosed spinal pain may be treated with mobilization techniques while progress is observed. The presence of any underlying serious lesion would appear unlikely if the patient improves. However, if symptoms are exacerbated therapy should be discontinued while further investigations are carried out.

Rarely successful

Patients with pain due to postural disturbances, the stiff-back syndrome (Stoddard, 1969), or severe degrees of acute lumbago (especially when associated with a marked lumbar kyphosis) are rarely helped by passive-movement techniques.

Contraindications

Diseases of the vertebral column

The rheumatic and orthopaedic conditions that form the basis of these conditions are discussed in Chapter 18. They include:

(1) Trauma, such as fractures, dislocations and spondylolysis.
(2) Infections.
(3) Inflammatory disease due to spondyloarthritis or rheumatoid arthritis.
(4) Metabolic bone disease, such as osteoporosis.
(5) Tumours—benign or malignant.
(6) Developmental anomalies.

Neurological lesions

Compression of neurological structures such as the spinal cord or cauda equina represents an absolute contraindication to any form of manual therapy, as does lumbar-canal stenosis. Manual therapy is also contraindicated in patients who have a severe degree of nerve-root pressure with a neurological deficit due to an intervertebral-disc prolapse; or in those patients who have evidence of compression of two nerve roots in the cervical spine.

Arterial compression

Evidence of vertebral-artery compression is an absolute contraindication; cases have been reported of occlusion of this artery after either manipulation or traction.

Psychogenic causes

Patients whose symptoms are primarily psychogenically determined should never be treated with any of the physical methods of therapy, including manual-therapy techniques.

26 Spinal traction

Spinal traction plays an important role in the therapy of many spinal conditions. Since it produces a vertical distraction force to the spine it may be classified as one form of passive-movement technique in which mobilization takes place in a vertical direction. The general principles applicable to its use are discussed in this chapter, and specific techniques for the lumbar, cervical and thoracic spines are discussed in their relevant sections.

Methods of application

Traction may be continuous, sustained, intermittent or rhythmic; it may be directed vertically, horizontally, or at an angle (in flexion, extension or neutral); it may be applied either manually or by one of numerous mechanical apparatuses, which usually employ weights, pulleys, or are motor driven.

Continuous traction is applied for several days or more with the patient in bed. Sustained traction implies traction lasting minutes or hours. Intermittent variable traction, using weights of 2 kg or more, is gradually applied, held momentarily, then gradually released. This is followed by a momentary rest before traction is reapplied. This cycle, repeated for varying periods and times for the 'hold' and 'rest' periods, may be used once or twice a day.

Mechanism of action

Several theories have been advocated to explain its mechanism of action.

LONGITUDINAL MOVEMENTS

The main mechanism of its action is apparently to provide a form of mobilization technique in which longitudinal movements are applied to the intervertebral joint complex. For this reason the main indications for its use in the relief of spinal pain are those already discussed in Chapter 25.

REST

It provides rest to the area being treated. Painful hip disease may be relieved with bed rest and continuous leg traction. Continuous spinal traction applied to the patient on bed rest has too small a weight to produce any distractive force but it may succeed by enforcing extra rest (Youel, 1967).

OVERCOMING MUSCLE SPASM

It may overcome muscle spasm. In patients with either peripheral or spinal joint lesions this would appear to be of only minor benefit.

Separation of joint surfaces

It is used to separate joint surfaces, and in the spine this is often considered to be its main mechanism. Thus de Seze estimated that a pull of 113 kg widened the intervertebral space by 1.5 mm, and Cyriax claims to have measured a maximum manual pull of 136 kg. Evidence to support this mechanism has been produced by measuring superimposed X-ray figures, but such experiments are open to gross errors in interpretation.

Mathews (1968) used epidurography to outline the posterior aspects of the discs and applied strong traction for half an hour. Eleven patients were investigated and three were reported upon. In two of these, 54.45 kg traction produced a distraction of 2 mm in each lumbar disc space. Mathews also reported that this method allowed the extent of the disc bulge to be reduced and eliminated the bulging in the wall of the dural sac. These findings are difficult to interpret with this technique.

Nachemson and Elfstrom (1970) used intravital discometry to study vertical traction in two normal subjects. They showed a step-wise reduction in intradiscal pressure with increasing loads. Judovich and Nobel (1957) studied the mechanics of lumbar traction, especially the effects of body friction and the weights of different part of the body— approximately half the body weight is below L3–4. A force of at least one quarter of the body weight is necessary to overcome resistance.

Distraction of prolapsed nuclear material

The representation that traction could succeed in producing sufficient distraction to prolapsed disc nuclear material to return it into its normal anatomical confines is clearly fanciful.

Uses

The indications for the uses of traction in each spinal region will be considered in the relevant section. In general, its main use has been for limb pain of spinal origin, and it does appear that symptoms are relieved while traction is being applied.

However, clinical trials have not been able to demonstrate any definite, prolonged benefit from its use.

Precautions

Traction should always be applied gently at first in the cervical and thoracic regions. The strength and safety of the pull can be assessed by palpating between interspinous processes, and the weight applied is considered to be adequate when movement is felt to take place there. The patient's symptoms are reassessed at this weight, and traction is reduced if these are aggravated. Progression is made either by increasing the strength of the traction or by increasing the amount of treatment time. The rate of progression is guided by constant reassessment of the patient's symptoms and signs.

In the lumbar spine the first treatment should be at a weight just sufficient to produce movement at the intervertebral joint being treated, usually with a weight of about 10 kg. If stronger traction is applied the patient may have difficulty in standing upright when traction is ceased because of the development of severe central low-back pain.

In patients with cervical or lumbar nerve-root pressure the amount of traction should not completely relieve pain, for with greater weights pain is nearly always exacerbated. This gentle traction is usually quite safe, and treatment may be slowly progressed by increasing the length of time of treatment. Then, as symptoms subside, the strength of traction may also be increased.

Contraindications and complications

The contraindications and complications are similar to those already described for the use of mobilization techniques, since traction should be considered as one form of spinal mobilization that now employs long-axis extension as its technique. Traction is contraindicated in patients with hypermobility syndromes involving the spine or sacroiliac joints.

27 The management of lumbar syndromes

The lumbar syndromes to be discussed in this chapter are divided into:

(1) Intervertebral-disc prolapse.
(2) Other disc degenerative lesions.
(3) Disorders of spinal movements:
    (a) Acute lumbago.
    (b) Hypomobility lesions.
    (c) Hypermobility lesions.

Management of lumbar intervertebral-disc prolapse

The initial management of a patient with a disc prolapse is determined by the severity of the lesion, which is assessed clinically by the degree of the patient's pain and the presence of neurological involvement. In this way, the condition may be classified as being either severe or moderate (*see Figure 27.1*).

Lumbar-disc prolapse of severe degree

In patients with a severe degree of involvement, management may be divided into initial, subsequent, and aftercare and prophylaxis.

Initial management

REST
This is essential. The patient needs complete bed rest; this may be possible at home, but since this is often difficult to obtain successfully for optimum treatment the patient should be admitted to hospital. The rationale of bed rest is twofold. Firstly, movement maintains the inflammatory reaction and oedema present around the nerve root and makes pain difficult to control. Secondly, as Nachemson and Morris (1964) demonstrated, the horizontal position produces the lowest intradiscal pressure, certainly much less than during sitting or standing.

Posture in bed is important. The patient is allowed to adopt as comfortable a position as possible to take tension off the inflamed nerve. This is usually best achieved by flexing the knees and hips in the Fowler's position or by lying on the side. The patient may need to be fed or may lie on his side to eat, but is not permitted to sit for meals. However, he is allowed up to a bedside toilet, as this is less stressful than having to struggle on to a bed pan.

An alternative method of resting the lumbosacral area is to immobilize the patient in a plaster jacket. This has the disadvantage of being most uncomfortable to wear, but at least allows the patient to remain mobile. An epidural injection of corticosteroid, described below, is usually given before the jacket is applied.

MEDICATION
Simple analgesics should be given in sufficient quantities to ensure pain relief and allow sleep, and there may be a need for sedation to allay anxiety. Anti-inflammatory agents are also given to control any inflammatory component present, even though one trial (Goldi, 1968) failed to show any efficacy.

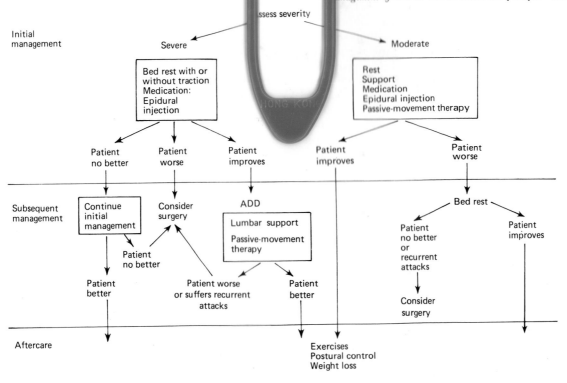

Figure 27.1 Management of lumbar intervertebral-disc prolapse

TRACTION

Traction applied either to each leg or through a pelvic harness may be used with the patient in bed. It may not be possible to use this continuously at first if pain is severe, though after a few days it may be so used. The strength of traction used does not produce any lumbar distraction but it may help to keep the patient immobilized, thus providing some relief of pain and muscle spasm. It may also be of psychological benefit, since it appears that something positive is being done.

The patient lies supine with the bed either horizontal or with the foot raised 25 cm. Fowler's position may be used in the initial stages and is particularly useful in those patients with a marked lumbar kyphosis. A pelvic belt is placed on the patient and then fitted to a spreader by ropes. From the spreader a rope passes over a pulley at the foot of the bed with weights attached to its end. Skin traction is best not used. The initial weight is 7 kg, which may be increased by 1 kg daily up to 10 kg. Traction is maintained for up to 3 weeks while the patient is rested in bed.

CORTICOSTEROID INJECTIONS

To ease the local painful inflammatory reaction an epidural injection of corticosteroid may be given either by the lumbar route or through the sacral canal. Soon after hydrocortisone was found suitable as a local injection, attempts were made to inject it near inflamed nerve roots. Reports of its use appeared first in the European literature (Lievre, Bloch–Michel and Attall, 1953) and in 1961 Goebert *et al.* reported its successful use in 113 patients. There have since been several reports on its successful use. Seghal, Tweed and Gardner (1961) reported that no complications followed the intrathecal injections of methylprednisolone into animals. A modification of this technique was reported by Warr *et al.* (1972), who treated 500 patients with epidural injections followed by manipulation under anaesthesia and found that 63 per cent had relief lasting at least 6 months. Subsequently, Burn and Langdon (1974) demonstrated that the period of relief that was produced corresponded with the duration of the corticosteroid's action.

A well-conducted double-blind trial of 120 patients with lumbar nerve-root compression that assessed the effect of an extradural corticosteroid injection of 80 mg methylprednisolone after 3 months (Dilke, Burry and Grahame, 1973) demonstrated pain relief and earlier return to normal occupation in most patients without any significant complications. It is essential that the injection be given extradurally only and that it is discontinued if the dura is pierced (Corrigan, Carr and Tugwell, 1982). The technique is similar to that of a lumbar puncture, using a disposable lumbar-puncture set and scrupulous aseptic technique. The patient lies curled up on the painful side and the injection is given at either the L3–4 or L4–5 level. The needle should be felt to lie free in the epidural space and various techniques (e.g. the hanging-drop method) have been described to ensure this. An injection of methylprednisolone 80 mg is then given and the patient is kept in bed for 2 days.

This procedure is best used in patients who have disc prolapse with evidence of nerve-root compression. The best results are obtained in those patients with a recent onset of severe back and leg pain. The injection may be repeated once or twice at weekly intervals if necessary. It may also be used in cases where a definitive diagnosis has not yet been made but where a disc prolapse is suspected. The injection must never be given in the presence of any nearby skin infection.

Complications are quite rare, but the patient's pain may be exacerbated for one or two days. Serious infective complications, including tuberculosis and cryptococcal meningitis, although excessively rare, have been reported.

Trans-sacral Approach   The epidural space lies between the two layers of dura; an outer or periosteal layer, and an inner or dural layer. This space, which is continuous from the foramen magnum to the sacral hiatus, also contains the vertebral venous plexus and fat. The dural sac usually terminates at the S2 level and the spinal cord at about L1. The sacrum comprises four fused vertebrae with a fifth vertebra remaining unfused and ending as two projections or cornua. The opening of the sacral hiatus—normally covered over by a firm, elastic ligament—lies between these two cornua. This hiatus, often the site of a skin dimple, may be identified between the readily palpable cornua on either side.

A solution of up to 40–50 ml of 1% lignocaine (Xylocaine) without adrenaline is used, to which 80 mg of methylprednisolone is added. The injection is best given in hospital with the patient lying prone and as relaxed as possible. The skin is thoroughly sterilized and a 19-gauge needle is inserted at the midline. The thumb and finger of the left hand are placed over the cornua to help guide the direction of the needle. As the ligament

is pierced there is a sensation of 'giving', and if the needle is angled slightly downwards it can then be felt to lie free within the sacral canal. If it impinges on bone the needle is withdrawn and slightly angled. If it lies outside the canal the subcutaneous tissue is seen and felt to swell with the injection of fluid (*see Figure 27.2*). Normally the injection is felt to run in without resistance. It is given slowly, over at least 10 minutes, with repeated aspirations to ensure the absence of any blood or CSF.

The patient is warned that a sensation of warmth and usually some exacerbation of pain may be produced and is asked to report any light-headedness or giddiness. The pulse rate and blood pressure should be monitored during the injection. If any untoward reaction is experienced the injection is stopped.

Indications—The best results with this technique are obtained in cases with severe degrees of sciatic pain of recent origin with or without neurological signs; the more severe the pain, the greater the chance of success. In patients with either a postero-lateral disc protrusion or bilateral leg pain this is often the best single method of providing pain relief but it can also be a useful technique in patients with back pain alone. Old age and pregnancy are not contraindications to its use.

Contraindications—The injection is contraindicated in people who have a sensitivity to local anaesthetic or who have any nearby skin infection.

Precautions on injection are as follows:

(1) Strict asepsis is necessary.
(2) The syringe must be constantly aspirated to ensure that no blood or CSF is withdrawn. The injection is ceased if the theca is punctured and CSF obtained, or else if blood is aspirated.
(3) The injection is given slowly.
(4) Side effects are anticipated by monitoring the pulse and blood pressure.
(5) The patient stays at rest for approximately 20 minutes after the injection and is then allowed to move about.

The injection may be repeated if necessary 1 week later and may be repeated several times provided that there is some degree of improvement. In at least 50 per cent of cases with sciatica there is marked relief of pain and increased mobility. Pain may be exacerbated after the injection though never for more than one or two days, so patients may be reassured that their condition will not be worsened. Its mechanism of action is unknown. Since the duration of the improvement

ures, both of which are intended to ease pain and provide an increase in the range of spinal mobility. These techniques may be continued provided that there is no exacerbation of the patient's symptoms.

Support in a corset is used to help ease pain while allowing the patient to become more mobile. Its mechanism of action is uncertain but it is believed to produce its effect (Bartelink, 1957) by increasing the intra-abdominal pressure. Nachemson and Morris (1964) showed that the use of an inflatable corset could reduce the load on the lumbosacral disc by up to 25 per cent. The most practical form of support is usually a well-fitted corset containing semi-rigid steel bands moulded into the lumbar lordosis. Although it cannot completely immobilize the spine, such a corset may limit movement, especially at the extremes of range, and may be advantageous:

(1) If the abdominal or spinal muscles are weak. This may be found in patients with severe disc prolapse after they have been confined to bed for a time. It is preferable to have the patient mobile in a corset rather than continue to have a prolonged period of immobilization.
(2) If extensive radiological changes of disc degeneration are present.
(3) In obese patients with a pendulous abdomen, a support may alter the patient's centre of gravity, so preventing excessive lumbar lordosis.

The disadvantages of wearing such a support include the following:

(1) There is usually considerable patient resistance to wearing corsets unless it can be demonstrated that pain relief will follow.
(2) Patients may become psychologically dependent on them.

To summarize, supports may be used to alleviate pain but should not be used as the sole method of management. Abdominal and spinal isometric exercises should be performed while supports are worn, and supports should be discarded as soon as is practical.

Lumbar-disc prolapse of moderate degree

The therapeutic regimen is modified if the initial assessment indicates that a less severe degree of prolapse is present. This may be judged clinically by the presence of a lesser intensity of pain, which may also be of more gradual onset, or else by the absence of any marked neurological deficit.

Treatments now available include rest, medication, local injection and passive-movement techniques.

Rest from those activities known to exacerbate pain is still necessary. Continuous bed rest is no longer necessary but a corset may help to relieve pain while keeping the patient ambulant.

Anti-inflammatory and analgesic agents are used to provide some degree of pain relief, and extrathecal injections of corticosteroid are still indicated. Passive-movement techniques, such as traction and mobilization, are used to a much greater extent during this phase than in those cases of severe degree. The aim of these treatments is gradually to increase joint mobility and to lessen pain.

Aftercare and prophylaxis

In most patients, pain and restriction of movement usually improve after this treatment regimen. Management during this next stage consists of having the patient taught back exercises and being informed about the need for postural control and back care. It is most useful to have an articulated spine available to demonstrate to patients the basic principles of such back care. With this as a model the vertebral column can be likened to a chain and the patient shown that his degenerative joint constitutes a weak link in this chain. While being encouraged to lead as normal a life as possible, the patient is advised to avoid excessive strains on this weak link and to have an optimistic view of the long-term prognosis. The patient is much more likely to heed this advice if there is a history of recurrent attacks, or if there is radiological evidence of degenerative changes. It can also be explained that a weak link is likely to react poorly to sudden, jerky movements. Unfortunately, it is not possible to avoid all such movements, especially since they usually occur before the person becomes aware of them. However, to forewarn the patient helps him to understand the problem of recurrences. Obese patients must be encouraged to lose weight; to point out that the extra weight is an additional load on the spine may help to motivate the patient.

The exercise programme and instructions for care of the back during daily activities require an individually tailored and supervised physical re-education programme.

A common clinical problem is to determine the best management for a patient who has recovered from an attack of back pain but whose affected joint, on examination, then shows either decreased or increased mobility. While there is no direct evidence to support a theory that such a joint is liable to recurrent attacks of trouble, experience indicates that this is indeed the case. In either of these circumstances continued use of manipulative procedures is contraindicated: those patients with a painless restricted joint are given mobilizing exercises to perform morning and night; those with a hypermobile joint are given stabilizing exercises.

EXERCISES

Muscle strength may decrease after an attack of intervertebal-disc prolapse has led to enforced rest (Pederson, Petersen and Staffeldt, 1975).

Accordingly, it is reasonable to prescribe muscle strengthening exercises, even though weakness has not been proved to predispose to recurrences. Until pain ceases to be a problem, exercises have little chance of being successful and may exacerbate pain if undertaken too soon or enthusiastically. There is no evidence that the spine will become stiff if they are not commenced early.

Three types of exercises are available: isometric, flexion, or extension. Each has its rationale, each its devotees. However, two well-conducted, controlled clinical trials (Kendall and Jenkins, 1968; Lindstrom and Zachrisson, 1970) found that isometric exercises produced the best results without the side effects displayed by other methods. They are, therefore, advocated.

Isometric exercises   Isometric exercises have as the rationale for their use (Bartelink, 1957) the belief that increasing intra-abdominal and intrathoracic pressure helps to prevent increased intradiscal pressures.

A further advantage in using isometric exercises is that they are not as likely to provoke pain as those exercises involving the movements of flexion or extension. It seems strange that many patients in whom pain is reproduced on extension are nevertheless prescribed hyperextension exercises. Indeed, in people who have degenerative apophyseal-joint changes excessive spinal exercises are likely to result in synovitis. Nachemson (1975) has shown that both flexion and extension exercises increase the load on the lumbar spine to the same degree as standing and leaning forwards with weights in the hand.

Isometric exercises are easy to teach and to perform; but like all exercise programmes they need to be individually tailored, carefully taught, performed twice daily by patients and supervised regularly by the physiotherapist, who must make certain that they do not produce any exacerbation of symptoms. Their success, as with other exercise regimens, often depends on the ability of the teacher to convince the patient of their long-term benefit.

When it becomes evident that muscle control is returning the patient is encouraged to resume normal daily activities, not only to increase spinal mobility and improve disc nutrition but also for the positive psychological benefits. For this purpose swimming, walking and bike riding are ideal. The intention is to restore as much mobility as possible without the use of forced movements. Some exercises are unsuitable, and many patients suffer back pain after having enthusiastically taken up 5BX exercises or Yoga.

Spinal flexion exercises (Williams, 1955). These also have as their aim an increase in the strength of abdominal flexor muscles, reducing lumbar lordosis and increasing trunk stability. They have the further theoretical advantages of widening the intervertebral foramen by moving apophyseal joints, and they may stretch some of the 'tight' posterior structures. For similar reasons, hamstring stretching exercises are also used.

However, Nachemson and Elfstrom (1970) found that these exercises increased the intradiscal pressure by 100 per cent compared with standing. In opposing their use, Armstrong (1967) states that these exercises 'produce a permanently unstable and irritable joint'.

Spinal extension exercises   These have also been widely advocated (Kraus, 1956). However, in their trial Kendall and Jenkins demonstrated that these exercises provided least benefit and, in fact, resulted in an exacerbation of symptoms in most patients. This corresponds with the experiments of Nachemson (1975), who demonstrated a rise in intradiscal pressure on spinal extension.

POSTURAL CONTROL

Degenerative change in the spine may be exacerbated by repeated minor trauma from many of the activities of daily living involving repetitive spinal flexion and rotational strains, either with or without the lifting of heavy objects. The patients should be made aware of this as a problem and should also know such activities need to be avoided as much as possible.

The overweight patient should lose weight, for it can easily be demonstrated that excess weight will only provide more stress on the lumbar discs. Another piece of advice is to try to avoid fatigue, for if a patient is overtired and the fatigued muscles fail to support the lumbar joints, extra strain could be placed on these joints and render them prone to minor sprains.

SLEEPING POSTURE

A sagging mattress must be avoided. Since night and early-morning pain are often a problem for the patient, a firm foam or inner-spring mattress with bed-boards is indicated. It is obviously most difficult to control night-time posture, but it is often possible to position pillows to avoid the prone position with hyperextension. This can be especially advantageous in those with some restriction, painful or painless, of back extension. This posture may be achieved by placing a pillow under the hips when the patient lies face down. The position that affords most relief, however, would appear to be sleeping on the side with a supporting pillow under the flexed, uppermost knee.

SITTING

Sitting is often the worst problem for a patient, as there is increased intradiscal pressure during sitting (Nachemson and Morris, 1964). The length of the chair and type of back support is important, and the design should allow the knees to be lower than the hips and the feet to be placed on the floor.

The best sitting posture remains debatable. Cyriax advises sitting with the knees lower than the hips and a small pillow in the lumbar hollow to keep the lumbar spine in lordosis. Williams advises that having the knees higher than the hips with a support under the feet will help to maintain lumbar flexion. It seems that both of these positions may increase pain in some patients.

A position midway between these two extremes seems preferable. The knees may be kept lower than the hips and a pillow should be used, not to increase the lumbar lordosis but merely to support the back in mid-position. Forward bending from this position should be avoided as much as possible.

These points are illustrated by the problems of driving a car, as the design of car seats commonly maintains a position of lumbar flexion. Also, disc pressure has been shown to increase when the clutch pedal is depressed (Nachemson, 1975). To overcome this poor posturing the patient is advised to use a small pillow or rolled-up towel to support the lumbar spine, and to sit with a support under the buttocks to lift himself higher than the seat

and so lower his knees. Patients should be advised to avoid sitting in one chair with their legs extended onto another chair.

STANDING

Most patients with disc degeneration are more comfortable while standing than sitting, which confirms Nachemson's finding that on standing intradiscal pressure decreases by 29 per cent. Standing is often made easier if the patient is able to vary his position from time to time, or ease the strain on his back by supporting one foot on a stool. The patient should stand up straight and should not slump. If pelvic obliquity is present pain may be increased on standing and eased by a heel raise.

WORKING

The design of better industrial and household equipment to ease back strain is a large field of ergonomic research. Many work situations necessitate working in a position that maintains the spine near the limit of its range, e.g. housewives who spend a large amount of time in a flexed position. The formula to be used should be to 'bring work up to the patient's level'.

The best advice for those whose work involves heavy lifting would be to avoid it. However, this may be impossible and most authors agree that lifting a heavy weight from the floor should be done with the knees and hips flexed and the spine maintained erect, and that bending only from the hips is most dangerous. Nachemson and Elfstrom (1970) showed a rise in intradiscal pressure with forward bending while the knees are kept straight. This pressure is markedly increased if a weight is being lifted. However, there is no firm agreement about the exact relationship of the spine during heavy activities. Cyriax advised that during heavy lifting the lumbar spine should be kept fully extended, whereas Williams advised that the person should make a conscious effort to have his spine fully flexed.

However, working with the back at the extreme of either range puts extra strain on the intervertebral joint and is more likely to exacerbate pain. The truth again lies between the two extremes, and as the patient lifts he should maintain or support his back in a position midway between flexion and extension. Many patients lifting take up this midway position as the natural one.

The patient is advised to use his thigh extensors and arm muscles as much as possible. As the patient commences to lift he first feels the heaviness and shape of the object to be lifted so that the weight can be transmitted progressively rather than in a sudden, jerky lift. If the weight, after having been lifted to the upright position, has to be placed to one side the patient is advised to move his feet around to face this area rather than to twist his body to put the weight down.

SUSTAINED WORKING POSITION
As an example of the problems of working in a sustained position, the example may be taken of a patient working at ground level, such as weeding a garden or polishing a floor by hand. Again, two different positions are advocated. One is that the patient should be on all fours with the body weight maintained forward over the hands and the lumbar spine held in a lordotic position. The opposite view is that the ideal position is sitting back on the feet so that the lumbar spine can be stretched forwards during the work. Once again, the best position appears to be midway between these two extreme views. If a person doing weeding is on all fours with the body weight supported forwards on one hand while working with the other hand, the spine can easily be maintained in a position midway between full flexion and extension.

Management of other disc degenerative lesions

Lumbar spondylosis

Patients with this condition are usually over 40, may be overweight, and their type of work may aggravate their disorder. They require rest from any known aggravating factors and should avoid those activities that involve excessive bending, such as gardening. Support in a corset may help to ease pain and restrict some of their activities.

Passive-movement techniques play a major role in the management of patients with this condition. Lumbar traction and spinal-mobilization techniques may be expected to relieve pain and increase mobility.

Carefully instituted isometric exercises are used to strengthen abdominal and back muscle groups. The overweight patient must lose weight and should be encouraged to exercise by walking or swimming within the limits of pain. Anti-inflammatory drugs are used in patients with evidence of the more severe degrees of degenerative apophy-

seal-joint changes in an attempt to reduce any associated synovitis.

In a few selected cases surgery may be indicated. However, the degenerative changes usually involve several discs in people of advancing age, and so the role of surgery is limited. In patients with sciatica an operation to decompress the nerve-root canal may be indicated and may include a partial facetectomy.

Isolated disc resorption

Conservative treatment, as outlined above, may settle the patient's symptoms. However, when the type of occupation places an excessive postural strain on the back the patient may need to be advised to seek new employment. In severe degrees of this condition surgery is usually necessary, and the technique then indicated is either a unilateral or bilateral nerve-root decompression (Crock, 1970).

Vertebral instability

The patient with this condition usually presents with a moderately severe degree of back pain that tends to be constantly present but may be modified by the adoption of certain postures. The aim of treatment is to control pain, improve postural control, and attempt to increase the control of the spinal muscles. Hence a combination of various therapies will be indicated.

Pain may be relieved by analgesics and by advising the patient to obtain extra rest for the back and avoid postures and movements known to exacerbate pain. This applies particularly to prolonged bending and lifting. Pain may also be relieved with a suitable support, such as a lumbar corset, which has the added advantage of allowing the patient to remain mobile. Passive-movement techniques, such as spinal mobilization, are also used for pain relief, but the more forcible manipulative techniques are rarely necessary. Isometric exercises to strengthen back and abdominal muscles and exercises to correct any postural fault, including hamstring tightness, are important.

Injection techniques that may be used include epidural injections of local anaesthetic and corticosteroid or, at times, infiltration of locally tender extraspinal structures, such as ligaments. However, these do not often produce any long-lasting relief.

Surgery may be indicated if pain is severe,

prolonged and unresponsive to conservative treatment, but the patient who can be so helped requires careful selection. Surgery will only be indicated, therefore, in a small proportion of cases.

Canal stenosis

Operative decompression of the lumbar spinal canal is an eminently successful surgical procedure in those patients with a canal stenosis and severe claudicant symptoms. In patients whose symptoms are less severe, or who have a contraindication to operation, management to relieve symptoms should consist of:

(1) Extra rest to the lumbar spine, including period of bed rest in hospital if necessary.
(2) Extradural injections with corticosteroids.
(3) Use of a lumbar support.
(4) Loss of weight if the patient is obese.

By these methods symptoms may be alleviated and the patient can be kept mobile.

Management of disorders of spinal movement

Acute lumbago

This condition may be of a moderate degree or else so severe as to render the patient incapable of movement.

The patient with severe lumbago is best treated by complete bed rest for several days in a position of comfort—with analgesics, sedation and local heat (such as a hot water bottle) for pain relief.

Manipulation is contraindicated because it may exacerbate the condition and because of the problems of properly positioning the patient. However, one mobilization technique that has a place in treatment during the early stages—even though it is virtually impossible to examine back movements—is the use of gentle, rhythmical manual traction applied to the patient's legs for 1–2 minutes. As the patient's movements begin to improve other mobilization techniques may be added. An epidural injection may be used to provide pain relief.

With more moderate degrees of involvement the patient is more mobile; mobilization techniques are then the treatment of choice, usually combined with analgesics or anti-inflammatory drugs. The patient may have learnt to use a form of mobilization technique, such as hanging suspended from an overhead beam for a few moments.

Hypomobility lesions

In hypomobility lesions of the lumbar spine mobilization and manipulative techniques are the treatment of choice and should provide relief of pain and restore the restricted range of intervertebral-joint movement in at least 90 per cent of cases.

Injections of local anaesthetic and corticosteroid into locally tender areas are of most use in patients with fibrositis who have referred pain and tenderness in localized areas. In those patients who do not respond adequately to mobilization techniques, these locally tender areas should be infiltrated since they probably contribute to the perpetuation of the pain. Medication with anti-inflammatory drugs rarely produces any great benefit but analgesics may be used as required. Mobilizing exercises are indicated if the condition has been present for a long time or is recurrent.

Prolonged rest and use of supports are contraindicated in this condition as they tend to increase the degree of restriction in the spinal joint. Medication only rarely produces any benefit; traction, which usually makes the patient's symptoms worse, and surgery are contraindicated.

Hypermobility

Patients with this syndrome who present with back pain are difficult to manage since the underlying hypermobile condition cannot be influenced by therapy, and pain tends to be recurrent. Isometric strengthening and stabilizing exercises form the main basis of treatment and at times a support may also be used to relieve pain. Mobilization techniques are indicated when a painful restriction of intervertebral movement within the hypermobile range can be demonstrated.

28 Manipulative therapy in the lumbar spine

Mobilization (*see Table 28.1*)

Many techniques of mobilization have been described for the lumbar spine and only the five most commonly used will be described here:

(1) Rotation.
(2) Posteroanterior central pressure.
(3) Posteroanterior unilateral vertebral pressure.
(4) Transverse pressure.
(5) Longitudinal movement.

Rotation

This is the most common effective mobilization technique used in the lumbar spine.

Starting position

The patient lies on his side with his head on a pillow.

The localization of this movement to one area in the lumbar spine is obtained by the degree of rotation, attained by appropriate positioning of the patient's thorax and pelvis and by positioning the lumbar spine towards either flexion or extension by flexion or extension of the hip (*see Figure 28.21*).

Method

An oscillatory movement is produced by the therapist's left hand, which rotates the patient's pelvis while the right hand is used to stabilize the thorax. For the upper lumbar spine, rotation is used with the spine in minimal extension; for

Table 28.1 Indications for lumbar-spine mobilization techniques

Technique	Main indications
Rotation	This is usually the first technique indicated and is especially useful in patients with unilateral pain
Posteroanterior central vertebral pressure	Patients with midline pain or with some radiation to either side; spondylosis
Posteroanterior unilateral vertebral pressure	Unilateral pain particularly arising from the middle or upper lumbar spine
Transverse vertebral pressure	Unilateral pain especially arising from the upper lumbar spine
Straight-leg raising	Pain and restricted movement in the pain-sensitive elements in the vertebral canal and foramen
Longitudinal movement:	
Using two legs	Bilateral pain arising from lower lumbar region
Using one leg	Unilateral pain arising from lower lumbar region
Lumbar traction	If symptoms are of gradual onset; if pain is not aggravated by active movements; spondylosis

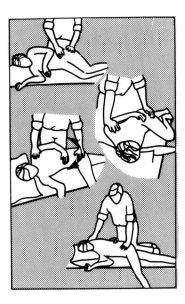

Figure 28.1 Mobilization of the lumbar spine: rotation

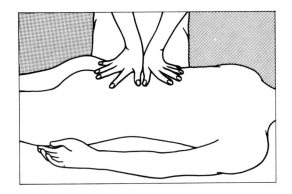

the lower lumbar spine, rotation is used with the spine towards flexion.

Indications

This is the most useful technique for patients with unilateral back or leg pain and in patients who have central-back pain but with a restriction of movement to one side alone.

Posteroanterior central vertebral pressure

Starting position—The patient lies prone with the arms by the side and head turned to one side. The therapist stands on the left side and places the pisiform area of his left hand over the spinous process and reinforces it with pressure from the right hand.

Method—An oscillating movement is obtained by the therapist rocking his upper trunk up and down, pressure being transmitted through shoulder and arms (*see Figure 28.2*).

Indications—This technique is indicated especially in those patients who have midline lumbar pain with some radiation out to both sides. Consequently it is most often of value in patients with a mechanical derangement of the lumbar

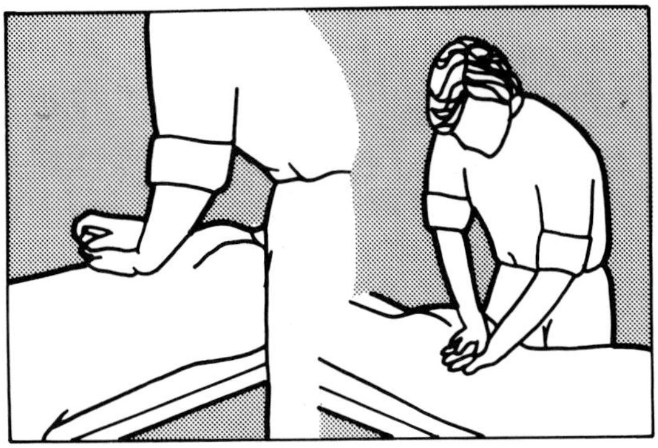

Figure 28.2 Mobilization of the lumbar spine: posteroanterior central vertebral pressure

intervertebral joint and is particularly of value in patients with lumbar spondylosis.

Posteroanterior unilateral vertebral pressure

Starting position—The patient lies prone with the arms to the side and the head turned to one side. The therapist stands on the side that is to be treated with thumbs placed lateral to the spinous process at the appropriate level (*see Figure 28.3*).

Method—By positioning the shoulders directly over the hands, pressure can be transmitted by movement of the trunk to the thumbs and so the thumbs themselves do not need to move.

Indications—This method is particularly useful in hypomobility lesions involving the upper or middle lumbar spine associated with localized back pain and muscle spasm.

Figure 28.3 Mobilization: posteroanterior unilateral vertebral pressure

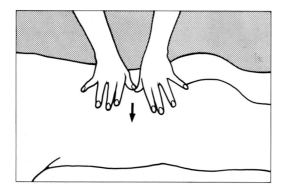

Figure 28.4 Mobilization: transverse vertebral pressure

Transverse vertebral pressure

Starting position—The patient lies prone with arms by the side and head turned to one side while the therapist stands to the right side with thumbs against the right side of the vertebra to be mobilized (*see Figure 28.4*).

Method—Pressure is applied through the thumbs against the spinous process in an oscillatory manner. The range of movement produced by this movement is greater at L1 than at L4.

Indications—This technique is used for unilateral lumbar pain but is more useful for upper than for lower lumbar spinal pain.

Longitudinal movement

This is a useful and gentle technique in which the therapist applies a rhythmical longitudinal movement to one or both of the patient's legs. This technique is especially useful in patients who have a sudden onset of severe pain, either in the lower lumbar midline or radiating to one side, and who may not be able to be positioned for any alternative mobilization technique.

Manipulation

Manipulation techniques are classified as being either:

(1) Non-specific; that is, applied to an area of the spine; or

(2) Specific, in which movement is localized to one intervertebral segment only.

Non-specific techniques

These are an extension of the mobilization techniques that have already been described in which a rapid thrust is now applied at the limit of the normal range. The two most important techniques to be considered are rotation and posteroanterior pressure.

Rotation

Starting position—The therapist stands on the right side of the couch with the patient supine. His left hand steadies the patient's left shoulder and his right hand positions the left hip and knee into flexion at a right angle. He rotates the patient's pelvis to the right by pulling the left knee across the body and down towards the floor (*see Figure 28.5*).

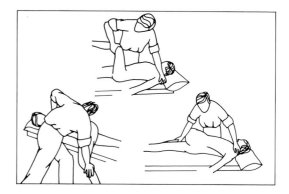

Figure 28.5 Manipulation of the lumbar spine: rotation

The therapist next grasps the posterolateral aspect of the patient's upper calf with his right hand and applies counter-pressure against the shoulder with his left hand. By suitable positioning of the patient's underneath leg, the lumbar spine may be placed into position of either flexion or extension.

Method—With the patient suitably positioned, an oscillatory rotational movement is supplied by each hand, then a sudden downward and rotary thrust is added to the leg while maintaining a strong counter-pressure to the shoulder; it is essential for this movement to produce a rotation of the pelvis and spine and not just an adduction movement of the leg.

Posteroanterior pressure

Starting position—With the patient lying prone the therapist uses the pisiform bone of his right hand to stretch the intervertebral joint to its limit.

Method—By suddenly increasing the pressure on the hands, a movement of very small range is produced. To increase the effectiveness of this movement, the patient's trunk or legs may be supported in a position of extension (*see Figure 28.6*).

Specific techniques

Lumbar rotation

Starting position—The therapist stands facing the patient, who lies on the right side with the left knee and hip flexed. The patient's lower right leg is then moved into sufficient flexion to position the appropriate lumbar intervertebral joint midway between its range of flexion and extension. The

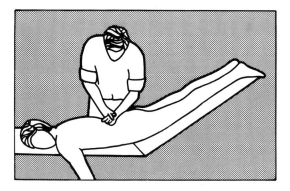

Figure 28.6 Manipulation of the lumbar spine: posteroanterior vertebral pressure

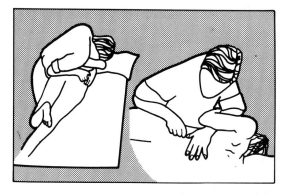

Figure 28.7 Manipulation: rotation of intervertebral joints

therapist then rotates the patient's thorax by pulling on the right arm. He leans over the patient with his left forearm against the patient's shoulder and his right upper forearm behind the left hip. His left thumb presses downwards against the left side of the spinous process of the upper vertebra of the joint to be manipulated. At the same time, his right middle finger pulls upwards against the spinous process of the lower vertebra (*see Figure 28.7*).

Method—The patient is rocked back and forth with the therapist's forearms until the maximum rotary stretch is applied. At the same time, the pressure against the spinous processes is increased until the joint is felt to be tight. The manipulation is performed by an increased push through both forearms while suddenly increasing the pressure against the spinous processes.

Lumbar traction

STARTING POSITION

The patient first of all stands up and a belt is firmly fixed around the thorax. The patient then lies down and a second belt is applied around the pelvis. It is important to ensure that no clothing is caught under either of these belts. The patient then lies either prone or supine on the traction couch. If supine the hips and knees may both be flexed. For maximal effect to be obtained, the intervertebral joint being treated should be positioned midway between its position of flexion and extension. The belts are then attached by straps to fixed points beyond the ends of the couch. Before traction is applied, these straps must be tightened to remove all looseness from the harness.

METHOD

The site and degree of the patient's pain is first determined. Traction is then applied from the head end, from the foot end, or from both ends. If a roll-top traction couch is not being used, care must be taken to eliminate friction between the patient and the couch. The physiotherapist does this by raising and lowering the patient's thorax and pelvis alternately to ensure that the stretch being applied between the belts is not lost by friction between the patient's body and the couch. A friction-free couch offers considerable advantage.

At first a maximum of 13 kg should be used for a period not exceeding 10 minutes. A careful watch should be kept for low-back symptoms caused by the traction, even if these are only induced by movement of the lumbar spine or coughing. If the patient experiences low-back pain the duration and pressure of this first treatment should be reduced. If 13 kg can be applied the patient's leg pain should be reassessed after 10 seconds.

PROGRESS

One of the following courses of action should then be taken:

(1) If severe symptoms are completely relieved the strength should be reduced by at least half, and the duration should not exceed 5 minutes to prevent a marked exacerbation of symptoms.
(2) If symptoms are only slightly relieved by 13 kg traction the strength may be increased to approximately 20 kg and the duration to 10 minutes. However, if 20 kg then completely relieves symptoms the strength should be reduced below 18 kg.
(3) If symptoms remain unchanged the traction should be increased to 20 kg and sustained for 10 minutes.
(4) If the symptoms are exacerbated traction should be reduced and its duration limited to 5 minutes.

While traction is being released slowly, the patient should gently tilt the pelvis from side to side. If pain is experienced with such movement traction should be held until the pain disappears. After the traction is removed, the patient should rest a few minutes before standing, especially after the first treatment. The patient should also be warned that it is normal for the back to feel strange for approximately 2 hours.

METHOD OF PROGRESSION

On the day after the first treatment the patient's symptoms and signs are assessed and compared with those present before traction to determine whether treatment should be repeated and if so how graduated. Signs may be assessed immediately after the first traction, but flexion is often more limited then. One way to gauge the success of traction is to note whether the weight known to produce pain can be increased at subsequent treatments without producing discomfort.

If during the first treatment the symptoms become exacerbated but remain unchanged after reducing the strength, traction must be discontinued. If, however, symptoms and signs do not deteriorate, traction can be reinstituted and an assessment then made of the strength that can be applied without increasing the symptoms. It is a good sign if a greater strength can be applied.

When there is a relief of symptoms on the first day, progression is guided mainly by the severity of any temporary exacerbation after treatment. During the first three or four treatments improvement will probably be small but noticeable, and treatment should be increased in time, not strength. When no exacerbation follows treatment, the weight can be gradually increased.

Otherwise strength and time can be increased together. The usual strength used is between 30 and 45 kg but with a slow rate of progress at lower strength traction up to 65 kg may be necessary. In general the length of treatment need not exceed 15 minutes, since longer periods do not produce any further progress.

The scale measurement is valuable mainly as a record. Strength should not be the controlling guide to treatment but is referred to only when traction has been set.

Intermittent variable traction can be used for the lumbar spine as in other areas of the vertebral column—its duration, strength and indications being similar to other forms of traction.

PRECAUTIONS

No soreness should be felt with the lower strengths

Table 28.2 Selection sequence of techniques for the lumbar region

Unilateral symptoms	Bilateral symptoms
1. Rotation or posteroanterior central vertebral pressure	1. Posteroanterior central vertebral pressure
	2. Rotation
For upper lumbar region:	For upper lumbar region:
1. Transverse vertebral pressure	1. Transverse vertebral pressure
2. Traction	2. Traction
For lower lumbar region:	For lower lumbar region:
1. Traction	1. Traction
2. Longitudinal movement	2. Longitudinal movement

of traction, with the exception of discomfort from the harness. After traction has been applied the patient should attempt alternate flattening and arching of the lumbar spine and coughing to test for any back discomfort.

The first session of traction is used in the form of a trial run to avoid the embarrassing (though harmless) situation where a patient has difficulty regaining his feet after excessive traction.

INDICATIONS

(1) Any symptoms of gradual onset whether localized to the lumbar area or referred into the leg and not produced by trauma may be treated successfully by traction.

(2) Back pain associated with lumbar spondylosis usually responds well to gentle traction or intermittent variable traction.

(3) Back pain with a normal range of active movement in the lumbar spine usually responds better to traction than manipulation.

(4) Traction is indicated when no further progress can be obtained by use of mobilization techniques.

(5) It may be necessary to precede traction with manipulation, particularly with painless intervertebral-joint stiffness. If traction does not result in any further progress it is best to revert to mobilization techniques, even if previously unsuccessful.

29   The sacroiliac joint

The sacroiliac joint is a synovial joint formed between the medial surface of the ilium and the lateral aspect of the upper sacral vertebrae. However, the sacroiliac joint is unique in that the space formed between the ilium and sacrum above this synovial joint is joined by a strong interosseous ligament. This fibrous joint accounts for about a third of the vertical distance between these two bones. The sacrum is wedge shaped so that its upper portion, or base, is wider than the lower portion, or apex. This gives the sacrum the appearance of being wedged between the two iliac bones. The articular surface of the sacrum is shaped like a letter L lying on its side with its upper, more vertical, limb being shorter than its lower, more horizontal, limb (*see Figure 29.1*). The articular surfaces are slightly irregular and interlocked, so providing increased stability, and a depression formed at the junction of the upper and middle thirds of the sacrum corresponds to a prominent protuberance on the ilium. The bony surfaces are lined by articular cartilage, which is thicker on the sacral side of the joint, and the joint is surrounded by a capsule that is lined by a synovial membrane.

The sacrum and ilium are connected by two sacroiliac ligaments which lie anteriorly and posteriorly to the joint. The anterior ligament is thin and weak but the posterior ligament is thick and strong and joins the roughened tuberosities on the sacrum and ilium dorsal to the joint surface. The stability of the sacroiliac joint primarily depends on this ligament, for the erector spinae muscle group neither spans nor controls this joint.

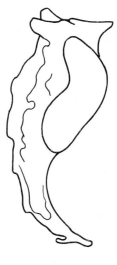

Figure 29.1 The sacroiliac joint. The articular surface of the sacrum is shaped like a letter L lying on its side

The main function of the sacroiliac joint is to transmit body weight but, as discussed below, the joint also has a small but important range of movement. The strong posterior sacroiliac ligaments are necessary to provide stability and prevent the tendency for the upper sacrum to be driven forwards and downwards into the pelvis during weight-bearing.

Movements

There has been considerable controversy and speculation about the role of movement in this joint, but there seems no doubt that the normal range of sacroiliac joint movement, although only a few millimetres, is important (Grieve, 1976). These movements are of importance in pregnancy when, enhanced by the action of the hormone relaxin, they are accompanied by a 4-mm increase in the width of the symphysis pubis (Young, 1940). Brooke (1924) described two movements, a gliding movement and a rotation of the sacrum. These slight movements also took place during lumbar-spine movements and Brooke correctly considered that this sacroiliac movement played an essential role in the normal functional movements of the lumbar spine.

Recent experiments using several different techniques to demonstrate sacroiliac movements have been described. Weisl (1955) used cineradiography in living subjects; Colachis *et al.* (1963) inserted wires into the iliac spines of medical students; and Frigerio, Stowe and Howe (1973) used a computerized X-ray technique in cadavers and living subjects. These experiments did not confirm the rotatory movements described by Brooke, but rather a nodding type of movement in the sacrum, in that the sacral promontory can move forwards and backwards between the iliac bones. During spinal flexion, or on standing up from lying down, the sacral promontory moves ventrally so that the anteroposterior diameter of the pelvic inlet is reduced and the apex of the sacrum moves in a dorsal direction. At the same time a movement takes place in the iliac bones, which become approximated, and in the ischial tuberosities, which move apart (Kapandji, 1974).

Alternatively, on spinal extension or on lying down, opposite movements occur so that the base of the sacrum moves dorsally and the apex of the sacrum moves ventrally, increasing the antero-posterior diameter of the pelvic inlet. At the same time a movement takes place in the iliac bones, which move apart, and in the ischial tuberosities, which become approximated (Kapandji, 1974). All authors agree that the range of movement is small and that there is a large individual and sex variation. Similar movements occur while climbing stairs or standing on one leg and are combined with movement in the pubis. For example, when standing supported on the right leg, the pubis on the right side moves forward in relation to the left pubis. Age changes in the joint result in an obliteration of the joint space by fibrous bands, which may develop to form a bony ankylosis (Sashin, 1930).

Sacroiliac pain

Pain arising in the sacroiliac joint is normally described as being a dull ache and is characteristically experienced in the buttock. It may also be referred to the groin or the posterior aspect of the thigh and rarely radiates below the knee. Pain may also be referred into the lower abdomen. Pain is then felt in the iliac fossa and is usually associated with a localized area of deep tenderness over the iliacus muscle, known as Baer's point. Such pain and tenderness often causes confusion with intra-abdominal lesions (Norman, 1968). Since the pelvis is formed into a bony ring, the patient may also experience pain anteriorly over the pubic symphysis or adductor tendon origin. In patients with inflammatory sacroiliitis, there is often a history of buttock pain that alternates from one side to the other. It is usually worse at night, is associated with stiffness of the back and may be unrelated to posture.

Characteristically, in patients with sacroiliac disorders neurological symptoms, such as paraesthesias or numbness, are absent but at times they may report a dull, heavy feeling in the leg.

When assessing patients with sacroiliac pain it must be realized that pain felt in this area may be referred from either the lower lumbar spine or the hip joint. Accordingly, clinical examination of both of these areas is necessary before conducting a formal test of the sacroiliac joint. For many years it was considered that sacroiliac sprain, described by Goldthwaite in 1905, was the most common cause of low-back pain. However, this was in most instances an example of referred pain and tenderness from degenerative or hypomobility lesions of the lumbosacral joint. Experimental injections of hypertonic saline into the ligaments around the lumbosacral joint can reproduce this referred pain and tenderness over the sacroiliac area. Hence this concept of sacroiliac sprain fell into disfavour, although it should be remembered that mechanical lesions of this joint, described below, do occur and may produce pain.

In patients with mechanical lesions of the sacroiliac joint the pain is usually unilateral, and pain can be exacerbated by movements that stress the sacroiliac joint. Finally, it should be remembered that this area is a common site for secondary malignant deposits or Paget's disease.

Examination

(1) Inspection.
(2) Sacroiliac tests.
(3) Palpation.

Inspection

The patient's general posture is first inspected; patients with unilateral sacroiliac pain often tend to stand or sit with the body weight supported on the opposite side. Any asymmetry of the skin creases or gluteal folds is looked for. The pelvic level is then assessed by measuring the leg length and by palpating the bony prominences of the pelvis. The examiner first crouches behind the patient and places his hands at the top of the iliac crests with one thumb on each posterior superior iliac spine; then while kneeling in front of the patient he places his hands along the patient's iliac crests with the thumbs on the anterior superior iliac spines.

The relative positions of the posterior superior iliac spines should be reassessed with the patient sitting down. In patients with unilateral sacroiliac disorders, these prominences are often found to lie at different levels, and usually the spine on the painful side is found to be at a lower level than the other one.

However, if the patient is asked to bend forwards their position usually becomes reversed so that the spine that previously lay at a lower level will now come to lie higher than the opposite one. Although its mechanism of production is uncertain, this sign is usually considered to indicate the presence of a mechanical sacroiliac lesion.

Sacroiliac tests

Movement in the sacroiliac joint is produced by a series of passive movements designed to stress the joint and reproduce the patient's pain. The numerous tests that have been devised to test the sacroiliac joints are some proof of their inadequacy. It must be remembered that the tests also stress other potentially pain-producing areas so that false-positive and false-negative tests are not uncommon.

The first three tests are performed with the patient lying face downwards. The remaining five tests are performed with the patient lying supine:

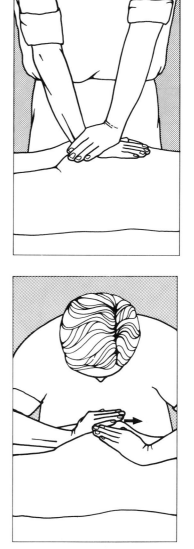

Figure 29.2 *(a)*

Figure 29.2 *(b)*

(1) With the patient lying prone, a rhythmical oscillatory pressure is applied to the apex of the sacrum by the examiner. It is achieved by pressure over the sacrum with the heel of the examiner's hand, the arm being kept fully extended. This springing movement produces a shearing movement across the sacroiliac joints and, although it also produces movement in the lumbosacral joint, is usually the most reliable of these tests (*see Figure 29.2(a)*).

(2) The sacroiliac joint may be stressed by stabilizing the ilium with one hand and then moving the sacrum in a cephalad direction with the other hand (*see Figure 29.2(b)*).

(3) This test may then be repeated by stabilizing the ischial tuberosity with one hand and moving the sacrum caudally with the other (*see Figure 29.2(c)*).

(4) The patient lies supine and pressure is applied by the examiner's hand against each anterior superior iliac spine, as though the examiner were trying to spread them apart (*see Figure 29.2 (d)*).

(5) The patient lies in the same position as in (4) and the iliac crests are compressed, as though squeezing them together (*see Figure 29.2 (e)*).

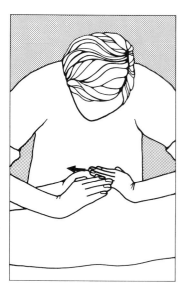

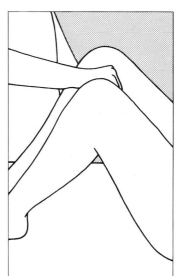

Figure 29.2 (*c*)

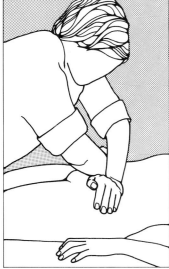

Figure 29.2 (*d*)

Figure 29.2 (*e*)

Figure 29.2 (*f*)

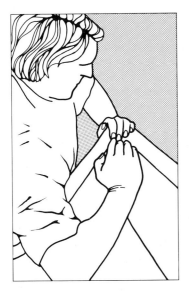

(g)

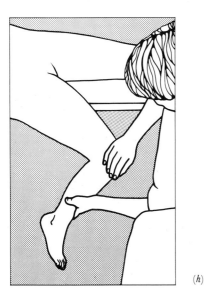

(h)

Figure 29.2 Sacroiliac tests.
(*a*) Rhythmical oscillatory pressure applied over the sacrum. (*b*) The ilium is stabilized by one hand and the sacrum moved cephalad with the right hand. (*c*) The ilium is stabilized by one hand and the sacrum is moved caudally with the left. (*d*) Pressure is applied against each anterior iliac spine to spread them apart.
(*e*) Pressure is applied to the iliac crests to compress them. (*f*) Isometric contraction of the hip adductors. (*g*) Isometric contraction of the hip abductors. (*h*) Passive extension of the hip

(6) The patient lies supine with the hips and knees flexed to 90 degrees. The adductors of the hip are isometrically contracted by attempting to squeeze the examiner's hand placed between the knees (*see Figure 29.2 (f)*).

(7) The patient lies in the same position as in (6) and the examiner fully resists the patient's attempt to spread the knees apart, so producing an isometric contraction of the hip abductors (*see Figure 29.2 (g)*).

(8) The patient lies on his back at the edge of the couch and the examiner takes the leg and hip backwards into full extension (*see Figure 29.2 (h)*).

Palpation

It is customary to palpate these joints for the presence of any tenderness, but the synovial portion of the joint lies deep to the overlying ilium and is inaccessible to direct palpation. Tenderness in this area usually represents a referred area of tenderness from disorders of the lower lumbar spine. In long-standing disorders of the sacroiliac joint, thickening of tissue overlying the dorsal sacroiliac ligaments may be found.

Sacroiliac disorders

Disorders of the sacroiliac joint may be classified as being:

(1) Inflammatory.
(2) Infectious.
(3) Mechanical.
(4) Degenerative.
(5) Osteitis condensans ilii.

Inflammatory disease

Inflammatory disease of the sacroiliac joint is most commonly associated with the seronegative group of spondyloarthritis and may be due to:

(1) Ankylosing spondylitis.
(2) Reiter's disease.
(3) Psoriatic arthritis.
(4) Arthritis associated with inflammatory bowel disease, such as ulcerative colitis or Crohn's disease.
(5) Still's disease.
(6) Behçet's disease.

X-ray evidence of the presence of sacroiliitis is necessary before diagnosis can be confirmed, and so the diagnosis must remain presumptive until the appropriate radiological changes are present. Sometimes these may take several years to develop and the X-ray changes in the early stages may be difficult to interpret accurately. There are several technical problems in obtaining a satisfactory view of these joints. Careful positioning of the patient is necessary to obtain an adequate view of the entire length of the joint.

The early X-ray changes of sacroiliitis appear in the lower half of the joint and involve especially the iliac side, since this has the thinner cartilaginous surface. Osteoporosis with demineralization occurs around the joint margins, which leads to a loss of the subchondral bone, which appears as a white line of increased density in the normal joint X-ray. The joint loses its normally well-defined contours as its margin becomes blurred and in some areas develops an apparently increased widening while in other areas it becomes narrowed and irregular. This irregularity is subsequently increased by the appearance of erosions along the joint margins and the presence of areas of bone condensation or sclerosis adjacent to the joint margin producing a mottled or 'moth-eaten' appearance. As the joint cartilage is lost and repair takes place, fibrous bands bridge the joint and lead to a fibrous ankylosis, which subsequently becomes a bony ankylosis. The late stages in this disorder are characterized by complete bone fusion across the joint and ossification in the surrounding ligamentous supports of the joint.

Infections

Infections usually involve only one sacroiliac joint and are most commonly caused by tuberculous, brucellar or staphylococcal infections. However, they now occur more rarely than in previous years.

In the early stages X-rays are usually normal and of no help in diagnosis, but at this stage a bone scan is often positive. Subsequently, X-rays show erosive, destructive changes in the joint and tomography may be indicated to define these changes. Needle biopsy, either closed or open, is usually necessary to confirm the diagnosis and to identify the causative organism.

Mechanical lesions

Mechanical lesions may be due to hypomobility or hypermobility of the sacroiliac joint.

Hypomobility lesions

These remain as quite a small but relatively important cause of lower back pain. They usually occur in young people and may be associated with certain activities that involve movements that place a rotational stress on the sacroiliac joint, such as golfing, tennis or ballet dancing. This lesion may also follow pregnancy, childbirth or trauma. It may also be associated with certain structural faults, such as an asymmetrical development of the pelvis, or unequal leg length (Wiltse, 1971).

Tests of sacroiliac movement should reproduce the patient's pain. Treatment by one of the passive-movement techniques, described at the end of this chapter, is usually eminently successful.

Hypermobility lesions

Hypermobility lesions of the sacroiliac joint are also rare and occur in one of two situations. The first is secondary to instability of the symphysis pubis, which occurs predominantly in athletes (Harris and Murray, 1974). This condition may be complicated by a mechanical lesion of one or both sacroiliac joints and may also be associated with an osteitis condensans ilii. The second occurs in young females, usually during or soon after pregnancy. The patient presents with sacroiliac pain that is made worse by standing or walking. The treatment of hypermobility is extremely difficult and manual-therapy techniques usually exacerbate the symptoms.

Treatment consists of rest, analgesics and anti-inflammatory agents; a sacroiliac belt may help to provide pain relief.

Degenerative changes

These may be expected to occur in the articular cartilage of these synovial joints (Resnick, Niwayama and Georgen, 1975, 1977). Degenerative changes first involve the iliac surface, where the cartilage is thinner than on the sacral surface. The cartilage changes are similar to those in peripheral joints with, ultimately, a fibrous ankylosis of the joint cavity.

These changes are reflected in the X-ray appearances as loss or irregularity of the joint space, subchondral sclerosis and osteophyte formation. Cystic and erosive changes are rarely seen.

The osteophytes may form on the inferior surfaces of the joint and so are easily recognized on X-ray, but they may also appear on the superoanterior joint aspect, where they appear as dense bony deposits and may give the appearance of ankylosis of the joint.

Degenerative changes are increasingly more common with advancing age and may occur secondary to disorders in which movement of the joint is decreased. This occurs in people who are immobilized, such as paraplegics, or patients with diseases of the hip joint. In patients with unilateral hip disease it is usual to find degenerative changes in the contralateral sacroiliac joint.

Osteitis condensans ilii

This is characterized by a condensation of bone on the iliac side of the sacroiliac joint. The diagnosis is made by X-ray. Its nature is uncertain but it most likely represents a bony reaction to unequal stress in this joint. It has also been considered to be only a coincidental radiological finding, which is not related to the patient's symptoms. It occurs mostly in young adults, more commonly in females—especially after childbirth, when complaints of pain in the back or sacroiliac area are common. Accordingly, it may be difficult to determine whether the X-ray changes present are responsible for the patient's symptoms.

The radiological picture of osteitis condensans ilii is usually characterized by a well-defined area of bone sclerosis and increased density adjacent to the sacroiliac joint along the inner and lower border of the ilium. The sacroiliac joint itself is normal, and it is extremely rare to find a similar change on the sacral surface of the joint. Osteitis condensans may, however, be bilateral and is then usually symmetrical.

The course of this disease is variable and can be prolonged, but ultimately spontaneous resolution may occur. Treatment consists of reassurance, analgesics, correction of any postural problem that may be present and, if necessary, a sacroiliac belt may be prescribed.

Passive-movement techniques

Mobilization

The three commonly used mobilization techniques for the sacroiliac joint are:

(1) Posteroanterior pressure.
(2) Backward rotation of the iliac crest.
(3) Forward rotation of the iliac crest.

The technique chosen is usually the one that reproduces the patient's pain.

Posteroanterior pressure

Starting position—The patient lies prone with the arms by the sides. The therapist stands by the patient's left side and places his left hand over the sacrum, reinforcing it with his right hand. His shoulders need to be positioned over the hands.

Method—Posteroanterior pressures are applied to the dorsal surface of the sacrum using small oscillations. The direction of this posteroanterior pressure may be inclined cephalad, caudad, towards the right or the left side, or in any combination of these directions. These may be complemented by an equal and opposite pressure over the adjacent ilium.

Backward rotation of the iliac crest

Starting position—The patient lies on the right side and the therapist, standing in front, places his left hand over the anterior superior iliac spine with the heel of his right hand against the posterior surface of the left ischial tuberosity. By leaning over the patient both the therapist's forearms are pointed in opposite directions but are maintained parallel (*see Figure 29.3*).

Method—The therapist holds the patient's pelvis firmly between his hands and rocks his body so that the ischial tuberosity moves posteroanteriorly and the anterior superior iliac spine moves anteroposteriorly, thus producing a backwards rotation of the iliac crest.

Forward rotation of the iliac crest

Starting position—This is similar to that described for the previous technique, except that in this

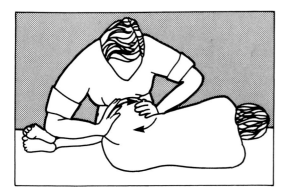

Figure 29.3 Backward rotation of iliac crest

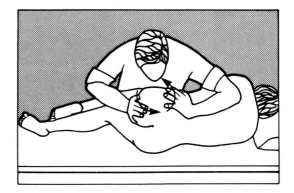

Figure 29.4 Forward rotation of iliac crest

movement the therapist places his left hand on the posterior surface of the iliac crest and the heel of his right hand under the ischial tuberosity, reaching as far anteriorly as possible.

Method—Holding the pelvis firmly between his hands the therapist moves the anterior superior iliac spine posteroanteriorly and the ischial tuberosity anteroposteriorly by means of a swinging movement of his trunk (*see Figure 29.4*).

Sacroiliac manipulation

The technique for manipulation of the sacroiliac joint also involves rotation of the lumbar spine (*see Figure 29.5*) and the technique used is identical with that described for a rotational manipulation of the lumbar spine.

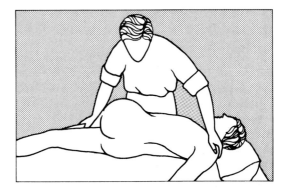

Figure 29.5 Lumbar rotation for manipulation of the sacroiliac joint

30 The cervical spine

The basic vertebral structure (with an anterior body and a posterior neural arch) applies in the lower cervical spine—that is, from C3 to C7—and the cervical mobile intervertebral segment, as in the lumbar spine, comprises an anterior cartilaginous joint and the two posterior apophyseal joints (*see Figures 30.1 and 30.2*). However, the anterior joint is modified by the presence of the neurocentral joints which abut across the posterior margin of the vertebral body.

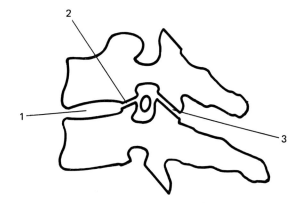

Figure 30.2 The lateral view of the cervical spine. The mobile intervertebral segment comprises the disc (1) and neurocentral joint (2) in front and the apophyseal joint (3) behind

Neurocentral joints

These small joints are also known as the joints of Luschka, uncovertebral, or lateral interbody joints. For many years there has been debate on whether they represent true synovial joints or pseudarthroses. It seems likely that they are formed from spaces in the posterolateral region of the intervertebral disc that develop as the result of movement, and that they aid in stability of the vertebrae. They become lined by synovial tissue and may undergo degenerative changes as part of the process of spondylosis. The osteophytic outgrowths that subsequently develop may then encroach upon the nearby transverse foramina, through which runs the vertebral artery.

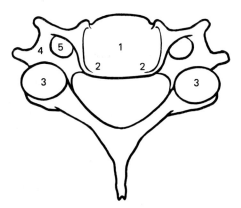

Figure 30.1 Cervical vertebra viewed from above. The mobile intervertebral segment comprises the disc (1) and neurocentral joints (2) in front and two apophyseal joints (3) behind. The transverse process (4) also contains a foramen (5), through which the vertebral artery passes

The upper cervical spine

The upper cervical spine comprises the atlas (C1) and the axis (C2), which have a distinct structure that is adapted to their different functions.

The atlas is shaped like a ring, with an anterior and posterior arch. The anterior arch articulates on its posterior aspect with the odontoid process of the axis. The atlas lacks a vertebral body but has two lateral masses, each of which bears a superior and an inferior articular process. The superior articular process, which is concave from side to side and from back to front, articulates with the occipital condyle to form the occipito-atlantal joint. Its convex inferior articular process articulates with a convex articular process on the upper surface of the axis to form the lateral atlantoaxial joint (*see Figure 30.3*).

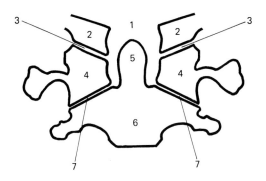

Figure 30.3 The C1–2 region: (1) foramen magnum; (2) occipital condyles; (3) atlanto-occipital joint; (4) lateral mass of C1; (5) odontoid process; (6) body of C2; (7) lateral atlantoaxial joint

The anterior portion, or body, of the axis carries a central portion, known as the odontoid process or dens, which articulates with the posterior aspect of the anterior arch of atlas and forms the anterior atlantoaxial joint. On its lateral aspect are two convex articular processes, which articulate with the lateral masses of the atlas to form the lateral atlantoaxial joints.

The posterior arch of the axis is formed by two pedicles and laminae; the inferior articular process, which articulates with the superior articular process of C3, arises from the inferior surface of the pedicle.

Cervical movements

In the relatively small area of the cervical spine, 35 joints are found. For the purpose of describing its movements, however, the neck may be divided into an upper cervical spine, comprising the atlanto-occipital and the atlantoaxial joints, and a lower cervical spine from C3 to C7.

Atlanto-occipital joints

Two physiological movements take place at the atlanto-occipital joints: flexion–extension and lateral flexion.

Flexion–extension of the atlanto-occipital joint produces a nodding movement of the head as the occiput tilts backwards and forwards on the concave surface of the upper facets of the lateral mass of the atlas.

Lateral flexion in this joint occurs as the occiput glides over the concave superior articular process of the lateral mass of the atlas and is of only a few degrees in range.

It is generally agreed that active rotation does not occur in this joint but, because of the shape of its articular facets, a small range of passive rotation is possible.

Atlantoaxial joints, C1–C2

The atlantoaxial joints are comprised of the two lateral atlantoaxial joints and a central joint formed between the anterior arch of the atlas and the odontoid process of the axis. Two physiological movements take place at these joints, namely rotation and flexion–extension.

Rotation, the principle movement, takes place by a pivoting movement of the atlas around the immobile odontoid and is also accompanied by a movement in the lateral atlantoaxial joints, so that one moves forwards and the other backwards. As the atlas rotates, so do the atlanto-occipital joints and the head. This movement is limited by the alar ligaments, which are check ligaments running from the odontoid to the occiput.

Flexion–extension of the atlantoaxial joints occurs at the lateral atlantoaxial joints, which are most unusual in that both surfaces are convex, so that this movement involves both a rolling and a sliding movement of the two articular facets.

It is generally agreed that active lateral flexion does not occur in the atlantoaxial joints but that a small range of passive movement is possible.

Lower cervical joints, C3–C7

Three movements are possible between C3 and C7: flexion–extension, lateral flexion and rotation.

During flexion the upper vertebral body tilts and slides anteriorly over the lower body and, as in the lumbar spine, is accompanied by an appropriate movement in the apophyseal joint. Similarly, during extension the upper vertebral body tilts and slides posteriorly, accompanied by a movement in the apophyseal joint.

Lateral flexion and rotation of the lower cervical vertebrae are really combined movements, as one cannot occur without a degree of the other. The reason for this is that, after only a few degrees of lateral flexion, the apophyseal joints come into apposition and so force the vertebrae into rotation towards the same side.

Conversely, after a few degrees of rotation, apposition in the apophyseal joints force the vertebrae into lateral flexion towards the same side.

The figures given for the normal range of cervical movement, and for the contribution to this range by the various cervical joints, vary widely and there is a large variation according to the patient's age and sex. Average figures for a normal male are given as a guide.

Flexion–extension occurs at the atlanto-occipital, atlantoaxial and lower cervical joints. The total range is approximately 45 degrees of flexion and 60 degrees of extension, of which about 50 degrees occurs in the upper cervical spine.

Lateral flexion occurs at the atlanto-occipital and the lower cervical joints. The range is approximately 45 degrees to either side, of which about 8 degrees occurs in the atlanto-occipital joint.

Rotation occurs at the atlantoaxial and lower cervical joints. The range is approximately 80 degrees to either side, of which about 25 degrees occurs in the upper cervical spine.

31 Examination of the cervical spine

(1) Inspection: Observation of the patient's posture, build, gait, and head movements.
(2) Active movements: Tests for flexion, extension, lateral flexion and rotation. Observation of range, reproduction of pain, and rhythm.
(3) Auxiliary testing:

   (a) Over-pressure.
   (b) Rapid movements.
   (c) Sustained pressure.
   (d) The quadrant positions.

(4) Passive movements:

   (a) Test the passive range at each joint in flexion, extension, lateral flexion and rotation.
   (b) Test the accessory movements at C1, C2 and the lower cervical spine.

(5) Palpation.
(6) Neurological testing of upper and lower limbs.
(7) General medical examination and vertebral-artery tests.
(8) Radiological examination.

Inspection

The patient's posture is observed, and may provide clues to diagnosis. With torticollis the head is held laterally flexed to one side, usually away from the painful side. With cervical nerve-root pressure the patient often needs to hold a hand under the elbow of the affected limb to relieve tension, or occasionally gets relief by placing the hand on the head. If a patient stands with the head poked forward it tends to throw the C7 spinous process into prominence and may be associated with an overlying fat pad, or dowager's hump.

Active movements

Active movements are best tested with the patient seated to stabilize the trunk. The patient is first asked whether any symptoms are experienced in this position and to indicate their site. He is then asked to move the neck into full flexion, followed by extension, lateral flexion to either side and then rotation to either side. These movements are observed with the examiner first standing in front and then beside the patient and noting:

(1) The range of movement.
(2) Whether the patient's symptoms are reproduced.
(3) Disturbances of rhythm and the presence or absence of any protective deformity.

The normal range, usually measured in degrees, varies with age and build (*see* page 334).

If no pain is present at rest the patient is asked to move the head in the direction to be tested until pain is felt. If pain is present at rest the patient should be asked to move until the pain begins to increase. The range of movement achieved is noted. Then, provided that pain is not too severe, the patient is asked to move further into the range and report any difference in the severity, site or distribution of pain. This may involve an increase in the severity of pain or an increase in the area of its referral. If pain becomes too severe the movement is stopped and the patient's head is returned to the resting position; otherwise the patient continues to move to the limit of the available range, reporting any alteration in symptoms.

The movements should be repeated while the examiner observes their rhythm and the presence of any local restriction in movement. These are best viewed by standing in front of, and then to the side of, the patient.

Flexion

The examiner stands in front of the seated patient and asks the patient to bend the head forwards; the examiner then notes whether the head and/or neck tend to deviate to either side of the centre line. With the patient's head fully flexed, the examiner stands alongside the patient to look down on the muscular contour of the neck from the occiput to C7, noting any difference in the degree of prominence on either side of the spinous processes. If one side is higher than the other it indicates the presence of a rotational deformity.

The examiner next stands alongside the patient and asks the patient to flex the head forwards; again, the examiner notes whether the cervical spine is unrolling evenly from the head down to C7. If the pain arises from the lower cervical spine, with muscle spasm protecting this movement, this flexion movement will occur mainly in the upper cervical area and in the upper thoracic area.

Extension

Extension should first be assessed with the examiner standing in front of the patient to observe whether the head deviates to one side or the other. By countering any deviation and then comparing the range and the reproduction of any pain with the uncorrected movement in extension, the relationship between the deformity

and the patient's symptoms may be assessed. Extension should also be observed from the side, because at least 80 per cent of extension may occur due to movement in the upper cervical area, thus giving a false impression of the test movement.

If this type of restriction occurs the examiner should hold the patient's head extended to its limit and then apply pressure to attempt to move the lower cervical spine into extension. If this segment is the site of pain this movement will be restricted and the patient's pain will be reproduced or exacerbated.

Lateral flexion

This movement should be observed by the examiner standing in front of the patient and watching the contour of the side of the neck from the mastoid process to the C7 level. The presence of any restrictions of movement is visible on inspection if this examination is carried out carefully (*see Figure 31.1*). If a restriction is present over-pressure to stretch the particular segment is then applied to determine its relationship to the symptoms.

Rotation

Rotation should also be observed by standing in front of the patient and noting whether the patient tends to tilt the head forwards or backwards during the side movement. Countering the abnormal rotation will again relate the presence of the deformity to the patient's symptoms.

Clinical findings

A typical pattern of restriction is usually found in cervical hypomobility syndromes, in which a painful limitation of extension is usually also associated with a restriction of lateral flexion and

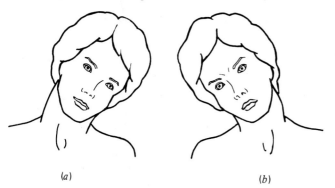

(a)   (b)

Figure 31.1 (*a*) Lateral flexion to the left is normal and is accompanied by a smooth curve in the right side of the neck. (*b*) Lateral flexion to the right is abnormal and is accompanied by a loss of the normal curve on the left side of the upper neck. This limitation is often easier to observe on repeated neck movements

rotation towards the painful side. Less commonly the pattern produced results in a restriction of movement in one direction only, or else in one away from the painful side.

Auxiliary tests

Symptoms arising from the cervical spine are reproduced by the above tests in most patients. But if the tests do not do so, and it still remains likely that symptoms arise from the neck, other measures should be used and assessed.
These are:

(1) Over-pressure.
(2) Repetition of test movements.
(3) Sustained pressure.
(4) The quadrant position.

Over-pressure

Over-pressure is applied by the examiner at the end of the painless range. It is controlled by producing small oscillatory movements at the limit of the range, which also allows the examiner to determine the end-feel of the movement.

Repetition of test movements

If pain is not provoked at the usual testing speed it may be necessary to perform the test movements repeatedly and at increasing speed. Pain may be reproduced if, for example, the patient is asked to rotate the neck quickly.

Sustained pressure

This is used especially in patients with arm pain to demonstrate the cervical origin of their symptoms. The neck is moved successively into the positions of extension, rotation and then lateral flexion towards the painful side. The head is moved either to the limit of the range or to the point where pain is experienced and then gentle pressure is applied and gradually increased for 10 seconds to determine whether pain is reproduced in the arm. Occasionally, pain is first felt as this movement is released or after it is released.

One further test involves compression applied to the head, with the neck held in slight extension and slight lateral flexion towards the painful side. This compression is applied slowly and progressed only in the absence of pain.

The quadrant position

The quadrant position both for the lower and upper cervical spine is tested to put the maximum stress on their intervertebral joints.

The lower cervical quadrant

In a patient who has left-sided pain the neck is tilted back until the lower cervical spine is fully extended and then laterally flexed to the left. While held in this combined position, rotation to the left side is added (*see Figure 31.2(a)*).

The upper cervical quadrant

Standing by the left side of the patient, the examiner guides the head into extension and applies pressure to localize the movement to the upper cervical joints. This is achieved by the examiner grasping the patient's chin in his left hand and the forehead in his right hand. At the same time, the patient's trunk should be stabilized by the examiner's arm from behind. The head is then held in extension and rotated to the left. The head is turned with oscillatory movements to the limit of the range of rotation. When the head is fully turned, it is then laterally flexed by tilting the crown of the patient's head in an oscillatory movement towards the examiner (*see Figure 31.2(b)*).

Passive movements

The two passive movements of the intervertebral joint complex to be tested are:

(1) The passive range at each individual joint; this is tested by feeling the movement between adjacent spinous processes and between articular pillars.
(2) The accessory movements, which are tested by applying pressure over the spinous processes and articular pillars.

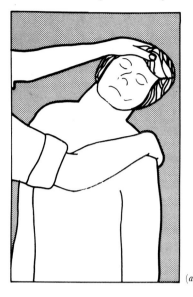

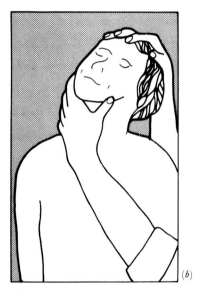

Figure 31.2 Cervical quadrant position: (*a*) lower; (*b*) upper

These tests assess pain and the range of movement, the end-feel of the range, the behaviour of pain and stiffness throughout the range, and the presence of any muscular spasm.

Passive range at individual joints

This is tested by the examiner moving the head and neck into flexion, extension, lateral flexion and then rotation while feeling for movement between adjacent spinal bone processes. Occipito-atlantal, atlantoaxial and the lower cervical joints are tested separately.

Atlanto-occipital joint

This may be tested in lateral flexion, rotation, and flexion–extension.

LATERAL FLEXION OF THE ATLANTO-OCCIPITAL JOINT

Starting position—The patient lies supine with the head projecting beyond the couch. The examiner, standing at the head of the couch, cradles the patient's occiput in his left hand and the patient's forehead in his right hand. The tip of his left thumb lies between the left transverse process of C1 and the adjacent mastoid process. Pressure is applied to the crown of the patient's head by the examiner's abdomen to central movement of the crown of the head (*see Figure 31.3*).

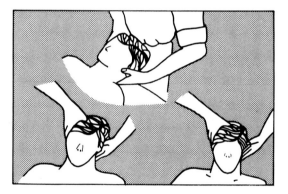

Figure 31.3 Lateral flexion at the atlanto-occipital joint

Method—Although the patient's head is to be laterally flexed to the right, the crown of the head must still remain near the midline. The examiner's hands and body tilt the head on the upper cervical area fully. The examiner's left thumb is positioned between the transverse process of C1 and the mastoid process.

As the head and neck are moved back and forth in the inner third (approximately 15 degrees) of the lateral flexion range, the thumb can feel the opening and closing of the gap between the two bony points of the transverse process of C1 and the mastoid process, and changes in tissue tension.

ROTATION OF THE ATLANTO-OCCIPITAL JOINT
The starting position is the same as that described
above for testing lateral flexion.

Method—When the patient's head has been
turned fully to the right the tip of the examiner's
left thumb is positioned between the left mastoid
process and the left transverse process of C1. The
patient's head is then rotated back and forth
through 20 degrees in the inner third of the range.
As maximum rotation is approached, the transverse process is felt to draw nearer to the mastoid
process and, as the head is brought back towards
the midline, the transverse process is felt to move
away from the mastoid process (*see Figure 31.4*).

FLEXION AND EXTENSION OF THE ATLANTO-
OCCIPITAL JOINT
Starting position—To feel this small amount of
nodding movement of the head the patient lies
supine with the head extending beyond the end
of the couch. The examiner cradles the patient's
head in his lap, holding the occiput in both hands

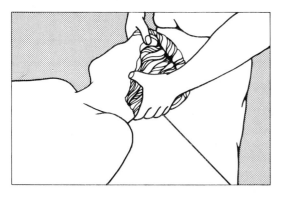

Figure 31.4 Rotation at the atlanto-occipital joint

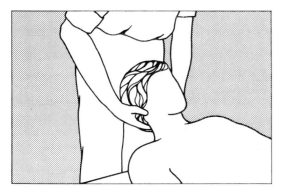

Figure 31.5 Flexion–extension at the atlanto-occipital joint

and placing the tips of his thumbs in contact
with the tip of each lateral mass of C1 and the
mastoid process (*see Figure 31.5*).

Method—The examiner rocks the base of the
patient's skull back and forth through a range of
approximately 20 degrees to produce the
nodding movement. The crown of the head
remains comparatively still. With the tips of his
thumbs the examiner can assess the small movement between the two bony points of each side.

Atlantoaxial joint

This is tested in rotation.

Starting position—To examine the range of rotation to the left between the first and second
cervical vertebrae, the patient is seated with the
examiner standing slightly behind the left shoulder. The examiner places his left hand over the
crown of the patient's head, with his little finger
and thumb spreading over the right and left
parietal areas, respectively, and his hand spread
backwards over the occiput. The hand should
spread to its maximum so that, with his left
forearm pointing vertically, the examiner has full
control of the patient's head. With his right hand
the examiner grasps the spinous process of C2
in a pincer grip between the tip of his index
finger and thumb (*see Figure 31.6*).

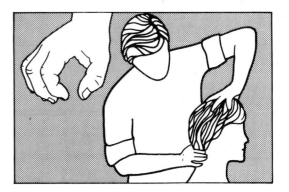

Figure 31.6 Rotation at the atlantoaxial joint

Method—The patient's head is rotated back and
forth from the midline to the left until the spinous
process is felt to move. The lamina of C2 on
the left is felt to move backwards against the
thumb, and the right lateral surface of the spinous
process moves against the pad of the index finger.
When this point has been reached the patient's
head is held still and the range of movement
assessed.

Lower cervical spine

Four movements of the cervical spine below C2 are assessed: flexion, lateral flexion, rotation, and extension.

C2–C7 FLEXION

Starting position—The patient lies supine with the head beyond the end of the couch, and the examiner crouches at the head of the couch, below the level of the patient. He holds the patient's occiput in the heel of his right hand with fingers and thumb over the crown of the head. The examiner then places his left hand against the left side of the patient's neck with the tip of the thumb between two spinous processes, and the tips of the index and middle fingers are placed over the anterior surface of the cervical transverse processes.

To test movement between C3 and C4 the thumb is placed between their spinous processes, with the index and middle fingers over the anterior surface of the left transverse process of C4 and C5 (*see Figure 31.7*).

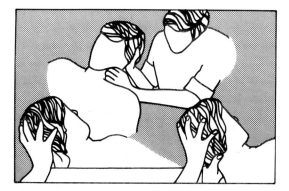

Figure 31.7 Flexion at C2–C7

Method—The patient's head is passively flexed by the examiner's right hand while the tip of his left thumb feels between the spinous processes for the amount of opening and closing that takes place as the head is moved backwards and forwards through a range of 15–20 degrees. To produce the maximum movement between C3 and C4, the vertebrae below C4 are stabilized by applying pressure against the anterior surface of the left transverse processes.

C2–C7 LATERAL FLEXION

Starting position—The patient lies supine, the head resting in the examiner's lap midway between the limits of flexion and extension for the joint being examined. In this position both lateral flexion and rotation are most free.

The examiner places the tip of his index finger deeply into the interlaminar space and supports the patient's occiput and neck with both hands (*see Figure 31.8*).

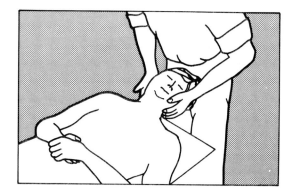

Figure 31.8 Lateral flexion at C2–C7

Method—Care is necessary to ensure that the joint being tested, and not the head alone, is moved. The examiner first laterally flexes the joint towards his immobile palpating finger, assessing the extent of closing in the interlaminar space. Movement in the opposite direction is then performed to assess the opening of the space.

C2–C7 ROTATION

Starting position—The starting position is as described above for lateral flexion, except that the index finger is carried laterally, so making a slightly broader contact with the margin of the apophyseal joint (*see Figure 31.9*).

Method—The head is pivoted away from the side, being palpated about its imaginary central axis. The examiner's hand produces the movement

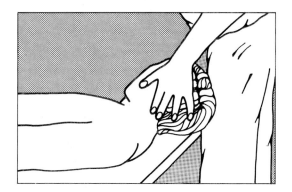

Figure 31.9 Rotation at C2–C7

in a steady, oscillatory fashion, down to, but not beyond, the joint. The palpating finger follows the movement of the joint to assess the extent of opening that occurs between the two adjacent articular processes.

C2–C7 EXTENSION

Starting position—The patient lies supine with the head resting in the examiner's lap. The examiner stands near the head, supporting underneath the patient's head and neck to the level of the joint being tested. He places the tips of both index fingers into the interlaminar space on each side, as described above for lateral flexion (*see Figure 31.10*).

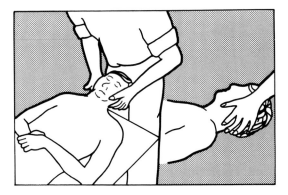

Figure 31.10 Extension at C2–C7

Method—The examiner extends the patient's head and neck down to the level being examined, while at the same time palpating with his fingertips for a closing down of the interlaminar space.

Accessory movements

These are tested using pressure against bony vertebral processes to localize a restricted and painful intervertebral joint. They are tested at C1 and C2 first, and then in the cervical spine.

Accessory movement of C1

POSTEROANTERIOR MOVEMENT

Position—The patient lies prone with the forehead resting on his hands.

Method—Posteroanterior pressures are applied by the examiner's thumbs, which are first placed centrally against the posterior tubercle of the atlas, and then laterally behind the atlanto-occipital joint (*see Figure 31.11*).

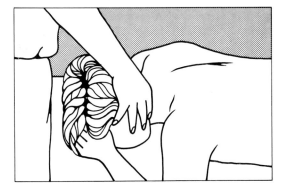

Figure 31.11 Test for accessory movements at C1. Posteroanterior pressure centrally over C1

TRANSVERSE MOVEMENT

Position—The patient's head is rotated first to the left side with the right arm by the side and the left arm level with the head, thus slightly raising the left shoulder and taking any strain off cervical rotation. In this position the lateral mass of C1 is easily palpable, as it has rotated with the head.

Method—Oscillatory pressures are applied by the thumbs directed transversely from the tip of the lateral mass of C1 on the left towards the tip of the lateral mass on the opposite side (*see Figure 31.12*).

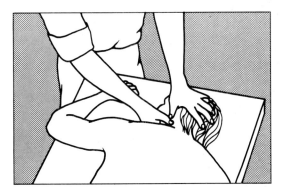

Figure 31.12 Transverse pressure against C1

Accessory movement of C2

Posteroanterior pressures against the spinous process of C2 are used first followed by posteroanterior pressure against the articular pillar of C2.

Position—The patient lies with the head resting on his hands (*see Figure 31.11*).

Method—The examiner applies posteroanterior pressures with his thumbs, which are placed on the posterior surface of the inferior articular process of the axis.

C2 may also be tested in rotation. For rotation to the left, the patient turns the head approximately 30 degrees to the left, resting the forehead in his hands. Posteroanterior pressure on the left articular process of C2 will then test the rotary movement between C1 and C2 (*see Figure 31.13*).

Accessory movement—lower cervical spine

Three tests of accessory movements are used routinely in the lower cervical spine:

(1) Posteroanterior pressures over the spinous process.
(2) Posteroanterior pressures over the articular pillar.

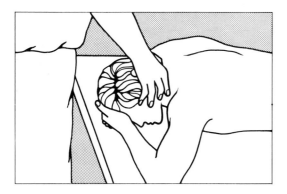

Figure 31.13 Test for the accessory movements of C2 in rotation

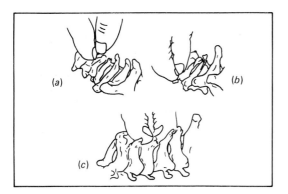

Figure 31.14 (*a*) Posteroanterior pressure on the spinous process; (*b*) posteroanterior pressure on the articular pillar; (*c*) transverse pressure on the lateral surface of the spinous process

(3) Transverse pressures against the lateral surfaces of the spinous process (*see Figure 31.14*).

The direction given to these pressures may be varied so that the posteroanterior pressure may also be directed towards the head or towards the feet. The direction taken by the posteroanterior pressure over the articular pillar may be further varied by directing the pressure laterally away from the spinous process, or else medially towards the spinous process.

The transverse pressure against the lateral surface of the spinous process may also be varied by inclining the direction of pressure either toward the feet or head, or across the back of the lamina so that the pressure is finally applied as a posteroanterior pressure against the articular pillar on the same side.

POSITION
The patient lies prone with his forehead resting on his hands and the chin tucked in, avoiding the fully flexed or extended position.

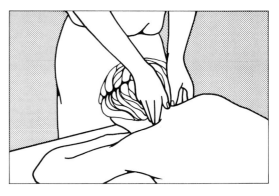

Figure 31.15 Central posteroanterior pressure over the spinous process

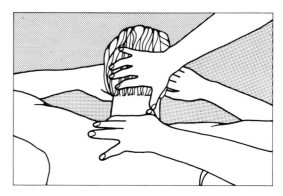

Figure 31.16 Transverse pressure against the lower cervical articular pillar

For posteroanterior pressures the examiner stands at the head of the patient and places his thumbs back to back over the spinous process and uses only gentle oscillatory pressure (*see Figure 31.15*).

For transverse pressures against the articular process the examiner then stands to one side and applies the pad of his thumb against the articular pillar (*see Figure 31.16*).

Palpation

The patient's neck is palpated to detect any alterations in the bony alignments, the presence of a cervical rib or muscle spasm. Areas of localized muscle spasm and tenderness are usually easily palpable around the scapula in the rhomboids, trapezius and levator scapulae muscles. Many of the bony prominences on the back of the skull and cervical vertebrae are easily palpable. In the occiput, the inion is easily felt as a bony lump in the midline of the occiput with the nuchal line radiating out on either side of it. These end in the prominent mastoid processes on either side. The spinous process of C1 is felt immediately

below the mastoid process and can be felt to move on rotating the head.

The spinous process of C1 is not normally palpable, and the first spinous process that is easily felt is that of C2. The spinous process from C3 to C7 can usually be palpated.

The apophyseal joints are also palpable below C2 and can be felt to move by placing the fingers over the side of the cervical spine approximately 2–3 cm away from the midline. The patient's neck needs to be fully relaxed, as these joints lie beneath the trapezius muscle. Osteophytic lipping and tenderness about their margin may be felt occasionally.

Neurological tests

A complete assessment of the central nervous system is necessary in all cervical disorders. Motor power, sensation and reflexes are tested in both upper and lower limbs.

Evidence of a lower motor-neurone lesion in the arm that produces muscular weakness is usually due to involvement of only one nerve root, and those of clinical significance are listed in *Table 31.1*.

Table 31.1 Muscular weaknesses in the arm produced from lower motor-neurone lesions

Movement	Main muscle involved	Nerve root	Method of testing
Abduction of arm	Deltoid	C5	The patient holds the arm abducted 45 degrees from the side while the examiner applies resistance to the lateral aspect of the arm just above the elbow
Elbow flexion	Biceps	C6	The patient holds the supinated forearm flexed at the elbow to 90 degrees. Resistance is applied against the anterior surface of the forearm just above the wrist
Elbow extension	Triceps	C7	The patient holds the elbow flexed to 90 degrees, resistance being applied against the dorsum of the forearm just above the wrist
Extension of thumb	Extensor pollicis longus	C8	The patient flexes the elbow to 90 degrees with forearm in mid-position and holds the extended thumb away from the palm and pointing towards the face. Resistance is directed against the thumbnail towards the little finger
Interphalangeal flexion	Flexor digitorum	C8	The patient flexes the elbow to 90 degrees with forearm in mid-position. The examiner stabilizes the forearm while the patient squeezes his fingers. Power of the long finger flexors is tested by resisting terminal interphalangeal flexion
Intrinsics		T1	The patient flexes the elbow to 90 degrees, extending the finger at the interphalangeal joints and flexing them at the metacarpo-phalangeal joints. The examiner places his finger between adjacent fingers of the patient in turn while the patient squeezes the extended fingers together

The girth of the arms is measured with a tape measure to record the presence of any muscle wasting.

Sensory disturbances to light touch and pin prick are sought in the dermatome distribution of the cervical nerves. Reflexes to be tested include the biceps jerk C5 and C6, the triceps jerk C7, and the supinator jerk C6 (*see Table 31.1*).

Finally, signs of an upper motor-neurone lesion, including the plantar responses, are tested for in the lower limbs.

General examination

A general medical examination, including the cardiovascular system and respiratory system, is mandatory. This includes palpation and ausculta-tion of the extracranial arteries, and a clinical test of the vertebral arteries.

Vertebral artery

In all patients with neck pain, but especially those who also complain of giddiness, an attempt should be made to assess the relationship between neck movements and the production of giddiness. This is done both by direct questioning and by testing neck movements.

Positioning is achieved by sustaining the three positions of extension and rotation to each side in turn. Dizziness may be experienced whilst this position is sustained or on its release. Alternatively, the examiner stands in front of the patient and holds the patient's head in his hands while the patient twists the trunk fully from side to side, with the feet remaining stationary. In this manner, the trunk is rotated beneath the motionless head. This eliminates the effect of inner-ear movement, hence dizziness produced during this test move-ment may be of cervical origin.

32 Cervical-disc degeneration

Disc degeneration commonly involves the cervical spine. This may be due to it having a greater range of movement than the lumbar or thoracic spines while supporting the weight of the head and being attached inferiorly to the relatively immobile upper thoracic segments and ribs. The normal lordotic curve in the cervical spine helps to localize these degenerative changes at the C5–6, C6–7 levels.

Cervical spondylosis is much more common clinically than lumbar spondylosis, whereas the incidence of acute cervical-disc prolapse is relatively much less common than lumbar-disc prolapse. This is due to anatomical differences. In the cervical spine the neurocentral joints occupy the posterolateral edges of the vertebrae so that the cervical discs do not extend as far posterolaterally as in the lumbar spine. The bony uncus may also provide some form of an anatomical barrier and the posterior longitudinal ligament,

thicker in the cervical than in the lumbar spine, provides stronger support.

The relationship of the nerve roots also varies, since the cervical roots do not run obliquely downwards across the disc as in the lumbar spine but are more laterally directed. Accordingly, they run behind the vertebral body and the neurocentral joint and are protected by what Ruth Jackson (1965) calls the 'silent zone'. The most severe degree of degenerative changes occurs in the C5–6 and C6–7 discs, with resultant narrowing of their corresponding intervertebral foramina. Accordingly, the nerve roots most commonly compressed are C6 and C7. The lower cervical nerve roots are the largest of the brachial plexus but the intervertebral foramina tend to be smaller here than in the other areas (Wilkinson, 1971).

Cervical spondylosis

Spondylosis is caused by degenerative changes in the discs, vertebrae and apophyseal joints which lead to osteophytic outgrowths that reduce the size of the intervertebral foramen and so may compromise the nerve roots (*see Figure 32.1*). The clinical syndrome involving the cervical spine is more common and severe than that of the lumbar spine and these differences are due to several additional features:

(1) The neurocentral joints. Degenerative changes in these joints with osteophytic outgrowths are common, further reducing the size of the intervertebral foramen, and are

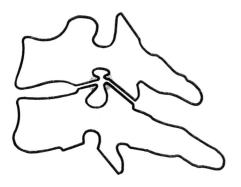

Figure 32.1 Osteophytic outgrowths from the neurocentral joint encroach upon the intervertebral foramen

often an important factor in the production of symptoms.

(2) Neural involvement. As in the lumbar spine, the nerve roots may be compressed or irritated. Frykholm (1951) first described nerve-root compression that resulted from thickening of the dural extension forming the root pouch. This root-sleeve fibrosis may also be responsible for other changes, such as constriction or sharp angulation of the nerve root, that render the nerve root more vulnerable to consequent inflammatory oedema. These findings were confirmed by Holt and Yates (1966), who also described the histology of increased amounts of connective tissue in the nerve tissue associated with axonal and myelin degenerative changes. Of importance in the cervical spine, but not present in the lower lumbar spine, is the possibility of spinal-cord compression and myelopathy. Besides direct involvement from the hard, protruding, posterior osteocartilaginous bars, occlusion of the anterior spinal artery may result in cord changes. Finally, neural tissue in the sympathetic chain may be involved.

(3) Vascular changes. The vertebral artery may be involved in its course through the transverse processes of the cervical vertebrae (*see Figure 32.2*).

(4) Surrounding soft tissues are more liable to be compressed and so produce symptoms.

Clinical presentations

Neck pain

The patient may present with neck pain commonly associated with stiffness. This is a dull, aching but often not particularly severe pain, which is often constantly present and made worse by sudden movements or most physical activities involving the neck. Pain is felt diffusely in the neck or in the interscapular region or shoulder. There is often a history of acute attacks that may have been minor or labelled 'fibrositis', in which pain or stiffness is felt in this same distribution. Pain may also be referred distally into the arms but the site of such pain does not always indicate the spinal level of the disc degeneration.

Arm pain

Pain in the arm in cases of cervical spondylosis may be either:

(1) Referred pain from the neck. This usually radiates into the extensor aspect of the upper arm only, though it may be felt at times anywhere in the limb. It may be associated with sensations of heat and cold in the limb, or with other dysthaesias that are not segmental.

(2) Due to nerve-root pressure. This usually follows minor trauma or overuse, commonly precipitated by activities involving extension of the head or excessive use of the arm—for example, after painting a ceiling. This is most likely due to an associated synovitis of the apophyseal joints, since evidence of a disc prolapse is usually absent. The C6 or the C7 nerve root is commonly involved, with or without neurological signs.

Headache

That headache may result from lesions of the cervical spine has been recognized in the medical literature since the beginning of this century (Holmes, 1913). Barré (1926) presented a detailed analysis of headache and vertigo in patients with neck lesions. More recently, it has been recognized

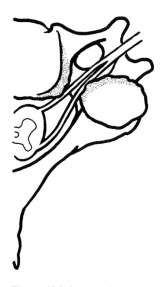

Figure 32.2 Osteophytic outgrowths from the apophyseal joint and vertebra may compress the intervertebral nerve or may even be large enough to encroach on the transverse foramen, with its vertebral artery

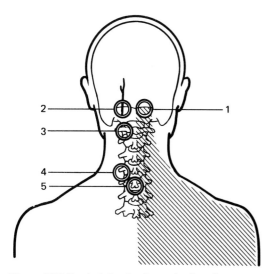

Figure 32.3 Cervical sites for the production of headache: (1) musculotendinous attachments; (2) compression of the greater occipital nerve; (3) atlantoaxial region, headache being due either to arthritis or to a hypomobility lesion; (4) involvement of the vertebral artery in the transverse foramen; (5) cervical spondylosis

that headache is a common feature of cervical spondylosis (Wilkinson, 1971) and that a similar type of headache is also caused by a hypomobility lesion of the upper cervical spine.

There are three other known causes for headache of cervical origin (*see Figure 32.3*):

(1) Arthritis of the atlantoaxial joints.
(2) Musculotendinous lesions of the attachment of the cervical muscles to the nuchal line.
(3) An entrapment neuropathy of the occipital nerves.

Finally, it is important to realize that migraine is quite disinct from these causes and will be discussed more fully below.

CLINICAL FEATURES
The type of headache associated with either cervical spondylosis or a hypomobility lesion of the upper cervical spine is usually so characteristic that the diagnosis should be suspected from the history alone. Pain is usually felt in the sub-occipital region either unilaterally or bilaterally, and radiates to the head, behind the eyes or into the face. In any individual patient the site and radiation of pain tends to remain constant. The pain, usually described as dull and aching or as a sensation of soreness, is often worse on arising in the morning or immediately after first

raising the head. When severe, pain may be felt also during the night and the patient may not be able to bear his head against a pillow. The headache usually eases as the day goes on but may be aggravated by neck and head movements or by jolting, as when riding in a bus. Some patients also notice that their headache can be relieved by posturing the neck. Head pain alone without neck pain is less common but does occur and is often associated with a feeling of neck stiffness.

In addition to head and neck pain, other symptoms may be present as the result of the lesion in the cervical spine. These include vertigo; vague symptoms, such as feelings of being generally unwell; nausea; depression; or a feeling of uncertainty. It may at times be difficult to differentiate these symptoms from psychosomatic disorders.

Clinical examination should confirm that neck movements reproduce the head pain. In patients with cervical spondylosis some degree of restriction of neck movements is to be expected, but in hypomobility lesions the overall physiological range may appear to be normal. However, testing the passive intervertebral movements in the upper cervical joints will reveal that their range is restricted, and that the patient's pain is reproduced. These signs may be present at one or more levels from C1 to C3 and be associated with local tenderness and thickening on palpation.

A common finding is for restriction of movement to be found at two levels but on opposite sides; for example, the right side of C1–2, and the left side at C2–3.

MECHANISM
The basis for these headaches is probably one of referred pain, and direct neural compression as the underlying cause need not be invoked. Referred pain is almost certainly the sole mechanism in hypomobility lesions, but with cervical spondylosis an additional factor may be alterations in neck posture that produce tension in the insertion of the cervical muscles. It has also been postulated that the cervical sympathetic nervous system may be involved but this would appear to be unlikely.

The sensory innervation of this area is derived from several sources:

(1) Branches from the sinuvertebral nerves arising from the upper three cervical. nerves carry sensory and sympathetic fibres and are dis-

tributed to the dura mater, periosteum and blood vessels in the floor of the posterior cranial fossa (Gardner, Gray and O'Rahilly, 1969).

(2) Afferent neurones of the fifth cranial nerve descend in its spinal tract and anastomose in the upper cervical cord with afferent fibres from the upper three cervical segments, which supply the joints and ligaments of the upper three vertebrae.

(3) The scalp is supplied mainly by branches of the posterior primary rami of the upper cervical nerves, which radiate as far as the frontal region (Bradley, 1977). The posterior primary ramus of C2 divides into a lateral and medial branch. The latter is known as the greater occipital nerve and it receives communications from the first and third cervical nerves. The anterior primary ramus of C2 also supplies the scalp. It may receive a branch from C3 and ascends as the lesser occipital nerve. The posterior primary ramus of the first cervical nerve (C1) mainly supplies the suboccipital muscles but it also supplies a filament to the greater occipital nerve. Kerr (1961) demonstrated that stimulation of the C1 dorsal nerve roots produced pain in the frontal and orbital regions.

(4) Smith (1969) described an experiment in which stimulation of the upper cervical sympathetic nerves produced pain in the head and face. This was experienced after division of the sympathetic nerve and stimulation of the proximal end of the divided nerve. It may also be relevant that sympathetic nerve fibres have been described as arising from as high as C5 in the spinal cord.

REFERRED PAIN

As already stated, the basis for this headache is referred pain. In common with other sites, the distance that the pain is referred reflects the severity of the underlying lesion. At first it may be considered unusual for referred pain to be distributed proximally rather than distally but this has been explained by Bradley (1977) on an evolutionary basis. In animals that walk on four legs the scalp, extending to the bridge of the nose, is supplied by nerves derived from the upper cervical vertebrae, and a similar arrangement persisted when humans assumed the upright position.

Experiments (e.g., Campbell and Parsons, 1944) with the use of injection of hypertonic saline

in the upper cervical area have been repeated. With injections at C1 pain is referred to the occipital and frontal areas, and at C2–3 pain is experienced in the neck and head.

Atlantoaxial arthritis

Both inflammatory and degenerative types of arthritis may involve the upper cervical spine and can then produce head pain. Arthritis of the atlanto-occipital or atlantoaxial joints may occur in patients with either rheumatoid arthritis or spondyloarthritis, and osteoarthritis may involve the lateral atlantoaxial joints.

The diagnosis of arthritis is confirmed by suitable X-rays of the atlantoaxial region.

Entrapment neuropathy

An entrapment neuropathy involving the occipital nerves has been well described. The greater occipital nerve is the medial branch of the posterior primary ramus of C2. It may be entrapped as it runs through the semispinalis capitis muscles or trapezius about 1 cm from the midline. It then crosses the nuchal line with the occipital artery and is distributed to the scalp as far as the frontal region (Bradley, 1977).

The cause of occipital-nerve entrapment may often be post-traumatic but it can also arise without a history of trauma, presumably due to entrapment in its course through the neck muscles. Mayfield (1954) described hyperextension injuries of the neck that produced damage to the C2 nerve root in its course between the atlas and axis and advocated surgery for their relief. De Palma and Rothman (1970) considered that the visual and auditory disturbances often associated with this injury may indicate an entrapment of the sympathetic nerves. The head pain that results from an entrapment neuropathy may be severe and intermittent and is often described as a burning, throbbing or piercing pain radiating from the neck up to the head. It is also often present at night. There may be associated hyperalgesia or paraesthesias of the scalp.

Symptoms can often be reproduced either by direct pressure over the nerve just distal to the nuchal line or by posturing the head. It may also be possible to demonstrate sensory disturbances over the skin of the scalp.

Musculotendinous lesions

Lesions of the musculotendinous attachment of the cervical muscles to the nuchal line of the skull may also result in head pain. One of three causes may then be present:

(1) Alteration in the patient's posture, which may itself be the result of an underlying hypomobility lesion or cervical spondylosis.
(2) An underlying tension state producing muscular tension in neck muscles. Patients with this cause may complain of neck or head pain alone, but more commonly complain of head and neck pain occurring together.
(3) Tendinitis may occasionally occur as the sole clinical finding without any evidence of these associated conditions.

Tendinitis in this area is evidenced by tenderness on palpation, which should also reproduce the patient's pain. The neck muscles should be contracted isometrically to determine whether pain is produced and infiltration of the locally tender area with local anaesthetic should relieve the patient's symptoms, at least temporarily.

Migraine

The clinical features of migraine are well known. They clearly present a different clinical picture to the type of headaches previously discussed and are not directly related to lesions of the cervical spine. Nevertheless, considerable confusion appears to exist about their relationship; this confusion may stem from several reasons.

Firstly, the diagnosis of migraine may have been incorrect. This tends to occur if the headache is severe, in which case a diagnosis of migraine may be incorrectly applied to a case of headache arising from the cervical spine. This appears to be the most common reason for reports in which migraine has been 'cured' after manipulation of the neck.

Secondly, migraine may occur coincidentally in the presence of a cervical lesion. It seems possible, then, that the neck lesion could be a non-specific triggering mechanism that will induce an attack of migraine. If so, treatment to the neck with mobilization techniques could help to stop an attack (Stoddard, 1969).

Thirdly, migraine may very rarely be produced by vertebral-artery compression in the neck, described by Dutton and Riley (1969) as cervical migraine. In their case report, a 54-year-old man complained of severe attacks of recurrent headaches of a migrainous nature. Arteriography during an attack demonstrated compression of the left vertebral artery caused by degenerative changes at the C6–7 level. Surgery relieved the compression and the patient was cured. In addition, patients with vertebrobasilar insufficiency due to atheroma may suffer headaches. These may occur in attacks and be associated with visual disturbances and vertigo (Bickerstaff, 1961).

Thus migraine is due to a disturbance of cranial blood flow and is rarely associated with disorders of the cervical spine. Accordingly, the failure of a trial of manipulation by Parker, Tupling and Pryor (1978) to diminish the frequency and duration of migraine attacks was entirely predictable.

Diagnosis of cervical headaches

Headache is common in patients with disorders of the cervical spine but no precise figures on its incidence are available. Investigations of the patient to exclude other potentially more serious causes of headache may be indicated but will not be considered here. It should be noted that Golding (1969) described four cases of posterior fossa tumours presenting with similar neck pain and headache. However, he points out that other diagnostic clinical features were also present.

The correct diagnosis of a headache arising from the cervical spine can usually be made on clinical grounds. It should be suspected from the patient's history and description of the characteristics of the headache, which have already been described. Other symptoms should be sought, including the relationship and influence of neck posture and movements; the presence of neck stiffness; and the influence of vibration, such as that caused by riding in a motor vehicle. A history of trauma to the neck may also be obtained. It is, however, essential to demonstrate the presence of appropriate neck signs before confirmation of the diagnosis can be achieved. This follows the plan of examination detailed in Chapter 31, during which the patient is questioned as to whether cervical movements reproduce the head pain. In patients with cervical spondylosis or rheumatoid arthritis active neck movements may be restricted.

Passive joint movements are then tested, while paying special attention to the use of passive intervertebral-joint movements of the upper cervical spine. A hypomobility lesion in this area may be demonstrated by a painful restriction in these movements with reproduction of the patient's pain and local joint tenderness on the side of the headache. Palpation of the attachments of the cervical muscles to the nuchal line is carefully carried out with the patient's neck relaxed. This is often best achieved by having the patient sit with the head flexed and supported on the arms, which are placed on the desk. In patients with an entrapment neuropathy, compression of the occipital nerve over the nuchal line should produce pain.

A full general examination should be carried out and X-rays of the head and neck, full blood counts, and an erythrocyte sedimentation rate are performed as a routine.

Facial pain

Facial pain, even in the absence of headache, may occur with lesions of the cervical spine. The pain is often deep seated, dull and aching. It is usually unilateral at first, tends to be constant in site, and may be made worse by neck and head movements or by straining. Facial pain may be associated with unusual sensations—such as a coldness in the face. Pain may be sited in the supraorbital region, behind the eyes, or around the ear. In the infraorbital regions this pain is often mistaken for sinusitis, thus forming the basis for cases of 'sinusitis' said to be cured by manipulation.

Vertigo

The causes of vertigo are complex and include disturbances of the inner ear, neurological lesions and vascular diseases.

Ryan and Cope (1955) suggested the term cervical vertigo for cases associated with neck pain and stiffness. Wing and Hargrave-Wilson (1974) reviewed 80 cases of cervical vertigo, most of whom were women between the ages of 40 and 60, in whom the only abnormal finding was a hypomobility lesion of the upper cervical spine. There was no history of neck trauma and they responded well to neck manipulation.

Clinical features of cervical vertigo

The patient describes a true vertigo with rotary movements of objects and a sense of falling to one side. Occasionally, nausea—coming on in attacks but usually lasting only a short time—is present.

These attacks are usually brought on by sudden changes in head position, and so are common whilst reversing a car or looking up in the shower. They are also precipitated after changing a position that has been maintained for a time, as when getting out of bed in the morning. There may be a short latent period between the neck or head movement and the onset of vertigo.

Pathogenesis

Vertigo due to cervical lesions is caused either by changes in the vertebral artery or by disorders of the musculoskeletal structures. The former is produced by obstruction of blood flow through the vertebral artery to the labyrinth and its neural connections. The most common cause of this is atheromatous changes in the artery, hence the increasing incidence with age. In such circumstances the efficiency of the vertebrobasilar system will depend on the anastomosis with the carotid system through the circle of Willis. Any alteration produced by atheromatous changes in the carotid system, or any congenital lesion affecting the calibre of either system, may result in symptoms.

Neck movements have also been implicated in causing an obstruction to the vertebral artery (de Kleijn and Nieuwenhuyse, 1927; Coburn, 1962; Husni, Bell and Storer, 1966). They would need to be extreme to cut off the blood supply in normal vertebral arteries, but movement can impair the blood supply in patients with atheroma or if degenerative changes in the cervical spine are present. Musculoskeletal disorders of the cervical spine may also cause vertigo, and four such conditions have been described.

Cervical spondylosis

Cervical spondylosis may cause an alteration in vertebral-artery flow because of kinking and distortion of the artery (Tatlow and Bammer, 1957; Bauer, Sheehan and Meyer, 1961; Powers, Drislane and Iandoli, 1963). Encroachment on the artery in its transverse foramen may be produced by osteophytes arising from the neurocentral joints or associated with lateral disc protrusions (Kovacs, 1955). Hutchinson and Yates (1956) examined 40 cadavers and showed that these osteophytic outgrowths produced compression and distortion of vertebral arteries. This occurred even with the head in the neutral position; these changes become more marked with head movement. Sheehan, Bauer and Meyer (1960) were able to demonstrate similar changes in patients with spondylosis by using vertebral angiography.

However, vertigo occurs in most cases of cervical spondylosis without any evidence of direct vertebral-artery compression. The cause of this is not known but it may be related to alterations in postural reflexes, as discussed more fully below.

Hypomobility lesion of the upper cervical spine

The essential clinical finding in this condition is a restriction in the range of passive intervertebral movements in one or more of the upper three cervical vertebrae. This restriction may involve rotation, flexion, extension or lateral flexion and is usually associated with spasm and tenderness in the upper cervical muscles. Although the basis for vertigo is unknown, two mechanisms have been suggested. The original theory of Barré (1926) and Lieou (1928) that a lesion of the cervical sympathetic nerves was responsible has now been discarded. The second theory depends on the fact that the upper cervical joints are richly supplied by mechanoreceptors responsible for joint proprioception. Impulses from these receptors provide tonic neck-righting reflexes, which are of major importance in the normal control of balance. They are carried along nerve fibres that connect to centres in the upper cervical cord and the brain stem. Cope and Ryan (1959) suggested that interference with these neck proprioceptive impulses that arise when musculoskeletal structures—such as neck joints, ligaments and muscles—are

stretched could produce vertigo. Thus it does seem most likely that these lesions of the upper cervical spine could produce an alteration in proprioceptive control and so cause vertigo.

Patients with either cervical hypomobility lesions or spondylosis could well have a disturbance of normal proprioception so that on movement of the neck a bombardment of afferent impulses into the spinal, cerebellum and vestibular nuclei produces a consciousness of disorientation of the body in space. Such a mechanism was considered likely to be present by Wing and Hargrave-Wilson (1974) and tends to be confirmed by clinical findings, as vertigo usually results after sustained movement towards the affected side.

Cervical trauma

Vertigo has been described either after direct trauma to the neck or after indirect trauma that produced sprains of the cervical spine after motor-vehicle accidents after which transient dizziness is a common complaint. However, if in such accidents the vertebral artery is damaged and produces ischaemic changes in the vertebrobasilar system then vertigo and, at times, deafness, may be produced (Pang, 1971).

Rheumatoid arthritis

Patients with rheumatoid arthritis involving the cervical spine may also complain of vertigo. This may follow atlantoaxial subluxation that produced distortion of the vertebral artery or more rarely be produced by an arteritis of this vessel (Webb, Hickman and Drew, 1968).

Scapular pain

Pain, which the patient usually describes as dull and aching or as occasionally throbbing or like a toothache, may be found in relation to the scapula, either in the interscapular region or felt over the upper scapular border. It may occur with or without neck pain on the same side.

An almost constant clinical finding is the presence of localized areas of tender, palpable thickening. They are readily palpable and usually disappear after manipulation of the appropriate spinal segment. They have also been referred to as 'trigger spots' or as fibrositis. Their origin is uncertain but it is presumed that they represent localized areas of muscle spasm, on the basis of mechanical derangement of the intervertebral joint with referred pain and tenderness.

Both the sixth and seventh cervical nerve roots and their posterior rami supply sensory fibres to posterior neck muscles, pectoralis major, latissimus dorsi and serratus anterior muscles besides the other trunk muscles. A lesion that produces irritation of these nerves may cause pain to be referred widely to the trunk, chest or even the lower back. Cloward (1963) has confirmed these findings.

Anterior chest pain

Ollie (1937) described the first large series that demonstrated the presence of anterior chest pain with cervical-spine lesions. In one-third of his 600 cases, chest pain was attributed to a spinal cause. There were subsequent numerous case reports in the literature before Davis (1957) documented the underlying spinal pathology with its clinical presentation.

The chest pain may be bilateral, substernal or felt in the anterior chest wall. Its character, site, severity and radiation can vary to a marked degree, and the pain may be related to exertion, posturing or breathing. Thus its importance may be in its simulation of disease, such as coronary artery or pulmonary disease, and in the avoidance of mis-diagnosis; it is equally as important to be sure that pain is *not* due to heart disease as it is to overlook it.

Such pain may arise from the spinal joints, two common causes being cervical spondylosis and hypomobility lesions. The essential feature in diagnosis is that the patient's type of pain will be reproduced on spinal movements or that local joint signs are found at an appropriate spinal level. The effect of treatment in easing or abolishing pain after several mobilization treatments also tends to confirm the diagnosis. Difficulty in diagnosis is increased in the elderly, when degenerative changes both in the coronary arteries and in the spine are common and so may be present together in the same patient. For this reason the presence of X-ray changes of degeneration in the cervical spine is not sufficient evidence to confirm the diagnosis of a spinal cause for chest pain.

Cervical myelopathy

Since the onset of cervical spondylosis is usually gradual, adjacent tissues also can gradually adjust so that symptoms are often absent or minimal. However, in the presence of large or multiple osteophytes or in patients with a narrowed spinal canal, symptoms of spinal-cord involvement may occur. The usual cause of this syndrome is the hard mass of bone and cartilage projecting from the posterior aspect of the vertebral body and indenting the spinal cord. The resultant syndrome is similar to that of a spinal-cord compression but may produce several different clinical presentations.

The onset is usually insidious, with symptoms arising from varying combinations of upper and lower motor-neurone lesions and sensory disturbances. The upper motor-neurone lesion affects the lower limbs, hence weakness of the legs is the most common presenting symptom. In the arms there are often sensory disturbances with pins and needles and numbness together with a sensation of weakness or of clumsiness.

A full neurological examination and assessment is essential. Reflex changes usually consist of increased tendon reflexes in the lower limbs with extensor plantar responses, whilst in the upper limb there may be an inverted radial reflex if the lesion is at the C5 level. The jaw jerk, a most useful sign to differentiate spinal from intracranial lesions, is positive only in the latter.

Nerve-root palsy

As a general rule, muscular wasting is not severe as a result of a radicular lesion in cervical spondylosis. However, severe muscle weakness and atrophy may occur in the absence of any sensory changes. The presumed basis for this is an anterior spinal-root compression from osteophytic encroachment in the intervertebral foramen. The most common site appears to be the C5 nerve root, which produces a paresis of shoulder muscles. The condition is usually painless, though pain may be present during the first 2 or 3 days. The paresis is associated with osteophytic encroachment on the C4–5 intervertebral foramen. The patient is usually elderly, presenting with weakness of shoulder movements, particularly abduction, whilst neck or arm pain or neck restriction are usually minimal or absent. Oblique neck X-rays confirm the presence of osteophytes. Most cases gradually improve over a long period of time.

Leg pain

Patients in whom the major complaint is of leg pain may show no evidence of lumbar intervertebral-disc changes but evidence of a marked degree of cervical spondylosis. The cervical origin of these cases was documented by Langfitt and Elliott (1967), who presented three examples of back and leg pain without any evidence of lumbar-disc disease but of severe degrees of cervical spondylosis. Bradshaw (1961) described such pain as being poorly localized and of a dull, aching or bursting character. This contrasts with sensory symptoms, such as numbness or paraesthesias, which are usually predominant features in cases of cervical spondylosis producing cervical-cord compression. But a similar basis of cord compression is proposed for the leg pain, which also helps explain the common occurrence of exaggerated lower limb tendon reflexes in such patients.

Pressure effects on surrounding soft tissues

Large anterior osteophytes—usually palpable as tender, bony protuberances—may produce pressure effects on surrounding soft tissues. Dysphagia has been documented. Examination with barium swallow showed indentation of the oesophagus and subsequent cure after levelling off of the osteophytes. Hoarseness can also be produced (Heck, 1956).

33 Cervical hypomobility lesions

Hypomobility lesions involving either the upper or lower cervical spine or both of these sites have many symptoms in common with those produced by cervical spondylosis.

Upper cervical spine

Lesions here may produce:

(1) Neck pain.
(2) Head pain.
(3) Face pain.
(4) Vertigo.

Neck pain is usually well localized and situated to one side of the upper cervical spine. The clinical features of headache, face pain and vertigo have already been considered.

Diagnosis depends on the ability either to reproduce the patient's symptoms or to produce a comparable degree of pain in an appropriate cervical-spine joint, together with finding a painful restriction in the range of passive intervertebral-joint movements. X-rays are normal for the patient's age.

Lower cervical spine

These may present as:

(1) Neck pain.
(2) Fibrositis.

(3) Torticollis.
(4) Shoulder pain.

Neck pain

Neck pain is common and usually well localized to one side. The essential clinical finding is a painful restriction of the active and passive range of movement in certain directions only. The most common pattern is a restriction of extension and of lateral flexion and rotation towards the painful side. Less commonly, movements away from the painful side are restricted and only rarely is flexion restricted. Ancillary tests using overpressure, sustained pressure or the quadrant position may be necessary if the active physiological range appears normal. Passive intervertebral-joint movements are found to be restricted in range and commonly reproduce the patient's pain. Tenderness and a sensation of thickening may be found over interspinous ligaments in the midline or over the apophyseal joints, and tender painful areas with palpable spasm are found around the scapula on the affected side. There are no abnormal neurological signs. X-rays are consistent with ageing changes alone, but it is usually impossible on the evidence of radiological changes to differentiate minor degrees of spondylosis from hypomobility syndromes.

Fibrositis

The features of fibrositis have already been considered. In the cervical spine, patients present with neck pain and stiffness, and tender localized areas of muscular spasm may be palpated above or medial to the scapula.

Torticollis

Torticollis is a descriptive title for a lateral deformity of the cervical spine. It is worthwhile retaining as a diagnostic term even though it represents several different clinical conditions. The most common form is acute torticollis, which represents a prime example of the hypomobility syndrome.

Acute torticollis

This common deformity occurs in patients, aged usually from about 15 to 30 years, who present with unilateral neck pain and deformity. In the sudden type of onset, the patient is either awakened by pain during the night or else feels that the neck becomes 'stuck' during a sudden movement during the day. There is sudden pain and immediate inability to return the head to its original position. Pain is usually felt unilaterally in the neck but may radiate either up to the head or down into the interscapular region. There are no neurological symptoms.

Examination reveals that the patient's head is held in lateral flexion to one side. This is usually flexed away from the painful side and rarely towards the painful side. This position of lateral flexion of the head is not usually associated with any element of head rotation. Both active and passive movements are found to be painfully limited. The usual pattern is a restriction of lateral flexion and rotation towards the painful side and loss of extension. An occasional variation is pain experienced at the end of the range of lateral flexion and rotation to the opposite side. The passive intervertebral movements and accessory movements are always found to be limited by pain and spasm.

More minor degrees of this condition usually resolve spontaneously but they also respond well to gentle mobilization techniques directed at the intervertebral space on the side of the pain. However, in the more severe degrees a full manipulation may be required to restore neck movement.

The basic underlying pathology is not known but its natural history and the age of onset would seem to differentiate it from a degenerative disc lesion. On clinical grounds all that can be determined is the presence of a mechanical derangement of intervertebral-joint movement. It is likely that more than one lesion could be responsible for this joint derangement, although lesions of apophyseal joints have been considered the most likely site.

Differential diagnosis—Cases of acute torticollis are readily differentiated from the four other types.

Congenital torticollis

This deformity is apparent soon after birth and consists of a lateral flexion of the neck due to a sternomastoid contracture in which the fibrous-tissue replacement is said to be due to ischaemia, which was possibly caused by the intrauterine position. A hard lump, the so-called sternomastoid tumour, is often visible. As the infant grows, facial asymmetry appears. Treatment consists of daily muscle stretching and over-correction—first of all by the physiotherapist, who can then teach this procedure to the parents. If this is not succeeding, the distal attachments of the muscle may be divided.

Traumatic torticollis

Fractures or fracture dislocations of the cervical spine may present with the same deformity and so must always be excluded by X-ray in children with torticollis.

Spasmodic torticollis

In this rare but distressing condition the patient suffers recurrent attacks of repeated, painless rotation or lateral flexion of the head.

The onset is gradual and occurs at about the age of 40, and the most common head movement is a rotation towards the left side. One interesting feature is that either the patient or the examiner can manually overcome the spasms. The aetiology of this condition is unknown, but several theories have been advanced to explain it. The bizarre clinical picture is reminiscent of hysteria and it is known that stress and tension often initiate or precipitate attacks. However, the type of attack is usually consistent and differs from hysterical torticollis, which is described below. Various neurological lesions, usually involving the extra-pyramidal system, have been described.

Management is difficult and many treatments have been advocated. Splinting with collars; muscle relaxants; manipulation; and surgery, such as division of the accessory nerve, have all been tried but only rarely provide relief. Stereotactic thalamic surgery has also been used, with some good results. More recently, electromyography has been used in an attempt to teach voluntary muscular control through feedback display with good results in seven of nine patients (Brudny, Grynbaum and Korein, 1974). Manipulative treatment plays no part in the treatment of these patients.

Hysterical torticollis

Hysterical torticollis, with its repetitive tic-like movement, is usually easy to diagnose. The patient usually forcibly hunches his shoulders while flexing the head to one side. On formal examination the patient usually does not move the neck in the direction in which the muscles can be felt to be rigidly contracted.

Shoulder pain

This may be present in three separate clinical situations:

(1) Pain may radiate from the neck above the scapula into the shoulder. Clinical examination then shows that shoulder movements are painless but that neck movements are painfully restricted and may reproduce the patient's shoulder pain.
(2) The patient may present with shoulder pain alone, without neck pain. In these cases the shoulder pain should be reproduced on neck movements.
(3) There is, however, another less common clinical setting involving shoulder pain in which shoulder movements are painful whilst neck movements are either clinically normal or only slightly painful. This is usually taken as sufficient evidence to implicate shoulder but not neck pathology. Nevertheless, a proportion of such cases will improve with treatment to the neck alone, usually traction and mobilization techniques to the C4–5, C5–6 area. If such improvement is to occur it will do so within one or two treatments, hence repeated neck treatments are unnecessary.

34   Cervical-disc prolapse

The patient with cervical-disc prolapse presents with severe pain, which is usually felt in the neck, scapula and down the arm but may be experienced at first only in the segmental distribution of the nerve. There may be a history of attacks of neck and interscapular pain and stiffness. Pain is made worse by neck movements, posturing or straining. Any neck movement may produce pain, especially extension or movement towards the affected side, and elevation of the shoulder. Pain may also be related to postural changes or maintaining certain positions, e.g. reading a book. Sudden straining, such as coughing or sneezing, is usually most painful. Pain is often present at night and disturbs sleep. The patient usually complains of pins and needles or paraesthesias in the dermatome of the affected nerve root.

Distribution varies according to the nerve root involved but precise anatomical localization can be difficult because of other factors, including a pre-fixed or a post-fixed brachial plexus.

With C5 nerve-root pressure pain is felt over the shoulder but may radiate down the arm. With C6 nerve-root pressure pain usually radiates into the scapular area, the shoulder and the lateral aspect of the arm down to the thumb and index finger. Sensory disturbances may be felt in the thumb or index finger. With C7 nerve-root pressure pain is felt over the upper border of the scapula, the shoulder and down the back of the arm and forearm to the middle fingers. Sensory changes are felt in the index and middle fingers. With C8 nerve-root pressure pain is felt in the shoulder and medial aspect of arm and forearm. Sensory changes are felt in the medial two fingers.

Examination

The diagnosis can usually be made in the presence of a disturbance of spinal mechanics and neurological signs. Signs of disturbed spinal mechanics include:

(1) Disturbances of posture; the neck is often held to the contralateral side and the affected arm may need to be supported by the opposite hand.
(2) Disturbances of movements; there is a loss of the normal range of movement, usually a painful limitation of extension with limited lateral flexion and rotation towards the painful side. Disturbances in the normal rhythm of cervical movements are common, e.g. during cervical rotation the neck may also be observed to move into flexion. Ancillary tests, e.g. sustained pressure or over-pressure to one side, are usually not needed to substantiate the diagnosis.

Neurological examination

A full neurological assessment of upper and lower limbs is mandatory. In the upper limb this involves tests for neurological deficits, including sensory, motor and reflex changes, on a segmental basis (see Table 34.1). In the lower limb upper motor-neurone involvement is evidenced by motor weak-

Table 34.1 Effects of cervical-disc prolapse

Spinal root	Muscles involved	Motor weakness	Reflex loss
C5	Deltoid, supraspinatus, infraspinatus and biceps	Glenohumeral abduction, glenohumeral lateral rotation and elbow flexion	Biceps jerk
C6	Biceps and supinator	Glenohumeral adduction, glenohumeral medial rotation and wrist supination	Biceps jerk and supinator jerk
C7	Triceps, pronators and flexor carpi radialis	Elbow extension, wrist pronation and wrist flexion	Triceps jerk
C8	Hand intrinsics, pronators, flexor digitorum and adductor pollicis	Wrist pronation, finger flexion and thumb adduction	—

ness or reflex changes, including alterations in plantar responses.

Variations in clinical presentation

(1) The degree of arm pain varies. It is usually severe but at times may be present as a dull ache without any associated neurological symptoms.

(2) There may be bilateral arm pain, due usually to a large central disc prolapse or, more rarely, to a bilateral disc prolapse.

(3) Distal arm pain with sensory disturbances such as numbness but without neck or proximal pain results in a clinical presentation similar to that of a peripheral entrapment neuropathy. An EMG with nerve conduction tests may also be necessary for elucidation.

(4) There may be neck pain alone, due to a central disc prolapse.

(5) A large central disc prolapse may produce cord compression.

35 Traumatic cervical syndrome

Motor-vehicle injuries involving either a rear-end or a head-on collision may produce considerable neck trauma, with resultant fractures, dislocations or soft-tissue injuries. The soft-tissue injuries involving ligaments, joint capsules, discs and muscles are affected by the direction of forces applied, their severity and the ability to limit neck movement by muscle bracing. Seat belts may aggravate the injury by limiting sudden movement to the cervical part of the spine.

Terminology of this condition remains a problem since the term 'whiplash', which has strong emotional overtones without any pathological connotation, is now firmly entrenched. This term was first used in 1928 by Crowe, who later stated that he regretted its widespread acceptance. Further, it is not even an accurate description of the mechanism of pathogenesis. Bosworth (1959) attacked the use of this term, pointing out that the action of the neck is not the same as in using a whip. Macnab (1964) used the term 'acceleration injury' because the car seat with its passenger is accelerated forwards. Since the resultant neck trauma occurs as the result of the abrupt forced stopping, the term 'deceleration injury' would appear even more appropriate. Damage, produced either by hyperextension or hyperflexion of the neck, varies according to whether the collision is rear end or head on.

Rear-end collision

The common story is that a stationary car, perhaps waiting for traffic lights to change, is hit from behind by another car, which may be travelling only slowly.

Sequence of events

(1) As the front seat is accelerated forwards, taking the lower part of the body with it, the neck and head are suddenly forcibly extended (*see Figure 35.1(a)*).
(2) Since no anatomical or mechanical barrier exists, the neck is hyperextended until (3).
(3) Reflex muscular contraction of the stretched anterior cervical muscles produces flexion of the head and neck until (4).
(4) The head returns to its original position.

Head-on collision

In this the car and its occupants are brought to a sudden halt.

Sequence of events

(1) The neck and head continue in the path of the original movement and produce a sudden hyperflexion injury (*see Figure 35.1(b)*).
(2) In this a mechanical barrier is produced when the chin reaches the anterior chest wall.
(3) Reflex muscular contraction now results in extension of the head and neck until (4).

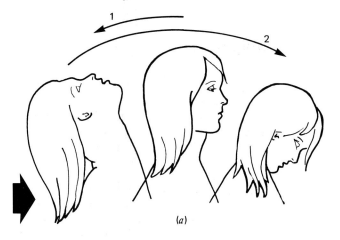

(a)

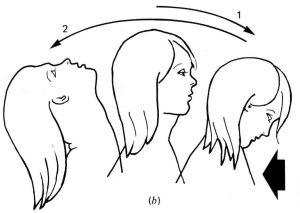

(b)

Figure 35.1 Mechanism of production of the traumatic cervical syndrome: (*a*) rear-end collision; (*b*) head-on collision

(4) Finally the head returns to its original position.

If the head is held in rotation on impact—as, for example, when the patient is talking to the other front-seat occupant—further rotation and side bending may be produced.

Site of damage

Injury to soft tissues may include ligaments, disc or apophyseal joints, neck-muscle tears or haematomas involving especially the sternomastoid. It is usual to find clinical involvement of the upper or mid-thoracic spine in many cases. Temporomandibular joint pain is also common.

Injury to the vertebral artery and its sympathetic nerve supply can cause a wide range of eye, ear and vestibular symptoms. Damage can also result to the spinal cord or nerve roots.

Firm pathological evidence of the type of injury produced is usually lacking in humans, but similar lesions have been produced in experimental animals, in whom tears of the anterior longitudinal ligament may be associated with disruption of the disc. Bailey (1963) demonstrated that the disc substance may be compressed or disrupted by this injury with bulging of the disc after a tear of the anterior longitudinal ligament.

Clinical findings

It is not particularly common for the patient to experience any severe degree of pain immediately after the accident and pain usually begins some hours later. Pain and stiffness are usually then intense, often radiating up into the head or down across the shoulders into the arms. Headaches are common whatever the site of neck damage. Neurological symptoms are usually absent. The patient is most unwilling to move the neck and marked muscle spasm can be detected.

In time, symptoms due to disturbance of the surrounding soft tissues or the autonomic system (Ueka and Ueda, 1969) may result in headaches, vertigo, tinnitus, visual disturbances, hoarseness, dysphagia, a strange feeling of uncertainty or even depression. Neck pain may radiate up into the head, chest or across the shoulders to the upper arm, though it is only rarely felt more distally. Evidence of nerve-root pressure is not common but disruption of the sympathetic chain may result in a Horner's syndrome.

Natural history

Assessment of the natural history of these lesions is clouded by the common problems of litigation and psychogenic overlay to symptoms. Macnab (1964), arguing in favour of an organic cause to such symptoms, reported a series of 266 cases followed up 2 or more years after they had had their legal claims settled. Of these cases, 145 were available for review, 121 still being symptomatic. Even if it were assumed that all other patients were symptom free, at least 45 per cent of patients still had residual neck problems. Macnab also commented that when other severe injuries had been sustained in the same accident they were not associated with a litigation neurosis or chronic symptoms, unlike those in the neck.

The natural history is influenced not only by the number, extent and site of the lesions but also by the age and sex of the patient and by the clinical state of the spine before the accident. Sequelae, due to disc damage, may develop many years after the injury.

Diagnosis

Diagnosis rests upon a full and detailed history of the mechanism of injury. This includes a description of the speed of the cars and force of impact; damage sustained by the cars, such as to the back of the seat or seat moorings or steering wheel; details of related injuries, such as lacerations or bruising and whether a seat belt was being worn. However, the occupants of a stationary car suddenly forced forward a few feet are more liable to serious injury than those in a car slowly rolled forwards over a long distance.

Although X-rays taken soon after the accident are usually normal for the patient's age, and while they do not demonstrate soft-tissue changes, nevertheless they are essential to show any associated bone damage or instability. Ultimate loss of disc space with osteophyte formation is common. Tomography of the cervical spine taken in flexion and extension is a most useful technique to reveal abnormality of segmental movement, often with disc bulging and calcification in surrounding soft tissue after haematoma formation.

Management

Initial care

Management of these injuries remains difficult and controversial. In the overall management of the patient it is necessary to be aware of such psychogenic overlay in the patient as anxiety, depression and fear related to the extent of the injury, and the significance of widespread symptoms and implications for the future, since most activities of daily living involving neck movements are painful.

The patient should be informed that the injury involves soft tissues and that the natural process of repair takes many months to complete. Rest is essential. If damage is sufficient this may need to be achieved by rest in bed for a few days. Subsequently rest is best achieved with a soft felt collar with the neck maintained in a non-painful posture, usually one of slight forward flexion. This is contrived by having the collar narrow at the front and wide at the back to avoid neck extension. The collar is usually worn constantly for about 6 weeks before the patient is gradually weaned off it.

Although the collar does not provide complete immobilization, it is usually sufficient to provide some degree of pain relief. For this reason it can also be worn at night. Analgesics, sedation and muscle relaxants may be used but heat and traction are only of limited value. If heat is used ultrasonics are generally preferred. Traction is given with the patient lying with slight neck flexion with 2–3 kg of weight. Manual methods including mobilization and manipulation are contraindicated at this stage.

Subsequent course

The patient should be advised that complete control of pain is often unlikely for a considerable time but, provided that forced or extreme neck movements are avoided, the pain associated with most daily activities does not necessarily represent any worsening of the underlying process. The patient must be carefully taught how to live within the means of the altered spinal mechanics, usually by avoiding excessive neck flexion or extension. The collar can still be used intermittently, particularly whilst engaged in activities known to produce pain or else at the end of the day and through the night. Mobilization techniques with posteroanterior pressure may now usefully be used provided that they do not exacerbate pain, but

forcible manipulation is almost never indicated. Mobilization is followed by heat and isometric neck exercises within the limits of pain.

Locally tender areas, usually found in muscles or at the musculotendinous attachment to the occiput, may be infiltrated with local anaesthetic and corticosteroid injections.

Surgery

In the absence of cervical fractures or fracture–dislocations, surgery in the early stages is not indicated. However, in those patients who develop subsequent evidence of cervical instability or the presence of neurological deficits, surgery may be indicated.

Prevention

The provision of head rests to the back of car seats is of undoubted benefit. They need to be made as an extension of the seat to provide stability and they need to project further forward than do most presently available head rests to prevent any backward movement of the head if the car is hit from behind. The use of the newer type of seat belts has not resulted in any decreased incidence of this injury and indeed could result in increased damage in hyperflexion injuries of the neck.

36 Management of cervical syndromes

Assessment and management of the total patient, as outlined for patients with lumbar spinal disorders, is of equal importance in cervical disorders (*see Table 36.1*). Symptoms and signs range in severity from minor to severe and treatment needs to be adjusted accordingly. Some patients complain of a grating or creaking sensation in the neck and only require reassurance about their ultimate prognosis. The vast majority of patients with cervical disorders will respond to a suitably organized therapeutic regimen and surgery needs to be considered in only a small percentage of the overall population. Finally, it should be noted that in the neck symptoms of pain and stiffness due to cervical spondylosis and to hypomobility lesions are more common than in the lumbar spine and usually respond well to mobilization techniques. Treatments available include:

(1) Rest: bed rest and support in a collar.
(2) Physical therapy:

    (a) Manual therapy—mobilization, manipulation, and traction.
    (b) Other physical therapies—heat and exercises.

Table 36.1 Management of cervical syndromes

Clinical syndrome	Management	Of doubtful or limited value	Contraindications
Cervical spondylosis	Rest, mobilization, traction, medication, heat, and injections	Surgery	
Cervical myelopathy	Rest; possibly surgery		Manipulation
Cervical-disc prolapse:			
Severe degree	Rest, medication, traction, possibly surgery	Mobilization	Manipulation
Moderate degree	Rest, medication, traction, and mobilization		
Aftercare and prophylaxis	Support, postural control, and exercises		
Hypomobility syndrome:			
Neck pain, acute torticollis, headaches, and vertigo	Mobilization, manipulation, and traction		
Fibrositis	As above, injections, and medication	Exercises	
Traumatic cervical syndrome:			
Early	Rest and analgesics	Heat and traction	Mobilization and manipulation
Late	Rest, analgesics, and exercises	Heat, traction, and mobilization	
Rheumatic diseases	Specific therapy		Manipulation

(3) Medication: analgesics and anti-inflammatory drugs.
(4) Injections.
(5) Surgery.
(6) Aftercare and prophylaxis.

Cervical spondylosis

Patients with cervical spondylosis usually present because of pain, and their symptoms may be related to certain neck movements. Activities that precipitate these symptoms commonly involve neck extension, often combined with lateral flexion to the side, such as painting ceilings, or after sporting activities, such as golf. The presumed basis for symptoms in these circumstances is a synovitis involving the apophyseal joints. Consequently, a reasonable treatment programme should provide as much rest to the neck as possible. This may be achieved by protecting the neck from movements known to exacerbate the patient's pain, by the use of a collar, and by suitable adjustments to the patient's work, rest or sleeping habits. Only in those patients with severe nerve-root pain or intractable neck pain is complete bed rest with traction indicated.

Collars

The main indication for the use of a collar is for the relief of pain. The aim is not to immobilize the neck completely, since cineradiographs have demonstrated this to be impossible. However, the collar does inhibit spontaneous movements, particularly of the lower cervical spine. Although patients are nearly always averse to wearing them at first, they can be persuaded to use them if it can be demonstrated that they do provide pain relief.

Collars may be made of rubber, felt or Plastozote; may have a brace with a chin cup or a support incorporated; and may be worn all the time, at night only, or when the patient undertakes any exertion or activity known to exacerbate the pain. It is important that the collar is so made that the neck is maintained in slight flexion and to use the simplest form of collar consistent with providing relief. A felt collar with the front cut lower than the back, incorporated in a stockingette to tie at the front, is usually sufficient. The chin cup is an essential component of collars worn by patients whose disorder is of the upper cervical spine.

Mobilization techniques

Mobilization techniques, including traction, should be tried in all patients having no evidence of neural involvement. Since the more gentle techniques usually provide good results, manipulations are not often required. The application of these techniques is considered in Chapter 37.

Medication

An inflammatory component may be present in cases of cervical-disc prolapse or if there is a synovitis involving the apophyseal joints. In these cases, anti-inflammatory drugs may be used for their anti-inflammatory and analgesic effects. Alternatively, analgesic drugs may be used for pain relief but there is no evidence that muscle relaxants are of any value.

Injections

Injections of local anaesthetic and corticosteroid into locally tender, painful areas around the scapula or at muscle attachments around the nuchal line are often useful, though they commonly produce temporary relief only. The presumed basis for the successful action of these injections is relief of a pain–spasm–pain cycle in which a locally painful area maintains the reflex pattern. Injections into the locally tender area may then help to relieve this cycle.

Surgery

Since nearly all patients with cervical spondylosis respond to these conservative measures, the role and results of surgery in these cases are difficult to evaluate. Most patients often suffer minimal symptoms or else attacks of neck and/or arm pain that respond to conservative therapy. Similarly, there are long periods of remission and exacerbation, which may be due to activities possibly causing a synovitis in the apophyseal joints after unaccustomed activities or may appear for no adequate reason. Surgery would obviously not be considered in these patients nor in elderly patients with widespread degenerative processes.

Operation should be considered in those patients with severe or recurrent symptoms, unresponsive to adequate conservative regimens or in those with severe or progressive neural involvement unresponsive to conservative treatment, for example:

(1) Spinal-cord compression. The cord is compromised by posterior osteocartilaginous bars often associated with an hypertrophic ligamentum flavum and narrowed spinal canal.
(2) Nerve-root pressure. The lower nerve roots are compressed by osteophytic outgrowths that reduce the size of the intervertebral foramen.
(3) Vertebral-artery compression by osteophytes.

The choice of operative technique lies between an anterior or a posterior approach to the cervical spine and myelography is usually indicated for adequate preoperative assessment. The more recently developed anterior approach permits disc excision, removal of osteophytes and interbody fusion. A review of 65 cases successfully treated with this approach has been presented by Jacobs, Krueger and Leivy (1970). The C5–6 and C6–7 discs were responsible for 82 per cent of their cases and about one-third of patients had multiple levels. However, the posterior approach either through a laminectomy or a facetectomy allows the nerve root to be examined and decompressed.

In a facetectomy the apophyseal joint is removed to relieve the nerve-root pressure; this removal may be combined with a division of the dural nerve-root sleeve or division of adhesions between the disc prolapse and osteophytic protrusions (Frykholm, 1951). In patients who have a progressive cervical myelopathy, a laminectomy may suffice to increase spinal-cord mobility and in the short term produces considerable relief.

Aftercare and prophylaxis

(1) Avoidance of movements known to produce symptoms.
(2) Postural control.
(3) Exercises.

Avoidance of movements

An assessment should be made of the patient's work and recreational habits so that he can attempt to avoid aggravating movements, best achieved by an occupational therapist. If excessive neck flexion at work represents a problem the patient should be advised to sit or adjust the work level as much as possible. Car driving that involves rotation and often excessive vibration of the unsupported neck is invariably a problem. Extension of the neck, as occurs in hanging clothes on the line and in sporting activities, should be avoided until the neck has recovered normal and painless mobility.

Posture

It may be necessary to modify the patient's posture during sleep, at work or leisure. Neck posture during sleep is dependent on the type of pillow. A test to determine its correct consistency may be performed easily by pushing one's fist into the pillow, so making a hollow in it. Then after removing the fist the hollow should remain for a time. This occurs with pillows filled with feather or down. The hollow is not maintained with a rubber pillow, which resumes its original shape as soon as the fist is removed.

A pillow should support both the neck and the head so that its height should be adjusted to the patient's posture. For example, in a patient with a deformity of the neck, it is preferable to support the head with two pillows rather than one. The shape of the pillow also should be varied to increase its support. One example is a pillow made with down and separated into two compartments. The smaller part supports under the head when the patient lies down and the larger, denser portion is used for support under the cervical spine (Jackson, 1971).

Posture at work should be reviewed to determine whether positions involving prolonged flexion or extension or the holding of heavy weights can be avoided. If patients find that symptoms are exacerbated only after sitting and holding a book or after watching television in a slumped or unsupported posture the use of a collar may be most helpful.

Exercises

While pain remains the patient's major symptom, exercise therapy is most unlikely to provide any benefit. Indeed, many patients continue to perform exercises, even though painful, in the mistaken belief that they are preventing future stiffness. However, when pain has settled exercises are especially of value in maintaining any increase in the range of movement achieved with additional physical therapy. The exercise regimen should involve mobility exercises into flexion, extension, lateral flexion and rotation and should be progressed in range provided that they do not provoke pain. Patients often find it useful to perform these exercises daily while standing under a hot shower.

Cervical-disc prolapse
(see Figure 36.1)

(1) If prolapse is of severe degree, initial management is:

   (a) Bed rest.
   (b) Traction.
   (c) Medication.

Subsequent management:

   (a) If the condition worsens or fails to improve surgery should be considered.
   (b) If it improves collar, traction and mobilization techniques should be added.

(2) If of moderate degree:

   (a) Rest.
   (b) Collar.
   (c) Traction.
   (d) Mobilization techniques.
   (e) Medication.

(3) Aftercare and prophylaxis:

   (a) Postural control.
   (b) Exercises.

Initial management

The clinical severity is first of all classified according to the degree of the patient's pain and the presence or absence of any neurological symptoms and signs as being either of a severe or a moderate degree. In severe degrees, with severe neck and arm pain or if there is any neurological deficit, complete rest in bed is usually indicated. This may be achieved either in hospital or home. The patient is made as comfortable as is possible and the neck may be postured in a position of ease with the aid of pillows as necessary. While in bed the neck should be immobilized in a collar or with traction.

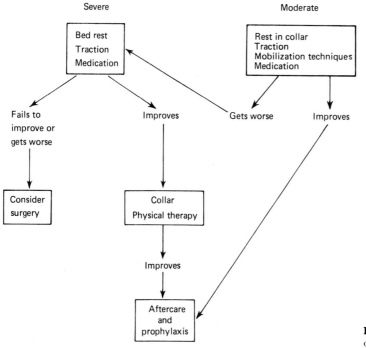

Figure 36.1 Assessment and management of cervical-disc prolapse

Hospital traction

The patient is supported in a half-lying position with pillows, one pillow supporting the head and neck. For patients with C6 or C7 nerve-root pain the neck is flexed slightly on the trunk and the head is then supported in a neutral position on the upper neck. The halter is then adjusted on the patient's head so as to maintain this position when traction is applied.

Initial weights used are small, approximately 2–3 kg. They may be increased by 0.5–1 kg daily up to a maximum of 5 kg. The amount of time that the patient should spend in traction varies; 1 hour on traction and half an hour off, repeated throughout the waking hours, may be all that is required. The total length of time over which traction needs to be maintained is usually 2–3 weeks. An alternative method that may be used is intermittent traction, which is given daily after a careful assessment has been made for any alteration in the spinal and neurological signs.

Medication

Three types of drug therapy are used; analgesics to ease pain; sedatives or muscle relaxants to help keep the patient immobilized; and anti-inflammatory drugs. Any form of manipulative procedure at this stage is contraindicated.

Subsequent course

In most patients pain should settle after 2–3 weeks on this regimen. As the pain eases, the patient is allowed out of bed in a collar. At this stage manual-therapy techniques are usually of considerable benefit and consist of cervical traction and mobilization techniques, both aimed at gently restoring movement in the cervical joint. These are usually given daily or on alternate days by the physiotherapist and may be maintained or progressed according to the patient's progress. Surgery may be considered in those patients who do not respond. There are three main indications for surgery:

(1) Severe pain that cannot be controlled by conservative measures.
(2) Neurological deficit not responding to conservative treatment.

(3) Central disc protrusion with cord compression.

Myelography is usually indicated first to confirm the site of the involved level. Surgical treatment, as previously considered, consists of either inter-body fusion or else a foraminotomy or facetectomy using a posterior approach.

Cervical-disc prolapse of moderate degree

If on the original assessment of the patient the symptoms and signs do not indicate a severe degree of involvement and there is no evidence of a severe degree of neurological deficit this treatment regimen may be modified accordingly. The patient does not need to be immobilized in bed but may use a collar for pain relief, is advised to obtain as much rest for the neck as possible and to refrain from activities known to aggravate the pain. Analgesics and anti-inflammatory drugs are again given as necessary. Manual-therapy techniques to be used include traction, usually given as intermittent variable traction and mobilization techniques.

Patients with this condition usually respond most satisfactorily to these measures over approximately 4–6 weeks.

Aftercare and prophylaxis

The regimen now adopted is similar to that outlined above for patients with cervical spondylosis.

Hypomobility syndromes

Mobilization and/or manipulative techniques are the treatment of choice for cervical hypomobility lesions; especially in those patients with neck pain or with pain referred distally, as they usually respond to a few treatment sessions. A similar result may be expected in those patients with shoulder pain referred from hypomobility lesions of the cervical spine.

Actue torticollis is best treated with mobilization techniques. In most patients these techniques, performed away from the painful side, will produce restoration of movement usually after a few treatments. In those few cases in which this produces little improvement, manipulation is indicated.

Headache

The treatment of headaches of cervical origin varies according to the type of underlying neck lesion, as classified in Chapter 33.

Hypomobility lesions of the upper cervical spine respond well to mobilization or occasionally to manipulative techniques; substantial relief may be expected after a few treatments, even when symptoms have been present for a considerable length of time. Traction may be necessary in those patients who do not respond. Pain relief may also be obtained from the use of collars, which may be worn especially at night to ease the typical early-morning pain. Exercises have no role to play in the treatment of the headache itself, but isometric exercises may be prescribed after the use of manual therapy techniques.

Headaches associated with cases of cervical spondylosis usually respond well to traction and manipulative therapy. A collar may also be useful, especially in cases where the head or neck pain is severe or a problem at night. Locally tender areas around the musculotendinous attachments to the skull may also be infiltrated with local anaesthetic and corticosteroid if the patient is slow to respond to these other methods. While it is not common to have a cervical fusion performed because of the headaches alone, it is not uncommon for patients who have undergone such surgery to report that their headache has now been cured.

In patients with headaches associated with arthritis of the upper cervical joints, management should consist of the use of a collar and general medical management of their disease. Very occasionally they may benefit from an injection of local anaesthetic and corticosteroid into a locally tender area and again their headaches may be relieved after the use of surgery. Traction and exercises are contraindicated.

Headaches due to an entrapment neuropathy of the occipital nerve should be treated in the first instance by rest, collar and injections around the course of the nerve entrapment in the upper cervical muscles. Occasionally mobilization techniques can also help to provide temporary relief. However, if these measures are not successful or if the problem becomes recurrent surgery with division of the nerves will be indicated and should be curative.

In patients with musculotendinous insertion lesions the best treatment is injection of local anaesthetic and corticosteroid into the locally tender area; these may be repeated from time to time as indicated. Manual-therapy techniques are indicated in those cases in which there is an associated hypomobility lesion of the cervical spine and may be combined with injection therapy. At times a collar is also needed for relief of pain.

Vertigo

Vertigo due to hypomobility lesions of the cervical spine responds extremely well to mobilization or traction in most cases. This was also the finding of Wing and Hargrave-Wilson (1974). Such treatment is never applied to cases in which there is a mechanical obstruction to the vertebral artery.

37 Manipulative therapy in the cervical spine

Therapy will be considered as either mobilization, manipulation or traction, involving either the upper or the lower cervical spine.

Mobilization

Mobilization techniques used in the upper cervical spine differ from those in the lower spine.

Mobilization of the upper cervical spine

In the upper cervical spine the main techniques are:

(1) Longitudinal movement.
(2) Posteroanterior central pressure.
(3) Posteroanterior unilateral pressure.

Longitudinal movement

Starting position—The patient lies supine with the head supported over the end of the couch, the neck midway between full extension and flexion and the head in a straight line. The therapist stands at the head of the couch and supports the patient's head in his right hand with the fingers spread out over the patient's occiput to behind the left ear and the thumb placed behind the right ear. He grasps the patient's chin with his left hand with his forearm alongside the patient's face (*see Figure 37.1*).

Method—An oscillatory movement is produced

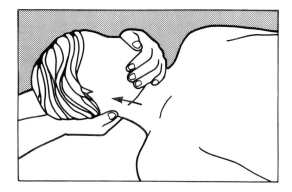

Figure 37.1 Cervical mobilization: longitudinal movement

in the patient's intervertebral joints by a gentle longitudinal pull that elongates the neck. This is produced by the therapist's forearms together with a slight backwards movement of his body and then followed by a controlled relaxation back to the starting position.

Posteroanterior central vertebral pressure

The patient lies prone with the chin tucked in. The therapist stands at the patient's head with the thumb-tips held back to back over the upper cervical vertebra to be mobilized and with the fingers around the patient's neck (*see Figure 37.2*).

The spinous process of C2 is usually easy to palpate but the spinous processes of C1 and C3 are usually difficult to palpate. The oscillatory pressure should be very gentle.

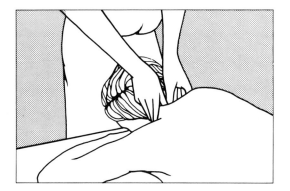

Figure 37.2 Cervical mobilization: posteroanterior central vertebral pressure

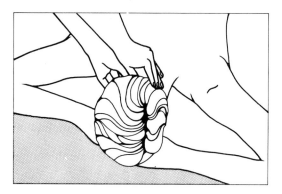

Figure 37.3 Cervical mobilization: posteroanterior unilateral vertebral pressure

Posteroanterior unilateral vertebral pressure

In the upper cervical spine, posteroanterior unilateral pressure applied to C2 with the patient's head kept straight mobilizes the C2–3 joint (*see Figure 37.3*).

If the patient's head is rotated to the left and a similar pressure applied to the left side of C2, the C1–2 joint is mobilized in rotation. In this position C1 is fully rotated to the left on C2 so that posteroanterior pressure on the left articular pillar of C2 further increases this rotation.

Starting position—The patient lies prone with the head turned to the left and supported in the patient's palms. The therapist stands at the patient's head with the tips of his opposed thumbs against the left articular pillar of C2. The long axis of each thumb is directed posteroanteriorly and tilted slightly towards the head.

Method—Movement produced by the therapist's trunk and arm action is transmitted to the thumbs. The mobilization created by posteroanterior pressure against C2 increases the rotation between C1 and C2.

Indications—The main indication for these three techniques is unilateral upper cervical pain or head pain arising from C1–2.

Mobilization of the lower cervical spine

Seven techniques are used.

Longitudinal movement

The patient lies supine with his head in the neutral position over the end of the couch and supported by the therapist's hands. The therapist grasps the patient's occipital area in his right hand and supports the patient's chin with his left hand so that his left forearm lies along the left side of the patient's face (*see Figure 37.4*).

METHOD
Oscillatory movements elongating the patient's neck are produced at the intervertebral joints by a gentle longitudinal movement of the forearm and body.

INDICATIONS
(1) This procedure is particularly useful for most painful cervical conditions, as it gains the patient's confidence. It also serves as a prognostic guide as patients who improve markedly with this procedure are likely to respond quickly to most therapeutic techniques.
(2) Torticollis.

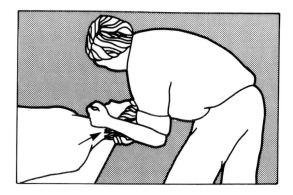

Figure 37.4 Mobilization of the lower cervical spine: longitudinal movement

Posteroanterior central vertebral pressure

STARTING POSITION
The patient lies prone with forehead resting on the hands and the chin slightly tucked in. The therapist stands at the patient's head, thumbs in contact with the spinous process to be mobilized and fingers straddling the neck (*see Figure 37.5*).

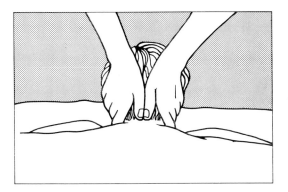

Figure 37.5 Mobilization of the lower cervical spine: posteroanterior central vertebral pressure

METHOD
Pressure is applied through the thumbs by movement of the therapist's arms and trunk.

INDICATIONS

(1) Midline or unilaterally distributed pain.
(2) Cervical spondylosis.
(3) Severe muscle spasm.

Posteroanterior unilateral vertebral pressure

STARTING POSITION
The patient lies prone with the forehead resting on the hands and the therapist stands to the side of the patient's head with his thumbs back to back on the articular pillar of the side to be mobilized (*see Figure 37.6*).

METHOD
Oscillatory pressure is directed posteroanteriorly against the articular process.

INDICATIONS
(1) Patients with unilateral neck pain.
(2) Cervical spondylosis.

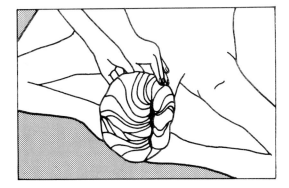

Figure 37.6 Mobilization of the lower cervical spine: posteroanterior unilateral vertebral pressure

Lateral flexion

STARTING POSITION
The patient lies supine with head and neck over the end of the couch. To produce lateral flexion to the right, the therapist stands alongside the patient's right shoulder, his right arm lying across the shoulder. The patient's head is then laterally flexed. The movement can be localized to one intervertebral level by pressure of the palmar surface of the left index finger against the articular pillar (*see Figure 37.7*).

METHOD
The therapist produces oscillatory movement by rocking his hips from side to side with a forward movement of the right side of his pelvis. The patient's head is firmly held to the therapist's body. For the upper cervical regions the patient's head is held in the neutral flexion–extension position, while for the lower cervical regions the head is held slightly flexed.

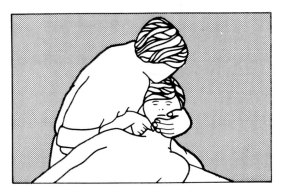

Figure 37.7 Mobilization of the lower cervical spine: lateral flexion

INDICATIONS
(1) Patients with unilateral pain in the neck, head, scapula or arm.
(2) Patients with painfully restricted cervical rotation.

Transverse vertebral pressure

STARTING POSITION
The patient lies prone with the head on the hands and the chin tucked in. The therapist stands on the patient's right side with the pad of his thumbs against the right side of the spinous process (*see Figure 37.8*).

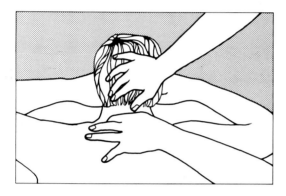

Figure 37.8 Mobilization of the lower cervical spine: transverse vertebral pressure against spinous processes

METHOD
Gentle pressure is needed since only a small oscillation can be produced.

INDICATIONS
(1) Patient's with cervical pain, especially if unilateral and well localized.
(2) Cervical spondylosis.

Rotation

STARTING POSITION
The patient lies with the head and neck over the end of the couch. To rotate the patient's head to the left, the therapist crouches at the end of the couch, his right hand supporting the patient's head, his left hand under the chin and left arm lying alongside the head (*see Figure 37.9*).

METHOD
Rotation of the patient's head is produced by an arm movement and moved by a synchronous

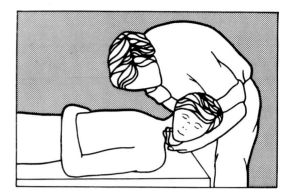

Figure 37.9 Mobilization of the lower cervical spine: rotation

action of both hands. For the upper cervical spine, the patient's neck is held on the same plane as the body; the lower the cervical level to be mobilized the greater the degree of neck flexion necessary.

INDICATIONS
This highly valuable technique is usually the first chosen for patients with unilateral neck pain.

Anteroposterior unilateral vertebral pressure

STARTING POSITION
The patient lies supine without a pillow to support the head. The therapist stands by the patient's head with both thumbs over the transverse process of the vertebra to be mobilized, fingers spread around the adjacent neck area (*see Figure 37.10*).

METHOD
The oscillatory anteroposterior pressures are per-

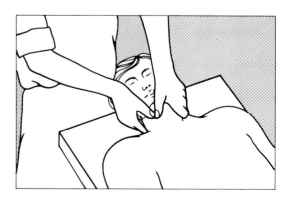

Figure 37.10 Mobilization of the lower cervical spine: anteroposterior unilateral vertebral pressure

formed very gently by the therapist's arms and trunk. The anterior neck muscles make direct contact with the transverse process rather difficult, so the thumbs must be carefully positioned.

INDICATIONS
Pain that is felt in the front or side of the neck and is reproduced by anteroposterior pressures.

Manipulation

Non-specific techniques

Rotation

The starting position is illustrated in *Figure 37.9*.

METHOD
This technique is never performed as a large movement by putting the neck through a full range from the central position. Rather, the head and neck are rotated to the limit of their range and then a quick rotary movement is given through a further 3–4 degrees.

Specific techniques

Atlanto-occipital joint

ROTATION
Starting position   The patient lies supine with the therapist standing towards the left shoulder, the patient's chin in his right hand and the atlas grasped by his left hand. The patient's head is

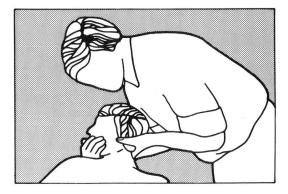

Figure 37.11 Manipulation of the atlanto-occipital joint: rotation

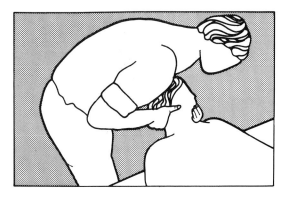

Figure 37.12 Manipulation of the atlantoaxial joint: rotation

rotated to the right until about 20 degrees short of full rotation (*see Figure 37.11*).
Method   Sudden rotation of the patient's head to the right through a few degrees by the therapist's right hand is effected while the left hand rotates the patient's atlas to the left.

Atlantoaxial joint

ROTATION
Starting position   The patient lies supine, head over the end of the couch. The therapist holds the patient's chin and head in his left arm and rotates the head through 40 degrees. C2 is firmly cradled by supporting the left articular pillar with the metacarpophalangeal joint of the therapist's index finger and support of the right transverse process of C2 with his left thumb. He then stands behind the patient's head with his left elbow pointed towards the floor (*see Figure 37.12*).
Method   The manipulation is carried out by a small rotary movement of the head to the left by the operator's left hand together with a small-amplitude unilateral posteroanterior thrust against the left side of C2 as it is rotated by the operator's right hand.

Lower cervical spine

LATERAL FLEXION
Starting position   The patient lies supine with the head over the end of the couch and the chin supported by the therapist's left arm.
   The therapist places the proximal phalanx of his right index finger against the articular pillar.

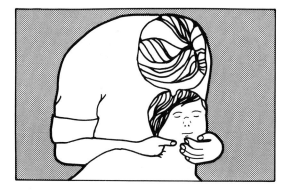

Figure 37.13 Manipulation of the lower cervical spine: lateral flexion

The patient's neck is displaced to the left and the head is laterally flexed to the right. The head is next rotated to the left by the therapist's left hand until the joint is felt to be at full stretch. The therapist's forearm is kept in line with the plane of the apophyseal joint (*see Figure 37.13*).

Method Applying an equal pressure with his left arm on the head and neck, the therapist gives a sudden thrust with his right index finger to stretch the apophyseal joint.

ROTATION

Starting position The patient lies supine with the neck and head extending beyond the end of the couch. The therapist at the head of the couch places his right hand under the head with the palmar surface of his index finger against the articular pillar of the vertebra forming the upper segment of the joint to be manipulated. The patient's chin is grasped by his left hand and the head is comfortably supported.

The patient's head is turned to the left by the

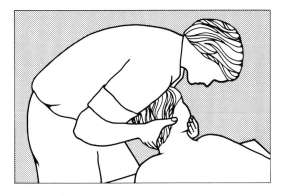

Figure 37.14 Manipulation of the lower cervical spine: rotation

left hand until the articular pillar is felt to move under his right index finger. The vertebrae above his index finger are held together in such a way that all of them move as a unit with the patient's head (*see Figure 37.14*).

Method The patient's head is sharply rotated to the left through a tiny range with the therapist's right index finger emphasizing the movement at the one joint being manipulated.

Cervical traction

Starting position

The joint to be treated should be positioned approximately midway between its position of flexion and extension; this position is influenced by:

(1) The presence of structural alterations in the cervical spine due to disease, congenital anomalies or trauma.
(2) The site of pain. If the lower cervical spine is involved the neck is positioned more towards flexion; for the upper spine it is positioned in the neutral position.
(3) The rate of subsequent improvement.

Whether the patient sits or lies down for treatment is governed by his comfort and the ease of administration. In general, traction in neutral for the upper cervical spine is best given with the patient sitting and traction in flexion for the lower cervical spine is best given with the patient lying down. Traction may be given either in the neutral position or in flexion.

Traction in neutral

Starting position

The patient sits comfortably slumped in a chair, with the back and arms supported and the head halter adjusted so that traction lifts the head off the neck in a neutral position. The occipital strap is used to lift under the occiput, not under sub-occipital structures (*see Figure 37.15*).

After determining the site and severity of the patient's symptoms the therapist places the tip of the index or middle finger against the side of the interspinous space of the affected joint.

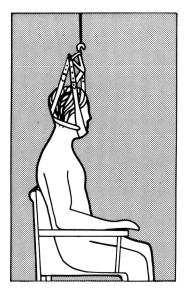

Figure 37.15 Cervical traction in neutral: starting position

Traction is then applied and relaxed in an oscillatory movement, very gently at first but gradually increasing, until movement in the interspinous space can be felt with the minimum of pressure. The patient's symptoms are reassessed after 10 seconds. Subsequent alterations are influenced if:

(1) Severe symptoms are completely relieved. The pressure is reduced by half for less than 5 minutes to minimize any exacerbation.
(2) Symptoms have been partly relieved. Traction should be maintained at this level for 5 minutes with severe pain and 10 minutes for more moderate degrees of pain.
(3) The symptoms have not altered; the amount of traction can be increased by a small amount for 10 minutes.
(4) Symptoms are made slightly worse, then the weight is halved.

If symptoms persist the head–neck relationship is changed by altering the harness or sitting position before reapplying gentler traction.

If the symptoms still persist one of two courses remain; either traction is discontinued or gentle traction is maintained for up to 5 minutes. If this produces some degree of improvement traction can be continued but if symptoms become worse then traction is discontinued.

The position chosen for treatment is governed not by the relief of symptoms but by the move-

ment produced at the relevant intervertebral joint. However, the amount and duration of traction is guided by any alteration of symptoms. Whether traction is indicated and whether the position, weight and duration chosen are correct are indicated by any changes in symptoms and signs induced by the treatment. When traction has been applied in the chosen position it should not be altered in an attempt to influence symptoms.

Method of progression

Treatment is guided by a continuous reassessment of symptoms and signs. Changes in techniques, as with mobilization, are guided by the patient's movements after treatment and also by the improvement between treatments.

Treatment of a patient with severe pain should be progressed very slowly by small increases in duration of the traction rather than weight. When there is little or no reaction from treatment the weight also can be increased gradually. However, if initial symptoms are moderate, progression can be both by poundage and by duration. The total treatment time is rarely more than 15 minutes, since longer periods do not produce better results. Traction should be discarded after four treatments if symptoms and signs remain unchanged.

The amount of traction given will be governed by a careful assessment of symptoms and signs before, during and after traction. The application of pressure is first governed by the movement at the intervertebral segment being treated; 4 kg traction applied to a 102-kg patient will produce less movement than in a 42-kg patient.

Traction in flexion

Starting position

The patient lies comfortably on the back, one or two pillows supporting the neck in slight flexion on the trunk so that the joint being treated will be midway between flexion and extension. It may be advisable to flex the hips and knees to rest the lower back. The halter is applied and the occipital strap positioned. Because the patient rests the head on this strap on the pillows, it will remain in position while the side straps and chin strap are being adjusted. To ensure that the harness is correctly adjusted the physiotherapist applies some traction via the spreader bar while ensuring

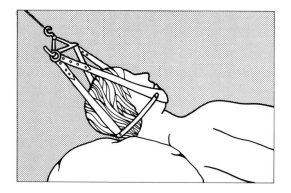

Figure 37.16 Cervical traction in flexion: starting position

that the head–neck relationship remains constant (*see Figure 37.16*).

Method

The operator alternately applies and relaxes pressure through the pulley system while watching and palpating for movement at the relevant inter-vertebral level. Pressure is sustained at the lowest value needed to produce joint movement. After approximately 10 seconds the patient's symptoms are reassessed. Subsequent treatment is as de-scribed for traction in neutral.

Complications

(1) A common problem with strong cervical traction is discomfort or pain in the patient's temporomandibular joints. This pain may be relieved by an alteration of the position of the straps or by placing a pad between the patient's molars. However, traction of this magnitude should not be required.
(2) Thoracic or lumbar pain may be induced by cervical traction.
(3) Traction in neutral may induce nausea usually only after prolonged or strong traction or with excessively apprehensive patients.
(4) Patients may experience a feeling of giddiness on release of traction, therefore the traction should be released slowly and the patient allowed to rest for a time.
(5) Traction in flexion can produce a burning feeling or pain in the suboccipital area; if so the harness is adjusted to extend the head slightly on the upper neck while maintaining the lower neck in flexion.

Table 37.1 Indications for cervical-spine mobilization techniques

Technique	Main indications
Longitudinal movement	Acute torticollis
Posteroanterior central vertebral pressure	Bilateral pain, spondylosis, torticollis, and other minor derangements
Posteroanterior unilateral vertebral pressure	Unilateral pain particularly arising from middle or upper cervical spine
Transverse vertebral pressure	Unilateral pain especially due to spondylosis
Anteroposterior unilateral vertebral pressure	Unilateral pain
Rotation	This is usually the first technique used for unilateral pain
Lateral flexion	Unilateral pain associated with restriction of lateral flexion or of rotation
Traction*	All cervical problems, and severe arm pain with restricted neck movement

*Neutral traction is used for upper cervical lesions, flexion for lower cervical lesions, and intermittent variable traction for cervical spondylosis

Table 37.2 Sequence of selection of techniques for the cervical region

Unilateral symptoms	Bilateral symptoms
1. Posteroanterior unilateral vertebral pressure or rotation	1. Posteroanterior central vertebral pressure
2. Traction	2. Posteroanterior unilateral vertebral pressure on both sides
3. Lateral flexion or transverse vertebral pressure	3. Longitudinal movement
	4. Traction
	5. Rotation

Indications for cervical traction (*see Tables 37.1 and 37.2*)

(1) Traction is of value in almost all cases of pain arising from the cervical joints. However, the rate of improvement in symptoms and signs is slower than that in the mobilization techniques.
(2) Patients with an arm pain and restriction of lateral flexion and rotation of the neck towards the painful side are best treated by traction in flexion.

(3) Traction is the treatment of choice in those patients with recent neurological changes.
(4) When intervertebral-joint movement is restricted traction may be ineffective unless preceded by manipulation.
(5) Intermittent variable cervical traction can be applied in neutral or in flexion for similar indications, using the same weights and duration of treatment. But with severe symptoms the amount of movement should be decreased with longer hold and rest periods. As symptoms abate the rest period can be reduced and the hold period maintained for approximately 3–5 seconds.

38   The thoracic spine

Lesions of the thoracic joints are a common source of pain, which may be experienced in any part of the chest wall and can closely mimic the symptoms of visceral disease.

Thoracic and chest pain

Thoracic pain may arise from visceral or musculo-skeletal disorders. The various organic diseases involving heart, lungs and mediastinal structures will not be discussed. Musculoskeletal disorders are also an important common cause of disability. At times their symptomatology closely mimics that of visceral disease, e.g. angina, which can then lead to incorrect diagnosis and treatment. Clearly it is equally as important to be certain that chest pain is not due to underlying visceral disease as it is to overlook its presence. Further confusion may arise because pain originating either in musculoskeletal structures or from an underlying visceral disease is often aggravated by breathing, coughing or posture. It is important to recognize the musculoskeletal origin of such pain, since it is often amenable to treatment.

The most common cause of musculoskeletal chest pain is that referred from the thoracic or lower cervical intervertebral joints. To confirm their diagnosis it is necessary to reproduce the patient's pain by appropriate testing. However, in the older age groups many patients suffer degenerative changes involving both musculo-skeletal structures and coronary arteries. If these two conditions are present in the same patient great difficulty may be experienced in determining the exact cause of pain.

Moreover, it is not an infrequent finding that a patient who has suffered a previous coronary occlusion may subsequently develop chest-wall pain. If, after appropriate tests, coronary-artery disease does not appear to be the cause of pain such symptoms are often considered psychogenic. However, in these patients it is often possible to demonstrate the presence of a hypomobility lesion of the thoracic spine and, after appropriate manipulative treatment, pain is relieved. The reason for the development of this hypomobility lesion is not understood, although an abnormal viscerosomatic reflex has been postulated.

Examination of thoracic spine

(1) Inspection: observation of patient's posture, build and gait.
(2) Active movements: testing of flexion, lateral flexion and rotation. Observation of range, rhythm, and reproduction of pain.
(3) Auxiliary tests:
    (a) Over-pressure.
    (b) Movements repeated quickly.
    (c) Sustained pressure.
    (d) Cervical-spine movements.
(4) Passive movements:

    (a) Passive range at each joint.
    (b) Accessory movements.
(5) Test costovertebral and costochondral joints and intercostal movement.

(6) Palpation.
(7) Neurological testing.
(8) General medical examination.
(9) Radiological examination.

Inspection

Spinal deformity due to either a kyphosis, scoliosis, or a combination of both should be readily apparent. Kyphosis may be smooth and rounded; the most common cause in adolescents is Scheuermann's disease and in the elderly disc degeneration. A localized kyphosis is usually produced by one or more collapsed thoracic vertebrae, which in the elderly are often associated with osteoporosis.

Scoliosis is gauged from the line of the spinal processes, minor deviations being relatively common. Scoliosis may also be evident from asymmetry of musculoskeletal structures, including the shoulder levels and relative prominence of one scapula and rib cage. In the presence of a structural scoliosis these deformities become more prominent on forward flexion.

Active movements

Movements of the thoracic spine form part of a continuous co-ordinated pattern with lumbar-spine movements and so they are assessed together. The patient is tested first while standing and is asked if any symptoms are experienced in this position. The patient is then asked to flex and then extend the spine, followed by lateral flexion and then rotation to both sides. The normal active range of lateral flexion, extension and rotation is approximately 30 degrees and of flexion, approximately 90 degrees. Flexion may be measured as the distance the finger-tips reach from the floor, and side bending by the distance of the fingers from the knees, but it is more important to observe the relative movement of the spinous processes and record any loss of range (*see Figure 38.1*). Rotation is tested by having the patient bend forward to 45 degrees with the hands behind the head and feet together. He then rotates fully to right and left. Rotation should be further tested with the patient seated and the trunk alternatively in flexion and then extension. Over-pressure can easily be applied in this position and may be necessary to reproduce the patient's pain.

Note is taken of the range of each of these movements, whether symptoms are reproduced,

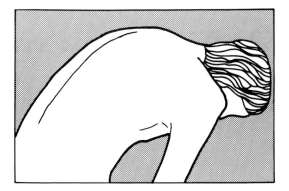

Figure 38.1 Limitation in the range of forward flexion at two levels of the thoracic spine: between about T5 and T8 forward flexion is very limited, whereas between T10 and L1 the movement appears less limited

disturbances in the normal synchronous rhythm and the presence of any muscle spasm.

Disturbance of range

Thoracic hypomobility syndromes are common, and the usual pattern of disturbance is a painful restriction on lateral flexion and/or rotation towards the painful side, associated with a restriction of either flexion or of extension.

Auxiliary tests

If these movements do not reproduce the patient's pain, auxillary tests that may do so include:

(1) Over-pressure, with small oscillatory movements, applied by the examiner at the end of the painless range in each direction.
(2) Performing the test movements repeatedly and at increasing speed.
(3) Application of sustained pressure at the limit of the range of relevant movements for some 10 seconds.
(4) Neck movements should always be tested to exclude those examples in which pain is referred from the lower cervical intervertebral joints. It should be remembered that neck flexion may exacerbate any thoracic pain, even in those cases in which pain arises from thoracic spinal joints.

Passive movements

The passive movements of the intervertebral joint to be tested are the passive range at each individual joint level, by feeling movement between the adjacent spinous processes; and accessory movements.

Passive range at individual joints

The passive movements of flexion and extension, lateral flexion and rotation are tested separately in the upper (T1–T4) and lower (T5–T11) spines.

T1–T4 FLEXION–EXTENSION
The patient lies on his right side and the examiner stands in front. The patient's head is grasped by the examiner's left hand and moved into flexion and extension while thoracic intervertebral movement is felt by the middle finger of his right hand placed between the spinous processes (*see Figure 38.2*).

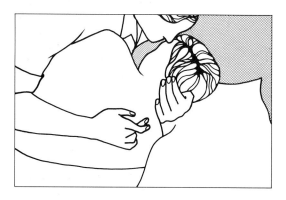

Figure 38.2 Intervertebral movement between T1 and T4 (flexion–extension)

T1–T4 LATERAL FLEXION
The patient lies on his right side near the edge of the couch, with his head resting on pillows. The examiner stands facing the patient, the head cradled in his left arm. He leans across the patient to palpate the insterspinous space: lateral flexion is obtained by lifting the patient's head and neck upwards (*see Figure 38.3*).

T1–T4 ROTATION
The starting position is as above. It is difficult to produce rotation alone without at the same time producing some degree of flexion or lateral

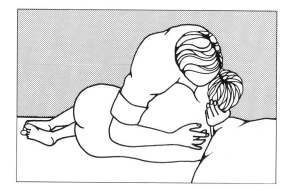

Figure 38.3 Intervertebral movement between T1 and T4 (lateral flexion)

flexion, but the rotation movement may be felt by placing the index finger on the side of the patient's interspinous space. The examiner cradles the patient's head and rotates the lower cervical spine towards him by elevating the scapula to its highest point, with counter-pressure applied over the thorax. This movement is difficult to achieve accurately (*see Figure 38.4*).

T5–T11 FLEXION–EXTENSION
This is tested with the patient sitting with the hands clasped behind the head. The examiner, standing by the left side, places his left arm under the patient's left upper arm to grasp the right upper arm. He places his right hand across the spine just below the level to be tested and, with the pad of the tip of the middle finger in the far side of the interspinous space, palpates between adjacent spinous processes.

To test flexion, he lowers the trunk from the neutral position until movement can be felt under his right middle finger. The patient is then

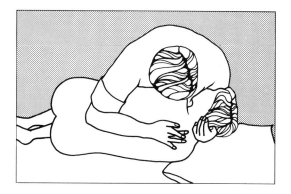

Figure 38.4 Intervertebral movement between T1 and T4 (rotation)

returned to the neutral position by lifting under the arms and so producing an oscillatory movement through an arc of approximately 20 degrees.

Extension is similarly produced by the examiner assisting trunk extension with the heel and ulnar border of his right hand and maintaining the pad of his middle finger between adjacent spinous processes. Movement at only one joint is examined so that large trunk movements are unnecessary.

T5–T11 LATERAL FLEXION

The patient sits with the hands clasped behind the neck while the examiner stands side on behind the patient's left side and reaches with his left arm to hold behind the right shoulder. He grips the patient's trunk firmly between his left arm and his left side. As the movement extends below T8 this grasp is moved to the patient's lower scapular area. The examiner places the heel of his right hand on the left side of the patient's back and places the tip of the pad of his flexed middle finger in the far side of the interspinous space of the joint to be tested (*see Figure 38.5*).

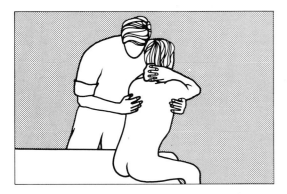

Figure 38.5 Intervertebral movement between T5 and T11 (lateral flexion)

The examiner laterally flexes the patient's trunk towards him with the heel of his right hand, and laterally flexes the upper trunk by lifting his left arm and pressing downwards with his left axilla. Interspinous movement is palpated through the pad of his middle finger.

T5–T11 ROTATION

This is tested with the patient lying on his right side with hips and knees flexed while the examiner, standing in front of the patient, leans over the trunk and cradles the pelvis between his right side and his right upper arm. The examiner's forearm is then in line with the patient's spine

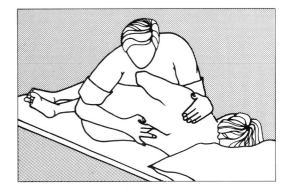

Figure 38.6 Intervertebral movement between T5 and T11 (rotation)

and he places his hand at the level to be moved. The pad of the right middle finger palpates the under-surface of the interspinous space. His left hand grasps as far medially as possible over the patient's suprascapular area with his forearm over the sternum (*see Figure 38.6*).

The patient's trunk is repeatedly rotated back and forth by the examiner's left forearm and hand through an arc of approximately 25 degrees, and the palpating finger follows the patient's trunk movement. When movement occurs at the joint being examined the upper spinous process will be felt to press into the pad of the upwardly directed middle finger.

Accessory movements

These passive movements are produced by the pressure of the thumbs against the two accessible bony vertebral processes, the spinous process and the transverse process. Spinous processes are tested using posteroanterior and transverse pressures, which may be varied by angling the direction of the pressure towards the head or feet. This is then followed by posteroanterior pressures against the transverse processes. Similar tests have been described in detail for the cervical and lumbar spines.

The costovertebral joints

The costovertebral joints and intercostal movements are tested by an oscillatory posteroanterior pressure. This is applied by the thumbs over the angle of the rib, which can be varied by directing the pressure in a cephalic or caudal direction, to attempt to reproduce the patient's pain.

Palpation

The spinous processes of C7 and T1 are easily palpated. The upper four thoracic spinous processes tend to be somewhat horizontal, but the next four run obliquely downwards, their tip at the level of the lower border of the subadjacent vertebra.

The transverse processes of the thoracic vertebrae are usually readily palpable with the patient lying prone. The region of the costotransverse joint, formed by a facet on the rib articulating with the transverse process, is palpable two finger-breadths laterally to a spinous process. The angle of the rib is found at the lateral border of the spinal extensor muscles. The scapula is easily palpable; its spine lies subcutaneously at the level of T3 and its lower angle lies opposite the spine of T7. Anterior structures such as the sternoclavicular joint, manubrium sterni, ribs and costochondral junctions are subcutaneous and so readily identifiable.

The thoracic spine is palpated for any alteration in bony alignment, muscle spasm and any localized tenderness which may be felt over the supraspinous ligaments or to the side of the interspinous space. Tapping sharply with the finger or a percussion hammer on the spinous processes, with the patient standing fully flexed, often elicits local tenderness over an affected level.

Neurological testing

Neurological testing should not be confined to testing sensation over the skin of the dorsal spine, and a full neurological assessment of upper and lower limbs is necessary. A general medical examination is always performed and X-rays are taken. Routine radiological examination includes AP and lateral X-rays of the thoracic spines and chest X-ray.

Classification

Classification of the causes of musculoskeletal thoracic pain is made according to the structures involved:

(1) Thoracic spine:
  (a) Intervertebral-disc lesions.
  (b) Hypomobility lesions.
  (c) Vertebral disease.
(2) Lower cervical spine.
(3) Thoracic joints:
  (a) Sternoclavicular.
  (b) Manubriosternal.
  (c) Costovertebral.
  (d) Costochondral.
  (e) Xiphoid.
  (f) Scapulothoracic.
(4) Muscular.

Thoracic intervertebral-disc lesions

These are relatively uncommon, possibly because of the relative thinness of the discs, whose mobility is limited by the splinting action of the rib cage.

Disc prolapse

Prolapse of a thoracic intervertebral disc is rare. Love and Schorn (1965), in a review of 61 surgical cases, found the most common site of prolapse to be between T11 and T12. Symptoms include local back pain and radicular pain. Evidence of cord compression—with resultant sensory loss, upper motor-neurone lesion and bladder symptoms—is frequent. A single disc was involved in all but one of their 61 cases.

Senile kyphosis

This common condition is responsible for the round shoulders with the forward carriage of the head, associated with advancing age. It occurs in older patients of either sex and is associated with severe degeneration of the mid-thoracic intervertebral discs. The principal radiological changes are seen to involve the anterior part of these discs with loss of disc space.

Senile kyphosis is usually asymptomatic but some patients present with severe, aching pain that has been present for many years, is worse after activity, disturbs sleep at night and tends to be episodically worse and difficult to control effectively with analgesics.

Pain relief is difficult; analgesics, exercise, postural control, use of a brace or mobilization techniques usually provide only temporary or partial relief.

Localized degenerative disc lesions

These are relatively uncommon. There is a higher incidence in people whose occupation involves repeated thoracic rotation—for example, professional golfers. Nerve-root involvement may occur, with pain radiating around the chest wall following the line of the rib, which may sometimes be associated with paraesthesias or numbness over the same distribution. Pain is made worse by movement and is often worse on lying down.

Treatment is difficult. Manipulation rarely helps, although there is sometimes slow response to traction and gentle mobilization techniques combined with some form of back support.

Thoracic hypomobility syndromes

Thoracic pain is usually most commonly felt as pain on either side of the midline, often radiating out along the chest wall for a few inches, or localized to one side of the spine. It may, however, be felt more diffusely over several thoracic intervertebral levels.

A thoracic hypomobility syndrome may also present with chest-wall pain. The patient may present with back pain, which either radiates around the chest or is felt to pass through from the back, but pain may occur as chest-wall pain alone without any accompanying back pain. Pain is of sudden onset, may at times be severe and, when aggravated by breathing or activity, be difficult to differentiate from underlying visceral disease. It may be found anywhere around the chest wall, but the most common site for this type of referred pain to be experienced is anteriorly over the costochondral region. Since pain in this anterior site may also be caused by a localized lesion of the costochondral junction, it may be difficult at times to differentiate the cause of the patient's symptoms. Also, in those patients in whom pain does arise from thoracic hypomobility syndrome, examination often reveals a localized area of pain and tenderness in the costochondral region, which is also due to referred pain and tenderness.

Finally, patients in whom the only clinical finding is a thoracic hypomobility lesion may present with lower back pain at any level in the lumbar spine. The hypomobile segment is most commonly found at the lowermost thoracic joint but may at times be even higher. Possible mechanisms for this type of lumbar pain may be on the basis of muscle spasm or as referred pain.

Examination

Routine testing of active movements reveals a limited range of intervertebral movement, usually with painful limitation of either flexion or extension, combined with a restriction of rotation and/ or of lateral flexion towards the painful side. This hypomobile segment, visible during movement, may also be associated with either a localized area of scoliosis or an arc of pain felt in the midrange of spinal flexion. The diagnosis is confirmed clinically on passive movement when intervertebral movements in the affected restricted segment reproduces the patient's pain.

Tenderness over interspinous ligaments and localized muscle spasm to one side of the affected segment confirm these findings.

Management

This depends on the clinical findings. A hypomobility syndrome producing back, or back plus chest-wall, pain is treated by mobilization of the affected segment, usually requiring only a few sessions for marked relief. In patients with both back and costochondral pain it may be difficult to determine the primary cause. The best treatment then is to mobilize the thoracic intervertebral joint first and subsequently assess the anterior pain. However, in a proportion of patients it will also be necessary to inject the locally tender anterior area with local anaesthetic and corticosteroid before complete relief is obtained.

The T4 syndrome

This refers to a common group of symptoms associated with the finding of a hypomobility lesion at the T4 level. The patient often complains of arm pain or a vague discomfort in the arm associated with paraesthesias that do not follow any dermatome pattern. Diffuse posterior neck pain may also be present in some patients. Hypomobility at the T3–T4, T4–T5 or T5–T6 level is the only positive sign that can be elicited, and mobilization or manipulation of this involved area almost always relieves symptoms after three or four treatments. The mechanism of its production is unknown but an associated disturbance of autonomic nerve control has been postulated.

Lower cervical spine

Pain referred from the cervical spine is most commonly felt between or above the scapulae. It may, however, be felt anywhere over the upper anterior chest wall; occasionally it is episodic or related to exertion, when it is difficult to distinguish from angina.

Thoracic joints

Sternoclavicular joint

Pain from this joint may be referred into the upper costochondral region. It may follow degenerative changes or be associated with an inflammatory synovitis due to rheumatoid arthritis or spondyloarthritis (*see* Chapter 7).

Manubriosternal joint

The manubriosternal joint is usually classified as a cartilaginous joint, but in approximately 30 per cent of people a synovial cavity is present. Inflammatory lesions occur both in spondyloarthritis and in rheumatoid arthritis. The most common is ankylosing spondylitis, with joint erosion and bony sclerosis leading ultimately to bony fusion.

The costovertebral joint

This may be involved in either inflammatory or degenerative joint disease. Complaints of pain in this region are common early in ankylosing spondylitis due to synovitis, and examination reveals local tenderness and a reduced chest expansion, a measurement that can also be used to assess the progress of this disease.

Degenerative changes may also occur, though they are usually asymptomatic and are often only a chance X-ray finding. They commence in the fourth decade, but symptoms such as localized pain and tenderness usually only result after some form of local trauma. Nathan *et al.* (1964) found degenerative changes in about half of 345 skeletons and in 17 per cent of 100 random chest X-rays examined. They related the distribution of these lesions to anatomical factors, so that the joints with a single facet (1, 11 and 12) have a much higher incidence of degenerative changes than the remainder, which have two hemi-facets. They also found the inferior rather than the superior joint facets to be the usual site of involvement.

Treatment with mobilization techniques and/or injections of local anaesthetic and corticosteroids into the joints is usually quite successful in relieving symptoms.

Costochondral joints

The upper seven ribs articulate anteriorly with the sternum through their costal cartilages. The costochondral junction forms a fibrocartilaginous joint in which the rib and cartilage are slotted in together. With the exception of the first rib, these costal cartilages also articulate with the sternum through a synovial sternocostal joint. The eighth, ninth and tenth ribs articulate through their costal cartilage with the rib above it, but the last two ribs are unattached.

PAIN IN THE UPPER COSTOCHONDRAL REGION
Pain of musculoskeletal origin in the upper costochondral region can arise from four sources: it may be referred, be due to polyarthritis, be post traumatic, or be due to Tietze's syndrome.

The most common cause of upper costochondral pain is referred pain from thoracic or cervical spinal lesions, as described above.

Inflammatory polyarthritis, such as in rheumatoid arthritis or spondyloarthritis, may at times produce pain in the synovial sternocostal joint.

Pain, which is usually associated with some degree of prominence of one or two costochondral joints, is not uncommon. It may occur after a burst of coughing or after local trauma. This lesion is often wrongly diagnosed as a Tietze's syndrome. What makes this condition confusing is that it may at times also be associated with a thoracic hypomobility syndrome. Treatment consists of local corticosteroid injections, thoracic mobilization and reassurance about its benign nature.

All of these first three conditions are often confused, particularly by over-anxious patients, with visceral diseases such as malignancy or cardiovascular disease.

Tietze's syndrome   This rare condition, described by Tietze in 1921, consists of a painful tender swelling, usually involving one of the upper costal cartilages. Until 1962 only 290 cases of this condition had been described in the literature (Levey and Calabro, 1963). It occurs mainly in young adults who complain of upper chest pain made worse by activity or sudden strain, such as coughing. In more than half the cases, the second costochondral junction of either side is involved; the next most common is the third costal cartilage, but other cartilages and the sternoclavicular joints have been implicated. The attack lasts usually for some days but may last for years or recur at intervals. The condition is benign, there are no systemic manifestations nor any relationship to the inflammatory diseases. The pathogenesis is unknown, but the suggestion that this condition may represent only a variety of post-traumatic prominence of the costochondral junction is most unlikely. Biopsy taken of the costal cartilage is normal, though minor inflammatory changes have been described in the surrounding perichondrium (Landon and Malpas, 1959).

Tietze's syndrome needs to be differentiated from other causes of pain and swelling in the costochondral areas. Post-traumatic causes include callus formation after a fracture; congenital deformities; infections, including tertiary syphilis; primary tumours, including multiple myeloma; and secondary deposits, especially from the thyroid, breast, bronchus, kidney or prostate. X-rays in a patient with Tietze's syndrome are normal and so differentiate it from these other conditions.

PAIN IN THE LOWER COSTOCHONDRAL REGION
Pain may also be felt in the lower costochondral region of the eighth, ninth or tenth ribs. This may be a referred pain from lesions in the thoracic spine but traumatic lesions are also quite common. The latter may arise from either direct or indirect trauma and produce a painful clicking of the costochondral junction. This condition is also known colloquially as a slipping or clicking rib. It produces a sharp stabbing or dull aching pain, localized in the epigastrium or hypochondrium, which is usually worse with movement but can also occur at rest.

Diagnosis of this condition may be made by palpating the tender area over the lower costochondral region, which may be associated also with a palpable clicking.

This condition rarely resolves spontaneously but may respond to local infiltration with local anaesthetic and corticosteroid and the use of anti-inflammatory drugs. If these fail a cure may be obtained by resecting the anterior rib margins.

Xyphoid process

Pain here is commonly post traumatic, but it may be a neurotic symptom. A painful tenderness of this structure occurring as a separate entity has been described, but it is doubtful if it does exist.

Scapulothoracic joint

The gliding plane between the scapula and thorax, lined by thin muscles, is necessary for the considerable range of scapular movement. Two lesions are described here: snapping scapula and scapulocostal tendinitis.

SNAPPING SCAPULA
The patient, who is usually young, presents with pain along the medial scapular border that is associated with a loud cracking or snapping sound as the scapula is abducted. The patient soon learns its performance as a trick movement and may neurotically click the shoulder back and forth. Pain is felt as a dull ache, usually constantly present along the medial border of the scapula, and the patient often does not associate the pain with the disturbance of scapular movement.

Examination often reveals that the patient has a generalized hypermobility syndrome. Shoulder examination reveals the abnormality of scapular movement, which may be felt and seen as the scapula moves. With full abduction of the scapula, tenderness may be palpated along its medial edge.

X-rays should include a lateral view of the scapula, which may at times detect an underlying bony abnormality such as an osteoma or a bony spur on the scapular border.

Treatment—The patient should avoid his trick movement. The tender areas in the muscle may be infiltrated with local anaesthetic and corticosteroid, which provide at least temporary relief. If a local bony abnormality can be demonstrated, and if symptoms persist, local bone resection usually proves curative.

SCAPULOCOSTAL TENDINITIS
Localized pain and tenderness, sometimes quite severe, may be found along the upper part of the medial scapular border. Pain usually gets worse as the day goes on or after use of the shoulders. It is commonly found in typists or sportsmen and may be associated at times with postural faults or sagging shoulders. However, the constancy of the site, its localized nature and the ability to reproduce the pain on resisted scapular movements make it more likely to be due to tendinitis than to postural disturbance alone.

Treatment consists of avoiding those movements known to produce pain, deep-friction massage, local injections of local anaesthetic and corticosteroid into the tender area, and re-education exercises.

Muscular lesions

Injuries to the chest-wall muscles are not common but may involve the serratus anterior, intercostal muscles or the musculotendinous origins of abdominal muscles. They may be produced by muscular exertion but can also be produced by attacks of violent coughing. Treatment designed to stretch these involved muscles plus the use of injections of local anaesthetic and corticosteroid is usually successful.

One not uncommon condition is a periodic attack of a sudden, sharp, momentary, cramp-like muscular pain in the anterior chest wall, which often follows a sudden movement or slouching in a chair. Its mechanism is unknown but it seems possible, by its nature, that it is caused by a mechanical derangement in a costal joint.

Postural pain

Muscular pain may also be experienced without any underlying lesion of the cervical or thoracic joints and is related to postural changes. The patient is usually a female, often middle aged, who complains of stiffness and tenderness of muscle groups related to the shoulder girdle and thorax. The pain usually becomes worse as the day goes on and the patient is often conscious that pain may be related to postural activities, such as sitting for prolonged periods, typing or other types of continuous work. Pain may also be made worse by fatigue, emotional stress or, at times, by changes in the weather. This same pain pattern has also been described in females with a postural sagging of the shoulder girdles or in those with large, pendulous breasts.

Ancillary tests such as X-rays and blood tests are normal, but other conditions—such as psychogenic rheumatism, hypomobility and hypermobility lesions—must be excluded.

These patients are treated by simple measures—such as reassurance, heat, analgesics, muscle-bracing exercises and injections of local anaesthetic and corticosteroid into locally tender areas.

39 Manipulative therapy in the thoracic spine

Mobilization techniques
(*see Tables 39.1 and 39.2*)

Three techniques are commonly used:

(1) Posteroanterior central vertebral pressure.
(2) Transverse vertebral pressure.
(3) Posteroanterior unilateral vertebral pressure.

Table 39.1 Manipulation of the thoracic spine—sequence of selection of techniques

Unilateral symptoms	Bilateral symptoms
(1) Posteroanterior central vertebral pressure	(1) Posteroanterior central vertebral pressure
(2) Transverse vertebral pressure	(2) Transverse vertebral pressure to each side
(3) Posteroanterior unilateral vertebral pressure	(3) Traction
(4) Traction	

Table 39.2 Indications for thoracic-spine mobilization techniques

Technique	Main indications
Posteroanterior central vertebral pressure	Bilateral pain, poorly defined or widespread unilateral pain
Transverse vertebral pressure	Unilateral pain
Posteroanterior unilateral vertebral pressure	Unilateral pain
Traction	Widely distributed pain, especially if associated with disc degeneration; or hypomobility lesions

Posteroanterior central vertebral pressure

Starting position

The patient lies prone.

Upper thoracic spine—The therapist stands at the patient's head with the pads of the thumbs placed over the spinous process. He leans over so that pressure is directed initially at right angles to the area being mobilized (*see Figure 39.1 (a)*).

Mid-thoracic spine—The therapist stands by the patient's side with his thumbs placed along the spine, pointing towards each other. The fingers spread out on either side of the vertebral column (*see Figure 39.1 (b)*).

Lower thoracic spine—The direction of pressure must initially be at right angles to the body surface at the level being treated, so that his shoulders are either over the thoracic spine or sacrum (*see Figure 39.1 (c)*).

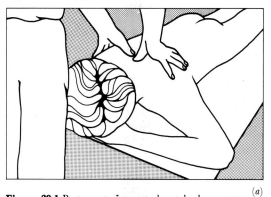

(a)

Figure 39.1 Posteroanterior central vertebral pressure: (a) upper thoracic; (b) mid-thoracic; and (c) lower thoracic

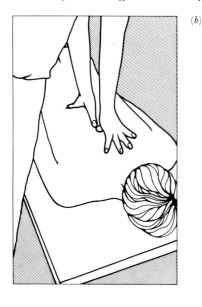

(b)

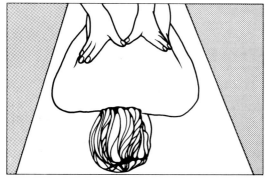

Figure 39.1 (*contd.*)

(c)

Method

Oscillatory pressure on the spinous process is produced by the therapist's body and then transmitted through the arms to the thumbs. This pressure must be achieved by the body weight, not by the thumbs themselves.

Indications

This is the most important technique used in the thoracic spine and may be used in all cases of thoracic pain, but it is of most value in patients having midline or bilateral pain.

Transverse vertebral pressure

Starting position

The patient lies prone. The therapist stands on the right side at the level of the vertebra to be mobilized with his thumbs against the side of the spinous process and fingers spread over the chest wall. One thumb is reinforced by placing the other thumb over it (*see Figure 39.2*).

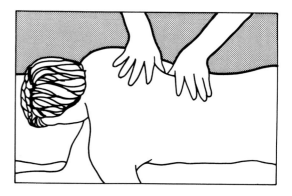

Figure 39.2 Transverse vertebral pressure: thoracic region

Pressure is applied through trunk movement. The upper thoracic region is readily accessible but has only limited movement, whereas the lower thoracic region is easily moved without requiring much pressure. The mid-thoracic spinous processes are relatively inaccessible.

Indications

This technique is used for unilateral thoracic pain and may need to be combined with mobilization of the rib.

Posteroanterior unilateral vertebral pressure

Starting position

The patient lies prone, the head to one side and arms over the sides of the couch. For the lower thoracic spine, the therapist stands by the patient's side with the pads of the thumbs pointing towards each other over the transverse process. Pressure is applied in a direct line through the shoulders

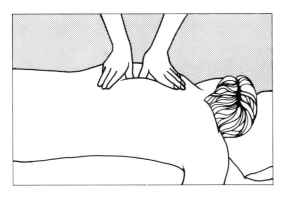

Figure 39.3 Posteroanterior unilateral vertebral pressure: thoracic region

and arms and at right angles to the body (*see Figure 39.3*).

Method

The oscillation is produced by the operator's trunk movements and firm pressure from the thumbs. Only a little movement can be obtained by this mobilization.

Indications

The indication is unilateral thoracic pain.

Manipulation

Non-specific technique — posteroanterior pressure

With the patient lying prone the therapist, using the pisiform bone of his right hand against the patient's spinous process, stretches the intervertebral joint to its limit and then produces a sudden movement of very small range.

Specific techniques

Rotation

Starting position—The patient sits on the edge of the couch, hugs his arms to the chest and turns the trunk to the left. The therapist reaches around with his left arm to the patient's right side, cradling the left shoulder in his axilla. With his

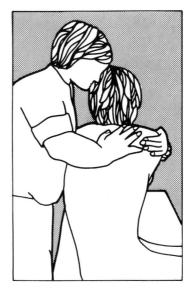

Figure 39.4 Rotation of intervertebral joints T3–T10 (mid-thoracic area)

right hand he puts pressure over the line of the ribs (*see Figure 39.4*).

Method—This is produced by a synchronous movement of the therapist's trunk together with pressure through the right hand. With his trunk he produces an oscillatory movement at the limit of the range of rotation. Manipulation consists of an over-pressure at the limit of the range.

Posteroanterior central pressure

Starting position—The patient lies supine with hands linked behind the head. The therapist stands by the right side with his right hand made into a fist by flexing middle, ring and little fingers

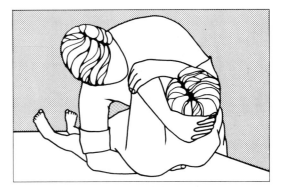

Figure 39.5 Posteroanterior central pressure on intervertebral joints T3–T10

into the palm but leaving the thumb and index finger extended. The patient's lower spinous process is then grasped between the terminal phalanx of the therapist's middle finger and the palmar surface of the head of the first metacarpal. The patient is then lowered until the therapist's right hand is wedged between the patient and the couch, with the therapist's forearm projecting laterally. The patient's elbows are grasped and the upper trunk gently moved back and forth in flexion and extension to obtain the mid position of this movement (*see Figure 39.5*).

Method—Manipulation consists of a downward thrust by the therapist directed through the patient's elbows and upper arms.

Thoracic traction

Traction can be administered to the thoracic spine as readily as it can to the cervical and lumbar areas, and the guiding principles are similar. However, thoracic traction is less often successful than in either of the other two areas, which may be partly due to the presence of the thoracic cage which limits the degree of movement. The main principle is to position the vertebral column so that the joint being treated is relaxed in a position midway between all of its ranges. The amount of pressure used is guided at first by the movement in the joint, and further changes in tension are made in response to changes in the patient's symptoms (as outlined previously for the cervical traction). Further treatment is guided by any changes in the patient's symptoms and signs, as has been already discussed with cervical traction.

Upper thoracic spine

Starting position

The patient lies on his back with one or two pillows under the head to flex the neck so that the intervertebral level to be treated is positioned midway between flexion and extension. A cervical halter is then applied, as has been described for cervical traction in flexion. If the traction needs to be very strong it may be necessary to apply some form of counter-traction. A belt fitted around the pelvis is attached to the foot end of the couch

to stabilize the distal end of the vertebral column. The halter is then attached to its fixed point so that the angle of its pull on the neck will be approximately 45 degrees from the horizontal. The angle used varies with the degree of kyphosis present in the upper thoracic spine but should allow the thoracic intervertebral joint to be stretched longitudinally in a position midway between its limit of flexion and extension. The hips and knees may be flexed to relieve the strain on the patient's lower back while the traction is being applied.

Method

Traction may be adjusted from either or both ends, but whatever type of adjustment is used care must be taken to ensure that friction between the patient's trunk and the couch is reduced to a minimum. This can be achieved while traction is being applied by gently allowing it to relax back into a new position. Friction is virtually eliminated by use of a couch with its surface in two halves that are free to roll longitudinally. Releasing the traction is relatively easy but should be done slowly.

Lower thoracic spine

Starting position

Traction is usually more effective with the patient supine, but may also be used with the patient prone. For the lower thoracic spinal conditions, a thoracic belt similar to that used for lumbar traction replaces the cervical halter.

The thoracic belt is applied above the spinal level being treated to hold the chest and is then attached to its fixed point. The direction of the pull is longitudinal in the line of the patient's trunk, but pillows may be used to adjust the position of the spine so that the joint being stretched is relaxed midway between flexion and extension.

Method

Traction is applied from either end or from both ends but care is necessary to reduce friction to a minimum. This may be achieved with a roll-top couch. The traction is released gradually and the patient is allowed to rest for a time before standing up.

Intermittent variable traction can also be used in the thoracic spine and the times for 'rest' and 'hold' periods are similar to those used for the cervical spine.

Local variations

Positioning of the patient is controlled by the degree of thoracic kyphosis, which varies considerably in each patient, especially in the upper thoracic spine. Theoretically the direction of pull should be at right angles to the upper and lower surfaces of the intervertebral disc of the level that is being stretched.

Precautions

The patient must be checked to ensure that the traction does not cause any low-back pain.

As with cervical traction in flexion it is possible that the head halter used in the upper thoracic traction may cause occipital headache, but this can be prevented as previously described.

Indications

Mobilization techniques are usually used before traction but if these fail traction can be used and may still prove successful. It is of most value in patients with a wide distribution of thoracic pain due either to hypomobility lesions or to disc degeneration, even when complicated by neurological changes or nerve-root pain.

Part III—Bibliography

Adams, C. B. T. and Logue, V. (1971) Studies in cervical spondylotic myelopathy, I, II, III. *Brain*, **94**, 557.

Adams, I. D. (1976) Osteoarthosis and sport. *Clinics in Rheumatological Disease*, **2**, 523.

Adams, P., Davies, G. T. and Sweetnam, P. (1970) Osteoporosis and the effects of aging on bone mass in elderly men and women. *Quarterly Journal of Medicine*, **39**, 601.

Adson, A. W. (1951) Cervical ribs: Symptoms, differential diagnosis and indications for section of the insertion of the scalenus anticus muscle. *Journal of the International College of Surgeons*, **16**, 546.

Ahlback, S., Bauer, G. C. H. and Bohne, W. H. (1968) Spontaneous osteonecrosis of the knee. *Arthritis and Rheumatism*, **11**, 705.

Aichroth, P. M. (1971) Osteochondritis dissecans of the knee. *Journal of Bone and Joint Surgery*, **53B**, 440.

Alexander, R. (1965) The aetiology of primary protrusio acetabuli. *British Journal of Radiology*, **38**, 567.

Alm, A., Liljedahl, S. and Stromberg, B. (1976) Clinical and experimental experience in reconstruction of the anterior cruciate ligament. *Orthopedic Clinics of North America*, **7**, 181.

American Academy of Orthopedic Surgeons (1965) *Joint Motion: Method of Measuring and Recording*, Revised Edn., Chicago.

Andrews, J. R. (1977) In discussion on the diagnosis of chronic anterolateral instability of the knee. *American Journal of Sports Medicine*, **5**, 104.

Appel, H. (1970) Late results after meniscectomy in the knee joint. *Acta Orthopaedica Scandinavica Supplement*, **133**.

Apley, A. G. (1977) *A System of Orthopaedics*, 5th Edn. London: Butterworths.

Armstrong, J. R. (1967) *Lumbar Disc Lesions*. London: Livingstone.

Arner, O., Lindholm, A. and Orell, S. R. (1958) Histological changes in subcutaneous rupture of the Achilles tendon. *Acta Chirurgica Scandinavica*, **116**, 484.

Aronson, H. A. and Dunsmore, R. H. (1963) Herniated upper lumbar discs. *Journal of Bone and Joint Surgery*, **45A**, 311.

Auld, A. W., Perlmutter, I. and Dooley, D. M. (1969) Normal leg raising tests with herniated lumbar disk. *Journal of the American Medical Association*, **207**, 2104.

Backhouse, K. M. (1968) The mechanics of normal digital control in the hand and an analysis of the ulnar drift of rheumatoid arthritis. *Annals of the Royal College of Surgeons of England*, **43**, 154.

Backhouse, K. M. (1969) Mechanical factors influencing normal and rheumatoid metacarpophalangeal joints. *Annals of Rheumatic Disease*, **28**, 15.

Backhouse, K. M. (1972) Extensor expansion of the rheumatoid hand. *Annals of Rheumatic Disease*, **31**, 112.

Bailey, R. W. (1963) Cervical intervertebral disc lesions in fractures and dislocations. *Journal of Bone and Joint Surgery*, **45A**, 461.

Ball, J. (1971) Enthesopathy of rheumatoid and ankylosing spondylitis. *Annals of Rheumatic Disease*, **30**, 213.

Banna, A. and Kendall, P. H. (1964) Spontaneous haemarthrosis of the shoulder joint. *Annals of Physical Medicine*, **7**, 180.

Barnes, C. G. and Currey, H. L. F. (1967) Carpal tunnel syndrome in rheumatoid arthritis. *Annals of Rheumatic Disease*, **26**, 226.

Barr, J. S., Kubik, C. S. and Molloy, M. K. (1967) Evaluation of end results in treatment of ruptured lumbar intervertebral discs with protrusion of nucleus pulposus. *Surgery, Gynecology and Obstetrics*, **125**, 250.

Barré, M. (1926) Sur un syndrome sympathetique cervicale posterieur et sa cause frequent; l'arthrite cervicale. *Revue Neurologie*, **33**, 1246.

Barry, P. J. and Kendall, P. H. (1962) Corticosteroid infiltration of the extradural space. *Annals of Physical Medicine*, **6**, 267.

Bartelink, D. L. (1957) The role of abdominal pressure in relieving the pressure on the lumbar intervertebral discs. *Journal of Bone and Joint Surgery*, **39B**, 718.

Bartschi-Rochaix, W. W. (1949) *Migraine Cervicale*. Berne: Huber.

Basmajian, J. V. (1974) *Muscles Alive. Their Function Revealed by Electromyography*, 3rd Edn. Baltimore: Williams and Wilkins.

Basmajian, J. V. and Stecko, G. (1963) Role of the muscles in the arch support of the foot. An electromyographic study. *Journal of Bone and Joint Surgery*, **45A**, 1184.

Basmajian, J. V. and Lovejoy, J. F. (1971) Functions of the popliteus muscle in man. *Journal of Bone and Joint Surgery*, **53A**, 557.

Bateman, J. E. (1978) *The Shoulder and Neck*, 2nd Edn. Philadelphia: W. B. Saunders.

Bauer, R., Sheehan, S. and Meyer, J. S. (1961) Arteriographic study of cerebrovascular disease. Cerebral symptoms due to kinking, tortuosity and compression of carotid and vertebral arteries in the neck. *Archives of Neurology and Psychiatry*, **4**, 119.

Bayer, A. S., Chow, A. W., Louie, J. S. and Guze, L. B. (1977) Sternoarticular pyoarthrosis due to Gram-negative bacilli. *Archives of Internal Medicine*, **137**, 1036.

Beck, E. L. and McGlamry, E. D. (1973) Modified Young tendsuspension technique for flexible flatfoot. *Journal of the American Pediatrics Association*, **63**, 582.

Bennett, G. A., Waine, H. and Bauer, W. (1942) Changes in the knee joint at various ages. *New York Commonwealth Fund*, **4**.

Bennett, G. E. (1959) Elbow and shoulder lesions of baseball players. *American Journal of Surgery*, **98**, 484.

Berry, R. J. (1961) Genetically controlled degeneration of the nucleus pulposus in the mouse. *Journal of Bone and Joint Surgery*, **43B**, 387.

Bick, E. M. (1963) Vertebral osteophytosis in the aged. *Clinical Orthopaedics and Related Research*, **26**, 50.

Bickerstaff, E. R. (1961) Impairment of consciousness in migraine. *Lancet*, **1**, 1057.

Biemond, A. and de Jong, J. M. B. (1969) On cervical nystagmus and related disorders. *Brain*, **92**, 437.

Blackwood, H. J. J. (1963) Arthritis of the mandibular joint. *British Dental Journal*, **115**, 317.

Blakey, P. R., Happey, F., Naylor, A. and Turner, R. L. (1962) Protein in the nucleus pulposus of the I.V. disc. *Nature (London)*, **195**, 73.

Bland, J. H., Buskirk, F. W. V., Tampas, J. P., Brown, E. and Clayton, R. (1965) A study of roentgenologic criteria for rheumatoid arthritis of the cervical spine. *American Journal of Roentgenology*, **95**, 949.

Blazina, M. E. and Saltzman, J. S. (1969) Recurrent anterior subluxation of the shoulder in athletes. *Journal of Bone and Joint Surgery*, **51A**, 197.

Blazina, M. E., Fox, J. M. and Carlson, J. G. (1974) Basketball injuries. In *Medical Aspects of Sport*. Chicago: American Medical Association.

Bloch, J. and Fischer, F. K. (1961) *Acta Rheumatologica*, No. 2. Basel: Documenta Geigy.

Bluestone, R., Bywaters, E. G. L., Hartog, M., Holt, P. J. L. and Hyde, S. (1971) Acromegalic arthropathy. *Annals of Rheumatic Disease*, **30**, 243.

Bocher, J., Mankin, H. J., Berk, R. N. and Rodnan, G. P. (1965) Prevalence of calcified meniscal cartilage in elderly persons. *New England Journal of Medicine*, **272**, 1093.

Bose, K. and Chong, K. C. (1976) Clinical manifestations and pathomechanics of contracture of the extensor mechanism of the knee. *Journal of Bone and Joint Surgery*, **58B**, 478.

Bosworth, D. M. (1959) Whiplash. *Journal of Bone and Joint Surgery*, **41A**, 16.

Bosworth, D. M. (1965) Surgical treatment of tennis elbow: A follow-up study. *Journal of Bone and Joint Surgery*, **47A**, 1933.

Boyd, H. B. and McLeod, A. C. (1973) Tennis elbow. *Journal of Bone and Joint Surgery*, **55A**, 1183.

Boyle, J. A. and Buchanan, W. W. (1971) *Clinical Rheumatology*. Oxford: Blackwell Scientific Publications.

Bradley, E. L. (1973) The anterior tibial compartment syndrome. *Surgery Gynaecology and Obstetrics*, **136**, 289.

Bradley, K. (1977) *Communication to the Australian Association of Manipulative Medicine*. (Unpublished observations.)

Bradshaw, P. (1957) Some aspects of cervical spondylosis. *Quarterly Journal of Medicine*, **26**, 177.

Bradshaw, P. (1961) Pain caused by cervical spondylosis. *Rheumatism*, **17**, 2.

Brain, W. R. and Wilkinson, M. (1967) *Cervical Spondylosis*, 1st. Edn. London: Heinemann.

Brattstrom, H. and Granholm, L. (1976) Atlanto-axial fusion in rheumatoid arthritis. *Acta Orthopaedica Scandinavica*, **47**, 619.

Brewer, B. J. (1962) Athletic injuries: The musculotendinous unit. *Clinical Orthopaedics and Related Research*, **23**, 30.

Brewerton, D. A. (1965) In *Progress in Clinical Rheumatology*, p. 56. Ed. Dixon, A. St. J. London: Churchill.

Brewerton, D. A., Sandifer, P. H. and Sweetnam, D. R. (1963) 'Idiopathic' pes cavus. *British Medical Journal*, **ii**, 659.

Bridgman, J. F. (1972) Periarthritis of the shoulder and diabetes mellitus. *Annals of Rheumatic Disease*, **31**, 69.

British Association of Physical Medicine (1966) Pain in the neck and arm: A multicentre trial of the effects of physiotherapy. *British Medical Journal*, **i**, 253.

British Medical Journal (1977) Painful shoulders and painful arcs. *British Medical Journal*, **6092**, 913.

British Medical Journal (1978) Persistent tennis elbow. *British Medical Journal*, **i**, 565.

British Medical Journal (1979) Muscle compartment syndrome. *British Medical Journal*, **ii**, 818.

Broadhurst, R. W. and Buhr, A. J. (1959) The pulled elbow. *British Medical Journal*, **i**, 1018.

Brodal, A. (1969) *Neurological Anatomy in Relation to Clinical Medicine*, 2nd Edn. London: Oxford University Press.

Brodey, P. A. and Wolff, S. M. (1975) Radiographic changes in the sacroiliac joint in familial mediterranean fever. *Radiology*, **114**, 331.

Brogadir, S. P., Schimmer, B. M. and Myers, A. R. (1979) Spectrum of gonococcal arthritis—dermatitis syndrome. *Seminars in Arthritis and Rheumatism*, **8**, 177.

Brooke, R. (1924) The sacroiliac joint. *Journal of Anatomy*, **58**, 299.

Browne, J. E., Stanley, R. F. and Tullos, H. S. (1977) Acromioclavicular joint dislocations. *American Journal of Sports Medicine*, **5**, 258.

Brudny, J., Grynbaum, B. B. and Korein, J. (1974) Spasmodic torticollis. *Archives of Physical Medicine and Rehabilitation*, **55**, 403.

Bulgen, D. Y., Hazleman, B. L. and Voak, D. (1976) HLA.B27 and frozen shoulder. *Lancet*, **i**, 1042.

Bulos, S. (1973) Herniated intervertebral lumbar disc in the teenager. *Journal of Bone and Joint Surgery*, **52B**, 432.

Bunnell, S. (1955) Surgery of the rheumatic hand. *Journal of Bone and Joint Surgery*, **37A**, 759.

Burke, G. L. (1964) *Backache from Occiput to Coccyx*. W. E. G. MacDonald: Vancouver.

Burn, J. M. B. and Langdon, L. (1970) Lumbar epidural injection for the treatment of chronic sciatica. *Rheumatism and Physical Medicine*, **10**, 368.

Burn, J. M. B. and Langdon, L. (1974) Duration of action of epidural methylprednisolone. *American Journal of Physical Medicine*, **53**, 29.

Burry, H. C. (1971) The pathology of painful heel. *British Journal of Sports Medicine*, **6**, 9.

Burry, H. C. (1978) Pathogenesis of some traumatic and degenerative disorders of soft tissue. *Australian and New Zealand Journal of Medicine*, **8**, Suppl. **1**, 163.

Burry, H. C. and Pool, C. J. (1973) Central degeneration of the Achilles tendon. *Rheumatism and Rehabilitation*, **12**, 177.

Bussere, A., Mielants, H., Veys, E. M. and Van den Jeught, J. (1975) Avascular necrosis and its relation to lipid and purine metabolism. *Scandinavian Journal of Rheumatology*, **4**, Supplement 8, 40.

Bywaters, E. G. L. (1981) *Rheumatoid Involvement of the Thoracic Spine*. Presented at the *ILAR Congress*, Paris.

Bywaters, E. G. L. and Dixon, A. St. J. (1965) Paravertebral ossification in psoriatic arthritis. *Annals of Rheumatic Disease*, **23**, 313.

Bywaters, E. G. L., Dorling, J. and Sutor, J. (1970) Ochronotic densification. *Annals of Rheumatic Disease*, **29**, 563.

Bywaters, E. G. L., Doyle, F. H. and Oakley, N. (1966) Senile hyperostotic ankylosing spondylitis in diabetes mellitus. *Arthritis and Rheumatism*, **9**, 495.

Cabaud, H. E. and Slocum, D. B. (1977) The diagnosis of chronic anterolateral rotary instability of the knee. *American Journal of Sports Medicine*, **5**, 99.

Calabro, J. J. (1975) Juvenile rheumatoid arthritis: A general review and report of 100 patients observed for fifteen years. *Seminars in Arthritis and Rheumatism*, **5**, 257.

Caldwell, J. W. and Krusen, E. M. (1962) Effectiveness of cervical traction in treatment of neck problems; Evaluations of various methods. *Archives of Physical Medicine and Rehabilitation*, **43**, 214.

Calin, A. and Fries, J. F. (1975) Striking prevalence of ankylosing spondylitis in 'healthy' W27 positive males and females. *New England Journal of Medicine*, **293**, 835.

Calin, A., Porta, J., Fries, J. F. and Schurman, D. J. (1977) Clinical history as a screening test for A.S. *Journal of the American Medical Association*, **237**, 2613.

Caroit, M., Djian, A., Hubault, A., Normandin, C. and de Seze, S. (1963) Duex cas de capsulite rétractile de la hanche. *Revue Rheumatologie*, **30**, 784.

Carrera, G. F., Haughton, V. M., Syversten, A. and Williams, A. L. (1980) Computerised tomography of the lumbar facet joints. *Radiology*, **134**, 145.

Carter, M. E. (1963) Sacro-iliac joints in juvenile rheumatoid arthritis. In *Radiological Aspects of Rheumatoid Arthritis*. Amsterdam: Excerpta Medica.

Cavagna, G. A., Dusman, B. and Margaria, R. (1968) Positive work done by a previously stretched muscle. *Journal of Applied Physiology*, **24**, 21.

Cawley, M. I. D., Chalmers, T. M., Kellgren, J. H. and Ball, J. (1972) Destructive lesions of vertebral bodies in ankylosing spondylitis. *Annals of Rheumatic Disease*, **31**, 345.

Chakravorti, B. G. (1969) Arterial supply of the cervical spinal cord and its relation to cervical myelopathy in spondylosis. *Annals of the Royal College of Surgeons*, **45**, 232.

Chamberlain, M. A. and Corbett, M. (1970) Carpal tunnel syndrome in early rheumatoid arthritis. *Annals of Rheumatic Disease*, **29**, 149.

Champion, D. (1969) Gouty tenosynovitis and carpal tunnel syndrome. *Medical Journal of Australia*, **i**, 1030.

Chandler, G. N. and Wright, V. (1958) Deleterious effect of intra-articular hydrocortisone. *Lancet*, **ii**, 661.

Charnley, J. (1951) Orthopaedic signs in the diagnosis of disc protrusions. *Lancet*, **i**, 189.

Charnley, J. (1974) Surgical treatment of osteoarthritis of the hip. In *VII Congress de la Societe Internationale de Chirurgie Orthopaedique et de Traumatologie*, p. 784.

Chrisman, O. D. and Gervais, R. F. (1962) Otologic manifestations of the cervical syndrome. *Clinical Orthopaedics and Related Research*, **24**, 34.

Chrisman, O. D., Mittnacht, A. and Snook, G. A. (1964) A study of the results following rotatory manipulation in the lumbar intervertebral disc syndrome. *Journal of Bone and Joint Surgery*, **46A**, 517.

Clarke, G. R. (1972) Unequal leg length. *Rheumatism and Physical Medicine*, **11**, 385.

Clarke, G. R., Willis, L. A., Stenner, L. and Nicholls, P. J. R. (1974) Evaluation of physiotherapy in treatment of osteoarthritis of the knee. *Rheumatism and Rehabilitation*, **13**, 190.

Clein, L. J. (1975) Suprascapular entrapment neuropathy. *Journal of Neurosurgery*, **43**, 337.

Cleland, L. G., Bowey, R. R., Henderson, D. R. F. and Milazzo, S. C. (1976) Spontaneous osteonecrosis of the medial femoral condyle. *Medical Journal of Australia*, **ii**, 92.

Close, J. R., Inman, V. T., Poor, P. M. and Todd, F. N. (1967) The function of the subtalar joint. *Clinical Orthopaedics and Related Research*, **50**, 159.

Cloward, R. B. (1952) Anterior herniation of a ruptured lumbar invertebral disk: Comments on the diagnostic value of diskogram. *Archives of Surgery*, **64**, 457.

Cloward, R. B. (1963) Lesions of the intervertebral disk and their treatment by interbody fusion method. *Clinical Orthopaedics and Related Research*, **27**, 51.

Coburn, J. (1962) Vertebral artery involvement in cervical trauma. *Clinical Orthopaedics and Related Research*, **24**, 61.

Codman, E. A. (1934) *The Shoulder*. Boston: T. Todd.

Colachis, S. C., Warden, R. E., Bechtol, C. D. and Strohm, B. R. (1963) Movement of the sacro-iliac joint in the adult male. *Archives of Physical Medicine and Rehabilitation*, **44**, 490.

Colcher, A. E. and Hursh, A. M. W. (1952) Pre-employment low back X-ray survey: A review of 1,500 cases. *Industrial Medicine and Surgery*, **21**, 319.

Collette, J. and Ludwig, E. G. (1968) Low back disorders. An examination of the stereotype. *Industrial Medicine and Surgery*, **37**, 685.

Collins, D. H. (1959) *The Pathology of Articular and Spinal Disease*. London: Arnold.

Collis, J. S. (1963) *Lumbar Discography*. Springfield, Ill.: Thomas.

Conlon, P., Isdale, I. C. and Rose, B. S. (1966) Rheumatoid arthritis of the cervical spine. *Annals of Rheumatic Disease*, **25**, 120.

Coonrad, K. W. and Hooper, W. R. (1973) Tennis elbow: Natural history, conservative and surgical management. *Journal of Bone and Joint Surgery*, **55A**, 1177.

Cope, S. and Ryan, G. M. S. (1959) Cervical and otolith vertigo. *Journal of Laryngology and Otology*, **73**, 113.

Copeman, W. S. C. (1978) In *Textbook of Rheumatic Diseases*, Ed. Scott. J. T. Edinburgh: Churchill-Livingstone.

Corrigan, A. B. (1965) The pulled elbow. *Medical Journal of Australia*, **ii**, 167.

Corrigan, A. B. and Fitch, K. D. (1972) Complications of jogging. *Medical Journal of Australia*, **ii**, 363.

Corrigan, A. B., Carr, G. and Tugwell, S. (1982) Intraspinal corticosteroid injections. *Medical Journal of Australia*, **1**, 224.

Costen, J. B. (1934) Syndrome of ear and sinus symptoms dependent upon disturbed function of the temporomandibular joint. *Annals of Otolaryngology*, **43**, 1.

Costen, J. B. (1936) Neuralgia associated with disturbed function of temporomandibular joint. *Journal of the American Medical Association*, **107**, 252.

Costill, D. L., Fink, W. S. and Habansky, A. J. (1977) Muscular rehabilitation following knee surgery. *Physician Sports Medicine*, **5**, 71.

Coventry, M. B. (1953) Problem of painful shoulder. *Journal of the American Medical Association*, **15**, 177.

Coventry, M. B. and Tapper, E. M. (1972) Pelvic instability. *Journal of Bone and Joint Surgery*, **54A**, 83.

Cox, J. S., Nye, C. E., Schaefer, W. W. and Woodstein, I. J. (1975) The degenerative effects of partial and total resection of the medial meniscus in dogs' knees. *Clinical Orthopaedics and Related Research*, **109**, 178.

Crain, D. C. (1961) Interphalangeal osteoarthritis characterized by painful inflammatory episodes resulting in deformity of the proximal and distal articulations. *Journal of the American Medical Association*, **175**, 1049.

Crelin, E. S. (1973) A scientific test of the chiropractic theory. *American Scientist*, **61**, 574.

Crock, H. (1970) A reappraisal of intervertebral disc lesions. *Medical Journal of Australia*, **i**, 983.

Cross, M. J. (1974) Current concepts of knee anatomy. *Bulletin of the Postgraduate Committee in Medicine, University of Sydney*, **4**, 127.

Cuddigan, J. H. P. (1973) Quadriceps femoris strength. *Rheumatism and Rehabilitation*, **12**, 77.

Cyriax, J. (1978) *Textbook of Orthopaedic Medicine. Vol. 1. Diagnosis of Soft Tissue Lesions*, 7th Edn. London: Ballière Tindall.

Dandy, D. J. and Poirier, H. (1975) Chondromalacia and the unstable patella. *Acta Orthopaedica Scandinavica*, **46**, 695.

D'Arcy, J. (1978) Pes anserinus: Transportation for chronic anteromedial rotational instability of the knee. *Journal of Bone and Joint Surgery*, **60B**, 66.

Darcy, K., Ansell, B. M. and Bywaters, E. G. L. (1978) A family with primary protrusio acetabuli. *Annals of Rheumatic Disease*, **37**, 53.

Darlington, L. G. and Coomes, E. N. (1977) The effects of local steroid injection for supraspinatus tears. *Rheumatism and Rehabilitation*, **16**, 172.

Darracott, J. and Vernon-Roberts, B. (1971) The bony changes in chondromalacia patellae. *Rheumatology and Physical Medicine*, **XI**, 175.

Davidson, C., Wojtulewski, J. A., Bacon, P. A. and Winstock, D. (1975) Temporo-mandibular joint disease in ankylosing spondylitis. *Annals of Rheumatic Disease*, **34**, 87.

Davidson, E. A. and Woodhall, B. (1959) Biochemical alterations in herniated I.V.D. concomitant with aging. *Journal of Biological Chemistry*, **234**, 2951.

Davis, D. (1957) Radicular syndromes with emphasis on chest pain simulating coronary disease. Chicago: Medical Year Book Publishers.

Debyre, J., Patte, D. and Elmelik, E. (1965) Repair of rupture of the rotator cuff of the shoulder with a note on advancement of the supraspinatus tendon. *Journal of Bone and Joint Surgery*, **47B**, 36.

Dehaven, K. E., Dolan, W. A. and Mayer, P. J. (1979) Chondromalacia patellae in athletes. *American Journal of Sports Medicine*, **7**, 5.

de Kleijn, A. and Nieuwenhuyse, P. (1927) Schwindelanfalle und Nystagmus bei einer Bestimenten Stellung des Kopfes. *Acta oto-laryngologica (Stockholm)*, **11**, 155.

Delmas, J. (1947) Comment atteninaire les fibres preganglion du membre superieur. *Coz. Med. de France*, **54**, 7033.

de Palma, A. F. (1950) *Surgery of the Shoulder*. Philadelphia: J. B. Lippincott.

de Palma, A. F. (1957a) *Degenerative Changes in the Sternoclavicular and Acromioclavicular Joints in Various Decades*. Springfield: Thomas.

de Palma, A. F. (1957b) The painful shoulder. *Postgraduate Medical Journal*, **21**, 368.

de Palma, A. F. and Marone, P. (1959) Spondylolysis following spinal fusion. *Clinical Orthopaedics and Related Research*, **15**, 208.

de Palma, A. F. and Subin, R. (1965) Study of the cervical syndrome. *Clinical Orthopaedics and Related Research*, **38**, 135.

de Palma, A. F. and Rothman, R. H. (1970) *The Intervertebral Disc*. Philadelphia: Saunders.

Desai, A. D. and Dastur, H. M. (1967) Phenobarbitone and the shoulder–hand syndrome. *British Medical Journal*, **ii**, 173.

de Sèze, A. (1955) Les attitudes antalgiques dans la sciatique discoradiculaire commune. Etude clinique et radiologique; interprétation pathogènique. *Seminar Hôpital, Paris*, **31**, 2291.

Devas, M. B. (1965) Stress fractures of the femoral neck. *Journal of Bone and Joint Surgery*, **47B**, 728.

Devas, M. B. (1970) Stress fractures in athletes. *Journal of the Royal College of General Practitioners*, **19**, 34.

Devas, M. B. (1975) *Stress Fractures*. Edinburgh: Churchill-Livingstone.

Dick, W. C. (1978) In *Drug Treatment of Rheumatoid Arhthritis in Copeman's Textbook of the Rheumatic Diseases*, p. 404. Ed. Scott, J. T. Edinburgh: Churchill-Livingstone.

Dickinson, P. H., Coutts, M. B., Woodward, P. E. and Handler, D. (1966) Tendo Achilles bursitis. *Journal of Bone and Joint Surgery*, **48A**, 77.

Dieppe, P. A., Huskisson, E. C., Crocker, P. and Willoughby, D. A. (1976) Apatite-deposition disease: A new arthropathy. *Lancet*, **i**, 266.

Dilke, T. F. W., Burry, H. C. and Grahame, R. (1973) Extradural corticosteroid injection in the management of lumbar nerve root compression. *British Medical Journal*, **ii**, 635.

Dillane, J. B., Fry, J. and Kalton, G. (1966) Acute back syndrome: A study from general practice. *British Medical Journal*, **iii**, 82.

Dingle, J. T. (1973) The role of lysosomal enzymes in skeletal tissues. *Journal of Bone and Joint Surgery*, **55B**, 87.

Di Stefano, V. J. (1980) Function, post-traumatic sequelae, and current concepts of management of knee meniscus injuries. *Clinical Orthopaedics and Related Research*, **151**, 143.

Dixon, A. St.J. (1963) The sacro-iliac joint in adult rheumatoid arthritis. In *Radiological Aspects of Rheumatoid Arthritis*. Amsterdam: Excerpta Medica.

Dixon, A. St.J. (1965) Factors in the development and presentation of osteoarthritis of the knee. In *Progress in Clinical Rheumatology*, p. 313. London: J. and A. Churchill.

Djian, A., Denis, A., Annonier, C. and Baudoin, P. (1967) La radiopodometrie. *Acta Rheumatologica*, **4**, 194.

Dobyns, J. H., O'Brien, E. T., Linscheid, R. L. and Farrow, G. M. (1972) Bowler's thumb—diagnosis and treatment. *Journal of Bone and Joint Surgery*, **54A**, 751.

Doran, D. M. L. and Newell, D. J. (1975) Manipulation in the treatment of low back pain—A multicentre study. *British Medical Journal*, **ii**, 161.

Doyle, F. H., Gutheridge, D. H., Joplin, G. F. and Fraser, R. (1967) An assessment of radiological criteria used in the study of spinal osteoporosis. *British Journal of Radiology*, **40**, 241.

Drennan, D. B., Fahey, J. J. and Maylahn, D. J. (1971) Important factors in achieving arthrodesis of the Charcot knee. *Journal of Bone and Joint Surgery*, **53A**, 1180.

Duncan, H., Frame, B. and Frost, H. (1969) Regional migratory osteoporosis. *Southern Medical Journal*, **62**, 41.

Duthie, R. and Harris, C. (1969) A radiographic and clinical survey of the hip joints in seropositive rheumatoid arthritis. *Acta Orthopaedica Scandinavica*, **40**, 346.

Dutton, C. B. and Riley, L. H. (1969) Cervical migraine: Not merely a pain in the neck. *American Journal of Medicine*, **47**, 141.

Dwosh, I. L., Resnick, D. and Becker, M. A. (1976) Hip involvement in ankylosing spondylitis. *Arthritis and Rheumatism*, **19**, 683.

Dwyer, F. C. (1959) Osteotomy of the calcaneum for pes cavus. *Journal of Bone and Joint Surgery*, **41B**, 80.

Dyson, M., Pond, J. B., Joseph, J. and Warwick, R. (1968) The stimulus of tissue generation by means of ultrasound. *Clinical Science*, **35**, 273.

Ebringer, R., Cooke, D., Cawdell, D. R., Cowling, P. and Ebringer, A. (1977) Ankylosing spondylitis: Klebsiella and HLA B27. *Rheumatism and Rehabilitation*, **16**, 190.

Edelson, J. C. and Nathan, H. (1977) Meralgia paresthetica. *Clinical Orthopaedics and Related Research*, **122**, 255.

Edgar, M. and Park, W. (1972) Induced pain patterns on passive straight leg raising in low lumbar disc prolapse. *Journal of Bone and Joint Surgery*, **54B**, 749.

Edwards, P. W. (1969) Peroneal compartment syndrome. *Journal of Bone and Joint Surgery*, **51**, 123.

Ehrlich, G. E. (1972) Inflammatory osteoarthritis I. The clinical syndrome. *Journal of Chronic Diseases*, **25**, 371.

Ehrlich, G. E. (1972) Inflammatory osteoarthritis II. The superimposition of rheumatoid arthritis. *Journal of Chronic Diseases*, **25**, 635.

Elftman, H. (1960) Transverse tarsal joint and its control. *Clinical Orthopaedics and Related Research*, **16**, 41.

Ellis, W. (1973) Rubella arthritis. *British Medical Journal*, **ii**, 549.

Ellsasser, J. C., Reynolds, F. C. and Omohundro, J. R. (1974) The nonoperative treatment of collateral ligament injuries of the knee in professional football players. *Journal of Bone and Joint Surgery*, **56A**, 1185.

Elves, M. W., Bucknill, T. and Sullivan, M. F. (1975) *In-vitro* inhibition of leucocyte migration in patients with intervertebral disc lesions. *Orthopedic Clinics of North America*, **6**, 59.

Epstein, J. A. (1960) Diagnosis of painful neurological disorders. *Journal of Neurosurgery*, **17**, 991.

Eriksson, E. (1976) Sports injuries of the knee ligaments; Diagnosis, rehabilitation and prevention. *Medical Science and Sports*, **8**, 133.

Evans, D. L. (1953) Recurrent instability of the ankle. *Proceedings of the Royal Society of Medicine*, **46**, 343.

Ewer, E. G. (1953) Manipulation of the spine. *Journal of Bone and Joint Surgery*, **35A**, 347.

Farfan, H. F. (1973) *Mechanical Disorders of the Low Back*. Philadelphia: Lea and Febiger.

Farfan, H. F. and Sullivan, J. D. (1967) The relation of facet orientation to intervertebral disc failure. *Canadian Journal of Surgery*, **10**, 179.

Farfan, H. F., Cossett, E. J. W., Robertson, G. H., Wells, R. V. and Kraus, H. (1970) The effects of torsion on the lumbar intervertebral joints: The role of torsion in the production of disc degeneration. *Journal of Bone and Joint Surgery*, **52A**, 468.

Farfan, H. F., Osteria, V. and Lamy, C. (1976) The mechanical etiology of spondylolysis and spondylolisthesis. *Clinical Orthopaedics and Related Research*, **117**, 40.

Fassbender, H. G. (1975) *Pathology of Rheumatic Diseases*. New York: Springer-Verlag.

Feagin, J. A. (1979) The syndrome of the torn anterior cruciate ligament. *Orthopedic Clinics of North America*, **10**, 81.

Feagin, J. A., Abbot, H. G. and Roukous, J. R. (1972) The isolated tear of the anterior cruciate ligament. *Journal of Bone and Joint Surgery*, **54A**, 1340.

Fearnley, G. R. (1951) Ulnar deviation of the fingers. *Annals of Rheumatic Disease*, **10**, 126.

Fearnley, M. E. and Vadasz, I. (1969) Factors influencing the response of lesions of the rotator cuff of the shoulder to local steroid injections. *Annals of Physical Medicine*, **X**, 53.

Feldman, F., Johnson, A. M. and Walter, J. F. (1974) Acute axial neuroarthropathy. *Radiology*, **111**, 1.

Ferguson, A. H. and Gingrich, R. M. (1957) The normal and abnormal calcaneal apophysis and tarsal navicular. *Clinical Orthopaedics and Related Research*, **10**, 87.

Fessel, W. J. (1975) *Rheumatology for Clinicians*. New York: Stratton Intercontinental Medical Books.

Fetto, J. F. and Marshall, J. L. (1979) Injury to the anterior cruciate ligament producing the pivot shift sign. *Journal of Bone and Joint Surgery*, **61A**, 710.

Ficat, P. and Hungerford, D. S. (1977) Disorders of the patellofemoral joint. Baltimore: Williams and Wilkins.

Filtzer, D. L. and Bahnson, H. T. (1959). Low back pain due to arterial obstruction. *Journal of Bone and Joint Surgery*, **41B**, 244.

Fisk, J. (1975) The straight leg raising test. *New Zealand Medical Journal*, **542**, 557.

Fitch, K. D. and Gray, S. D. (1974) Indomethacin in soft tissue sports injuries. *Medical Journal of Australia*, **i**, 260.

Flatt, A. E. (1974) *The Care of the Rheumatoid Hand*, 3rd Edn. St. Louis: C. V. Mosby.

Fleming, A., Dodman, S., Beer, T. C. and Crown, S. (1976) Personality in frozen shoulder. *Annals of Rheumatic Disease*, **35**, 456.

Foerster, O. (1933) Dermatomes in man. *Brain*, **56**, 1.

Ford, F. R. and Clark, D. (1956) Thrombosis of the basilar artery due to manipulation of the neck. *Bulletin of the Johns Hopkins Hospital*, **98**, 37.

Forestier, J. and Lagier, R. (1971) Ankylosing hyperostosis of the spine. *Clinical Orthopaedics and Related Research*, **74**, 65.

Forestier, J. and Rôtes-Querol, J. (1950) Senile ankylosing hyperostosis of spine. *Annals of Rheumatic Disease*, **9**, 321.

Forrest, A. J. and Wolkin, S. M. (1974) Masked depression in men and low back pain. *Rheumatology and Rehabilitation*, **13**, 148.

Foss, M. U. L. and Byers, P. D. (1972) Bone density, osteoarthrosis of the hips and fracture of the upper end of the femur. *Annals of Rheumatic Disease*, **31**, 259.

Frankel, C. J. (1959) Medical-legal aspects of injuries to the neck. *Journal of the American Medical Association*, **169**, 216.

Frankel, V. H. (1977) The Terry-Thomas sign. *Clinical Orthopaedics and Related Research*, **129**, 321.

Franks, A. S. T. (1969) Temporomandibular joint in adult rheumatoid arthritis. *Annals of Rheumatic Disease*, **23**, 138.

Freeman, M. A. R. (1965) Instability of the foot after

injuries to the lateral ligament of the ankle. *Journal of Bone and Joint Surgery*, **47B**, 669.

Freeman, M. A. R. (1967) Instability of the foot following ligament injuries at the ankle. *Proceedings of the Royal Society of Medicine*, **60**, 532.

Freeman, M. A. R. and Wyke, B. D. (1964) Articular contributions to limb muscle reflexes. *Journal of Physiology (London)*, **171**, 21.

Freeman, M. A. R. and Wyke, B. D. (1967) Articular reflexes at the ankle joint. *British Journal of Surgery*, **54**, 990.

Freeman, M. A. R. and Wyke, B. D. (1976) The innervation of the ankle joint. *Acta Anatomica*, **68**, 321.

Freeman, M. A. R., Dean, M. R. E. and Hanham, I. W. F. (1965) The etiology and prevention of functional instability of the foot. *Journal of Bone and Joint Surgery*, **47B**, 678.

Freiberg, A. H. (1914) Infraction of the second metatarsal bone, a typical injury. *Surgery, Gynecology and Obstetrics*, **19**, 191.

Friberg, S. (1948) Anatomical studies on lumbar disc degeneration. *Acta Orthopaedica Scandinavica*, **19**, 222.

Friedenberg, Z. B. and Miller, W. T. (1963) Degenerative disc disease of the cervical spine. *Journal of Bone and Joint Surgery*, **45A**, 1171.

Friedmann, E. (1963) Rupture of the distal brachii tendon. *Journal of the American Medical Association*, **184**, 182.

Frigerio, N. A., Stowe, R. R. and Howe, J. W. (1974) Movement of the sacro-iliac joint. *Clinical Orthopaedics and Related Research*, **100**, 370.

Froimson, A. I. (1971) Treatment of tennis elbow and forearm support band. *Journal of Bone and Joint Surgery*, **53A**, 183.

Frykholm, R. (1951a) Lower cervical nerve roots and their investments. *Acta Chirurgica Scandinavica*, **101**, 457.

Frykholm, R. (1951b) Lower cervical vertebrae and intervertebral discs. Surgical anatomy and pathology. *Acta Chirurgica Scandinavica*, **101**, 345.

Frykholm, R. (1951c) Cervical nerve root compression from disc degeneration and root sleeve fibrosis. *Acta Chirurgica Scandinavica Supplement*, **160**.

Galway, R. D. (1972) Pivot shift syndrome. *Journal of Bone and Joint Surgery*, **54B**, 558.

Galway, R. D., Beaupre, A. and McIntosh, D. L. (1972) Pivot shift: A clinical sign of symptomatic anterior cruciate insufficiency. *Journal of Bone and Joint Surgery*, **54B**, 763.

Gardner, E., Gray, D. J. and O'Rahilly, R. (1969) *Anatomy*, 3rd Edn. Philadelphia: Saunders.

Gardner, R. C. (1970) Tennis elbow: Diagnosis, pathology and treatment: Nine severe cases treated by a new reconstructive operation. *Clinical Orthopaedics and Related Research*, **72**, 248.

Gaughwin, C. (1982) The Patello-femoral joint. An evaluation of Zohlern's sign and survey in fulfilment of Graduate Diploma in Advanced Manipulation Therapy, South Australian Institute of Technology, Australia.

Ghosh, P., Taylor, T. K. S., Yarroll, J. M., Braund, K. G. and Larsen, L. H. (1975) Genetic factors in the maturation of the canine intervertebral disc. *Research in Veterinary Science*, **19**, 304.

Giannestras, N. J. (1973) *Foot Disorders, Medical and Surgical Management*, 2nd Edn. Philadelphia: Lea and Febiger.

Gibson, T., Burry, H. C., Poswillo, D. and Glass, J. (1977) Effect of intra-articular corticosteroid injections on primate cartilage. *Annals of Rheumatic Disease*, **36**, 74.

Gill, G. G., Manning, J. G. and White, H. L. (1955) Surgical treatment of spondylolisthesis without spine fusion; excision of loose lamina with decompression of nerve roots. *Journal of Bone and Joint Surgery*, **37A**, 493.

Ginsburg, J. H. and Ellsasser, J. C. (1978) Problem areas in the diagnosis and treatment of ligament injuries of the knee. *Clinical Orthopaedics and Related Research*, **132**, 201.

Glenn, W. V., Rhodes, M. L. and Altschuler, E. M. (1979) Multiplanar display computerized body tomography—applications in the lumbar spine. *Spine*, **4**, 282.

Glick, E. M. (1966) A radiological comparison of the hip joint in rheumatoid arthritis and ankylosing spondylitis. *Proceedings of the Royal Society of Medicine*, **59**, 1229.

Glick, J. M., Milburn, L. J., Haggerty, J. F. and Nishimoto, D. (1977) Dislocated acromio-clavicular joint. Follow-up study of 35 unreduced acromic-clavicular dislocations. *American Journal of Sports Medicine*, **5**, 264.

Glinz, W. (1978) Arthroscopy in articular cartilage injury. In *The Knee: Ligament and Articular Cartilage Injuries*, Ed. Hastings, D. E. New York: Springer-Verlag.

Glover, J. R., Morris, J. G. and Khosla, T. (1974) Back pain: A randomised clinical trial of rotational manipulation of the trunk. *British Journal of Industrial Medicine*, **31**, 59.

Goddard, M. D. and Reed, J. D. (1965) Movements induced by straight-leg raising in the lumbo-sacral roots. *Journal of Neurology, Neurosurgery and Psychiatry*, **28**, 12.

Goebert, H. W., Jallo, S. J., Gardner, W. J. and Wasmuth, C. E. (1961) Painful radiculopathy treated with epidural injections. *Current Research in Analgesic and Anaesthesia*, **40**, 130.

Gofton, J. P. (1971) Studies in osteoarthritis of the hip. Part III. Congenital subluxation and osteoarthritis of the hip. *Canadian Medical Association Journal*, **104**, 911.

Gofton, J. P. and Trueman, G. E. (1971) Studies in osteoarthritis of the hip: Part II. Osteoarthritis of the hip and leg-length disparity. *Canadian Medical Association Journal*, **104**, 791.

Goldenberg, D. L. and Cohen, A. S. (1976) Acute infectious arthritis. *American Journal of Medicine*, **60**, 369.

Golding, D. N. (1969) Cervical and occipital pain as presenting symptoms of intracranial tumour. *Annals of Physical Medicine*, **10**, 1.

Goldman, S., Linscheid, R. L. and Bickel, W. H. (1969) Disruption of the tendo achillis. *Proceedings of the Mayo Clinic*, **44**, 28.

Golub, B. S. and Silverman, B. (1969) Transforaminal ligaments of the lumbar spine. *Journal of Bone and Joint Surgery*, **51A**, 947.

Gondos, B. (1968) Roentgen abnormalities in diabetic osteopathy. *Radiology*, **91**, 6.

Goodfellow, J. (1966) Aetiology of hallux rigidus. *Proceedings of the Royal Society of Medicine*, **59**, 821.

Goodfellow, J., Hungerford, D. S. and Zindel, M. (1976) Patellofemoral joint mechanics and pathology. *Journal of Bone and Joint Surgery*, **58B**, 287.

Gowers, W. R. (1904) Lumbago. Its lessons and analogues. *British Medical Journal*, **i**, 117.

Graham, W. (1960) In *Arthritis and Allied Conditions*, 6th Edn., Ed. Hollander, J. L. Philadelphia: Lea and Febiger.

Grant, A. E. (1964) Massage with ice (cryokinetics) in the treatment of painful conditions of the musculoskeletal system. *Archives of Physical Medicine and Rehabilitation*, **45**, 233.

Gray, H. (1973) *Anatomy of the Human Body*, Ed. Goss, C. M. Philadelphia: Lea and Febiger.

Gray, E. and Basmajian, J. (1968) Electromyography and

cinematography of leg and foot (normal and flat) during walking. *Anatomical Reviews*, **16**, 1.

Green, D. and Joynt, R. J. (1959) Vascular accidents to the brain stem associated with neck manipulation. *Journal of the American Medical Association*, **170**, 522.

Grieve, G. P. (1976) The sacro-iliac joint. *Physiotherapy*, **62**, 383.

Griffen, C. J. and Harris, R. (1975) *The Temporomandibular Joint Syndrome*. Basle: Karger.

Gucker, T. (1965) In *Therapeutic Exercise*. Ed. Licht, A. B. Maryland: Waverly Press.

Gunn, C. C. and Milbrandt, W. E. (1976) Tennis elbow and the cervical spine. *Canadian Medical Association Journal*, **114**, 803.

Hadley, L. (1936) Apophyseal subluxation. *Journal of Bone and Joint Surgery*, **1B**, 428.

Hajkova, Z., Sterda, A. and Skrha, F. (1965) Hyperostotic spondylosis and diabetes mellitus. *Annals of Rheumatic Diseases*, **24**, 536.

Hakelius, A. and Hindmarsh, J. (1972) The comparative reliability of pre-operative diagnostic methods in lumbar disc surgery. *Acta Orthopaedica Scandinavica*, **43**, 239.

Hakstian, R. W. and Tubiana, R. (1967) Ulnar deviation of the fingers. *Journal of Bone and Joint Surgery*, **49A**, 299.

Harcke, H. T. (1978) Bone imaging in infants and children. *Journal of Nuclear Medicine*, **19**, 324.

Harris, N. H. and Murray, R. O. (1974) Lesions of the symphysis in athletes. *British Medical Journal*, **iv**, 211.

Harris, R. I. (1965) Rigid valgus foot due to a talocalcaneal bridge. *Journal of Bone and Joint Surgery*, **37A**, 169.

Harris, R. I. and Beath, T. (1948) Hypermobile flatfoot with short tendo achilles. *Journal of Bone and Joint Surgery*, **30A**, 116.

Harris, R. I. and Beath, T. (1948) Aetiology of peroneal spastic flatfoot. *Journal of Bone and Joint Surgery*, **30B**, 624.

Harris, R. I. and Macnab, I. (1954) Structural changes in lumbar intervertebral discs. *Journal of Bone and Joint Surgery*, **36B**, 304.

Harrison, M. H. M. and Turner, M. H (1974) Containment splintage for Perthes' disease of the hip. *Journal of Bone and Joint Surgery*, **56B**, 199.

Hart, F. D. (1955) Ankylosing spondylitis. *Annals of Rheumatic Disease*, **14**, 77.

Hart, F. D. (1968) The stiff aching back. The differential diagnosis of ankylosing spondylitis. *Lancet*, **i**, 740.

Hartviksen, K. (1962) Ice therapy in spasticity. *Acta Neurologica Scandinavica*, **38**, Suppl. **3**, 79.

Harvey, W., Dyson, M., Pond, J. B. and Grahame, R. (1975) The stimulation of protein synthesis in human fibroblast by therapeutic ultrasound. *Rheumatology and Rehabilitation*, **14**, 237.

Hazleman, B. L. (1972) The painful stiff shoulder. *Rheumatology and Physical Medicine*, **X1**, 8, 413.

Head, H. (1920) *Studies in Neurology*. London: Oxford University Press.

Heck, C. V. (1956) Hoarseness and painful deglutition due to massive cervical exostoses. *Surgery, Gynecology and Obstetrics*, **102**, 657.

Heinz, G. J. and Zavala, D. C. (1977) Slipping rib syndrome: Diagnosis using the hooking manoeuvre. *Journal of the American Medical Association*, **237**, 794.

Helfet, A. J. (1974) *Disorders of the Knee*. Philadelphia: J. B. Lippincott.

Hench, P. S. and Boland, E. W. (1946) Chronic arthritis and other rheumatic diseases among soldiers of the United States Army. *Annals of Internal Medicine*, **24**, 808.

Henderson, D. R. F. (1975) Vertebral atlanto-axial subluxation in rheumatoid arthritis. *Rheumatism and Rehabilitation*, **14**, 1, 31.

Hendry, N. G. (1958) The hydration of the nucleus pulposus and its relation to intervertebral disc derangement. *Journal of Bone and Joint Surgery*, **40B**, 132.

Henning, C. and Egge, L. (1977) Cast brace treatment of acute unstable lateral ankle sprain. *American Journal of Sports Medicine*, **5**, 252.

Henry, J. H. and Crosland, J. W. (1979) Conservative treatment of patellofemoral subluxation. *American Journal of Sports Medicine*, **7**, 12.

Herbet, C. M., Lindberg, K. A., Jayson, M. I. V. and Bailey, A. J. (1975) Changes in the collagen of human intervertebral discs during aging and degenerative disc diseases. *Journal of Molecular Medicine*, **1**, 79.

Herlin, L. (1966) *Sciatic and Pelvic Pain due to Lumbo-sacral Nerve Root Compression*. Springfield: Thomas.

Hicks, J. H. (1953) The mechanics of the foot. I. The joints. *Journal of Anatomy*, **87**, 345.

Hicks, J. H. (1961)The three weight-bearing mechanisms of the foot. In *Biomechanical Studies of the Musculoskeletal System*. Springfield: C. Thomas.

Highton, T. (1972) Scanning electron-microscopic study of menisci. Communication to *The Second Seapal Conference*, Auckland, New Zealand.

Hilton, J. (1855) *Rest and Pain*. London: Bell and Sons.

Hilton, R. C., Ball, J. and Benn, R. T. (1976) Vertebral end-plate lesions (Schmorl's nodes) in the dorsolumbar spine. *Annals of the Rheumatic Diseases*, **35**, 127.

Hirsch, C. and Schajowicz, F. (1953) Studies on structural changes in the lumbar annulus fibrosus. *Acta Orthopaedica Scandinavica*, **22**, 184.

Hlavac, H. (1970) Compensated forefoot varus. *Journal of the American Podiatry Association*, **60**, 229.

Hockaday, J. M. and Whitty, C. W. M. (1967) Patterns of referred pain in the normal subject. *Brain*, **90**, 481.

Hollander, J. L. (1970) Intra-synovial coricosteroid therapy in arthritis. *Maryland State Medical Journal*, **19**, 62–6.

Hollander, J. L. and Horvath, S. M. (1949) The influence of physical therapy procedure on the intra-articular temperature of normal and arthritic subjects. *American Journal of Medical Science*, **218**, 543.

Holmes, G. (1913) Headaches of organic origin. *The Practitioner*, **90**, 968.

Holt, S. and Yates, P. O. (1966) Cervical spondylosis and nerve root lesions. Incidence at routine necropsy. *Journal of Bone and Joint Surgery*, **48B**, 407.

Hoppenfeld, J. (1976) *Physical Examination of the Spine and Extremities*. New York: Appleton-Century-Crofts.

Horal, J. (1969) The clinical appearance of low back disorders in the city of Gothenberg, Sweden. *Acta Orthopaedica Scandinavica Supplement*, **118**, 1.

Hoskinson, J. (1974) Freiberg's disease; Review of long-term results. *Proceedings of the Royal Society of Medicine*, **67**, 10.

Howard, F. M. and Fahey, T. (1974) Rotary subluxation of the navicular. *Clinical Orthopaedics and Related Research*, **104**, 134.

Howes, R. G. and Isdale, I. C. (1971) The loose back: An unrecognised syndrome. *Rheumatology and Physical Medicine*, **11**, 72.

Howse, A. J. G. (1964) Osteitis pubis in an olympic road walker. *Proceedings of the Royal Society of Medicine*, **57**, 88.

Hubbard, A. W. (1960) In *Science and Medicine of Exercise and Sports*, p. 7. Ed. Johnson, W. R. New York: Hanfer.

Hudgins, W. R. (1977) The crossed-straight leg raising test. *New England Journal of Medicine*, **297**, 1127.

Hughston, J. C. (1969) Subluxation of the patella in athletes. In *Symposium on Sports Medicine*, p. 162. St. Louis: C. V. Mosby.

Hughston, J. C. (1972) Reconstruction of the extensor mechanism for patellar subluxation. *Journal of Sports Medicine*, **1**, 6.

Hughston, J. C., Andrews, J. R., Cross, J. M. and Moschi, A. (1976) Classification of knee ligament instabilities. *Journal of Bone and Joint Surgery*, **58A**, 159.

Hult, L. (1954) Cervical, dorsal and lumbar syndromes. *Acta Orthopaedica Scandinavica Supplement*, **17**.

Hult, L. (1954a) *The Munkfors Investigation*. Copenhagen: Munksgaard.

Hult, L. (1954b) *Cervical, Dosal and Lumbar Spinal Syndromes*. Copenhagen: Munksgaard.

Huskisson, E. C., Dieppe, P. A., Tucker, A. K. and Cannell, L. B. (1979) Another look at osteoarthritis. *Annals of Rheumatic Disease*, **38**, 423.

Husni, E. A., Bell, H. S. and Storer, J. (1966) Mechanical occlusion of the vertebral artery. *Journal of the American Medical Association*, **196**, 475.

Hutchinson, E. C. and Yates, P. O. (1956) The cervical portion of the vertebral artery. A clinico-pathological study. *Brain*, **79**, 319.

Iggarashi, M., Miyatah, H., Alford, B. R., and Wright, W. K. (1972) Nystagmus after experimental cervical lesions. *Laryngoscope*, **82**, 1609.

Illingworth, C. M. (1975) Pulled elbow: A study of 100 patients. *British Medical Journal*, **ii**, 672.

Ingpen, M. L. and Burry, H. C. (1970) A lumbo-sacral strain syndrome. *Annals of Physical Medicine*, **10**, 270.

Inman, V. T. (1966) The human foot. *Manitoba Medicine Reviews*, **46**, 513.

Inman, V. T. (1969) Foot, ankle influence on the proximal skeletal structures. *Artificial Limbs*, **13**, 1.

Inman, V. T. (1976) *The Joints of the Ankle*. Baltimore: Williams and Wilkins.

Inman, V. T. and Saunders, J. B. de C. M. (1944) Referred pain from skeletal structures. *Journal of Nervous and Mental Diseases*, **99**, 660.

Inman, V. T. and Saunders J. B. de C. M. (1947) Anatomico-physiological aspects of injuries to the intervertebral disc. *Journal of Bone and Joint Surgery*, **29**, 2.

Inman, V. T., Saunders, J. B. de C. M. and Abbot, L. C. (1944) Observations on the function of the shoulder joint. *Journal of Bone and Joint Surgery*, **26A**, 1.

Insall, J. and Salvati, E. (1971) Patella position in the normal knee joint. *Radiology*, **101**, 101.

Isdale, I.C. (1970) Hip disease in juvenile rheumatoid arthritis. *Annals of Rheumatic Disease*, **29**, 603.

Isdale, I. C. and Corrigan, B. (1970) Backward luxation of the atlas. *Annals of Rheumatic Disease*, **29**, 6.

Ito, R. (1971) The treatment of low back pain and sciatica with epidural corticosteroids injection and its pathophysiological basis. *Journal of the Japanese Orthopaedics Association*, **45**, 769.

Jackson, J. P. (1968) Degenerative changes in the knee after meniscectomy. *British Medical Journal*, **ii**, 525.

Jackson, R. (1965) *The Cervical Syndrome*. Springfield: Thomas.

Jackson, R. W. (1967) Headache associated with disorders of the cervical spine. *Headache*, **6**, 175.

Jackson, R. W. and Abe, I. (1972) The role of arthroscopy in the management of disorders of the knee. *Journal of Bone and Joint Surgery*, **54B**, 310.

Jacobs, B. and Wade, P. (1966) Acromio-clavicular joint injury: An end result study. *Journal of Bone and Joint Surgery*, **48A**, 475.

Jacobs, B., Krueger, E. G. and Leivy, D. M. (1970) Cervical spondylosis with radiculopathy. *Journal of the American Medical Association*, **211**, 2135.

Jacobsen, J. (1977) Stress radiographical measurements of post-traumatic knee instability. *Acta Orthopaedica Scandinavica*, **48**, 335.

Jacobson, B. (1938) *Progressive Relaxation*. University of Chicago Press.

James, S. L., Bates, B. T. and Osternig, L. R. (1978) Injuries to runners. *American Journal of Sports Medicine*, **6**, 40.

Jayson, M. I. V. and Dixon, A. St. J. (1970) Intra-articular pressure in rheumatoid arthritis of the knee. I. Pressure changes during passive joint distension. II. Pressure changes during joint use. *Annals of Rheumatic disease*, **29**, 261 and 401.

Johnson, J. T. H. (1959) Frozen shoulder syndrome in patients with pulmonary tuberculosis. *Journal of Bone and Joint Surgery*, **41A**, 877.

Johnson, J. T. H. (1967) Neuropathic fractures and joint injuries. *Journal of Bone and Joint Surgery*, **49A**.

Johnson, L. C., Stradford, H. T., Geis, R. W., Dineen, J. R. and Kerley, E. (1963) Histogenesis of stress fractures. *Journal of Bone and Joint Surgery*, **45A**, 1542.

Johnson, R. J., Kettelkamp, D. B., Clark, W. and Leaverton, P. (1974) Factors affecting late results after meniscectomy. *Journal of Bone and Joint Surgery*, **56A**, 719.

Jones, R. A. C. and Thompson, J. L. G. (1968) The narrow lumbar canal. *Journal of Bone and Joint Surgery*, **50B**, 595.

Jones, R. E., Smith, E. C. and Reisch, J. S. (1978) Effects of medical meniscectomy in patients older than forty. *Journal of Bone and Joint Surgery*, **60A**, 783.

Jowsey, J. (1966) Quantitative microradiography. *American Journal of Medicine*, **40**, 485.

Jowsey, J. and Riggs, B. L. (1972) Assessment of bone turnover by microradiography and autoradiography. *Seminars in Nuclear Medicine*, **2**, 3.

Jowsey, J., Riggs, B. L., Kelly, P. J. and Hoffman, D. L. (1972) Effect of combined therapy with sodium fluoride, vitamin D and calcium in osteoporosis. *American Journal of Medicine*, **53**, 43.

Junghanns, H. (1939) *Pathologic der Wirbelsaule*, Vol. 4, p. 280. Berlin:

Kabat, H. (1965) Proprioceptive facilitation in therapeutic exercise. In *Therapeutic Exercise*, pp. 327. Ed. Licht, A. B. Baltimore: Waverly Press.

Kalliomaki, J. L., Viitanen, S. M. and Virtama, P. (1968) Radiological findings of sternoclavicular joints in rheumatoid arthritis. *Acta Rheumatologica Scandinavica*, **14**, 233.

Kapandji, I. A. (1974) *The Physiology of Joints*, Vols. **1**, **2** and **3**. Edinburgh: Churchill-Livingstone.

Kaplan, H. and Brooke, M. H. (1971) Histochemical study of muscles in rheumatic disease. *Procedures of 16th Interim Scientific Session of the Arthritis and Rheumatism Association, Washington, D.C.*

Karlson, S. (1939) Chondromalacia patellae. *Acta Chirurgica Scandinavica*, **83**, 347.

Kattan, K. R. (1973) Modified view for use of Roentgen examination of the sternoclavicular joints. *Radiology*, **108**, 8.

Katzberg, R. W., Dolwick, M. F., Bales, D. J. and Helms, C. A. (1979) Arthrotomography of the temporo-mandibular joint: New technique and preliminary observations. *American Journal of Roentgenography*, **132**, 949.

Kaye, J. J. and Freiberger, R. H. (1975) Arthrography of the knee. *Clinical Orthopaedics and Related Research*, **107**, 73.

Keegan, J. (1953) Alterations of the lumbar curve related to posture and seating. *Journal of Bone and Joint Surgery*, **35A**, 589.

Kellgren, J. H. (1938) Observations on referred pain arising from muscle. *Clinical Science*, **3**, 175.

Kellgren, J. H. (1939). On distribution of pain arising from deep somatic structures with charts of segmental pain areas. *Clinical Science*, **4**, 35.

Kellgren, J. H. and Moore, R. (1952) Generalised osteoarthritis and Heberden's nodes. *British Medical Journal*, **i**, 181.

Kelly, M. (1956) Pain due to pressure on nerves? Spinal tumours and the intervertebral disc. *Neurology*, **6**, 32.

Kelsey, J. L. (1975) An epidemiological study of acute herniated lumbar intervertebral discs. *Rheumatology and Rehabilitation*, **14**, 144.

Kemp, H. B. S. (1973) Perthes' disease: An experimental and clinical study. *Annals of the Royal College of Surgeons*, **52**, 18.

Kendall, P. H. and Jenkins, J. M. (1968) Exercises for back ache. A double-blind controlled trial. *Physiotherapy*, **54**, 154.

Kennedy, B. (1965) A muscle bracing technique utilising intra-abdominal pressure to stabilise the lumbar spine. *Australian Journal of Physiology*, **11**, 102.

Kennedy, J. C. and Fowler, P. J. (1971) Medial and anterior instability of the knee. An anatomical and clinical study using stress machines. *Journal of Bone and Joint Surgery*, **53A**, 1257.

Kennedy, J. C., Weinberg, H. W. and Wilson, A. S. (1974) The anatomy and function of the anterior cruciate ligament. *Journal of Bone and Joint Surgery*, **56A**, 223.

Kerr, F. W. L. (1961) A mechanism to account for frontal headaches in cases of posterior fossa tumours. *Journal of Neurosurgery*, **26**, 168.

Kersley, G. D., Mandel, L., and Jeffrey, M. R. (1950) Gout: An unusual case with softening and subluxation of the first cervical vertebra and splenomegaly. *Annals of Rheumatic Disease*, **9**, 282.

Kessell, L. and Watson, M. (1977) The painful arc syndrome. Clinical classification as a guide to management. *Journal of Bone and Joint Surgery*, **59B**, 166.

Key, J. A. (1945) Intervertebral disc lesions and the most common cause of low back pain with or without sciatica. *Annals of Surgery*, **121**, 534.

Khalili, A. A. (1974) Neuromuscular electrodiagnostic studies in entrapment neuropathy of the suprascapular nerve. *Orthopaedic Reviews*, **3**, 27.

Khan, M. A., Kushner, I. and Braun, W. E. (1977) Comparison of clinical features in HLA B27 positive and negative patients with ankylosing spondylitis. *Arthritis and Rheumatism*, **20**, 909.

King, J. W., Bradsford, H. J. and Tullos, H. S. (1969) Epicondylitis and osteochondritis of the professional baseball pitcher's elbow. In *Symposium on Sports Medicine*, p. 75. St. Louis: Mosby.

Kirby, N. G. (1970) Exercise ischaemia in the fascial compartment of soleus. *Journal of Bone and Joint Surgery*, **52B**, 738.

Kirk, J. A., Ansell, B. M. and Bywaters, E. G. L. (1967) The hypermobility syndrome. *Annals of Rheumatic Disease*, **26**, 419.

Kirk, J. A. and Kersley, G. D. (1968) Heat and cold in the physical treatment of rheumatoid arthritis of the knee. *Annals of Physical Medicine*, **9**, 270.

Knutsson, B., Lindh, K. and Telhag, H. (1966) Sitting—an electromyographic and mechanical study. *Acta Orthopaedica Scandinavica*, **37**, 415.

Knuttson, F. (1944) The instability associated with disc degeneration in the lumbar spine. *Acta Radiologica*, **25**, 593.

Kopell, H. P., and Thompson, W. A. L. (1963) *Peripheral Entrapment Neuropathies*. Baltimore: Williams and Wilkins.

Kopp, S., Carlsson, G. E., Hansson, T. and Oberg, T. (1976) Degenerative disease of the temporomandibular, metatarso-phalangeal and sternoclavicular joints: An autopsy study. *Acta Odontologica Scandinavica*, **34**, 23.

Koskoff, Y. D., Morris, L. E. and Lubic, L. G. (1953) Paraplegia as a complication of gout. *Journal of the American Medical Association*, **152**, 37.

Kovacs, A. (1955) Subluxation and deformation of cervical apophyseal joints; Contribution to aetiology of headache. *Acta Radiologica, Stockholm*, **43**, 1.

Kraus, H. (1956) *Principles and Practice of Therapeutic Exercises*. Springfield: Thomas.

Kraus, H. and Raab, W. (1961) *Hypokinetic Diseases*. Springfield: Thomas.

Krogdahl, T. and Torgensen, O. (1940) Die unco-vertebral gelenke und die arthrosis deformans unco-vertebralis. *Acta Radiologica*, **21**, 231.

Kuhlendahl, H. and Hensell, V. (1958) Nil nocere. *Munchener Medizinische Wochenschrift*, **100**, 1738.

Kuczynski, K. (1971) The synovial structure of the normal and rheumatoid digital joints. *The Hand*, **3**, 1.

Laban, M. M. and Meerschaert, J. R. (1975) Lumbosacral–anterior pelvic pain associated with pubic symphysis instability. *Archives of Physical Medicine and Rehabilitation*, **56**, 54B.

Lachmann, E. (1955) Osteoporosis: the potentialities and limitations of its roentgenologic diagnosis. *American Journal of Radiology*, **74**, 712.

Lagier, R. and Sitaj, S. (1974) Vertebral changes in ochronosis. *Annals of Rheumatic Disease*, **331**, 86.

Ladley, G. (1971) An investigation into the effectiveness of various forms of quadriceps exercise. *Physiotherapy*, **57**, 356.

Laing, D. R., Dailey, D. R. and Kirk, J. A. (1973) Ice therapy in soft tissue injuries. *New Zealand Medical Journal*, **78**, 155.

Lance, J. W. (1982) *Mechanism and Management of Headache*, 4th Edn. London: Butterworth.

Landon, J. and Malpas, J. S. (1959) Tietze's syndrome. *Annals of Rheumatic Disease*, **18**, 249.

Landsmeer, J. M. F. (1949) The anatomy of the dorsal aponeurosis of the human finger and its functional significance. *Anatomical Records*, **104**, 131.

Landsmeer, J. M. F. (1955) Anatomical and functional investigations of the articulation of the human finger. *Acta Anatomica*, **25**, Suppl. **24**.

Landsmeer, J. M. F. (1962) Power grip and precision holding. *Annals of Rheumatic Disease*, **21**, 164.

Langfitt, T. W. and Elliott, F. A. (1967) Pain in the back and legs caused by cervical spinal cord compression. *Journal of the American Medical Association*, **200**, 382.

La Rocca, H. and Macnab, I. (1969) Value of pre-employment radiographic assessment of the lumbar spine. *Canadian Medical Association Journal*, **101**, 383.

Laruelle, L. L. (1940) Les bases anatomiques du systeme autonome corticol et bulbo-spinal. *Revue Neurologie*, **72**, 349.

Lasègue (1864) Consideration sur la sciatique. *Archives of General Medicine*, **2**, 558.

Laskar, F. H. and Sargison, K. D. (1970) Ochronotic arthropathy. A review with four case reports. *Journal of Bone and Joint Surgery*, **52B**, 653.

Last, R. J. (1978) *Anatomy: Regional and Applied*, 6th Edn. Edinburgh: Churchill-Livingstone.

Lawrence, J. S. (1963) The prevalence of arthritis. *British Journal of Clinical Practice*, **17**, 699.

Lawrence, J. S. (1968) *Population Studies of the Rheumatic Diseases*. Amsterdam: Excerpta Medica.

Lea, E. B. and Smith, L. (1972) Non-surgical treatment of tendo achilles rupture. *Journal of Bone and Joint Surgery*, **54A**, 1398.

Leabhart, J. W. (1959) Stress fractures of the calcaneus. *Journal of Bone and Joint Surgery*, **41A**, 1285.

Leeming, J. T. (1973) Skeletal disease in the elderly. *British Medical Journal*, **iv**, 472.

Lees, F. and Turner, J. W. A. (1963) Natural history and prognosis of cervical spondylosis. *British Medical Journal*, **ii**, 1607.

Lelievre, J. (1970) Current concepts and correction in the valgus foot. *Clinical Orthopaedics and Related Research*, **70**, 43.

Lesquesne, M. (1967) *Diseases of the Hip in Adult Life*. Folia Rheumatologica. Basel: Geigy.

Lesquesne, M. and Forestier, F. (1961) La coxite primitive. *Vie Medicine*, **42**, 1679.

Lettin, A. W. F. (1967) Diagnosis and treatment of lumbar instability. *Journal of Bone and Joint Surgery*, **49B**, 520.

Leventhal, G. H. and Dorfman, H. D. (1974) Aseptic necrosis of bone in systemic lupus erythematosus. *Seminars in Arthritis and Rheumatism*, **4**, 73.

Levey, G. S. and Calabro, J. J. (1962) Tietze's syndrome. *Arthritis and Rheumatism*, **5**, 261.

Levy, L. F. (1967) Lumbar intervertebral disc disease in Africans. *Journal of Neurosurgery*, **26**, 31.

Lichtenstein, L., Scott, H. W. and Levin, M. H. (1956) Pathologic changes in gout—Survey of eleven necropsied cases. *American Journal of Pathology*, **32**, 871.

Lieou, Y.-C. (1928). *Syndrome Sympathique Cervical Postérieur et Arthrité Chromique de la Colonne Vertébrale Cervicale*. Strasbourg: Schuler and Mink.

Lievre, J. A., Bloch-Michel, H. and Attali, P. (1953) L'injection trans-sacrée. Etude clinique et radiolique. *Bull. Soc. Med Hop. Paris*, **73**, 1110.

Lindahl, O. (1966) Hyperalgesia of lumbar nerve roots in sciatica. *Acta Orthopaedica Scandinavica*, **37**, 367.

Lindahl, O. and Rexed, B. (1951) Histologic changes in spinal nerve roots of operated cases of sciatica. *Acta Orthopaedica Scandinavica*, **20**, 215.

Lindberg, T. (1963) Intervertebral calcinosis in childhood. *Annals of Paediatrics*, **201**, 172.

Lindblom, K. (1939) On pathogenesis of ruptures in the tendon aponeurosis of the shoulder joint. *Acta Radiologica*, **20**, 563.

Lindblom, K. (1948) Diagnostic puncture of intervertebral discs in sciatica. *Acta Orthopaedica Scandinavica*, **17**, 231.

Lindblom, K. and Rexed, B. (1948) Lumbar discs. *Journal of Neurosurgery*, **5**, 413.

Lindeman, S. H. (1885) Partial dislocation of the radial head peculiar to children. *British Medical Journal*, **ii**, 1058.

Lindstrom, A. and Zachrisson, M. (1970) Physical therapy on low back pain and sciatica. An attempt at evaluation. *Scandinavian Journal of Rehabilitation and Medicine*, **2**, 37.

Linscheid, R. L., Dobyns, J. H., Beabout, J. W. and Bryon, R. S. (1972) Traumatic instability of the wrist: Diagnosis, classification and pathomechanics. *Journal of Bone and Joint Surgery*, **54A**, 1612.

Livingston, M. C. P. (1971) Spinal manipulation causing injury. A three year study. *Clinical Orthopaedics and Related Research*, **81**, 820.

López-Ibor, J. J. (1972) Marked depression. *British Journal of Psychiatry*, **120**, 245.

Lotke, P. A. (1970) Ossification of the Achilles tendon. *Journal of Bone and Joint Surgery*, **52A**, 157.

Love, J. G. (1955) *Clinical Neurology*, Vol. **2**, p. 1398. New York: Hoeber-Harper.

Love, J. G. and Schorn, V. G. (1965) Thoracic intervertebral disc protrusion. *Journal of the American Medical Association*, **191**, 627.

Love, J. G. and Emmett, J. L. (1967) Asymptomatic protruded lumbar disc as a cause of urinary retention. *Proceedings of the Mayo Clinic*, **42**, 249.

Lucas, D. B. (1973) Biomechanics of the shoulder joint. *Archives of Surgery*, **107**, 425.

Lundquist, R. (1968) Subcutaneous partial rupture of Achilles tendon. *Acta Orthopaedica Scandinavica Supplement*, **113**.

McCarty, D. J. (1978) In *Arthritis and Allied Conditions*, 9th Edn. Philadelphia: Lea and Febiger.

McDougall, A. (1955) The os trigonum. *Journal of Bone and Joint Surgery*, **37B**, 257.

McEwen, C., Ditata, D., Lingg, C., Porini, A., Good, A. and Rankin, T. (1971) Ankylosing spondylitis and spondylitis accompanying ulcerative colitis, regional arteritis, psoriasis and Reiter's disease. *Arthritis and Rheumatism*, **14**, 291.

McGinty, J. B., Geuss, L. F. and Marvin, R. A. (1977) Partial or total meniscectomy? *Journal of Bone and Joint Surgery*, **59A**, 763.

McKibbin, B. and Ralis, Z. (1974) Pathological changes in a case of Perthes' disease. *Journal of Bone and Joint Surgery*, **56B**, 438.

McMurray, T. P. (1942) The semilunar cartilage. *British Journal of Surgery*, **29**, 407.

McMurray, T. P. (1950) Footballer's ankle. *Journal of Bone and Joint Surgery*, **32B**, 68.

Macnab, J. (1964) Acceleration injuries of the cervical spine. *Journal of Bone and Joint Surgery*, **46A**, 1797.

Macnab, I. (1969) Pathogenesis of symptoms in discogenic low back pain. *Proceedings of the A.A.O.S. Symposium on the Spine*. St. Louis: Mosby.

Macnab, I. (1971) The traction spur an indicator of segmental instability. *Journal of Bone and Joint Surgery*, **53A**, 663.

Macnab, I. (1973a) Management of low back pain. *Current Practice in Orthopaedic Surgery*, **5**, 241.

Macnab, I. (1973b) Rotator cuff tendinitis. *Annals of the Royal College of Surgeons of England*, **53**, 271.

McRae, D. L. (1956) Asymptomatic intervertebral disc protrusions. *Acta Radiologica*, **46**, 9.

Magill, H. K. and Aitken, A. P. (1954) Pulled elbow. *Surgery, Gynecology and Obstetrics*, **98**, 753.

Maigne, R. (1972). *Orthopaedic Medicine*. Springfield: Thomas.

Mair, W. G. P. and Druckman, R. (1953) The pathology of spinal cord lesions and their relation to the clinical factors in protrusion of cervical intervertebral discs. *Brain*, **76**, 70.

Maitland, G. D. (1973) *The Vertebral Column. Examination and Recording Guide*, 3rd Edn. Adelaide: Virgo Press.

Maitland, G. D. (1976). *Peripheral Manipulation*, 4th Edn. London: Butterworths.

Maitland, G. D. (1977). *Spinal Manipulation*, 2nd Edn.. London: Butterworths.

Maitland, G. D. (1979) *Musculo-skeletal Examination and Recording Guide*. Adelaide: Lauderdale Press.

Malawista, S. E., Seegmiller, J. E., Hathaway, B. E. and Sokoloff, L. (1965) Sacro-iliac gout. *Journal of the American Medical Association*, **194**, 954.

Malgaigne, J. F. (1847) *Traité des Fractures et des Luxations*. Paris: Baillière.

Mankin, H. J. (1975) Biochemical and metabolic abnormalities in degenerative arthritis. In *Surgical Management of Degenerative Arthritis of the Lower Limbs*. Philadelphia: Lea and Febiger.

Marbach, J. J. (1977) Arthritis of the temporo-mandibular joints and facial pain. *Bulletin of Rheumatic Diseases*, **27**, 918.

Marks, J. S. and Hardinge, K. (1979) Clinical and radiological features of spondylitic hip disease. *Annals of Rheumatic Disease*, **38**, 332.

Marshall, L. L. and Trethewie, E. R. (1973) Letter. *Lancet*, **ii**, 320.

Martel, W. (1968) Cervical spondylitis in rheumatoid disease. *American Journal of Medicine*, **44**, 441.

Martel, W. (1977) Pathogenesis of cervical discovertebral destruction in rheumatoid arthritis. *Arthritis and Rheumatism*, **20**, 1217.

Martel, W., Hayes, J. T. and Duff, I. F. (1965) The pattern of bone erosions in the hand and wrist in rheumatoid arthritis. *Radiology*, **84**, 204.

Maquet, P. G. J. (1976) *Biomechanics of the Knee*. Berlin: Springer-Verlag.

Mason, R. M., Murray, R. S., Oates, J. K. and Young, A. C. (1958) Prostatitis and ankylosing spondylitis. *British Medical Journal*, **i**, 748.

Matheson, A. T. (1960) Cauda equina syndrome. *British Medical Journal*, **i**, 570.

Matheson, A. T. (1966) The rarity of lumbar disc protrusion in the Rhodesian bantu. *Journal of Bone and Joint Surgery*, **48B**, 398.

Matthews, B. F. (1952) Collagen/chondroitin sulphate ratio of human articular cartilage related to function. *British Medical Journal*, **ii**, 1295.

Mathews, J. A. (1968) Dynamic discography: A study of lumbar traction. *Annals of Physical Medicine*, **7**, 275.

Mathews, J. A. (1974) Atlanto-axial subluxation in rheumatoid arthritis. A five year follow-up study *Annals of Rheumatic Disease*, **33**, 526.

Mathews, J. A. and Hickling, J. (1975) Lumbar traction—a double-blind control study. *Rheumatology and Rehabilitation*, **14**, 222.

Mathews, J. A. and Yates, D. A. H. (1969) Reduction of lumbar disc prolapse by manipulation. *British Medical Journal*, **iii**, 696.

Mattingly, S. (1968) Pain in the shoulder. *Annals of Physical Medicine*, **5**, 266.

Matsen, F. and Clawson, D. K. (1975) The deep posterior compartmental syndrome of the leg. *Journal of Bone and Joint Surgery*, **57A**, 34.

Maurer, R. C. and Larsen, I. J. (1970) Acute necrosis of cartilage in slipped femoral epiphysis. *Journal of Bone and Joint Surgery*, **52A**, 39.

Mayfield, F. H. (Ed.) (1954) *Symposium on Cervical Trauma*. *Clinical Neurosurgery*. New York.

Mayfield, G. W. (1977) Popliteus tendon tenosynovitis.

American Journal of Sports Medicine, **5**, 31.

Medical Journal of Australia (1971) The treatment of osteoporosis. *Medical Journal of Australia*, **ii**, 1156.

Medlar, R. C., Mandiberg, J. J. and Lyne, E. D. (1979) *The Long Term Follow-Up of Meniscectomies in Children*. San Francisco: American Orthotic Society for Sports Medicine.

Melzack, R. and Wall, P. D. (1965) Pain mechanisms: A new theory. *Science*, **150**, 971.

Mennell, J. McM. (1955) Manipulation and the treatment of low back pain. *Clinical Orthopaedics and Related Research*, **5**, 82.

Mensor, M. C. and Duvall, G. (1959) Absence of motion at the 4th and 5th lumbar interspaces in patients with and without low back pain. *Journal of Bone and Joint Surgery*, **41A**, 1047.

Michele, A. A. (1958) The flip sign in sciatic nerve tension. *Surgery*, **44**, 940.

Michele, A. A. (1963) *Ilio-psoas Development of Anomalies in Man*. Springfield: Thomas.

Michele, A. A., Davies, J. J., Grueger, F. J. and Lichtor, J. M. (1950) Scapulocostal syndrome (fatigue–postural paradox). *New York State Journal of Medicine*, **50**, 1353.

Miller, J. E. (1960) Javelin thrower's elbow. *Journal of Bone and Joint Surgery*, **42B**, 788.

Mills, G. P. (1928) Treatment of tennis elbow. *British Medical Journal*, **i**, 12.

Mitchell, P. E., Hendry, N. G. and Billewica, W. Z. (1961) Clinical background of intervertebral disc prolapse. *Journal of Bone and Joint Surgery*, **41B**, 237.

Mixter, W. J. and Barr, J. S. (1934) Rupture of intervertebral disc with involvement of spinal canal. *New England Journal of Medicine*, **211**, 210.

Moll, J. M. H. and Wright, V. (1971) Normal range of spinal mobility. *Annals of Rheumatic Disease*, **30**, 381.

Mooney, V. and Robertson, J. (1976) The facet syndrome. *Clinical Orthopaedics and Related Research*, **115**, 149.

Moore, M. (1952) Radiohumeral synovitis. *Archives of Surgery*, **64**, 501.

Morag, B. and Shahin, N. (1975) The value of tomography of the sternoclavicular region. *Clinical Radiology*, **26**, 57.

Morgan, F. P. and King, T. (1957) Primary instability of lumbar vertebrae as a common cause of low back pain. *Journal of Bone and Joint Surgery*, **39B**, 6.

Morris, H. (1882) Rider's sprain. *Lancet*, **ii**, 557.

Morris, J. M., Lucas D. B. and Bresler, B. (1961) Role of the trunk in stability of the spine. *Journal of Bone and Joint Surgery*, **43A**, 327.

Morris, L. H. (1943) Athlete's ankle. *Journal of Bone and Joint Surgery*, **25**, 220.

Morton, D. J. (1935) *The Human Foot. Its Evolution, Physiology and Functional Disorders*. New York: Columbia University Press.

Morton, T. G. (1876) Peculiar painful affliction of fourth metatarso-phalangeal articulation. *American Journal of Medical Science*, **71**, 37.

Moseley, H. F. and Goldie, I. (1963) The arterial pattern of the rotator cuff of the shoulder. *Journal of Bone and Joint Surgery*, **48B**, 780.

Muckle, D. S. (1973) Dislocation of the superior tibio-fibular joint—an unusual soccer injury. *British Journal of Sports Medicine*, **vii**, 365.

Muckle, D. S. (1980) A double blind trial of ibuprofen and aspirin in the treatment of soft itssue injuries sustained in professional football. *British Journal of Sports Medicine*, **14**, 46.

Mueller, S. and Sahs, A. L. (1976) Brain stem dysfunction related to cervical manipulation. *Neurology*, **26**, 547.

Murray, R. O. (1965) The aetiology of primary osteoarthritis of the hip. *British Journal of Radiology*, **38**, 810.

Murray, R. O. and Jacobson, H. G. (1971) *Radiology of Skeletal Disorders*. Edinburgh: Livingstone.

Murray-Leslie, C. and Wright, V. (1976) Radiological and clinical relationship between idiopathic carpal tunnel syndrome, humeral epicondylitis and cervical spine changes. *Annals of Rheumatic Disease*, **35**, 545.

Murtagh, J. E. (1978) Tennis elbow: Description and treatment. *Australian Family Medicine*, **7**, 1307.

Nachemson, A. (1960) Lumbar intradiscal pressure; experimental studies on post-mortem material. *Acta Orthopaedica Scandinavica Supplement*, **43**, 1.

Nachemson, A. (1966) Electromyographic studies on the vertebral portion of the psoas muscle. *Acta Orthopaedica Scandinavica*, **37**, 177.

Nachemson, A. (1975) Towards a better understanding of low back pain. A review of the mechanics of the lumbar disc. *Rheumatism and Rehabilitation*, **14**, 129.

Nachemson, A. and Morris, J. M. (1964) *In vivo* measurements of intradiscal pressure: Discometry, a method for determination of pressure in the lower lumbar discs. *Journal of Bone and Joint Surgery*, **46A**, 1077.

Nakazawa, K. and Takahashi, S. (1974) Analysis of the mandibular movements in temporomandibular joint disorders. *Bulletin of the Tokyo Dental College*, **15**, 143.

Nalebuff, E. A. (1969) Hand surgery and the rheumatoid patient. *Surgical Clinics of North America*, **49**, 787.

Napier, J. R. (1956) The prehensile movements of the human hand. *Journal of Bone and Joint Surgery*, **38B**, 902.

Nathan, H. (1962) Osteophytes of the vertebral column. *Journal of Bone and Joint Surgery*, **44A**, 243.

Nathan, H., Weinberg, H., Robin, G. C. and Aviad, I. (1964) Costovertebral joints. *Arthritis and Rheumatism*, **7**, 228.

Naylor, A. (1971) The biochemical changes in the human intervertebral disc in degeneration and nuclear prolapse. *Orthopedic Clinics of North America*, **2**, 2.

Naylor, A. (1974) The late results of laminectomy for lumbar disc prolapse. *Journal of Bone and Joint Surgery*, **56B**, 17.

Naylor, A. and Shentall, R. (1976) Biochemical aspects of intervertebral discs, in ageing and disease. In *The Lumbar Spine and Back Pain*, p. 317. Ed. Jayson, M. London: Sector Publishing.

Neer, C. S. (1972) Anterior acromioplasty for chronic impingement syndrome in the shoulder. *Journal of Bone and Joint Surgery*, **54A**, 41.

Neuwirth, E. (1952) Headaches and facial pains in cervical discopathy. *Annals of Internal Medicine*, **37**, 75.

Neviaser, J. S. (1945) Adhesive capsulitis of the shoulder. *Journal of Bone and Joint Surgery*, **27**, 211.

Newman, J. H. and Goodfellow, J. W. (1975) Fibrillation of head of radius as one cause of tennis elbow. *British Medical Journal*, **ii**, 328.

Newman, P. H. (1963) The etiology of spondylolisthesis. *Journal of Bone and Joint Surgery*, **45B**, 39.

Newman, P. H. (1968) The spine, the wood and the trees. *Proceedings of the Royal Society of Medicine*, **61**, 35.

Newman, P. H. (1973) Surgical treatment for derangement of the lumbar spine. *Journal of Bone and Joint Surgery*, **55B**, 7.

Newman, P. H. (1974) Spondylolisthesis. *Physiotherapy*, **60**, 14.

Newman, P. H. and Sweetnam, R. (1969) Occipito-cervical fusion. An operative technique and its indications. *Journal of Bone and Joint Surgery*, **51B**, 423.

Newton-John, H. F. and Morgan, D. B. (1968) Osteoporosis: Disease or senescence? *Lancet*, **i**, 232.

Nicholas, J. A. (1970) Injuries to the knee ligaments. Relationship to looseness and tightness in football players. *Journal of the American Medical Association*, **212**, 2236.

Nicholas, J. A. (1973) The five–one reconstruction for anteromedial instability of the knee. *Journal of Bone and Joint Surgery*, **55A**, 899.

Nicholas, J. A., Freiberger, R. H. and Killorian, P. J. (1970) Double contrast arthrography of the knee—its value in the management of 225 knee derangements. *Journal of Bone and Joint Surgery*, **52A**, 203.

Nicholas, J. A., Strizak, A. M. and Veras, G. J. (1976) A study of thigh muscle weakness in different pathological states of the lower extremity. *American Journal of Sports Medicine*, **4**, 241.

Nichols, P. J. R. (1960) Short-leg syndrome. *British Medical Journal*, **i**, 1863.

Nicoll, E. A. (1954) Miners and mannequins. *Journal of Bone and Joint Surgery*, **36B**, 171.

Noble, C. A. (1979) The treatment of iliotibial band friction syndrome. *British Journal of Sports Medicine*, **13**, 51.

Norman, G. F. (1968) Sacro-iliac disease and its relationship to lower abdominal pain. *American Journal of Surgery*, **116**, 54.

Norman, J. E. de B. (1975) Temporomandibular joint disorders: Diagnosis and treatment. *Medical Journal of Australia*, **ii**, 679.

Norris, C. W. and Eakins, K. (1974) Temporomandibular joint syndrome. *Laryngoscope*, **84**, 1466.

Norwood, L. A. and Cross, M. J. (1979) Anterior cruciate ligament: Functional anatomy of its bundles in rotary instabilities. *American Journal of Sports Medicine*, **7**, 23.

O'Donoghue, D. H. (1973a) Subluxating biceps tendon in the athlete. *Journal of Sports Medicine*, **1**, 20.

O'Donoghue, D. H. (1973b) Treatment of acute ligamentous injuries of the knee. *Orthopedic Clinics of North America*, **4**, 7.

O'Donoghue, D. H. (1984) *Treatment of Injuries to Athletes*. 4th edn. W. B. Saunders Co., Philadelphia.

Ollie, J. A. (1937) Differential diagnosis of pain in the chest. *Canadian Medical Association Journal*, **37**, 209.

Orova, S. (1978) Ilio-tibial band friction syndrome in athletes. *British Journal of Sports Medicine*, **12**, 69.

Orava, S. and Puranen, J. (1979) Athletes' leg pains. *British Journal of Sports Medicine*, **13**, 92.

Osgood, R. (1922) Radiohumeral bursitis, epicondylitis, epicondylalgia (tennis elbow). *Archives of Surgery*, **4**, 420.

Ottosson, L. (1978) Lateral instability of the ankle treated by a modified Evans procedure. *Acta Orthopaedica Scandinavica*, **49**, 302.

Outerbridge, R. E. (1964) Further studies on the etiology of chondromalacia patellae. *Journal of Bone and Joint Surgery*, **46B**, 179.

Outerbridge, R. E. and Dunlop, J. (1975) The problem of chondromalacia patellae. *Clinical Orthopedics of North America*, **110**, 177.

Paget, J. (1867) Cases that bonesetters cure. *British Medical Journal*, **i**, 1.

Paine, K. W. E. and Huang, P. W. H. (1972) Lumbar disc syndrome. *Journal of Neurosurgery*, **37**, 75.

Palmer, I. (1938) Injuries to the ligaments of the knee joint. *Acta Chirurgica Scandinavica Supplement*, **53**.

Pang, L. Q. (1971) Otological aspects of whiplash injuries. *Laryngoscope*, **81**, 1381.

Parker, G. B., Tupling, H. and Pryor, D. S. (1978) A controlled trial of cervical manipulation for migraine. *Australian and New Zealand Journal of Medicine*, **8**, 589.

Pauwels, F. (1973) *Atlas zur Biomechanik der Gesunden und Kranken Hufte*. Berlin: Springer.

Patrick, H. T. (1918) Rheumatic headache. *Journal of the American Medical Association*, **71**, 82.

Pearson, J. R. and Riddell, D. M. (1962) Idiopathic osteoarthritis of the hip. *Annals of Rheumatic Disease*, **21**, 31.

Pederson, O. F., Petersen, R. and Staffeldt, E. S. (1975) Back pain and isometric back muscle strength of workers in a Danish factory. *Scandinavian Journal of Rehabilitation Medicine*, **7**, 125.

Percy, E. C., Hill, R. D. and Callaghan, J. E. (1969) The sprained ankle. *Journal of Trauma*, **9**, 972.

Peter, J. B., Pearson, C. M. and Marmor, L. (1966) Erosive osteoarthritis of the hands. *Arthritis and Rheumatism*, **9**, 365.

Phalen, G. S. (1966) The carpal tunnel syndrome: 17 years experience in diagnosis and treatment of 654 hands. *Journal of Bone and Joint Surgery*, **48A**, 211.

Piggott, H. (1960) The natural history of hallux valgus in adolescence and early adult life. *Journal of Bone and Joint Surgery*, **42B**, 749.

Pipes, T. V. and Wilmore, H. H. (1975) Isokinetic *vs.* isotonic strength training in adult men. *Medical Science in Sports*, **7**, 262.

Plagenhoef, S. (1971) *Patterns of Human Motion. A. Cinematographic Analysis*. New Jersey: Prentice-Hall.

Plewes, L. W. (1956) Emergencies in general practice: Common dislocations. *British Medical Journal*, **i**, 1227.

Polley, H. F. and Hunder, G. G. (1978) *Rheumatological Interviewing and Physical Examination of the Joints*. Philadelphia: W. B. Saunders.

Poppen, N. K. and Walker, P. S. (1976) Normal and abnormal motion of the shoulder. *Journal of Bone and Joint Surgery*, **58A**, 195.

Posch, J. L. and Marcotte, D. R. (1976) Carpal tunnel syndrome: A review of 1201 cases. *Orthopaedic Reviews*, **5**, 25.

Post, M. (1978) *The Shoulder: Surgical and Non-surgical Management*. Philadelphia: Lea and Febiger.

Powers, S. R., Drislane, T. M. and Iandoli, E. W. (1963) The surgical treatment of vertebral artery insufficiency. *Archives of Surgery*, **86**, 60.

Pratt-Thomas, H. R. and Berger, K. E. (1947) Cerebellar and spinal injuries after chiropractic manipulation. *Journal of the American Medical Association*, **133**, 600.

Price, C. T. and Allen, W. C. (1978) Ligament repair in the knee with preservation of the meniscus. *Journal of Bone and Joint Surgery*, **60A**, 61.

Pringle, R. M., Protheroe, K. and Mukherjee, S. K. (1974) Entrapment neuropathy of the sural nerve. *Journal of Bone and Joint Surgery*, **56B**, 465.

Puranen, J. (1974) The medial tibial syndrome. *Journal of Bone and Joint Surgery*, **56B**, 712.

Radin, E. L. (1973) Biomechanics of the knee joint. *Orthopedic Clinics of North America*, **4**, 539.

Radin, E. L. and Paul, I. L. (1971) Importance of bone in sparing articular cartilage from contact. *Clinical Orthopaedics and Related Research*, **78**, 342.

Rassmussen, H. and Bordier, P. (1973) The cellular basis of metabolic bone disease. *New England Journal of Medicine*, **289**, 25.

Rathbun, J. B. and Macnab, I. (1970) The microvascular pattern of the rotator cuff. *Journal of Bone and Joint Surgery*, **52B**, 540.

Reeves, B. (1966) Arthrographic changes in frozen and post-traumatic stiff shoulders. *Proceedings of the Royal Society of Medicine*, **59**, 827.

Reginato, A. J., Schumacher, H. R., Jiminez, S. and Mauer, K. (1979) Synovitis in secondary syphilis. *Arthritis and Rheumatism*, **22**, 170.

Reneman, R. S. (1975) The anterior and the lateral compartment syndrome of the leg due to intensive use of muscles. *Clinical Orthopaedics and Related Research*, **113**, 69.

Resnick, D. (1976) Rheumatoid arthritis of the wrist. *Medical Radiology and Photography*, **52**, 50.

Resnick, D. and Niwayama, G. (1976) Radiographic and pathologic features of spinal involvement in diffuse idiopathic skeletal hyperostosis (DISH). *Radiology*, **119**, 559.

Resnick, D., Niwayama, G. and Georgen, T. G. (1975) Degenerative disease of the sacro-iliac joint. *Investigative Radiology*, **10**, 608.

Resnick, D., Niwayama, G. and Goergen, T. G. (1977) Clinical, radiographic and pathologic abnormalities in calcium pyrophosphate dihydrate deposition disease (CPPD): An analysis of 85 patients. *Radiology*, **122**, 1.

Resnick, D., Niwayama, G. and Goergen, T. G. (1977) Comparison of radiographic abnormalities of the sacro-iliac joint in degenerative disease and ankylosing spondylitis. *American Journal of Roentgenology*, **128**, 189.

Richardson, A. T. (1975) The painful shoulder. *Proceedings of the Royal Society Medicine*, **68**, 731.

Ricklin, P., Ruttmann, A. and Del Buono, M. S. (1971) *Meniscus Lesions: Practical Problems of Clinical Diagnosis: Arthrography and Therapy*. New York: Grune and Stratton.

Rinaldi, R. R. and Sabia, M. L. (1978) *Sports Medicine '78*. New York: Futura Publishing.

Ritchie, G. W. and Keim, H. A. (1964) A radiographic analysis of major foot disabilities. *Canadian Medical Association Journal*, **91**, 840.

Rockwood, C. A. and Eilert, R. E. (1969) Camptocormia. *Journal of Bone and Joint Surgery*, **51A**, 553.

Robbins, H. (1963) Anatomical study of the median nerve in the carpal tunnel and etiologies of the carpal tunnel syndrome. *Journal of Bone and Joint Surgery*, **45A**, 953.

Robichorv, J., Desjardins, J. P., Koch, M. and Hooper, C. E. (1974) The femoral neck in Legg–Perthes' disease. *Journal of Bone and Joint Surgery*, **56B**, 62.

Robillard, R., Gagnon, P. A. and Alarie, R. (1964) Diabetic neuroarthropathy. *Canadian Medical Association Journal*, **91**, 795.

Robinson, A. R. and Darracott, J. (1970) Chondromalacia patellae. *Annals of Physical Medicine*, **10**, 286.

Roles, N. C. and Maudesley, R. H. (1972) Radial tunnel syndrome: Resistant tennis elbow as a nerve entrapment. *Journal of Bone and Joint Surgery*, **54B**, 499.

Romanus, R. (1953) Pelvo-spondylitis ossificans in the male (ankylosing spondylitis) and genito-urinary infection: Study of 117 male patients. *Acta Medica Scandinavica*, **145**, Suppl. **280**.

Romanus, R. and Yden, S. (1955) *Pelvospondylitis Ossificans*. Copenhagen: Munksgaard.

Root, M. L., Orien, W. P., Weed, J. H. and Hughes, R. J. (1971) *Biomechanical Examination of the Foot*. Los Angeles: Clinical Biomechanics Corporation.

Rosati, L. M. and Lord, J. W. (1961) *Neurovascular*

Compression Syndromes of the Shoulder Girdle. New York: Grune and Stratton.

Rose, G. K. (1951) The painful heel. *British Medical Journal*, **ii**, 831.

Rose, G. K. (1962) Correction of the pronated foot. *Journal of Bone and Joint Surgery*, **44B**, 642.

Rosenhorn, M. and Pedersen, B. E. (1974) The significance of the coraco-clavicular ligament in experimental dislocation of the acrimio-clavicular joint. *Acta Orthopaedica Scandinavica*, **45**, 346.

Roub, L. W., Gumerman, L. A., Hanley, E. N., Clark, M. W., Goodman, M. and Herbert, D. L. (1979) Bone stress: A radionuclide imaging perspective. *Radiology*, **132**, 431.

Roydhouse, R. H. (1973) Whiplash and temporomandibular dysfunction. *Lancet*, **i**, 1394.

Ryan, G. M. S. and Cope S. (1955) Cervical vertigo. *Lancet*, **ii**, 1355.

Rydell, N. W. (1966) Forces acting on the femoral head prosthesis. A study of strain gauge supplied prosthesis in living persons. *Acta Orthopaedica Scandinavica, Supplement*, **88**.

Sachs, B. and Fraenkel, I. (1900) Progressive ankylotic rigidity of the spine. *Journal of Nervous and Mental Diseases*, **27**, 1.

St. Jacques, O. R. and Laurin, C. A. (1965) Normal variation of the talar tilt of the ankle in children. *Canadian Medical Association Journal*, **93**, 695.

Salter, R. B. (1973) The scientific basis for innominate osteotomy in the treatment of Legg–Perthes' disease. *Journal of Bone and Joint Surgery*, **55B**, 216.

Salter, R. B. and Zaltz, C. (1971) Anatomic investigation of the mechanism of injury and pathologic anatomy of 'pulled elbow' in young children. *Clinical Orthopaedics and Related Research*, **77**, 134.

Salter, R. B., Gross, A. and Hall, J. H. (1967) Hydrocortisone arthropathy. An experimental investigation. *Canadian Medical Association Journal*, **92**, 374.

Samilson, R. L. and Binder, W. F. (1975) Symptomatic full-thickness tears of the rotator cuff. *Orthopedic Clinics of North America*, **6**, 449.

Sashin, D. (1930) A critical analysis of the anatomy and pathological changes of the sacro-iliac joints. *Journal of Bone and Joint Surgery*, **12**, 891.

Saville, P. D. (1970) Observations on 80 women with osteoporotic spine fractures. In *Osteoporosis* New York: Grune and Stratton.

Scham, S. S. (1974) Manipulation of the lumbo-sacral spine. *Clinical Orthopaedics and Related Research*, **101**, 146.

Schatzker, J. and Dennal, G. F. (1968) Spinal stenosis, a cause of cauda equina compression. *Journal of Bone and Joint Surgery*, **50B**, 606.

Scheuermann, H. (1921) Kyphosis dorsalis juvenalis. *Orthopaedica Chirurgica*, **41**, 305.

Schmorl, G. (1930) Die Pathegenese der Juvenilen kyphose. *Fortchr. Geb. Rontgen*, **41**, 359.

Schmorl, G. and Junghanns, H. (1971) *The Human Spine in Health and Disease*. Translated by Besemann, E-F. London: Grune and Stratton.

Schwartz, L. and Chayes, C. M. (1966) In *Symposium on Temporomandibular Joint*. Dental Clinics of North America. Philadelphia: Saunders.

Seager, K., Bashir, H. V., Geczy, A. F., Edmonds, J. and De Vere-Tyndall, A. (1979) Evidence for a specific B27-associated cell surface marker on lymphocytes of patients with ankylosing spondylitis. *Nature (London)*, **277**, 68.

Seghal, A. D., Tweed, D. C. and Gardner, W. J. (1961) Laboratory studies after intrathecal corticosteroid. *Archives of Neurology*, **9**, 64.

Sever, J. W. (1912) Apophysitis of the os calcis. *New York State Journal of Medicine*, **95**, 1025.

Sgarlato, T. E. (1965) The angle of gait. *Journal of the American Podiatry Association*, **55**, 645.

Shah, J. S., Hampson, W. G. J. and Jayson, M. I. V. (1978) The distribution of surface strain in the cadaveric lumbar spine. *Journal of Bone and Joint Surgery*, **60B**, 246.

Shapiro, J. S. (1970) A new factor in the etiology of ulnar drift. *Clinical Orthopaedics and Related Research*, **68**, 32.

Sharp, J. (1954) Heredo-familial vascular and articular calcification. *Annals of Rheumatic Disease*, **13**, 15.

Sharrard, W. J. W. (1976) Knock knees and bow legs. *British Medical Journal*, **i**, 826.

Sheehan, S., Bauer, R. B. and Meyer, J. S. (1960) Vertebral artery compression in cervical spondylosis. *Neurology*, **10**, 968.

Shephard, E. (1951) Tarsal movements. *Journal of Bone and Joint Surgery*, **33B**, 258.

Shine, I. B. (1951) Hallux valgus. *British Medical Journal*, **i**, 1648.

Sicard, M. A. (1901) Les injections medicamenteuses extra-durales par voie sacro-coccygienne. *Compte Rendu des Séances de la Societé de Biologie*, **53**, 396.

Sims-Williams, H., Jayson, M. I. V. and Baddeley, H. (1978) Small spinal fractures in back pain subjects. *Annals of Rheumatic Disease*, **37**, 262.

Sims-Williams, H., Jayson, M. I. V., Young, S. M. S., Baddely, H. and Collins, E. (1978) Controlled trial of mobilisation and manipulation for patients with low back pain in general practice. *British Medical Journal*, **ii**, 1338.

Sinclair, D. B. and Houpt, J. B. (1976) *Spontaneous Osteonecrosis of the Knee. Communication to Australian Rheumatology Association* Melbourne.

Singh, A., Dass, R. and Hayreh, S. S. (1962) Skeletal changes in endemic fluorosis. *Journal of Bone and Joint Surgery*, **44B**, 806.

Singh, M., Riggs, B. L., Besbout, J. W. and Jowsey, J. (1973) Femoral trabecular pattern index for evaluation of spinal osteoporosis. *Mayo Clinic Proceedings*, **48**, 184.

Slater. R. A., Pineda, A. and Porter, R. W. (1965) Intradural herniation of lumbar intervertebral discs. *Archives of Surgery*, **90**, 266.

Slocum, D. B. and Larson, R. L. (1968) Rotary instability of the knee. *Journal of Bone and Joint Surgery*, **50A**, 211.

Slocum, D. B., James, S. L. and Singer, K. M. (1976) Clinical test for anterolateral rotary instability of the knee. *Clinical Orthopaedics and Related Research*, **118**, 63.

Slocum, D. B., Larson, R. L. and James, S. L. (1974) Late reconstruction of ligamentous injuries of the medial compartment of the knee. *Clinical Orthopaedics and Related Research*, **100**, 23.

Smith, B. H. (1969) Anatomy of facial pain. *Headache*, **9**, 7.

Smith, E. M., Juvinall, R. C., Bender, L. F. and Pearson, J. R. (1966) Flexor forces and rheumatoid metacarpophalangeal deformity. *Journal of the American Medical Association*, **198**, 160.

Smith, P. H., Benn, R. T. and Sharp, J. (1972) Natural history of rheumatoid cervical luxations. *Annals of Rheumatic Disease*, **31**, 431.

Smith, R. A. and Estridge, M. N. (1962). Neurological complications of head and neck manipulations. *Journal of the American Medical Association*, **182**, 528.

Smillie, I. S. (1967) Treatment of Freiburg's infraction. *Proceedings of the Royal Society of Medicine*, **60**, 29.

Smillie, I. S. (1974) *Diseases of the Knee Joint*. Edinburgh: Churchill-Livingstone.

Smith, R. J. and Kaplan, E. B. (1967) Rheumatoid deformities at the metacarpophalangeal joints of the fingers. *Journal of Bone and Joint Surgery*, **49A**, 31.

Smythe, H. A. and Moldofsky, H. (1978) Two contributions to understanding of the 'Fibrositis' syndrome. *Bulletin of Rheumatic Disease*, **28**, 1.

Soderberg, L. (1956) Prognosis in conservatively treated sciatica. *Acta Orthopaedica Scandinavica Supplement*, **21**, 1.

Sokoloff, L. (1969) *The Biology of Degenerative Disease*. University of Chicago Press.

Solomon, L. (1973) Drug induced arthropathy and necrosis of the femoral head. *Journal of Bone and Joint Surgery*, **55B**, 246.

Solomon, L. (1976) Patterns of osteoarthritis of the hip. *Journal of Bone and Joint Surgery*, **56B**, 176.

Souter, W. A. and Taylor, T. K. F. (1970) Sulphated acid mucopolysaccharide metabolism in the rabbit intervertebral disc. *Journal of Bone and Joint Surgery*, **52B**, 371.

Spangfort, E. V. (1972) The lumbar disc herniation. *Acta Orthopaedica Scandinavica Supplement*, **142**, 5.

Spencer, G. E. and Hernod, C. E. (1953) Surgical treatment of tennis elbow. *Journal of Bone and Joint Surgery*, **35A**, 421.

Spritzer, H. W., Weaver, A. L. and Diamond, H. S. (1969) Relapsing polychondritis: Report of a case with vertebral column involvement. *Journal of the American Medical Association*, **208**, 355.

Stack, H. G. (1962) Muscle function in the fingers. *Journal of Bone and Joint Surgery*, **44B**, 899.

Stahl, D. C. and Jacobs, B. (1967) The diagnosis of obscure lesions of the skeleton. *Journal of the American Medical Association*, **201**, 229.

Stecher, R. M. (1959) Heredity of the joint diseases. *Rheumatism*, **11**, 1.

Steinberg, C. L. R., Duthie, R. B. and Piva, A. E. (1962) Charcot-like arthropathy following intra-articular hydrocortisone. *Journal of the American Medical Association*, **181**, 851.

Steinberg, V. L. and Mason, R. M. (1959) Cervical spondylosis. Pilot therapeutic trial. *Annals of Physical Medicine*, **5**, 37.

Steinbrocker, O. (1968) Shoulder–hand syndrome: Present perspective. *Archives of Physical Medicine and Rehabilitation*, **49**, 388.

Steinbrocker, O. (1972) In *Arthritis and Allied Conditions*, p. 1461. Eds. Hollander, A. B. and McCarty, C. P. Philadelphia: Lea and Febiger.

Steinbrocker, O. and Argyros, T. G. (1974) Frozen shoulder: Treatment by local injections of depot corticosteroids. *Annals of Physical Medicine and Rehabilitation*, **55**, 209.

Steindler, A. (1955) Kinesiology of the human body under normal and pathological conditions. Springfield: Thomas.

Stewart, D. Y. (1962) Current concepts of the 'Barré syndrome' or the posterior cervical sympathetic syndrome. *Clinical Orthopaedics and Related Research*, **24**, 40.

Stewart, T. D. (1953) The age incidence of neural arch defects in Alaskan natives. *Journal of Bone and Joint Surgery*, **35A**, 937.

Stewart T. D. (1956) Examination of the possibility that certain skeletal characteristics predispose to defects in the lumbar neural arches. *Clinical Orthopaedics and Related Research*, **8**, 44.

Stilwell, D. L. (1956) The nerve supply of the vertebral column and its associated structures in the monkey. *Anatomical Record*, **125**, 139.

Stockman, R. (1920) *Rheumatism and Arthritis*. Edinburgh: Green.

Stoddard, A. (1969) *Manual of Osteopathic Practice*. London: Hutchinson.

Stoddard, A. (1972) Scheuermann's disease. In *Proceedings of the 6th International Congress of Physical Medicine*.

Stone, C. A. (1916) Subluxation of the head of the radius. Report of a case and anatomical experiments. *Journal of the American Medical Association*, **1**, 28.

Strange, F. G. St. Clair (1966) Debunking the disc. *Proceedings of the Royal Society of Medicine*, **59**, 952.

Stulberg, S. D. and Harris, W. H. (1976) Acetabular dysplasia and development of osteoarthritis in the hip. In *Proceedings of the Second Open Scientific Meeting of the Hip Society*.

Subotnick, S. I. (1975) *Podiatric Sports Medicine*. New York: Futura.

Sudeck, P. (1900) Uber die acute Entzundliche Knockenatzophie. *Archiv Klinika Chirurgica*, **62**, 147.

Sullivan, C. R. (1964) Spondylolysis and spondylolisthesis. *Manitoba Medical Review*, **11**, 81.

Suramo, I., Puranen, J., Heikkinen, E. and Vuorinen, P. (1974) Disturbed patterns of venous drainage of the femoral neck in Perthes' disease. *Journal of Bone and Joint Surgery*, **56B**, 448.

Swanson, A. B. (1968) Silicone rubber implants for replacement of arthritic or destroyed joints in the hand. *Surgical Clinics of North America*, **4B**, 1003.

Swanson, A. B. (1972) Implant arthroplasty for the great toe. *Clinical Orthopaedics and Related Research*, **85**, 75.

Swezey, R. L. (1972) Dynamic factors in deformities of the rheumatoid arthritic hand. *Bulletin of Rheumatic Diseases*, **22**, 649.

Sylven, B. (1951) On biology of nucleus pulposus. *Acta Orthopaedica Scandinavica*, **20**, 275.

Taillard, W. F. (1976) Etiology of spondylolisthesis. *Clinical Orthopaedics and Related Research*, **117**, 30.

Tanz, S. S. (1953) Motion of the lumbar spine: A roentgenologic study. *American Journal of Roentgenology*, **69**, 399.

Tapper, W. M. and Hoover, N. W. (1969) Late results after meniscectomy. *Journal of Bone and Joint Surgery*, **51A**, 517.

Tatlow, W. F. T. and Bammer, H. G. (1957) Syndrome of vertebral artery compression. *Neurology*, **7**, 331.

Taylor, T. K. S. and Akeson, W. H. (1971) Intervertebral disc prolapse. A review of morphologic and biochemic knowledge concerning the nature of prolapse. *Clinical Orthopaedics and Related Research*, **76**, 54.

Taylor, T. K. S. and Little, K. (1963) Calcification in the intervertebral disc. *Nature (London)*, **109**, 612.

Telhag, H. and Lindbergh, L. (1972) A method for inducing osteoarthritic changes in rabbits' knees. *Clinical Orthopaedics and Related Research*, **86**, 214.

Thorndike, A. (1959) Frequency and nature of sports injuries. *American Journal of Surgery*, **98**, 316.

Tini, P. G., Wieser, C. and Zinn, W. M. (1977) The transitional vertebra of the lumbo-sacral spine. *Rheumatism and Rehabilitation*, **16**, 180.

Tipton, C. M., Matthes, R. D., Maynard, J. A. and Carey, R. A. (1975) The influence of physical activity on ligaments and tendons. *Medical Science and Sports*, **7**, 165.

Toller, P. A. (1977) Use and misuse of intra-articular corticosteroids in the treatment of temporomandibular joint pain. *Proceedings of the Royal Society of Medicine*, **70**, 461.

Töndury, G. (1971) Functional anatomy of the small joints of the spine. *Annales de Médecin. Physique*, **15**, 2.

Trickey, E. L. (1976) Ligamentous injuries around the knee. *British Medical Journal*, **ii**, 1492.

Tullos, H. S. and King, J. W. (1973) Throwing mechanisms in sport. *Orthopedic Clinics of North America*, **4**, 709.

Tzaczuk, H. (1968) Tensile properties of human lumbar longitudinal ligaments. *Acta Orthopaedica Supplement*, **115**.

Tzaczuk, H. (1968) Electromyographic studies on the vertebral portion of the psoas muscle. *Acta Orthopaedica Scandinavica Supplement*, **115**, 16.

Ueke, T. and Ueda, F. (1969) Dysfunction of the autonomic nervous system in whiplash injury. *Journal of West Pacific Orthopedics Association*, **6**, 1.

Unsworth, A., Dowson, D. and Wright, V. (1971) Cracking joints. *Annals of Rheumatic Disease*, **30**, 348.

Urist, M. R. (1959) The treatment of dislocations of the acromio-clavicular joint. *American Journal of Surgery*, **98**, 423.

Vainio, K. (1965) The rheumatoid foot: A clinical study with pathological and roentgenolical comments. *Arch. Chir. Gyn. Fenn.*, **45**, Suppl. **1**.

Van Arsdale, W. H. (1889) On subluxation of the head of the radius in children with a resumé of one hundred consecutive cases. *Annals of Surgery*, **9**, 401.

Vaz, M., Wadia, R. S. and Gokhole, S. D. (1978) Another cause of a positive crossed-straight leg raising test. *New England Journal of Medicine*, **299**, 779.

Verbiest, H. (1954) Radicular syndrome from developmental narrowing of the lumbar vertebral canal. *Journal of Bone and Joint Surgery*, **36B**, 230.

Verbiest, H. (1955) Further experiences on the pathological influence of a developmental narrowness of the bony lumbar vertebral canal. *Journal of Bone and Joint Surgery*, **37B**, 576.

Vernon-Roberts, B. and Pirie, C. J. (1973) Healing trabecular microfractures in the bodies of lumbar vertebrae. *Annals of Rheumatic Disease*, **32**, 406.

Vernon-Roberts, B. and Pirie, C. J. (1977) Degenerative changes in the intervertebral discs of the lumbar spine and their sequelae. *Rheumatism and Rehabilitation*, **16**, 13.

Vernon-Roberts, B., Pirie, C. J. and Trenwith, V. (1974). Pathology of the dorsal spine in ankylosing hyperostosis. *Annals of Rheumatic Disease*, **33**, 281.

Vidigal, E., Jacoby, R. K., Dixon, A. St. J., Ratliff, A. H. and Kirkup, J. (1975) The foot in chronic rheumatoid arthritis. *Annals of Rheumatic Disease*, **34**, 292.

Vinstein, A. L. and Cockerill, E. M. (1972) Involvement of the spine in gout. *Radiology*, **103**, 311.

Von Luschka, H. (1850) *Die Nerven des Menschlichen Wirbelkanales*. Loupp: Tubingen.

Wadsworth, T. G. and Williams, J. R. (1973) Cubital tunnel external compression syndrome. *British Medical Journal*, **i**, 662.

Wang, C. J. and Walker, P. S. (1974) Rotary laxity of the human knee joint. *Journal of Bone and Joint Surgery*, **56A**, 161.

Ward, J. R., Dolowitz, D. A., Bankol, J. L., Smith, C. and Fingerle, C. O. (1963) Painful dysfunction of the temporomandibular joint. *Archives of Internal Medicine*, **112**, 693.

Warr, A. C., Wilkinson, J. A., Burn, J. M. B. and Langdon, L. (1972) Chronic lumbosciatic syndrome treated by epidural injection and manipulation. *The Practitioner*, **209**, 53.

Webb, F. W. S., Hickman, J. A. and Drew, D. St. J. (1968) Death from vertebral artery thrombosis in rheumatoid arthritis. *British Medical Journal*, **ii**, 537.

Weber, H. (1973) Traction therapy in sciatica due to disc prolapse. *Journal of the Oslo City Hospital*, **23**, 167.

Weddell, G. (1957) Referred pain. *Proceedings of the Royal Society of Medicine*, **50**, 581.

Weisl, H. (1955) The movements of the sacro-iliac joint. *Acta Anatomica*, **23**, 80.

Welfling, J. (1969) *Painful Shoulder*. Folia Rheumatologica. Basel: Documenta Geigy.

Weston, W. J. and Palmer, D. G. (1978) *Soft Tissues of the Extremities: A Radiological Study of Rheumatic Disease*. New York: Springer-Verlag.

Westrin, C. G. (1973) Low back sick listing. A neurological and medical investigation. *Scandinavian Journal of Social Medicine, Supplement*, **7**.

Wiberg, G. (1939) Studies of dysplastic acetabula and congenital subluxation of the hip joint. *Acta Chirurgica Scandinavica*, **83**, Suppl. **58**.

Wiberg, G. (1941) Roentgenographic and anatomic studies on the patello-femoral joint with special reference to chondromalacia patellae. *Acta Orthopaedica Scandinavica*, **12**, 319.

Wilkinson, M. (1971) *Cervical Spondylosis*, 2nd. Edn. London: Heinemann.

Williams, H. J. and Pugh, D. G. (1963) Vertebral epiphysitis. *American Journal of Roentgenology*, **90**, 1236.

Williams, J. G. P. (1971) Diagnostic pitfalls in the sportsman's knee. *Proceedings of the Royal Society of Medicine*, **64**, 640.

Williams, J. G. P. (1973) Lesions of tendon attachments. *Rheumatism and Rehabilitation*, **12**, 182.

Williams, J. G. P. and Sperryn, P. M. (Eds.) (1976) *Sports Medicine*. London: Edward Arnold.

Williams, P. C. (1955) Examination and conservative treatment to disc lesions of the lower spine. *Clinical Orthopaedics and Related Research*, **5**, 28.

Williams, P. C. (1965) *The Lumbosacral Spine*. New York: McGraw–Hill.

Willis, T. A. (1931) The separate neural arch. *Journal of Bone and Joint Surgery*, **13**, 709.

Wilson, J. N. (1967) A diagnostic sign in osteochondritis dissecans of the knee. *Journal of Bone and Joint Surgery*, **49A**, 477.

Wiltse, L. L. (1962) The aetiology of spondylolisthesis. *Journal of Bone and Joint Surgery*, **44A**, 539.

Wiltse, L. L. (1971) The effect of common anomalies at the lumbar spine upon disc degeneration and low back pain. *Orthopedic Clinics of North America*, **2**, 569.

Wing, J. B., Rubin, R. N. and Marshall, J. L. (1975) Mechanism of isolated anterior cruciate rupture. *Journal of Bone and Joint Surgery*, **57A**, 411.

Wing, L. W. and Hargrave-Wilson, W. (1974) Cervical vertigo. *Australian and New Zealand Journal of Surgery*, **44**, 275.

Woodhall, B. and Hayes, G. (1950) The well-leg raising test of Fajerstatjn in the diagnosis of ruptured lumbar intervertebral disc. *Journal of Bone and Joint Surgery*, **32A**, 1950.

Woods, G. W., Stanley, R. F. and Tullos, H. S. (1979) Lateral capsular sign: X-ray clue to a significant knee instability. *American Journal of Sports Medicine,* **7**, 27.

Woods, G. W., Tullos, H. S. and King, J. W. (1973) The throwing arm: Elbow joint injuries. *Journal of Sports Medicine,* **1**, 43.

Wright, S. (1961) *Applied Physiology,* 1st Edn. Revised by Keele, Neil and Jepson. London: Oxford University Press.

Wright, V. (1961) Psoriatic arthritis. *Annals of Rheumatic Disease,* **20**, 123.

Wright, V. and Reed, W. B. (1964) The link between Reiter's syndrome and psoriatic arthritis. *Annals of Rheumatic Disease,* **23**, 12.

Wright, V. and Watkinson, G. (1965) Sacro-iliitis and ulcerative colitis. *British Medical Journal,* **ii**, 675.

Wright, V. and Moll, J. M. H. (1971) Normal range of spinal mobility. *Annals of Rheumatic Disease,* **30**, 381.

Wright, V. and Dowson, W. (1975) Biomechanics and joint function. In *Current Topics in Connective Tissue Disease,* p. 115. Ed. Holt, P. J. L. Edinburgh: Churchill-Livingstone.

Wright, V. and Haq, A. M. M. M. (1976) Periarthritis of the shoulder. *Annals of Rheumatic Disease,* **35**, 213.

Wright, V., Dowson, D. and Longfield, M. D. (1969) Joint stiffness—its characteristics and significance. *Biomed. Engin.,* **4**, 8.

Wyke, B. (1967) The neurology of joints. *Annals of the Royal College of Surgeons of England,* **41**, 100.

Wyke, B. (1970) The neurological basis of thoracic spinal pain. *Rheumatism and Physical Medicine,* **10**, 356.

Yergason, R. M., (1931) Supination sign. *Journal of Bone and Joint Surgery,* **13**, 160.

Yocum, L. A., *et al.* (1979) Isolated lateral meniscectomy. *Journal of Bone and Joint Surgery,* **61A**, 338.

Youel, M. A. (1967) Effectiveness of lumbar traction. *Journal of Bone and Joint Surgery,* **49A**, 2051.

Young, C. S. (1939) Operative treatment of pes planus. *Surgery, Gynecology and Obstetrics,* **68**, 99.

Young, J. (1940) Rotation of the pelvis joints in pregnancy. *Journal of Obstetrics and Gynaecology,* **47**, 493.

Index

Page numbers in *italic* refer to illustrations.